Neurotrauma

Neurotrauma

A Comprehensive Book on Traumatic Brain Injury and Spinal Cord Injury

Edited by

Kevin K. W. Wang, PhD
Program for Neurotrauma, Neuroproteomics, & Biomarkers Research (NNBR)
Department of Emergency Medicine
University of Florida
Gainesville, FL, USA

and

Brain Rehabilitation Research Center (BRRC)
Malcom Randall VA Medical Center
North Florida/South Georgia Veterans Health System
Gainesville, FL, USA

OXFORD
UNIVERSITY PRESS

OXFORD
UNIVERSITY PRESS

Oxford University Press is a department of the University of Oxford. It furthers
the University's objective of excellence in research, scholarship, and education
by publishing worldwide. Oxford is a registered trade mark of Oxford University
Press in the UK and certain other countries.

Published in the United States of America by Oxford University Press
198 Madison Avenue, New York, NY 10016, United States of America.

CIP data is on file at the Library of Congress
ISBN 978–0–19–027943–1

9 8 7 6 5 4 3 2 1

Printed by Sheridan Books, Inc., United States of America

"I want to dedicate this book to my wife and best friend Alice.
I could not have completed this book without her amazing support,
proof-reading and patience with me.

Thank you, Alice!"
—— Kevin K.W. Wang

Contents

Section III: Neuroimaging and Biomarker Assessments in TBI

Section VII: Common Themes Between Traumatic Brain and Spinal Cord Injury

Foreword I

Although traumatic brain injury (TBI) has been a threat to mankind throughout history, the scope of the problem did not reach public consciousness until two media events that occurred exactly one month apart in 2007. A January 18, 2007, article in the *New York Times*[1] documented the (then) unusual pathologic findings in the brain of deceased football player Andre Waters and raised the specter of chronic traumatic encephalopathy instead of the phrase "Be tough, get back in there." One month later, a February 18, 2007, *Washington Post* article[2] documented the squalid lodging conditions of the unexpected onslaught of wounded service members returning from Afghanistan and Iraq and focused unprecedented attention on TBI and posttraumatic stress disorder (PTSD). The phrase "Invisible Wounds of War" was coined.

Much progress has been achieved in the care of more severe cases of TBI, particularly through the implementation of evidence-based guidelines for care in the intensive care unit, which has reduced mortality by approximately 50%.[3] However, the consequences of milder forms of TBI (including concussion) were largely ignored by the medical community, the military, and the public in general. As a result of media attention to this issue, the US Congress quickly reacted in 2007 by including $901 million in a supplemental appropriation for psychological health and TBI care and research. This was followed by annual appropriations of approximately $120 million to continue the research efforts. In addition, Congress directed the Veterans Administration and the National Institutes of Health to increase their efforts in this area. These federally funded efforts, along with a burgeoning interest by philanthropic organizations establishing numerous "brain science" institutions often affiliated with universities, have resulted in a broad renaissance in neuroscience, despite many of the large pharmaceutical companies exiting neurotherapeutic research.

In August 2012, President Obama issued an Executive Order entitled "Improving Access to Mental Health Services for Veterans, Service Members, and Military Families," which directed that "the Departments of Defense, Veterans Affairs, Health and Human Services, and Education, in coordination with the Office of Science and Technology Policy, shall establish a National Research Action Plan (NRAP)." In response, the NRAP was co-developed among these four federal agencies and was published by the White House on August 31, 2012.[4] The principal outcome of this plan has been to coordinate federal funding for research to "accelerate discovery of the causes and mechanisms underlying PTSD, TBI, and other co-occurring outcomes like suicide, depression, and substance use disorders." Several large multiagency-funded efforts were initiated as a result, some of which are documented in this volume. The results from this coordinated effort are now coming to fruition in the US Food and Drug Administration (FDA) clearance of a number of devices to aid in the diagnosis of TBI and the development of evidence-based guidelines for the management of TBI and PTSD.

The rapid pace of knowledge acquisition has been astounding given the relatively short duration of these efforts. However, the more we learn about the nervous system in health and in disease, the more we realize that there are still vast knowledge gaps to be filled.

This volume's thorough yet broad coverage of the current state of knowledge regarding neurotrauma including TBI and spinal cord injury by today's luminaries in the field will make it a valuable reference and resource for researchers, clinicians, and the public at large for many years to come.

Dallas Hack, MD, Colonel, US Army (Retired)
Cohen Veterans Bioscience

References

1. Swartz A. Expert ties ex-player's suicide to brain damage. *New York Times*, January 18, 2007. http://www.nytimes.com/2007/01/18/sports/football/18waters.html?_r=0. Accessed March 6, 2018.

2. Priest D, Hull A. Soldiers face neglect, frustration at army's top medical facility. *Washington Post*, February 18, 2007. http://www.washingtonpost.com/wp-dyn/content/article/2007/02/17/AR2007021701172.html. Accessed March 6, 2018.

3. Gerber LM, Chiu YL, Carney N, Härtl R, Ghajar J. Marked reduction in mortality in patients with severe traumatic brain injury. *J Neurosurg.* 2013 Dec;119(6):1583–90. doi: 10.3171/2013.8.JNS13276.

4. National Research Action Plan. https://obamawhitehouse.archives.gov/sites/default/files/uploads/nrap_for_eo_on_mental_health_august_2013.pdf. Accessed March 6, 2018.

Foreword II

Neurotrauma is a remarkable and timely book. Remarkable because it captures the excitement of recent scientific advances in brain and spinal cord injury research while also providing a historical framework and global perspectives. The editor, Kevin Wang, demonstrates his expertise in this field through his comprehensive selection and organization of topics. Plus, the book chapters, written by a diverse and widely acclaimed scientists, are informative and insightful.

Neurotrauma primarily focuses on traumatic brain injury, but also includes chapters on spinal cord injury. This enhances the learning experience because research from one field informs the other. The overlapping pathophysiology of these complex central nervous system injuries provides an opportunity to accelerate the development of targeted therapies when they present singly or as comorbid conditions. The inclusion of both pediatric and adult studies is another notable strength. For practical and ethical reasons, most clinical studies are limited to one age group or the other. However, scientifically, the transitions in age-dependent mechanisms of traumatic brain injury and recovery are poorly understood and unlikely to be so stark. A better understanding of these transitions is key to designing clinical trials with inclusion and exclusion criteria based on mechanisms of injury rather than arbitrary age cutoffs. Similarly, including research on acute and chronic stages of injury is essential for understanding the trajectory and for ultimately developing effective therapeutics.

We are on the threshold of major advances in healthcare, in part because of "big data" approaches to science. The vision of personalized medicine is becoming a reality. Large, comprehensive genetic and phenotypic data are emerging from clinical and preclinical neurotrauma research. These large datasets have the potential to be transformative, but their analysis and interpretation will require a solid understanding of what is currently known. This timely book takes us to the threshold of knowledge about neurotrauma. For those who want to cross the threshold, this book is highly recommended.

Ramona Hicks, PhD
Director, Science & Technology
One Mind
Seattle, Washington

Preface

This new book volume, simply titled *Neurotrauma*, aims to bring together the latest clinical practice and research in the field of two forms of trauma to the central nervous system: namely, traumatic brain injury (TBI) and spinal cord injury (SCI). Nationally, more 1.9 million Americans sustain a TBI annually. In parallel, there are an estimated 12,000 new cases of SCI in the United States annually. In addition, approximately 1.2 million people live with paralysis due to SCI. In recent years, dramatic advancements in the field have resulted in much improved outcomes for patients and higher standards of care. This volume brings together the latest research and clinical practice in the treatment of neurotrauma in a comprehensive but easy-to-follow format.

Our target readership is intentionally broad. It includes clinicians who are involved in caring for TBI in the emergency room, hospital, or neurointensive care unit or during patient rehabilitation; clinical research professionals; research nurses; and nonclinical academic researchers, such as research professors, research scientists, medical students, graduate students, and nurse specialists, as well as biomedical industry R&D scientists and clinical associates.

As editor of this volume, I want all readers to find a chapter or section on almost all aspects related to TBI or SCI. I also hope that they will encounter some areas they might be already familiar with. Yet, at the same time, I hope that they will also discover or rediscover other less familiar areas in neurotrauma that they have always wanted to learn more about. Last, I want to make this volume as layman-like and as easy to follow as possible so that it can also serve as a resource book for TBI or SCI patients or caregivers who want to better educate themselves about these conditions.

Kevin K. W. Wang

Contributors

Stephen T. Ahlers, PhD
Department of Neurotrauma
Operational and Undersea Medicine
   Directorate
Naval Medical Research Center
Silver Spring, Maryland

Hisham F. Bahmad, PhD
Department of Anatomy, Cell Biology,
   and Physiological Sciences
Faculty of Medicine
Postdoctoral Research Fellow
American University of Beirut
Beirut, Lebanon

Lijun Bai, PhD
Athinoula A. Martinos Center for
   Biomedical Imaging
Massachusetts General Hospital
Harvard Medical School
Charlestown, Massachusetts
and
Key Laboratory of Biomedical
   Information Engineering
Ministry of Education, Department of
   Biomedical Engineering
School of Life Science and Technology
Xi'an Jiaotong University
Xi'an, China

Zachary Bailey, BSc
Department of Biomedical Engineering
   and Mechanics
Virginia Tech
Blacksburg, Virginia

Andrew J. Baker, MD
Chief, Department of Critical Care, St.
   Michael's Hospital Medical
Director, Trauma and Neurosurgery
   Program, St. Michael's Hospital
Professor, Departments of Anesthesia and
   Surgery, University of Toronto
Toronto, Ontario, Canada

Nagaraja S. Balakathiresan, PhD
Department of Pathology
Uniformed Services University of the
   Health Sciences
Bethesda, Maryland

Codruta Birle Barle, PhD
RoNeuro Institute for Neurological
   Research and Diagnostic
Cluj-Napoca, Romania

Michael J. Bell, MD
Departments of Critical Care Medicine,
   Neurological Surgery, and Pediatrics
Safar Center for Resuscitation Research
University of Pittsburgh
Pittsburgh, Pennsylvania

Rachel Pardes Berger, MD, MPH
Department of Pediatrics
Children's Hospital of Pittsburgh
   of UPMC
Pittsburgh, Pennsylvania

Melany Betancourt-Loza
Institute of Neurology and Neurosurgery
Havana, Cuba

Manish Bhomia, PhD
Department of Pathology
Uniformed Services University of the
    Health Sciences
Bethesda, Maryland

Angela M. Boutté, PhD
Brain Trauma Neuroprotection and
    Neurorestoration Branch
Center for Military Psychiatry and
    Neuroscience
Walter Reed Army Institute of Research
Silver Spring, Maryland

Helen M. Bramlett, PhD
Department of Neurological Surgery
University of Miami Leonard M. Miller
    School of Medicine
Miami, Florida

Ross Bullock, MD, PhD
Department of Neurosurgery
University of Miami
Miami, Florida

Nicole Bye, PhD
Division of Pharmacy
School of Medicine
University of Tasmania
Hobart, Tasmania, Australia

Joseph A. Caruso, PhD
Institute of Environmental Health
    Sciences
Wayne State University
Detroit, Michigan

Ibolja Cernak, MD, PhD [ME, MHS]
Founder, STARR-C LLC (Stress,
    Trauma and Resilience Research
    Consulting) LLC
Philadelphia, Pennsylvania

Amit Chakrabarty, MD
Consultant Neurosurgeon
Eternal Hospital
Jaipur, India

Peng-Yuan Chang, MD
Department of Neurological Surgery
University of Miami
Miami, Florida

Jinhui Chen, PhD
Spinal Cord and Brain Injury
    Research Group
Department of Neurosurgery
Stark Neuroscience Research Institute
Indianapolis, Indiana

Mauricio Chinchilla, PhD
Institute of Neurology and Neurosurgery
Havana, Cuba

Jennifer Clarke, MD
Department of Pediatrics
Children's Hospital of Pittsburgh
    of UPMC
Pittsburgh, Pennsylvania

Anay Cordero-Eiriz, PhD
Neurobiology Department
Institute of Neurology and Neurosurgery
Havana, Cuba

Cezara Costin, PhD
RoNeuro Institute for Neurological
    Research and Diagnostic
Cluj-Napoca, Romania

S. A. Dambinova, DSc, PhD
Brain Biomarkers Lab
DeKalb Medical Center
Decatur, Georgia

Hansen Deng, BA
Department of Neurological Surgery
University of California
San Francisco, California

Ramon Diaz-Arrastia, MD, PhD
Department of Neurology
University of Pennsylvania Perelman
    School of Medicine
Penn Presbyterian Medical Center
Philadelphia, Pennsylvania

W. Dalton Dietrich, PhD
Department of Neurological Surgery
University of Miami Leonard M. Miller
   School of Medicine
Miami, Florida

James M. Ecklund, MD
Chairman of Neurosurgery
Inova Fairfax Hospital
Professor of Neurosurgery
Virginia Commonwealth University
and
Uniformed Services University of the
   Health Sciences
Bethesda, Maryland

Mario Estévez, MD, PhD
Institute of Neurology and Neurosurgery
Havana, Cuba

Shiqing Feng, MD
Department of Orthopedics
Tianjin Medical University General
   Hospital
Tianjin, China

Candace L. Floyd, PhD
Associate Professor and Director of
   Research, Department of Physical
   Medicine and Rehabilitation
University of Alabama at Birmingham
Birmingham, Alabama

Xiang Gao, MD
Spinal Cord and Brain Injury
   Research Group
Department of Neurosurgery
Stark Neuroscience Research Institute
Indianapolis, Indiana

James W. Geddes, PhD
Spinal Cord and Brain Injury
   Research Center
Biomedical & Biological Sciences
   Research Building (BBSRB)
University of Kentucky
Lexington, Kentucky

Thomas Gennarelli, MD
Medical College of Wisconsin
George Washington University
West Chester, Pennsylvania

Alexander V. Glushakov, PhD
Single Breath, Inc.
Gainesville, Florida

Olena Y. Glushakova, MS
Department of Neurosurgery
Virginia Commonwealth University
Richmond, Virginia

Sergio González-García, PhD
Neurobiology Department
Institute of Neurology and Neurosurgery
Havana, Cuba

Alina González-Quevedo, PhD
Neurobiology Department
Institute of Neurology and Neurosurgery
Havana, Cuba

Per-Olof Grände, MD, PhD
Department of Anesthesia and
   Intensive Care
Skåne University Hospital
Lund, Sweden

Allison Guettler, PhD
Department of Mechanical Engineering
Virginia Tech
Blacksburg, Virginia

Joy Guingab-Cagmat, PhD
University of Florida
Gainesville, Florida

Margalit Haber, PhD
Department of Neurology
University of Pennsylvania Perelman
   School of Medicine
Penn Presbyterian Medical Center
Philadelphia, Pennsylvania

Lauren A. Hanlon, PhD
Program in Neuroscience
Graduate School of Biomedical Sciences
   and Professional Studies
Drexel University
Philadelphia, Pennsylvania

Yan Hao, MD
Department of Orthopedics
Tianjin Medical University General
   Hospital
Tianjin, China

Ronald L. Hayes, PhD
Department of Neurosurgery
Virginia Commonwealth University
Richmond, Virginia
and
Banyan Biomarkers, Inc.
Alachua, Florida

Sarah C. Hellewell, PhD
Canadian Military and Veterans' Clinical
   Rehabilitation Research Program
Faculty of Rehabilitation Medicine
University of Alberta
Edmonton, Alberta, Canada

Helene Henson, MD
Executive, Rehabilitation Service Line
Michael E. De Bakey Veterans Affairs
   Medical Center
and
Professor, Department of Physical
   Medicine & Rehabilitation Medicine
Baylor College of Medicine
Houston, Texas

Zenaida Hernández-Díaz, PhD
Radiology Department
Institute of Neurology and Neurosurgery
Havana, Cuba

Jimmy W. Huh, PhD
Department of Anesthesiology and
   Critical Care
Children's Hospital of Philadelphia
Philadelphia, Pennsylvania

Kimbra Kenney, MD
Department of Neurology
Uniformed Services University of the
   Health Sciences
and
National Intrepid Center of Excellence
Walter Reed National Military
   Medical Center
Bethesda, Maryland

Barbara Knollmann-Ritschel, PhD
Department of Pathology
Uniformed Services University of the
   Health Sciences
Bethesda, Maryland

Firas Kobeissy, PhD
Departments of Psychiatry
University of Florida
Gainesville, FL, USA
Neuroscience Research Center
Faculty of Medical Sciences
Lebanese University
Beirut, Lebanon

John Paul G. Kolcun, MS
Department of Neurological Surgery
MD Candidate
University of Miami
Miami, Florida

Isha Kothari, PhD
Departments of Psychiatry
University of Florida
Gainesville, Florida

Michelle C. LaPlaca, PhD
Coulter Department of Biomedical
   Engineering
Associate Professor
Georgia Institute of Technology and
   Emory University School of Medicine
Atlanta, Georgia

Christine Leeper, MD
Department of Surgery
Children's Hospital of Pittsburgh
of UPMC
Pittsburgh, Pennsylvania

Harvey S. Levin, PhD
Research Scientist
Michael E. De Bakey Veterans Affairs
Medical Center and Professor
Department of Physical Medicine &
Rehabilitation Medicine
Baylor College of Medicine
Houston, Texas

Jianjun Li, MD
Capital Medical University School of
Rehabilitation Medicine and China
Rehabilitation Research Center
Center of Neural Injury and Repair
Beijing Institute for Brain Disorder
Beijing, China

Geoffrey S. F. Ling, MD, PhD
Interim Vice-Chair of Research, Inova
Fairfax Hospital
Professor of Neurology, Johns Hopkins
Medical Institutions
Professor of Neurology, Uniformed
Services University of the Health
Sciences
Falls Church, Virginia

Calixto Machado, PhD
Institute of Neurology and Neurosurgery
Havana, Cuba

Geoffrey T. Manley, MD, PhD
Department of Neurological Surgery
University of California
San Francisco, California

Amy J. Markowitz, JD
Department of Neurological Surgery
University of California
San Francisco, California

Elizabeth McNeil, PhD
Department of Biomedical Engineering
and Mechanics
Virginia Tech
Blacksburg, Virginia

Ahmed Moghieb, PhD
Department of Psychiatry
Postdoctoral Associate
University of Florida
Gainesville, Florida

Cristina Morganti-Kossmann, MC
Department of Epidemiology and
Preventive Medicine
Australian New Zealand Intensive Care
Research Centre
Monash University
Melbourne, Victoria, Australia
Department of Child Health, University
of Arizona College of Medicine –
BARROW Neurological Institute at
Phoenix Children's Hospital
Phoenix, Arizona
and
Lex Medicus PTY LTD
South Yarra, Victoria, Australia

J. D. Mullins, MD
Department of Surgery
Piedmont Hospital
Atlanta, Georgia

Dafin Muresanu, MD, PhD, MBA
Department of Clinical Neurosciences
Iuliu Hatieganu University of Medicine
and Pharmacy
and
RoNeuro Institute for Neurological
Research and Diagnostic
Cluj-Napoca, Romania

Ioana Muresanu, PhD
RoNeuro Institute for Neurological
Research and Diagnostic
Cluj-Napoca, Romania

Magnus Olivecrona, MD, PhD
Department of Anesthesia and
    Intensive Care
Örebro University
Örebro, Sweden

Zandra Olivecrona, MD, PhD
Department of Anaesthesiology and
    Intensive Care
Örebro University Hospital
Örebro, Sweden

**Linda Papa, MD, CM, MSc, CCPF,
    FRCP(C), FACEP**
Director of Academic Clinical Research
    and Attending Emergency Physician
Department of Emergency Medicine,
    Orlando Regional Medical Center
McGill University
Orlando, Florida
and
University of Central Florida College of
    Medicine
Clinical Associate Professor
Florida State University College of
    Medicine
Orlando, Florida

Eugene Park, PhD
Keenan Research Centre
St Michael's Hospital
Toronto, Ontario, Canada

Jesús Pérez-Nellar
Institute of Neurology and Neurosurgery
Havana, Cuba

G. K. Prusty, MCh
Professor of Neurosurgery
MGM Medical College
Kishanganj, India

Alexandru Rafila
Department of Microbiology and
    Epidemiology
University of Medicine and Pharmacy
    Carol Davila
Bucharest, Romania

Ramesh Raghupathi, PhD
Program in Neuroscience
Graduate School of Biomedical Sciences
    and Professional Studies
and
Department of Neurobiology and
    Anatomy
Drexel University
Philadelphia Pennsylvania
and
Veteran's Administration Medical Center
Coatesville, Pennsylvania

Rafael Rodríguez, PhD
Institute of Neurology and Neurosurgery
Havana, Cuba

Olivia Rosu, PhD
RoNeuro Institute for Neurological
    Research and Diagnostic
Cluj-Napoca, Romania

Richard Rubenstein, PhD
SUNY Downstate Medical Center
Department of Neurology
Brooklyn, New York

Randall S. Scheibel, PhD
Research Scientist
Michael E. De Bakey Veterans Affairs
    Medical Center and Professor
Department of Physical Medicine &
    Rehabilitation Medicine
Baylor College of Medicine
Houston, Texas

Bridgette D. Semple, PhD
Department of Medicine (Royal
    Melbourne Hospital)
The University of Melbourne
Melbourne, Victoria, Australia

Deborah Shear, PhD
Department of Medicine (Royal
  Melbourne Hospital)
The University of Melbourne
Brain Trauma Neuroprotection and
  Neurorestoration Branch
Center for Military Psychiatry and
  Neuroscience
Walter Reed Army Institute of Research
Silver Spring, Maryland

Riyi Shi, PhD
Department of Basic Medical Sciences
Weldon School of Biomedical
  Engineering
Purdue University
West Lafayette, Indiana

Kentaro Shimoda, MD
Department of Neurosurgery
Nihon University School of Medicine
Tokyo, Japan

Virendra Deo Sinha, Mch
Senior Professor and Head
Department of Neurosurgery
S. M. S. Medical College and Hospital
Jaipur, India

Dana Slavoaca, PhD
RoNeuro Institute for Neurological
  Research and Diagnostic
Cluj-Napoca, Romania

Paul M. Stemmer, PhD
Institute of Environmental Health
  Sciences
Wayne State University
Detroit, Michigan

Chuanzhu Sun, MD
Key Laboratory of Biomedical
  Information Engineering
Ministry of Education, Department of
  Biomedical Engineering
School of Life Science and Technology
Xi'an Jiaotong University
Xi'an, China

Dong Sun, MD, PhD
Department of Neurosurgery
Medical College of Virginia Campus
Virginia Commonwealth University
Richmond, Virginia

Wenjing Sun, PhD
Department of Neuroscience
Wexner Medical Center
Ohio State University
Columbus, Ohio

**Charles H. Tator, OC, MD, PhD,
  FRCSC, FACS**
Professor of Neurosurgery
University of Toronto, and Toronto
  Western Hospital
Director, Canadian Concussion Centre
Toronto Western Hospital
Toronto, Ontario, Canada

Andrea Tedeschi, PhD
Department of Neuroscience
Wexner Medical Center
Ohio State University
Columbus, Ohio

Karin Thompson, PhD
Director, PTSD Clinic, Mental
  Health Line
Michael E. De Bakey Veterans Affairs
  Medical Center
and
Associate Professor
Department of Psychiatry
Baylor College of Medicine
Houston, Texas

Maya Troyanskaya, MD
Research Scientist, Michael E. De Bakey
  Veterans Affairs Medical Center
and
Assistant Professor, Department of
  Physical Medicine & Rehabilitation
  Medicine
Baylor College of Medicine
Houston, Texas

Johan Undén, MD
Associate Professor
Department of Anaesthesiology and
  Intensive Care
Hallands Hospital, Halmstad
and
Skåne University Hospital
Lund, Sweden

Alex B. Valadka, MD
Department of Neurosurgery
Virginia Commonwealth University
Richmond, Virginia

Pamela VandeVord, PhD
Salem Veterans Affairs Medical Center
Blacksburg, Virginia
and
Department of Biomedical Engineering
  and Mechanics
Virginia Tech
Blacksburg, Virginia

Johannes Vester, PhD
Department of Biometry and Clinical
  Research
IDV Data Analysis and Study Planning
Krailling, Germany

Kevin K. W. Wang, PhD
Program for Neurotrauma,
  Neuroproteomics, & Biomarker
  Research
Department of Emergency Medicine,
  Psychiatry and Neuroscience
McKnight Brain Institute
University of Florida
Gainesville, Florida

Michael Y. Wang, MD, FACS
Departments of Neurosurgery &
  Rehabilitation Medicine
Miller School of Medicine
and
Lois Pope Life Center
University of Miami
Miami, Florida

Shan Wang, PhD
Key Laboratory of Biomedical
  Information Engineering
Ministry of Education, Department of
  Biomedical Engineering
School of Life Science and Technology
Xi'an Jiaotong University
Xi'an, China

Xiaoting Wang, MD
Spinal Cord and Brain Injury
  Research Group
Department of Neurosurgery
Stark Neuroscience Research Institute
Indianapolis, Indiana

Shanna Williams, MS OTR/L, CBIS
Tree of Life Services, Inc.,
Richmond, Virginia

Ethan A. Winkler, MD, PhD
Department of Neurological Surgery
University of California
San Francisco, California

Aaron T. Wong, BS
Department of Psychiatry
University of Florida
Gainesville, FL, USA

Kendra Woods, MD
Department of Critical Care Medicine
University of Pittsburgh
Pittsburgh, Pennsylvania

Ping Wu, MD, PhD
Department of Neuroscience and Cell
  Biology
University of Texas Medical Branch
Galveston
Beijing Institute for Brain Disorders
Capital Medical University
China

Mingliang Yang, MD
Department of Spinal and Neural
  Function Reconstruction
Capital Medical University School of
  Rehabilitation Medicine and China
  Rehabilitation Research Center, China
Center of Neural Injury and Repair
Beijing Institute for Brain Disorder
Beijing, China

Zhihui Yang, PhD
Department of Emergency Medicine
University of Florida
Gainesville, Florida

Shoji Yokobori, MD
Department of Emergency and Critical
  Care Medicine
Nippon Medical School
Tokyo, Japan

John K. Yue, BA
Department of Neurological Surgery
University of California
San Francisco, California

**Nathan D. Zasler, DABPM&R,
  FAAPM&R, FACRM, BIM-C,
  FIAIME, DAIPM, CBIST**
CEO & Medical Director, Concussion
  Care Centre of Virginia, Ltd. And
Tree of Life Services, Inc.
Professor, affiliate, Department of Physical
  Medicine and Rehabilitation
Virginia Commonwealth University,
Richmond, Virginia

Tian Zhu, MD
Department of Emergency Medicine
Assistant Professor
University of Florida
Gainesville, Florida

Jenna M. Ziebell, PhD
Wicking Dementia Research and
  Education Centre
University of Tasmania
Hobart, Tasmania, Australia
and
Department of Child Health
University of Arizona College of Medicine
Phoenix, Arizona
and
Barrow Neurological Institute at Phoenix
  Children's Hospital
Phoenix, Arizona

Section I

Severe Traumatic Brain Injury

History, Overview, and Human Anatomical Pathology of Traumatic Brain Injury

Kentaro Shimoda, Shoji Yokobori, and Ross Bullock

1

Introduction

This chapter discusses the history, epidemiology, and pathophysiology of traumatic brain injury (TBI), as well as its trends in morbidity, causes, and resulting economic damage. Although TBI has been recognized since ancient times, the overall picture of the condition varies from country to country and has changed over time. It is classified as either *primary* brain injury, meaning damage resulting from the instantaneous impact, and it may be also classified as a *secondary* brain injury because much of the damage evolves later, as a consequence of biological reactions after the initial incident. The best treatments and means of prevention depend on the classification of brain injury and understanding the pathological mechanisms, which will be discussed here in relation to how clinical, physiological, and imaging features are used to diagnose each variant of the disease.

History and Epidemiology of Traumatic Brain Injury

Few events in human life have the same capacity as TBI to reduce an individual from a vibrant independent person to a vegetative being dependent on others for every function of life. TBI is one of the oldest and commonest causes of medical distress in humans.

Injury to the cranium has been found in prehistoric human skeletal remains, which suggests that TBI has been a common medical condition for a long time. In the prehistoric age, between 10% and 50% of cranial injuries are associated with evidence of climactic stress and political/social instability.[1,2] Most of these injuries probably were the result of warfare because high-energy interpersonal violence was universal in early humans. In our industrialized society, TBI is also the leading cause of death and disability in persons under 40 years. This chapter discusses the incidence of TBI, trends in morbidity and mortality, shifts in causes of TBI, and economic burden on society.

In 2010, the US Centers for Disease Control and Prevention (CDC) reported that 2.5 million Americans were treated in an emergency department (ED), admitted to a hospital, or died due to TBI.[3] Of these people, approximately 87% were treated and released from an ED, 11% were hospitalized, and 2%—a total of 52,000—died. These likely underestimate the prevalence of TBI because they exclude patients with mild TBI who were treated in outpatient clinics and patients who received care at a federal facility, such as people in the US military or seeking care at a Veterans Affairs hospital.[3] Department of Defense data show that approximately 230,000 people serving in the

3

US military were diagnosed with a TBI from 2000 to 2011, which suggests that military personnel are at significant risk for TBI. CDC data from 1997 to 2007 reported an 8.2% reduction of mortality for TBI. TBI-related mortality decreased for people aged 0–44 years and significantly increased for people aged over 75 years.[4] In addition, three times as many TBI-related deaths occurred among males as among females, and non-Hispanic American Indian/Alaska Native persons have the highest mortality among ethnicities. Major causes of TBI were firearms (34%), motor vehicle accidents (31%), and falls (17%). Additionally, firearm-related death rates were highest in persons aged 15–34 years and older than 75 years. Motor vehicle–related death rates were highest among persons aged 15–24 years. In comparison, fall-related death rates were highest in persons aged more than 75 years. Thus, special strategies for prevention of TBI are needed for specific age groups, ethnicities, and causes.

Trends in Pediatric Traumatic Brain Injury

TBI is one of the commonest causes of death and long-term disability in the pediatric age range.[5] Children are more vulnerable to TBI and have longer recovery periods than do adults.[6] TBI-related deaths account for approximately one-third of all injury-related deaths in the United States, and a high incidence in adolescents has been reported.[4] According to CDC data, children aged less than 4 years, adolescents aged 15–19 years, and adults over 65 years of age are most likely to sustain a TBI.[3] An estimated 500,000 children younger than 14 years annually visit an ED for TBI.[7] In 2000, children and adolescents younger than 17 years had approximately 50,000 TBI-related hospitalizations at a cost of acute medical treatment estimated at more than $1 billion.[8] Falls are the leading cause of TBI for children less than 4 years of age. In addition, fall-related TBI for children less than 14 years of age increased 62% from 2002 to 2006 according to CDC data.[3] Data from the US Nationwide Inpatient Sample investigating TBI for people between the ages of 10 and 19 years from 2005 to 2009 showed that the leading causes of TBI are motor vehicle accidents (35%) for adolescents and falls (22%) for children aged 10–13 years. Annual TBI hospitalizations for adolescents decreased from 75.5 to 59.3 persons per 100,000 people from 2005 to 2009. Incidence of motor vehicle accident-related TBI decreased from 27.6 to 20.2 persons per 100,000 people. Firearms have higher rates of hospitalization and death for adolescent TBI than do motor vehicle accidents.[9] The decrease of adolescent TBI might be due to development of motor vehicle technology such as seat belts, airbags, and automatic braking systems. Although wearing helmets and providing safe environments can reduce the severity of TBI, preventing fall-related TBI is a big issue for pediatric TBI.

Recently, TBIs occurring during sports and recreation have been better recognized in adolescents. During 2001–2009, approximately 170,000 people annually were treated in an ED for sports concussion and recreation-related TBI,[10] of whom 70% were children aged 10–19 years. The most frequent activities leading to TBI-related ED visits are bicycling, football, playground activities, basketball, and soccer. According to CDC data, from 2001 to 2009, the estimated number of sports- and recreation-related TBI visits to an ED increased 62%, from 153,375 to 248,418, and the estimated rate of TBI visits increased 57%, from 190 to 298 per 100,000 population. To reduce the frequency and severity of TBI, prevention strategies should include increased recognition of TBI risk, use of appropriate techniques and protective equipment, and quicker response to TBI incidents.

Trends in Elderly Traumatic Brain Injury

Elderly people are increasing globally, and solving the problem of elderly TBI is becoming a big challenge.[11] The number of US individuals older than 65 will reach 71 million in 2030 and approximately 88.5 million in 2050.[12] In Pennsylvania, the incidence of elderly TBI has approximately doubled in the past 18 years, and the highest numbers of TBI occurred in persons aged 83–90 years.[13] The number of TBI-related ED visits has been increasing faster than population growth for older adults. Annual costs of hospitalization for TBI treatment of individuals older than 65 exceed approximately $2 billion.[14] Elderly brains have widespread atrophy and neuronal loss, reduced synaptic density, and decreased neural plasticity.[15,16] In addition, older adults often have several medical complications that worsen outcome from TBI, such as diabetes, hypertension, and chronic renal failure. Compared with younger people, older people tend to have slower functional recovery rates, longer hospital stays, greater in-hospital mortality, and lower functional status at discharge.[17] The possibility that older people are more vulnerable to more secondary complications after TBI is consistent with research indicating that younger people are more frequently seen in EDs and discharged, while older people more often require hospital admission for TBI of similar severity. Furthermore, anticoagulants and antiplatelet treatments increase the incidence of intracranial hemorrhage, which is associated with a worse outcome.[18] Although young patients with TBI are often injured in motor vehicle accidents, elderly people more often fall at home, which can cause severe TBI and death. Fall risk factors for older adults are imbalance, frailty, joint disorders, chronic medical conditions, and medication interactions.[19] In the Netherlands from 1986 through 2008, fall-related injuries in adults older than 65 doubled in all age groups, and the greatest number of fall-related injuries occurred in persons aged 85 years and older.[20] Incidence of trauma-related hospitalization following falls is rapidly increasing in the elderly population of the Netherlands. Using known effective strategies is expected to slow the rise of morbidity and mortality and optimize the quality of life and functional outcome for elderly people following TBI.[21,22]

Pathology of Traumatic Brain Injury

The major prognostic factor after TBI is the severity of the primary brain injury. Following impact, a delayed secondary brain injury cascade is set in progress. The two combine to determine outcome.

Primary brain injury itself is mostly unavoidable except by behavior modification, such as the use of seat belts; therefore, prevention should be the primary strategy of practical TBI "treatment."

In contrast, the main focus for medical treatment of TBI should be the prevention of secondary brain injury. Therefore, adequate understandings of the pathology of this secondary injury is needed in the management of TBI patients.

Classification of TBI: Primary and Secondary, Focal and Diffuse

Both primary and secondary brain damage can be further classified by *focal* and *diffuse* mechanisms (Table 1.1). The distinction between focal and diffuse injuries is historically derived from the absence or presence of mass lesions on imaging evaluations such as computed tomography (CT). This distinction has now evolved to consider the pathological mechanisms imparted by the trauma in regions local to and remote from the point of impact. Although these classifications are widely accepted, most TBIs consist of a heterogeneous admixture of focal and diffuse damage. Because focal and diffuse pathological processes are often intermingled (Figure. 1.1)—making it difficult to distinguish focal, diffuse, primary, and secondary categories—it is useful to consider them separately for the purpose of understanding TBI pathophysiology (Table 1.1).

Diffuse Axonal Injury: Best Example of Diffuse Brain Injury

The clearest representative of primary diffuse injury is diffuse axonal injury (DAI). DAI was first defined as a clinical syndrome in patients who were not conscious from the time of trauma, who had histopathological evidence of axonal damage in many white matter areas of the brain, and who were without major intraparenchymal mass lesions. DAI is usually caused by shearing forces leading to widespread tearing of axons and small vessels.[23] Areas commonly affected include axons in the brainstem, parasagittal white matter near the cerebral cortex, and corpus callosum.[24]

DAI is now recognized to typically involve a more progressive, slower response involving a transient, traumatically induced, neurochemically magnified disruption of the axonal membrane and its associated ion channels over the course of 24 hours in humans causing uncontrollable calcium influx.[25] These mechanisms induce a subsequent failure of axoplasmic transportation, pooling of intraaxonal contents, and separation of the axon from its distal part, thus creating a "retraction ball" of axoplasm. This disconnecting process occurs over the course of 24–72 hours from the traumatic impact and is termed *delayed* or *secondary axonotomy*.

Table 1.1:
Neuropathological classification of TBI

	Diffuse Brain Injury	Focal Brain Injury
Primary brain injury	Diffuse axonal injury Petechial white matter hemorrhage with diffuse vascular injury	Focal cortical contusion Intracerebral hemorrhage Extracerebral hemorrhage
Secondary brain injury	Delayed neuronal injury Diffuse brain swelling Diffuse ischemic injury Diffuse hypoxic injury Diffuse metabolic dysfunction	Delayed neuronal injury Focal brain swelling Focal ischemic injury Focal hypoxic injury Regional metabolic dysfunction

In TBI cases, several types of injury coexist at the same time; for example, nerve and vessel injury, diffuse and focal injury.

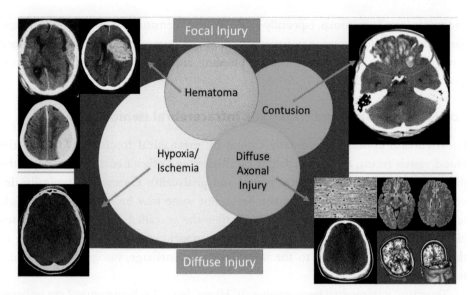

Figure 1.1 Schematic illustration of the intermingled pathophysiology in admixture of focal and diffuse damage. For easy understanding, the pathophysiology of traumatic brain injury is largely divided into focal and diffuse injury. Epidural hematoma, subdural hematoma, and intraparenchymal hematoma are included in focal injuries. Ischemic and axonal injuries are in the category of diffuse injury.

Brain Swelling

Brain swelling occurs in almost all patients with severe brain injury. This high incidence is a major reason for neurointensive care management of these patients; because brain swelling may cause delayed intracranial hypertension and death, aggressive management improves mortality.[26]

The causes of brain swelling after severe head injury are multifactorial. There is now clear evidence that the majority of early brain edema, both global and focal, is cytotoxic rather than vasogenic. In humans studied with both gadolinium-enhanced magnetic resonance imaging (MRI) and pertechnetate-enhanced single-photon emission computed tomography (SPECT) scans, vasogenic edema with opening of the blood–brain barrier is only seen at later time points around contusions, and not at all in patients with diffuse, nonfocal injuries.[27–29]

Hypoxic-Ischemic Brain Damage

The majority of patients who die after severe TBI will demonstrate at autopsy severe and widespread ischemic neuronal damage if the brain is examined microscopically. This maybe laminar necrosis or cortical infarction, with loss of all neurons in the area involved, as seen especially in the occipital lobe after transtentorial herniation. In less severe nonfatal TBI, pyknotic shrinkage and death of variable numbers of neurons is almost always seen, especially in vulnerable areas of the brain such as hippocampus and cerebellum. This has been well documented in those few patients who later die due to unrelated causes, such as pulmonary embolus or myocardial infarct, and also in animal models of TBI. Similar zones of infarcted neurons are always seen around contusions and under large hematomas, especially acute subdural hematoma. This cerebral ischemic damage is especially common in patients with lung injury and in those with prolonged shock due to intraabdominal or external bleeding, and it has been shown to be associated with dramatically worse outcome.

Cortical Contusion and Traumatic Intracerebral Hemorrhage

Focal cortical contusion is usually caused by mechanical forces that damage the blood vessels (veins, arteries, or larger capillaries) and other neural structures of the pia and underlying parenchyma (neural and glial cells). Contusions typically develop on the inferior surface on the brain, but some may be due to hemorrhagic lesions in the deeper structures of the brain—the so-called *gliding contusions* associated with DAI.[30] Contusions often increase in size over hours to days owing to the evolving events related to the interplay of hemorrhage, vasogenic edema, and ischemic necrosis.

Traumatic intracerebral hemorrhages (ICH) are defined as hematomas 2 cm or larger not in contact with the surface of the brain. The pathology of ICH is due to rupture of the intrinsic blood vessels, typically in deep white matter tracts or basal ganglia at the time of impact. Damage to multiple small blood vessels may result in the coalescence of many smaller hemorrhages. Hemorrhage sometimes will expand with time, and the rate and extent of increase in volume are related to factors such as the type and size of injured vessel, blood pressure, and the underlying bleeding tendency. Delayed traumatic intracerebral hemorrhage (DTICH) is one of the causes of neurological deterioration after TBI, and increase in intracranial hemorrhage has been reported in up to 51% of patients on repeated CT scan in the first 24 hours.[31,32]

Epidural Hematoma

Epidural hematoma (EDH), occurring between the dura and skull, is most frequently found in the temporoparietal regions, where the middle meningeal arteries have been damaged by fracture.[33]

The size of the hematoma depends on the diameter of the injured vessels and how tightly the dura is adherent to the skull. The dura mater of infants is firmly adherent to the developing skull, and the meningeal vessels are not embedded in the skull, as is often the case in later life. Thus, epidural hematomas are not common under the age of 2 years. Deformation of the more elastic skulls of adolescents or young adults may strip the dura mater from the bone and thus produce an epidural hematoma more easily in younger adults. With increasing age, the meningeal vessels become embedded in the bone layer and are at a greater risk for being damaged with skull fracture.

The unique clinical symptom of epidural hematoma is the "lucid interval." This occurs typically after trivial or mild injury but results in delayed coma due to brain compression. On the other hand, one-third of patients have other significant brain injuries such as cerebral contusions, subdural hematomas, and lacerations, and such patients may experience no lucid interval and be unconscious from the time of impact.

Subdural Hematoma

Subdural hematomas (SDHs), the commonest type of mass lesion, are usually caused by rupture of the veins that bridge the subdural space, where they connect the superior surface of the cerebral hemispheres to the sagittal sinus. Thin bilateral films of blood in the subdural space are common in acute fatal head injury, and, in about 13% of cases, the hematoma is "pure" with very little evidence of other brain damage. Because blood can spread freely throughout the subdural space, SDHs tend to cover the entire hemisphere and are more extensive than EDHs, usually 200–300 mL versus 60–100 mL for EDH. Some SDHs are arterial in origin, with the hemorrhage stemming from a cortical artery, and these typically occur with contusions.

The reported mortality rate of traumatic SDH varies from 30% to 90%, with the lower mortality rates occurring in patients who are operated within 4 hours of injury.[34]

The severity of the underlying brain injury determines the outcome even when surgery is done promptly. Outcome has been correlated with neuropathologic studies showing ischemic brain damage in the hemisphere underlying the hematoma. An important factor leading to this ischemic damage is raised intracranial pressure (ICP) producing impaired cerebral perfusion. Increasing ICP reduces the volume of cerebral blood circulation. Unfortunately, removal of the SDH may result in the immediate reversal of global ischemia, and this abrupt reduction of mass lesion sometimes induces "reperfusion injury."[35–37] Previous experimental and clinical studies have shown that SDH and its removal may be considered as ischemic/reperfusion (I/R) injury.[38–40]

Conclusion

Although more than 60,000 research studies have been published on TBI, the main focus of treatment, as discussed elsewhere in this book, is supportive care and removal or decompression of mass lesions. This is because no specific therapeutic agent has yet been proved, through the rigors of clinical testing, to be safe and effective for clinical use. Only by understanding the diverse pathophysiology mechanisms of TBI can new and effective therapies be directed at the primary injuries and the secondary injury cascades that develop in TBI. The following chapters address many facets of this process.

References

1. Tung TA. Trauma and violence in the Wari empire of the Peruvian Andes: warfare, raids, and ritual fights. *Am J Phys Anthropol.* Jul 2007;133(3):941–956.

2. Torres-Rouff C, Costa Junqueira MA. Interpersonal violence in prehistoric San Pedro de Atacama, Chile: behavioral implications of environmental stress. *Am J Phys Anthropol.* May 2006;130(1):60–70.

3. Faul M, Likang Xu, Wald MM, et al. Traumatic brain injury in the United States: emergency department visits, hospitalizations, and deaths 2002–2006. https://www.cdc.gov/traumaticbraininjury/pdf/blue_book.pdf, accessed June 1 2018.

4. Coronado VG, Xu L, Basavaraju SV, et al. Surveillance for traumatic brain injury-related deaths—United States, 1997–2007. *MMWR Surveill Summ.* May 6, 2011;60(5):1–32.

5. Guice KS, Cassidy LD, Oldham KT. Traumatic injury and children: a national assessment. *J Trauma.* Dec 2007;63(6 Suppl):S68–80; discussion S81–66.

6. McCrory P, Meeuwisse WH, Aubry M, et al. Consensus statement on concussion in sport: the 4th International Conference on Concussion in Sport held in Zurich, November 2012. *Br J Sports Med*. Apr 2013;47(5):250–258.

7. Langlois JA, Thomas KE. *Traumatic Brain Injury in the United States: Emergency Department Visits, Hospitalizations, and Deaths*. Atlanta, GA: Centers for Disease Control and Prevention, National Center for Injury Prevention and Control; 2006. https://www.cdc.gov/traumaticbraininjury/pdf/blue_book.pdf

8. Schneier AJ, Shields BJ, Hostetler SG, Xiang H, Smith GA. Incidence of pediatric traumatic brain injury and associated hospital resource utilization in the United States. *Pediatrics*. Aug 2006;118(2):483–492.

9. Asemota AO, George BP, Bowman SM, Haider AH, Schneider EB. Causes and trends in traumatic brain injury for United States adolescents. *J Neurotrauma*. Jan 15, 2013;30(2):67–75.

10. Nonfatal traumatic brain injuries related to sports and recreation activities among persons aged ≤19 years—United States, 2001–2009. *MMWR Morb Mortal Wkly Rep*. Oct 7, 2011;60(39):1337–1342.

11. Shimoda K, Maeda T, Tado M, Yoshino A, Katayama Y, Bullock MR. Outcome and surgical management for geriatric traumatic brain injury: analysis of 888 cases registered in the Japan Neurotrauma Data Bank. *World Neurosurg*. Dec 2014;82(6):1300–1306.

12. Vincent GK, Velkoff, VA. The next four decades: the older population in the United States: 2010–2050. *Curr Population Rep*. 2010 May; 1125–38.

13. Ramanathan DM, McWilliams N, Schatz P, Hillary FG. Epidemiological shifts in elderly traumatic brain injury: 18-year trends in Pennsylvania. *J Neurotrauma*. May 1, 2012;29(7):1371–1378.

14. US department of Health and Human Service, Agency for Healthcare research and quality. H-CUPnet, healthcare cost and utilization project. https://hcupnet.ahrq.gov/#setup. Accessed July 1 2018.

15. Fjell AM, Walhovd KB. Structural brain changes in aging: courses, causes and cognitive consequences. *Rev Neurosci*. 2010;21(3):187–221.

16. Dijkers M CJ, Hibbard M. The consequences of TBI in the elderly: a systematic review. *Brain Inj Professional*. 2008;5:14–18.

17. Ott MM, Eriksson E, Vanderkolk W, Christianson D, Davis A, Scholten D. Antiplatelet and anticoagulation therapies do not increase mortality in the absence of traumatic brain injury. *J Trauma*. Mar 2010;68(3):560–563.

18. Brewer ES, Reznikov B, Liberman RF, et al. Incidence and predictors of intracranial hemorrhage after minor head trauma in patients taking anticoagulant and antiplatelet medication. *J Trauma*. Jan 2011;70(1):E1–5.

19. Cefalu CA. Theories and mechanisms of aging. *Clin Geriatr Med*. Nov 2011;27(4):491–506.

20. Hartholt KA, Van Lieshout EM, Polinder S, Panneman MJ, Van der Cammen TJ, Patka P. Rapid increase in hospitalizations resulting from fall-related traumatic head injury in older adults in The Netherlands 1986–2008. *J Neurotrauma*. May 2011;28(5):739–744.

21. Gillespie LD, Robertson MC, Gillespie WJ, et al. Interventions for preventing falls in older people living in the community. *Cochrane Database Syst Rev*. 2012;9:CD007146.

22. Kannus P, Sievanen H, Palvanen M, Jarvinen T, Parkkari J. Prevention of falls and consequent injuries in elderly people. *Lancet*. Nov 26, 2005;366(9500):1885–1893.

23. Moenninghoff C, Kraff O, Maderwald S, et al. Diffuse axonal injury at ultra-high field MRI. *PLoS One*. 2015;10(3):e0122329.

24. Meythaler JM, Peduzzi JD, Eleftheriou E, Novack TA. Current concepts: diffuse axonal injury-associated traumatic brain injury. *Arch Phys Med Rehabil.* Oct 2001;82(10):1461–1471.

25. Pettus EH, Christman CW, Giebel ML, Povlishock JT. Traumatically induced altered membrane permeability: its relationship to traumatically induced reactive axonal change. *J. Neurotrauma.* Oct 1994;11(5):507–522.

26. Yokobori S, Yamaguchi M, Igarashi Y, et al. Outcome and refractory factor of intensive treatment for geriatric traumatic brain injury: analysis of 1165 cases registered in the Japan Neurotrauma Data Bank. *World Neurosurg.* 2016 Feb;86:127–133.e1. doi:10.1016/j.wneu.2015.09.105. Epub 2015 Oct 13.

27. Bullock R, Butcher S, McCulloch J. Changes in extracellular glutamate concentration after acute subdural haematoma in the rat: evidence for an "excitotoxic" mechanism? *Acta Neurochir. Suppl. (Wien).* 1990;51:274–276.

28. Lang DA, Hadley DM, Teasdale GM, Macpherson P, Teasdale E. Gadolinium DTPA enhanced magnetic resonance imaging in acute head injury. *Acta Neurochir. (Wien).* 1991;109(1-2):5–11.

29. Todd NV, Graham DI. Blood–brain barrier damage in traumatic brain contusions. *Acta Neurochir. Suppl. (Wien).* 1990;51:296–299.

30. Sganzerla EP, Tomei G, Rampini P, et al. A peculiar intracerebral hemorrhage: the gliding contusion, its relationship to diffuse brain damage. *Neurosurg Rev.* 1989;12 Suppl 1:215–218.

31. Yokota H. Cerebral endothelial damage after severe head injury. *J Nippon Med Sch.* Oct 2007;74(5):332–337.

32. Yokota H, Naoe Y, Nakabayashi M, et al. Cerebral endothelial injury in severe head injury: the significance of measurements of serum thrombomodulin and the von Willebrand factor. *J. Neurotrauma.* Sep 2002;19(9):1007–1015.

33. Jamieson KG, Yelland JD. Extradural hematoma. Report of 167 cases. *J. Neurosurg.* Jul 1968;29(1):13–23.

34. Seelig JM, Becker DP, Miller JD, Greenberg RP, Ward JD, Choi SC. Traumatic acute subdural hematoma: major mortality reduction in comatose patients treated within four hours. *N Engl J Med.* Jun 18, 1981;304(25):1511–1518.

35. Miller JD, Bullock R, Graham DI, Chen MH, Teasdale GM. Ischemic brain damage in a model of acute subdural hematoma. *Neurosurgery.* Sep 1990;27(3):433–439.

36. Kuroda Y, Bullock R. Local cerebral blood flow mapping before and after removal of acute subdural hematoma in the rat. *Neurosurgery.* May 1992;30(5):687–691.

37. Burger R, Bendszus M, Vince GH, Solymosi L, Roosen K. Neurophysiological monitoring, magnetic resonance imaging, and histological assays confirm the beneficial effects of moderate hypothermia after epidural focal mass lesion development in rodents. *Neurosurgery.* Mar 2004;54(3):701–711; discussion 711–2.

38. Kuroda Y, Fujisawa H, Strebel S, Graham DI, Bullock R. Effect of neuroprotective N-methyl-D-aspartate antagonists on increased intracranial pressure: studies in the rat acute subdural hematoma model. *Neurosurgery.* Jul 1994;35(1):106–112.

39. Yokobori S, Gajavelli S, Mondello S, et al. Neuroprotective effect of preoperatively induced mild hypothermia as determined by biomarkers and histopathological estimation in a rat subdural hematoma decompression model. *J. Neurosurg.* 2013 Feb;118(2):370–380. doi:10.3171/2012.10.JNS12725. Epub 2012 Nov 9.

40. Yokobori S, Mazzeo AT, Hosein K, Gajavelli S, Dietrich WD, Bullock MR. Preconditioning for traumatic brain injury. *Transl Stroke Res.* Feb 2013;4(1):25–39.

Severe TBI in Military: Medical and Surgical Interventions

Geoffrey S. F. Ling and James M. Ecklund

2

Introduction

Traumatic brain injury (TBI) is a common combat casualty. In the modern wars of Operation Iraqi Freedom (OIF) and Operation Enduring Freedom in Afghanistan (OEF), TBI was so prominent that it was referred to as the "signature injury of the war."[1,2]

Historically, severe TBI has been considered a nonsurvivable injury. From the Viet Nam War experience, Bellamy noted that close to 15% of wounds incurred in combat were to the head.[3] He also reported that severe TBI patients contributed disproportionally more to those service members who either were killed in action (KIA) before reaching medical care or died of wounds (DOW) after reaching medical care. In Operation Desert Storm, again, even with many fewer casualties than in Viet Nam, head injury accounted for close to 15% of wounds incurred in combat.[4] Fortunately, far fewer patients who reached medical care died of their wounds. This was attributed to the better protection provided by Kevlar helmets and improvements in medical care.

In OIF and OEF, head injury accounted for about 30% of wounds incurred in battle.[5] Owens et al. reports data from the OIF/OEF Joint Theater Trauma Registry showing that there were fewer thoracic and abdominal injuries suffered by US service members.[5] This results in proportionally more TBI and extremity injuries. Given this change in injury pattern, it is concluded that modern body armor is protective of the chest and abdomen.[6–8] However, US military body armor does not protect either the arms or legs. Helmets only partially protect the head as the wearer has to be able to see, hear, and freely move his or her neck. Consequently, both TBI and extremity injury are disproportionally greater and thus become even more significant.

A growing appreciation of the significance of TBI among OIF and OEF service members began early in these conflicts. The Armed Forces Health Surveillance Center (AFHSC), using data analysis conducted by the Defense and Veterans Brain Injury Center (DVBIC), notes that TBI cases steadily increased over the course of these wars.[9] In 2001, there were 11,619 cases of TBI across all four military services.[9] The Army and Marines accounted for the majority of cases, as would be expected because they are the primary services involved in ground combat. In 2001, moderate to severe TBI were 16.3% of all cases. TBI numbers reached their peak in 2011. At that time, there were 32,829 TBI cases, of which 7.4% were moderate to severe.[9] Even in 2016, with OIF over and OEF forces reduced to less than 10,000 troops, there were 17,672 TBI cases, of which 13.5% were moderate to severe.[9] From this latter statistic, it is clear that, even when not at war, TBI risk remains significant for the military. This is likely due to the nature of combat arms training.

As TBI became more prominent, the Department of Defense (DoD) faced criticism that this condition was not being adequately met. However, civilian TBI care at that time was no better. Military healthcare providers typically take best civilian clinical practices and adapt them for the war environment. For moderate to severe TBI, this meant following the American Association of Neurological Surgeons (AANS) and Congress of Neurosurgery (CNS) clinical practice guidelines (CPGs) for managing severe TBI and applying them to military wartime medical practice.[10] This was, in fact, done.[11]

Where CPGs did not exist or were not appropriate for military medical practice, the DoD convened panels of clinical experts, both military and civilian, to create new CPGs. Examples are the CPG for "Guidelines for the Field Management of Combat-Related Head Trauma" and "VA/DoD Clinical Practice Guidelines for the Management of Concussion/Mild TBI."[12,13]

In one aspect of TBI, the military exceeded civilian practice, and that is in the clinical management of mild TBI or concussion. Data analysis by the AFHSC and DVBIC showed that mild TBI or concussion was much more prevalent than previously suspected. This was occurring at about the same time that the controversy arose surrounding the prevalence of mild TBI in professional sports. Recognizing how important mild TBI/concussion was becoming, in 2005, Admiral Mullen, then Chairman of the Joint Chiefs of Staff, ordered a team of military physicians to go into theater to determine the state of TBI care. This first Gray Team was composed of five military physicians who had all previously deployed to provide medical care in the war theaters. They also represented each branch of the military: Army (Col. Christian Macedonia, commander; Col. Todd Dombroski; Col. Geoffrey Ling), Navy/Marines (Cdr. James Hancock), and Air Force (Col. Michael Jaffee). The Gray Team moniker refers to both their senior ranks and brain cortex being gray matter.[14,15] Later there would be three more Gray Team missions with additional members.

The Gray Team had four total missions. The results of their findings led to the creation of an in-theater system of care for mild TBI. It began with mandatory TBI screening using the military acute concussion evaluation (MACE). Embedded in the MACE is the standardized assessment of concussion developed by McCrea et al. for professional sports.[16,17] This is an easy-to-use paper-and-pencil test that could be administered by military first providers. It should be emphasized that screening of patients suspected of having or being in an event (such as a bomb blast) where a TBI could occur was mandatory. Directive Type Memorandum (DTM) 09-033, in fact, was a general order that required this screening and applied to everyone in the US military.[18] Furthermore, it held leaders, not the patient, accountable. It was understood that a patient with a brain injury may not know that he or she was injured. Thus, it was incumbent on leaders to properly care for their subordinates.

Once a service member was identified as being "at-risk" of having suffered a mild TBI/concussion, he or she was referred to an advanced medical provider who would make the diagnosis based on history and physical and neurological exam. Treatment would then be provided at a Concussion Care or Restoration Center located near the battle front. Once recovered, the service member would be returned to duty. If recovery was prolonged, then they were referred to a military neurologist for further care.

Pathophysiology

TBI begins with a physical force to the head. If that force is sufficient to cause either an anatomical lesion and/or neurological dysfunction, then TBI has occurred. A formal definition of TBI endorsed by the DoD is a traumatically induced structural injury and/or physiological disruption of brain function as a result of an external force, indicated by new onset or worsening of at least one of the following clinical signs immediately following the event: any period of loss of or a decreased level of consciousness, any loss of memory for events immediately before or after the injury (posttraumatic amnesia), any alteration in mental state at the time of the injury (e.g., confusion, disorientation, slowed thinking, alteration of consciousness/mental state), neurological deficits that may or may not be transient, or intracranial lesion.[13]

There are two types of TBI. One is referred to as *closed head* because the skull remains intact. The other is *open* or *penetrating head TBI* because the skull is breached. The vast majority of TBI experienced by the military is closed head injury (>95%).[7]

In military closed head TBI, there are three main subtypes. They are blunt force, acceleration/deceleration, and explosive blast. Each subtype can occur with another. For example, a soldier who is exposed to explosive blast may be injured by the primary explosive shock wave but, at the same time, may also be blown off his feet and strike his head on the ground or a wall upon landing.[19]

In blunt force closed head TBI, an external force such as being struck by an object, causes the skull to move faster than the brain. This occurs because the brain is surrounded by fluid that gives it a higher moment of inertia. Thus, when the head is moving, the brain movement lags. As a consequence, the skull impacts the brain. Another closed head TBI is caused by rapid acceleration/deceleration of the head such as from a motor vehicle accident where the head is moving rapidly and suddenly comes to an abrupt stop from the collision. Again, the head is moving faster than the brain. The abrupt stop followed by rebound causes the skull to strike one side of the brain and then the other. This leads to *coup–contre coup* brain lesions.[19]

In OIF and OEF, the effectiveness of US troops in combat led the enemy to minimize direct contact. Instead they resorted to using improvised explosive devices (IEDs). As a result, a large percentage of TBI can be attributed to either closed head injury from explosive blast or penetrating head injury from IED fragments.

Explosive blast TBI is a recently identified closed head injury. This TBI occurs when an explosive shock wave impacts the head. When an IED detonates, the chemical reaction leads to superheating of surrounding air.[11] This creates a rapidly moving pressure wave of air known as the "shock wave" that expands outward from the detonation. If it encounters a head, it will couple to and transmit its forces into the brain. This leads to disruption of cellular activity and subsequent neurological injury.[19–21]

Penetrating head TBI occurs more commonly in military clinical cases than in civilian. During battle, service members are exposed to fragments from explosive devices or bullets. Gunshot wounds to the head are typically devastating injuries. Bullets are of small mass but are traveling with high velocity. A military 9 mm handgun round is about 7.5 g and has a muzzle velocity of 380 m/sec. If a handgun bullet strikes and enters the skull, it will create an injury track through the brain that is about the diameter of the round itself. Along its injury track, parenchyma, vasculature, and cerebrospinal fluid (CSF) spaces will all be disrupted. The neurological consequences will depend on which brain structures are violated. TBI from handgun rounds is rare among US service members because a standard issue US military helmet is able to withstand this bullet.[22,23]

Rifle bullets are much more injurious because they typically are moving much faster on impact than handgun rounds. The most common military rounds are the 7.62 mm bullet used by AK-47 rifle and the 5.56 mm bullet used by the M-16 or M-4 rifle. Of the two, the AK-47 round is larger but slower, with a weight of 7.9 g and muzzle velocity of 715 m/sec, which is more than twice that of a handgun round. The M-16 round is much smaller, with a weight of 3.6 g and a muzzle velocity of 990 m/sec or almost three times that of a handgun round. Because a rifle round is typically moving at supersonic speed on impact, the bullet creates a vacuum inside the head along its track when it penetrates the skull and moves through brain tissue. Air will rush in behind the bullet, forcing the brain tissue to rapidly expand and leading to a cavitating lesion that stretches and tears tissue. This means that the rifle bullet injury track is many times larger than the diameter of the bullet itself. In addition, the light weight of a rifle bullet may cause it to pitch and yaw after entering the skull, which also contributes to the very large injury track. The burden of brain damaged by rifle rounds is so severe that these are rarely survivable injuries. A US military helmet can degrade rifle round effectiveness but is not able to fully defeat it.[22,23]

Fragments from IEDs are typically larger than bullets and are moving much more slowly. The effective range of an IED fragment to penetrate an unprotected head is much less than a handgun bullet's range. Penetrating fragments can lead to injury tracks that are irregular. As with handgun rounds, neurological impairment will depend on which brain structures are violated. US military helmets are very effective at withstanding fragments.

TBI has two separate neuropathological phases. The first or primary phase is the injury that occurs directly from the traumatic event. This tissue damage happens immediately with and following the impact of the brain or penetration by the foreign body. This is followed quickly by the secondary injury phase, which takes place over the course of seconds to days following the primary phase. This process is a result of reactive oxygen species, inflammatory cascades, and excitatory amino acid releases. The neurophysiological consequences are tissue necrosis, cellular apoptosis of neurons, and cerebral edema. Cerebral edema is especially concerning because it can lead to increased intracranial pressure (ICP), which in turn compresses vascular and other structures leading to ischemia and thus exacerbating the injury state. Severe cerebral edema can cause brain herniation.[24]

Because primary injury happens so quickly, the best option is prevention. The military requires all combat troops to wear their helmets. Secondary injury occurs when there is opportunity for medical intervention. At present, there are no clinically available neuro-rescue or neuro-prophylaxis medications. Thus, treatment is largely supportive. The goals of therapy are to maintain the general physiology to meet the increased metabolic needs of the injured brain and prevent exacerbation of injury.[24]

Clinical Care

Clinical care begins on the battlefield. In 2005, the DoD in collaboration with the Brain Trauma Foundation issued "Guidelines for the Field Management of Combat-Related

Head Trauma" for prehospital management of combat-related TBI.[12] Care begins with the ABCs (airway breathing and circulation), Glasgow Coma Score (GCS) determination, and pupillary reactivity assessment. Severe TBI patients should have their airways secured using an oropharyngeal or similar device if needed. If their GCS is 8 or less, then endotracheal intubation is indicated. Oxygenation goal is pulse oximetry of 90% or more. Hyperventilation is not to be used routinely and is instead reserved only for situations when there is clinical evidence of brain herniation (e.g., unilaterally dilated pupil). Bleeding is to be arrested. All US military personnel in a combat zone carry tourniquets. Hemostatic agents such as and Hemcon and QuikClotR were developed for OIF and OEF.[25] Systolic blood pressure (SBP) should be kept greater than 90 mm Hg. Unlike civilian practice, prophylactic antibiotics can be considered if there is evidence of a skull fracture (i.e., penetrating head TBI) because, during battle, the opportunity for evacuation may be prolonged. Also, the use of sedating and analgesic medications is permitted because an injured service member struggling or crying out could be detrimental to his or her unit while they are actively engaged in combat with the enemy. If used, small incremental doses should be used to allow better clinical monitoring and to avoid exacerbating the patient's neurological condition (e.g., worsening ICP) and to minimize effects on ventilation and perfusion. Any patient with a GCS of 13 or less is to be evacuated directly to a medical treatment facility with a neurosurgeon.

Upon reaching a higher echelon of care, which in OIF and OEF is typically a combat support hospital, treatment is similar to what is available at a US-based Level 1 trauma center. The CPG for managing severe TBI is enacted.[10,26] In brief, these are maintaining ICP at less than 20 mm Hg, normal partial pressure of oxygen (Po_2) (80–100 mm Hg), normal partial pressure of carbon dioxide (Pco_2) (40 mm Hg), and normal body temperature. Blood pressure is maintained to a cerebral perfusion pressure (CPP) of greater than 70 mm Hg or, if an ICP monitor has not yet placed, mean arterial pressure (MAP) is maintained at greater than 70 mm Hg or a SBP of greater than 110 mm Hg. Hyperventilation to Pco_2 35 mm Hg is reserved only for evidence of sustained increase in ICP or clinical evidence of herniation. If used, the understanding is that hyperventilation is a temporizing measure. Thus the goal is to initiate other measures to reduce ICP and to return the patient to normal carbic state as soon as possible. An antiepileptic medication such as phenytoin or fosphenytoin will be administered for 7 days after injury and then discontinued. It will be continued or restarted if a seizure should occur. In the absence on contraindicated conditions (e.g., hemorrhagic shock), low-dose heparin is initiated within the first day after TBI. Mechanical compression devices are also used if available. Both are to prevent deep vein thrombosis, especially on long evacuation flights.

One important modification to the AANS/CNS GPG for managing severe TBI is preferred use of hypertonic saline in the Brain Code of mannitol, hyperventilation, and head elevation to 30 degrees. Military severe TBI casualties often also suffer from hemorrhagic shock due to extremity injury. Because of this, using the osmotic diuretic mannitol would lead to compromise of their already depleted intravascular volume and thus worsen their shock state. This in turn decreases CPP at a critical time when maintaining cerebral perfusion is paramount. Instead, hypertonic saline solution of 23.4% saline bolus (30 cc) followed by a continuous intravenous infusion of 3% hypertonic saline is to be used.[7,11] This approach increases the serum osmolarity, which helps reduce ICP without decreasing intravascular volume.[27,28]

Another military departure from civilian practice is the use of hemicraniectomy. This is a common option used by military neurosurgeons for severe military TBI casualties. Recognizing that evacuation from the war theater to a higher echelon of care either in the Germany or the United States takes a long time—up to 20 hours or more— this surgery is performed to allow better ICP control when these patients are under the care of critical care air transport (CCAT) teams. Although clinically expert, CCAT teams are resource limited while on board aircraft. A hemicraniectomy greatly simplifies ICP management. Although both the DECRA and RecueICP trials of hemicraniectomy did not show neurological benefit following hemicraniectomy versus medical management alone, hemicraniectomy performed in a war theater usually happens much sooner in the injury process than was reported in these two clinical trials (a couple of hours versus many more).[29,30] Whether earlier use of this surgical intervention is relevant to potential efficacy remains to be validated in a clinical trial. However, from a strictly clinical ICP management standpoint, hemicraniectomy is useful in a wartime evacuation paradigm when duration of transport is prolonged.[25,31]

One important clinical finding from the OIF and OEF experience is the risk of developing explosive blast–related vasospasm.[32] In a retrospective review of severe TBI OIF and OEF patients treated at Walter Reed Army Medical Center, close to 50% developed clinically relevant vasospasm. In contrast to aneurysmal subarachnoid vasospasm, the explosive blast–related TBI window of risk was 30 days versus 14 days. These patients responded well to "triple-H therapy" of induced hemodilution, hypervolemia, and hypertension. Patients recalcitrant to triple-H therapy underwent endovascular therapy with angioplasty and intraarterial pharmacological vasodilation with beneficial results.

Conclusion

Severe TBI management in a military theater of war begins with adapting best civilian clinical practices to this unique practice setting. When CPGs do not exist or are not appropriate, then the DoD convenes both military and civilian clinical experts to develop guidelines of care. During OIF and OEF, military clinicians contributed to the understanding and clinical management of TBI. They identified a new clinical condition, explosive blast TBI. New CPGs were created. The DoD TBI management system is the first large-scale, systemwide standardized approach to TBI care. It begins by empowering the military first provider with the MACE to identify patients at risk for TBI. Accountability is placed with leaders to be certain the system will be properly used. Once identified as being at-risk, the patient is referred to an advanced healthcare provider for diagnosis. When diagnosed, patients are triaged and evacuated to the appropriate level of in-theater care. This could be a concussion restoration or care center located at a forward operating base or to a combat support hospital where a neurosurgeon and/or neurologist is located. For severe TBI, medical care must begin as soon as possible, which means on the battlefield. Military first providers are guided by the CPG "Guidelines for the Field Management of Combat-Related Head Trauma." Patients must be triaged and evacuated to a combat support hospital with neurosurgical assets. There, an adapted version of the civilian "Guidelines for Managing Severe TBI" is used. For patients suffering from increased ICP, diffuse cerebral edema, and related effects, hemicraniectomy may be performed to optimize in-transport medical care. Later, if vasospasm should manifest, then hypervolemic, hypertensive, and hemodilution therapy is instituted. If this is insufficient, then endovascular intervention can be used with either angioplasty or intraarterial pharmacologic vasodilators. Medicine advances in time of war; because of OIF and OEF, the care of everyone with TBI, military and civilian, has improved.

Disclaimer

The opinions and views expressed herein belong only to the authors. They do not nor should they be interpreted as being those of or endorsed by the DoD, the Uniformed Services University of the Health Sciences, or any other agency of the federal government.

References

1. Warden D. Military TBI during the Iraq and Afghanistan wars. *J Head Trauma Rehabil.* 2006;21(5):398–402.

2. Warden DL, French L. Traumatic brain injury in the war zone. *N Engl J Med.* 2005;353(6):633–634.

3. Bellamy RF. The causes of death in conventional land warfare: implications for combat casualty care research. *Mil Med.* 1984;149(2):55–62.

4. Carey ME, Joseph AS, Morris WJ et al. Brain wounds and their treatment in VII Corps during Operation Desert Storm, February 20 to April 15. 1991. *Mil Med.* 1998;163(9):581–586.

5. Owens BD et al. Combat wounds in operation Iraqi Freedom and operation Enduring Freedom. *J Trauma.* 2008;64(2):295–299.

6. Okie S. Traumatic brain injury in the war zone. *N Engl J Med.* 2005;352(20):2043–2047.

7. Ling GS, Ecklund JM. Traumatic brain injury in modern war. *Curr Opin Anaesthesiol.* 2011;24(2):124–130.

8. Ling GSF, Ecklund JM. Neurotrauma from explosive blast. In Elsayed NM, Atkins JL, eds. Explosion and *blast-related injuries. Effects of explosion and blast from military operations and acts of terrorism.* Elsevier: New York: Elsevier; 2008:91–104.

9. DVBIC. DoD worldwide numbers TBI. 2016. http://dvbic.dcoe.mil/dod-worldwide-numbers-tbi.

10. The Brain Trauma Foundation. The American Association of Neurological Surgeons. Guidelines for the management of severe traumatic brain injury. *J Neurotrauma.* 2007;24(Suppl 1):S1–106.

11. Ling G, Bankak F, Armonda R et al. Explosive blast neurotrauma. *J Neurotrauma.* 2009;26(6):815–825.

12. Knuth T, Letarte P, Moores L et al. Guidelines for the Field Management of Combat-Related Head Trauma. New York: Brain Trauma Foundation; 2005;1–95. https://www.braintrauma.org/uploads/02/09/btf_field_management_guidelines_2.pdf

13. VA/DoD Clinical Practice Guideline for Management of Concussion/Mild Traumatic Brain Injury. *J Rehabil Res Dev.* 2009;46(6):CP1–68.

14. Weinberger S. Bombs' hidden impact: the brain war. *Nature.* 2011;477:390–393.

15. Hamilton J. All Things Considered: How a Team of Elite Doctors Changed the Military's Stance on Brain Trauma. Washington, DC: National Public Radio (NPR); 2016.

16. McCrea M. Standardized mental status assessment of sports concussion. *Clin J Sport Med.* 2001;11(3):176–181.

17. McCrea M, Kelly JP, Kluge J et al. Standardized assessment of concussion in football players. *Neurology.* 1997;48(3):586–588.

18. Department of Defense (DoD). DTM-09-033: Policy Guidance for Management of Concussion/Mild Traumatic Brain Injury in the Deployed Setting. Washington, DC: US Department of Defense; 2010.

19. Bandak FA, Ling G, Bandak A et al. Injury biomechanics, neuropathology, and simplified physics of explosive blast and impact mild traumatic brain injury. *Handb Clin Neurol.* 2015;127:89–104.

20. Lu J, Ng KC, Ling G et al. Effect of blast exposure on the brain structure and cognition in Macaca fascicularis. *J Neurotrauma,* 2012 May 1;29(7):1434–54.

21. Alford PW, Dabiri BE, Goss JA et al. Blast-induced phenotypic switching in cerebral vasospasm. *Proc Natl Acad Sci U S A.* 2011;108(31):12705–12710.

22. Ling G et al. Penetrating brain injury (PTBI) model: mathematical prediction and biological validation in rats. In Advanced Technology Applied to Combat Casualty Care. 2003. St. Petersburg, Fl. Abstract.

23. Moshang, E. and G. Ling. Combat Casualty Care and Penetrating Head Wound Injuries: Development of a Non-Ballistic Penetrating Traumatic Brain Injury (PTBI) Model Using Air Inflation Technique. in Advanced Technology Applied to Combat Casualty Care. 2002. St. Petersburg, Fl. Abstract.

24. Ling G, Ecklund J. Neuro critical care in modern war. *J Trauma.* 2007;62(6 Suppl):S102.

25. Ling G, Rhee S, Ecklund JM. Surgical innovations arising from the Iraq and Afghanistan wars. *Annu Rev Med.* 2010;61:457–468.

26. Carney N, Totten A, O'Reilly C et al. Guidelines for the Management of Severe Traumatic Brain Injury, 4th Edition. New York: Brain Trauma Foundation; 2016.

27. Suarez JI, Qureshi AI, Bhardwaj A et al. Treatment of refractory intracranial hypertension with 23.4% saline. *Crit Care Med.* 1998;26(6):1118–1122.

28. Koenig MA, Bryan M, Lewin JL 3rd et al. Reversal of transtentorial herniation with hypertonic saline. *Neurology.* 2008;70(13):1023–1029.

29. Cooper DJ, Rosenfeld JV, Murray L et al. Decompressive craniectomy in diffuse traumatic brain injury. *N Engl J Med.* 2011;364(16):1493–1502.

30. Hutchinson PJ, Kolias AG, Timofeev IS et al. Trial of decompressive craniectomy for traumatic intracranial hypertension. *N Engl J Med.* 2016;375(12):1119–1130.

31. Bell RS, Mossop CM, Dirks MS et al. Early decompressive craniectomy for severe penetrating and closed head injury during wartime. *Neurosurg Focus.* 2010;28(5):E1.

32. Armonda RA, Bell RS, Vo AH et al. Wartime traumatic cerebral vasospasm: recent review of combat casualties. *Neurosurgery.* 2006 Dec; 59(6):1215–25.

Pediatric Severe Traumatic Brain Injury Management

Kendra Woods and Michael J. Bell

3

Introduction

Severe traumatic brain injury (TBI) is the leading cause of death and disability in the developed world. Management of this disease has evolved over decades toward a step-wise approach to add therapies as the disease evolves. A central tenet of treating children with severe TBI is to minimize secondary injuries including intracranial hypertension (increased intracranial pressure [ICP]), cerebral hypoperfusion, hypoxia, and other systemic disturbances. Evidence-based guidelines were first published in 2003 and updated in 2012 to guide management strategies. Because the literature is insufficient, these guidelines cannot currently recommend many specific therapies for individual patients. It is hoped that future research will contribute to our understanding of the pathophysiology and characteristics of the disorder so more comprehensive and patient-specific treatments can be applied in the future. This review is intended to review the current management strategies and the evidence underpinning their use.

For several decades, TBI has been the leading cause of death in children in the United States. In 2005, trauma caused more than 7,000 deaths in children younger than 19 years of age, and TBI is thought to be responsible for more than 50% of these deaths.[1,2] Between 100,000 and 150,000 children suffer from severe TBI, and approximately 10–15% result in death or severe disability.[3] The burden of childhood TBI is expected to exceed $30 billion annually within the United States, and this estimate is only likely to grow as survivors continue to utilize resources through improvements in rehabilitation and outpatient care.[4,5] Despite this enormous burden to society, brain-specific therapies for TBI are limited.

An understanding of the pathogenesis of TBI is necessary to explore the therapies in current practice. Primary injury consists of damage to the brain itself, hematomas that occur around the brain (epidural/subdural), and other damage to the cranium and blood vessels of the brain. After the primary injury, pathological processes evolve over hours to days that can lead to worsening of the injury. These processes include alterations in cerebral blood flow, increases in cerebral swelling leading to increases in ICP, and increased brain metabolism (particularly from seizures and fevers) that can lead to inadequate tissue perfusion, among other cascades. In addition, secondary injuries such as hypoxemia and hypotension can exacerbate pathological processes that are already in motion. Most of contemporary neurotrauma care is intended to recognize these processes early and mitigate any secondary injuries as they arise.

The main physiological principle that underpins contemporary neurotrauma care for children is the Monro-Kellie doctrine. Decades ago, the relationship between the contents of the brain (brain parenchyma, arterial and venous blood, and cerebrospinal fluid [CSF]) and the overall volume of the cranial vault was recognized. Specifically, the pressure within the cranial vault is related to the contents of the brain and the cranial vault volume. As pathological contents—such as hematomas or swelling—increase, nonpathological contents of the vault are first extruded from the cranium to maintain normal pressure. These compensatory mechanisms are decreases in venous blood volume by increased venous drainage into the thorax and decreased CSF volume by movement of CSF to the spinal canal. As these compensatory mechanisms are overcome, increases in pathological volumes result in increases in pressure within the cranial vault. In the extreme, if this ICP exceeds mean arterial blood pressure (MAP), then there is no flow of blood to the brain and ischemia and death ensues. Finding thresholds of ICP that are associated with favorable outcome—generally now accepted as ICP of less than 20 mm Hg—has been a focal point of research. Moreover, maintaining cerebral perfusion pressure (CPP; the arithmetic difference between MAP and ICP) is also part of contemporary clinical care.

To a great extent, contemporary care includes minimizing the effects of pathological processes initiated by the primary injury and allowing the brain to recover function over time. To achieve this, strategies must be implemented to optimize oxygen and glucose delivery to the brain, and then brain-specific therapies need to be initiated to maximize benefits and minimize side effects of treatment. Since hypoxic-ischemic injury is common after severe TBI,[6–9] institution of mechanical ventilation with endotracheal intubation in children with severe TBI is necessary. Precise targets for oxygenation are arbitrary, with some recommending a Pao_2 of greater than 60–65 mm Hg and Sao_2 of greater than 90%. Others recommend targeting brain tissue oxygen tension (Pbo_2) for this important parameter. Resuscitation should have a goal of maintaining adequate blood pressure to provide cerebral perfusion and prevent secondary organ injuries. Evidence-based guidelines for the management of children with severe TBI have been published that summarize these goals for basic aspects of care.[10] The remainder of this review will concern itself with brain-specific therapies for children with severe TBI.

Mechanical Therapies: Surgical Evacuation

Surgical evacuation of hematomas and other pathological masses leads to lower ICP for two reasons: removing the mass leads to a lowered volume of the contents of the skull cavity and the removal of the bone effectively increases the size of the cranial vault. While decompressive surgery early after injury has been a mainstay of neurotrauma care for decades, precise recommendations for the timing of the procedure have remained elusive. Anecdotal reports from recent wars suggested that early decompressive surgery can result in improved outcomes as soldiers are evacuated outside of the combat theater. However, in a randomized controlled trial involving 27 children with severe TBI, early decompressive craniectomy resulted in decreased ICP for the first 48 hours after surgery, but no definitive improvement in outcome was proven[11]—mimicking a larger multicenter study in adults with severe TBI.[12]

Mechanical Therapies: Cerebrospinal Fluid Drainage

Drainage of CSF can be accomplished by the placement of a catheter in the cerebral ventricle or the lumbar spinal column. The rationale for either approach is the same: decrease the CSF volume within the cranial vault and thereby lower the pressure within the cranial vault. Shapiro and Marmarou developed the pressure–volume index (PVI) as a bedside procedure to measure intracerebral compliance.[13] To perform the maneuver, a small volume of sterile saline was instilled into the cerebral ventricle to determine the extent of ICP increase, with greater increases in ICP indicative of decreased cerebral compliance. In this landmark report, children with reduced PVI were at highest risk for intracranial hypertension. Like most other TBI therapies, definitive outcome studies for this therapy are lacking. James and colleagues demonstrated that intermittent drainage of CSF from an externalized drain caused a decrease in ICP for dozens of patients of varying ages.[14] However, this therapy alone was insufficient to control ICP as the injury evolved. Fortune and colleagues found that CSF drainage for intracranial hypertension led to a decrease in ICP that was associated with favorable effects on cerebral blood flow.[15] To illustrate the complexity of this decision, Jagannathan and colleagues reported that ventricular CSF drainage improved ICP and quality of life in children while also causing an increased incidence of meningitis (22%).[16] Nevertheless, CSF diversion via ventriculostomy remains a standard therapy for children with severe TBI.

In contrast to CSF diversion via ventriculostomy (a Tier 1 therapy for intracranial hypertension), lumbar drainage is a second-tier ICP therapy. The rationale for this secondary consideration of lumbar removal of CSF reflects the relative lack of evidence for the therapy and the concern that placement of such a device in children with noncommunicating hydrocephalous can lead to cerebral herniation. In the largest series, 16 children receiving lumbar drainage after failing Tier 1 therapies experienced decreased ICP and had a survival rate of 88%.[17] Nevertheless, how this therapy should be administered remains unclear with the current literature.

Therapeutic Maneuvers: Hyperventilation

As early airway support for stabilization of the child after TBI has been understood for decades, the level of ventilation that should be targeted has been a constant source of controversy. Physiologically, hyperventilation leads to cerebral vasoconstriction, ultimately leading to decreased cerebral blood volume and lowered ICP. However, the balance between supporting cerebral blood flow—which can be compromised by excessive hyperventilation—and ICP becomes a clinical challenge. Earlier studies demonstrated that a protocol that included aggressive hyperventilation could result in good neurological outcome, with the rationale for this approach being that excessive cerebral blood flow was common in children.[18] However, using xenon computed tomography (Xe-CT) scanning, others reported that cerebral ischemia was common early after severe TBI and questioned whether hyperventilation could exacerbate the injury.[19,20–23] As a result, brief periods of hyperventilation appear prudent as an emergency measure for acute herniation events, while protracted periods of hyperventilation appear to have a detrimental risk–benefit ratio. Tellingly, acute hyperventilation was extremely common in the largest randomized controlled trial performed in children with severe TBI to date.[24] In this study, hyperventilation (defined as P_{CO_2} <30 mm Hg) was employed in 40% of children in both the hypothermia and normothermia groups. So, despite little evidence for how to use this therapy, it remains a very commonly used strategy in trauma centers around the world.

Medications: Hyperosmolar Therapies

Hyperosmolar therapies can lower ICP by two alterations in cerebrohemodynamics. First, within seconds, the intravenous infusions of these agents leads to decreased blood viscosity and improved laminar flow through arterioles, thus leading to decreased vessel size without alterations in blood flow and decreased ICP. Second, the increase in serum osmolarity that occurs minutes after administration of these agents leads to fluid flux out of the brain and decreased ICP. This second mechanism is functional in brain regions where the blood–brain barrier is functioning normally. Similar to other TBI therapies, definitive studies regarding hyperosmolar therapies and outcomes are lacking, yet volumes of studies point to the beneficial role these agents play in treating children with TBI. James and colleagues[25] reported that a dose of mannitol of 0.5 g/kg resulted in decreased ICP in 78% of patients with a variety of central nervous system (CNS) pathologies (trauma, brain tumor, encephalopathy, and subarachnoid hemorrhage), while a larger dose of 1 g/kg was nearly universally effective (99%). Furthermore, Mendelow and colleagues demonstrated similar effects of mannitol on ICP with additional benefit noted to CPP and cerebral blood flow as well.[26] In the previously cited manuscript by Shapiro and Marmarou,[13] mannitol was shown to be effective in improving cerebrohemodynamics by changes in both ICP and PVI. Specifically, PVI increased and ICP decreased in almost all of the 22 children studied (the two nonresponders died from uncontrolled intracranial hypertension shortly after the study).

Direct comparisons between hyperosmolar solutions are largely lacking. Despite this, one of the only Level 2 recommendations in the current guidelines supports that hypertonic saline should be considered for intracranial hypertension. This recommendation stems from a randomized study of 18 children by Fisher and colleagues where a 25% decrease in ICP after 3% saline and no change in the normal saline group was observed.[27] Most recently, Shein and colleagues used a system that collected data every 5 seconds linked with the timing of medications for intracranial crises and found that hypertonic saline (3% saline) was superior to lowering ICP and maintaining CPP over fentanyl and pentobarbital.[2]. Unfortunately, in their analysis, this paper did not have sufficient doses of mannitol to adequately compare those two different solutions.

Complications of mannitol include concerns for hypovolemia due to diuresis as well as an association between mannitol use and renal failure at extremes of serum osmolarity. Peterson and colleagues reported successful treatment of intracranial hypertension with 3% saline to very high levels of sodium in a retrospective cohort of 68 children.[29] This group demonstrated improved outcomes based on trauma scores and found no adverse events despite serum sodium concentrations of greater than 180 meq/L in some cases. For the clinician caring for such children, it is clear that the hydration of children receiving mannitol and carefully monitoring sodium concentrations of children receiving hypertonic saline solutions—both as care is being escalated as well as when therapies are being withdrawn—should be very carefully monitored.

Medications: Barbiturates and Drug-Induced Coma

Barbiturates cause a decrease in metabolic activity in the brain, leading to decreases in necessary cerebral blood flow and decreases in blood volume within the brain to treat intracranial hypertension. At doses sufficient to induce coma, barbiturate use is associated with significant cardiovascular side effects including hypotension, vasoparesis, and decreased cardiac performance. Beneficial effects on ICP,[30] brain oxygenation,[31] and decreased excitotoxicity[32] in adults after severe TBI have been observed after barbiturate administration. However, the relationship between barbiturate use and outcome is difficult to establish. Pittman and colleagues found that pentobarbital decreased ICP in more than 50% of children with TBI yet could not identify a positive long-term outcome in the cohort. Because data supporting barbiturate therapy are so lacking, the current guidelines state that barbiturates may be considered, and, when considered, advanced hemodynamic monitoring should be used.

Experimental Therapies: Hypothermia

Therapeutic hypothermia may be the most well-studied intervention for children with severe TBI, and, unfortunately, the results have been relatively disappointing. Moderate hypothermia is defined as the maintenance of a core body temperature of 32–34°C, and this level of hypothermia has been used clinically for its lack of significant side effects and efficacy in animal models. In fact, therapeutic hypothermia has demonstrated efficacy in phase III trials for adults with cardiac arrest and neonates with perinatal asphyxia. Like pentobarbital coma, hypothermia's effect on ICP is believed to be decreasing cerebral metabolic rate, leading to decreases in cerebral blood flow and cerebral blood volume.

Clinical studies of hypothermia for TBI have almost universally proposed that the early application of hypothermia to the entire population of patients with severe TBI can lead to some improvement in overall outcome: mortality, Glasgow Outcome Scale (GOS), or some other measure of function. In adults with severe TBI, Marion and colleagues demonstrated that hypothermia for 24 hours led to improved neurological outcome at 6 months, particularly in patients who had the higher range of Glasgow Coma Scale (GCS) scores at enrollment.[33] Disappointingly, Clifton and colleagues failed to demonstrate any significant beneficial effect in a four-center study of 392 patients.[34]

For children with severe TBI, the results are also disappointing. Adelson and colleagues performed a phase II safety study in 48 children and found that hypothermia was safe and there was a trend toward a decrease in mortality at 3 months.[35] However, in a phase III trial, Hutchison and colleagues not only failed to show a benefit, but demonstrated a trend toward harm in the experimental group.[24] In this study, 225 children were randomized, and the hypothermia group had worse outcome (31% vs. 22%) which did not reach statistical significance. Adelson and colleagues used a longer period of hypothermia with slower rewarming in the Cool Kids Trial.[36] After randomizing 77 children, this trial also failed to demonstrate a beneficial effect of hypothermia and was stopped by the Data Safety Monitoring Board due to concerns regarding futility. Most recently, Beca and colleagues performed a phase II safety study of an extended period of hypothermia (72 hours) in 55 children in Australia/New Zealand.[37] While they found no differences in complications, they also found no beneficial effects of the therapy.

Conclusion

In summary, while the evidenced-based guidelines are not as robust as clinicians desire due to lack of evidence of proven therapies, substantial information is available to guide therapies in children with severe TBI. It is hoped that future research can establish higher levels of evidence and work toward personalizing the care of such children.

Disclaimer

Dr. Bell is supported by an National Institutes of Health (NIH) Grant (NS 081041). Neither Dr. Woods nor Dr. Bell has other relevant conflict of interests.

References

1. Kung H-C, Hoyert DL, Xu J, Murphy SL. Deaths: final data for 2005. *National Vital Statistics Reports.* 2008;56(10):1–121.

2. Faul MD, Xu L, Wald MM, Coronado VG. *Traumatic Brain Injury in the United States: Emergency Department Visits, Hospitalizations and Death 2002–2006.* Atlanta (GA): Centers for Disease Control and Prevention, National Center for Injury Prevention;2010.

3. Luerssen TG, Klauber MR, Marshall LF. Outcome from head injury related to patient's age. A longitudinal prospective study of adult and pediatric head injury. *J Neurosurg.* Mar 1988;68(3):409–416.

4. Cohadon F, Richer E, Castel JP. Head injuries: incidence and outcome. *J Neurol Sci.* Jul 1991;103 Suppl:S27–31.

5. Frankowski R, Annegers J, Whitman S. *Epidemiology and descriptive studies. Part 1. The descriptive epidemiology of head trauma in the United States.* Bethesda: National Institute of Health, NINDS;1985.

6. Cooper A, DiScala C, Foltin G, Tunik M, Markenson D, Welborn C. Prehospital endotracheal intubation for severe head injury in children: a reappraisal. *Semin Pediatr Surg.* Feb 2001;10(1):3–6.

7. Murray JA, Demetriades D, Berne TV, et al. Prehospital intubation in patients with severe head injury. *J Trauma.* Dec 2000;49(6):1065–1070.

8. Stocchetti N, Furlan A, Volta F. Hypoxemia and arterial hypotension at the accident scene in head injury. *J Trauma.* May 1996;40(5):764–767.

9. Winchell RJ, Hoyt DB. Endotracheal intubation in the field improves survival in patients with severe head injury. Trauma Research and Education Foundation of San Diego. *Arch Surg.* Jun 1997;132(6):592–597.

10. Kochanek PK, Carney NA, Adelson PD, et al. Guidelines for the Acute Medical Management of Severe Traumatic Brain Injury in Infants, Children and Adolescents: Second Edition. *Pediatr Crit Care Med.* 2012;13, No. 1 (Suppl):S1–S82.

11. Taylor A, Butt W, Rosenfeld J, et al. A randomized trial of very early decompressive craniectomy in children with traumatic brain injury and sustained intracranial hypertension. *Childs Nerv Syst.* Feb 2001;17(3):154–162.

12. Cooper DJ, Rosenfeld JV, Murray L, et al. Decompressive craniectomy in diffuse traumatic brain injury. *N Engl J Med.* Apr 21, 2011;364(16):1493–1502.

13. Shapiro K, Marmarou A. Clinical applications of the pressure-volume index in treatment of pediatric head injuries. *J Neurosurg.* Jun 1982;56(6):819–825.

14. James HE, Langfitt TW, Kumar VS. Analysis of the response to therapeutic measures to reduce intracranial pressure in head injured patients. *J Trauma*. Jun 1976;16(6):437–441.

15. Fortune JB, Feustel PJ, Graca L, Hasselbarth J, Kuehler DH. Effect of hyperventilation, mannitol, and ventriculostomy drainage on cerebral blood flow after head injury. *J Trauma*. Dec 1995;39(6):1091–1097; discussion 1097–1099.

16. Jagannathan J, Okonkwo DO, Yeoh HK, et al. Long-term outcomes and prognostic factors in pediatric patients with severe traumatic brain injury and elevated intracranial pressure. *J Neurosurg Pediatr*. Oct 2008;2(4):240–249.

17. Levy DI, Rekate HL, Cherny WB, Manwaring K, Moss SD, Baldwin HZ. Controlled lumbar drainage in pediatric head injury. *J Neurosurg*. Sep 1995;83(3):453–460.

18. Bruce DA, Langfitt TW, Miller JD, et al. Regional cerebral blood flow, intracranial pressure, and brain metabolism in comatose patients. *J Neurosurg*. Feb 1973;38(2):131–144.

19. Adelson PD, Clyde B, Kochanek PM, Wisniewski SR, Marion DW, Yonas H. Cerebrovascular response in infants and young children following severe traumatic brain injury: a preliminary report. *Pediatr Neurosurg*. Apr 1997;26(4):200–207.

20. Kiening KL, Hartl R, Unterberg AW, Schneider GH, Bardt T, Lanksch WR. Brain tissue pO2-monitoring in comatose patients: implications for therapy. *Neurol Res*. Jun 1997;19(3):233–240.

21. Muizelaar JP, Marmarou A, Ward JD, et al. Adverse effects of prolonged hyperventilation in patients with severe head injury: a randomized clinical trial. *J Neurosurg*. Nov 1991;75(5):731–739.

22. Schneider GH, von Helden A, Lanksch WR, Unterberg A. Continuous monitoring of jugular bulb oxygen saturation in comatose patients: therapeutic implications. *Acta neurochirurgica*. 1995;134(1-2):71–75.

23. von Helden A, Schneider GH, Unterberg A, Lanksch WR. Monitoring of jugular venous oxygen saturation in comatose patients with subarachnoid haemorrhage and intracerebral haematomas. *Acta Neurochir Suppl (Wien)*. 1993;59:102–106.

24. Hutchison JS, Ward RE, Lacroix J, et al. Hypothermia therapy after traumatic brain injury in children. *N Engl J Med*. Jun 5, 2008;358(23):2447–2456.

25. James HE. Methodology for the control of intracranial pressure with hypertonic mannitol. *Acta neurochirurgica*. 1980;51(3-4):161–172.

26. Mendelow AD, Teasdale GM, Russell T, Flood J, Patterson J, Murray GD. Effect of mannitol on cerebral blood flow and cerebral perfusion pressure in human head injury. *J Neurosurg*. Jul 1985;63(1):43–48.

27. Fisher B, Thomas D, Peterson B. Hypertonic saline lowers raised intracranial pressure in children after head trauma. *J Neurosurg Anesthesiol*. Jan 1992;4(1):4–10.

28. Shein SL, Ferguson NM, Kochanek PM, et al. Effectiveness of pharmacological therapies for intracranial hypertension in children with severe traumatic brain injury: results from an automated data collection system time-synched to drug administration. *Pediatr Crit Care Med*. Mar 2016;17(3):236–245.

29. Peterson B, Khanna S, Fisher B, Marshall L. Prolonged hypernatremia controls elevated intracranial pressure in head-injured pediatric patients. *Crit Care Med*. Apr 2000;28(4):1136–1143.

30. Eisenberg HM, Frankowski RF, Contant CF, Marshall LF, Walker MD. High-dose barbiturate control of elevated intracranial pressure in patients with severe head injury. *J Neurosurg*. Jul 1988;69(1):15–23.

31. Chen HI, Malhotra NR, Oddo M, Heuer GG, Levine JM, LeRoux PD. Barbiturate infusion for intractable intracranial hypertension and its effect on brain oxygenation. *Neurosurgery*. Nov 2008;63(5):880–886; discussion 886–887.

32. Goodman JC, Valadka AB, Gopinath SP, Cormio M, Robertson CS. Lactate and excitatory amino acids measured by microdialysis are decreased by pentobarbital coma in head-injured patients. *J Neurotrauma*. Oct 1996;13(10):549–556.

33. Marion DW, Penrod LE, Kelsey SF, et al. Treatment of traumatic brain injury with moderate hypothermia. *N Engl J Med*. Feb 20, 1997;336(8):540–546.

34. Clifton GL, Miller ER, Choi SC, et al. Lack of effect of induction of hypothermia after acute brain injury. *N Engl J Med*. Feb 22, 2001;344(8):556–563.

35. Adelson PD, Ragheb J, Kanev P, et al. Phase II clinical trial of moderate hypothermia after severe traumatic brain injury in children. *Neurosurgery*. Apr 2005;56(4):740–754; discussion 740–754.

36. Adelson PD, Wisniewski SR, Beca J, et al. Comparison of hypothermia and normothermia after severe traumatic brain injury in children (Cool Kids): a phase 3, randomised controlled trial. *Lancet Neurol*. Jun 2013;12(6):546–553.

37. Beca J, McSharry B, Erickson S, et al. Hypothermia for traumatic brain injury in children: a phase II randomized controlled trial. *Crit Care Med*. Jul 2015;43(7):1458–1466.

Treatment of Severe Traumatic Brain Injury in the Scandinavian Countries, with Special Emphasis on the Lund Concept

Magnus Olivecrona and Per-Olof Grände

4

Introduction

In the Nordic countries, severe traumatic brain injury (s-TBI) (Glasgow Coma Scale [GCS] ≤8) is treated only at centers with neurosurgical competence. Currently, there are two main guidelines, the Brain Trauma Foundation (BTF) guidelines with the latest version from 2016,[1] and the Lund concept (LC).[2,3] The LC predominates in Sweden and was clinically introduced at Lund University Hospital in 1992. The BTF guidelines were introduced in 1996[4] and are the most commonly used set of guidelines outside of Sweden.

The BTF guidelines are based on a meta-analytic approach using outcomes from clinical studies. These guidelines can be said to represent a *cerebral pressure perfusion (CPP)-targeted therapy*. When introduced, the guidelines were more or less a pure CPP-guided therapy with a recommendation that the lowest acceptable CPP was 70 mm Hg, maintained if necessary with frequent use of vasopressors.[4]

The Lund concept was a theoretical approach based on physiological principles of brain volume and brain perfusion regulation; it can be described as an *intracranial pressure (ICP)- and perfusion-targeted therapy*. It gave strict recommendations regarding ICP, CPP, fluid therapy, ventilation, sedation, nutrition, and the use of vasopressors and osmotherapy. In the 25 years following its introduction, the main components of the Lund concept have found strong support in experimental and clinical studies. In principle, the Lund concept has not changed since its introduction in 1992, with the exception that the venoconstrictor dihydroergotamine has been phased out from the concept due to possible adverse peripheral vasoconstrictor effects.[2,3] All outcome studies using the LC have been summarized and discussed in a recent review.[5]

At their introduction in 1996, the BTF guidelines differed considerably from the LC. Over the years, the BTF guidelines have gone through several updates and moved closer to the LC,[1,6] although there are still some major differences. The BTF guidelines from 2007[6] had changed their recommendations regarding CPP from higher than 70 mm Hg to 50–70 mm Hg, which is in the same range as suggested in the LC. The last versions of the BTF guidelines also recommend less frequent use of vasopressors and mannitol and the avoidance of active cooling[1,6]—all in line with the LC.[2] In the last version, the BTF guidelines recommend that a raised ICP should not be treated until greater than 22 mm Hg.[1] The Lund concept has instead recommended that ICP-reducing therapy should start as soon as possible after arrival at the intensive care unit independent of ICP in order to prophylactically counteract ICP elevations.[2,3]

Today, there is still a lack of convincing evidence-based support for both the BTF and the LC guidelines. In this sense, the guidelines are all equally deficient. However, there have been several smaller, single-center outcome studies using the LC indicating good outcome.[7–10] The study by Gerber et al.[11] also indicated good outcome when using the BTF guidelines. The LC has also been used in the treatment of people with severe life-threatening meningitis and brain edema in two outcome studies with favorable results.[12,13]

Because this is a summary of treatment of s-TBI in Scandinavia, we have chosen to focus more on the LC as these guidelines are more associated with Scandinavia.

Intracranial Pressure with the Lund Concept

Due to the rigid cranium which has only minor space for intracranial expansion, the volume-regulating mechanisms of the brain must be more effective than those of other organs of the body to avoid adverse alterations in ICP. In the normal brain with an intact blood–brain barrier (BBB), only water can pass through the capillary membrane passively. The transcapillary hydrostatic pressure force favoring filtration is balanced by a corresponding oncotic absorbing pressure force, formulated in the Starling formula for transcapillary fluid exchange.[14,15] Other solutes, such as sodium and chloride ions, can be transported over the membrane to a small degree only, with an energy-requiring active process of low capacity.[14]

In the intact BBB, water passing through the capillary membrane passively results in interstitial dilution. Filtration of water results in a decrease in interstitial crystalloid osmotic pressure from its normal value of about 5,500 mm Hg, thus creating an absorbing crystalloid osmotic counterpressure, and the filtration will very soon cease (Figure 4.1A). This explains why brain volume is kept relatively constant when the BBB is intact.

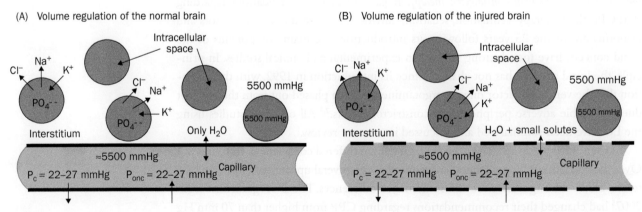

Figure 4.1 (A) Schematic illustration of a cerebral capillary in the normal brain with intact blood–brain barrier (BBB). The Starling forces (transcapillary hydrostatic and oncotic pressures) responsible for transcapillary fluid exchange are shown. Only water can pass through the intact BBB passively. (B) Cerebral capillary in the injured brain with disrupted BBB, in which the capillaries are passively permeable to water and small solutes. The Starling forces are also shown. For further details of the volume regulation mechanisms in the normal and injured brain, see text.

From Grände (2006), with permission.[2]

After an s-TBI, the BBB is disrupted in the sense that small solutes can pass through the capillary membrane passively. This is similar to the mechanisms for transcapillary fluid exchange in other organs of the body. An increase in transcapillary hydrostatic capillary pressure (e.g., after an increase in arterial pressure or precapillary vasodilation or a decrease in transcapillary oncotic pressure) will initiate filtration (Figure 4.1B). The filtrate moving to the brain interstitium will have approximately the same composition as that of plasma. Therefore no crystalloid counteracting force will develop, and the filtration will continue until stopped by the increase in ICP. This is the physiological explanation for development of vasogenic brain edema.[14]

Important hemodynamic characteristics of the brain are based on the fact that the brain is enclosed in a rigid cranium, as shown schematically in Figure 4.2. Hemodynamic effects of changes in arterial and venous pressure for an organ enclosed in a rigid shell have been investigated previously.[16,17] ICP for the normal brain is 8–11 mm Hg as compared to normal tissue pressure in the rest of the body, which is 0–2 mm Hg.[15] The brain is the only organ of the body with a significantly positive tissue pressure. This is no coincidence, since a positive ICP is essential for proper function of the normal brain, as will be explained later.

The venous pressure outside the dura (P_V in Figure 4.2) is close to 0 or negative at upright position. This means that there is a fall in pressure in the veins between the subdural and extradural spaces. As early as 1928, it was shown experimentally[18] that this pressure fall creates a venous collapse at a short distance before the veins leave the brain, creating a subdural venous outflow vascular resistance (R_{out} in Figure 4.2). This principle was confirmed experimentally on a skeletal muscle enclosed in a plethysmograph.[17,19,20] Venous pressure just before R_{out} (P_{out} in Figure 4.2) will change in parallel with the variation in ICP as the resistance created by the passive collapse (R_{out}) is directly related to the pressure fall (ICP − P_V) (Figure 4.2).[16,19]

The hydrostatic capillary pressure can increase by 4–5 mm Hg at most. The vasogenic brain edema can increase many times more than this. This *paradoxical event* is based on

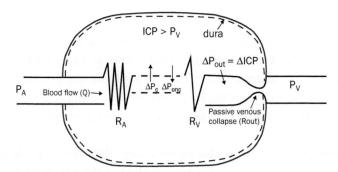

Figure 4.2 Hemodynamic consequences for the brain enclosed in the rigid dura/cranium. ΔPc is the transcapillary hydrostatic capillary pressure, ΔP$_{onc}$ the transcapillary oncotic pressure, P_A the arterial inflow pressure, Q the cerebral blood flow, R_A the arterial precapillary resistance, and R_V the venular resistance. ΔP$_{out}$ is transvascular pressure retrogradely to the subdural venous collapse (R_{out}). P_V is the extracranial venous pressure.

From Grände (2006), with permission.[2]

hemodynamic principles for an organ enclosed in a rigid shell, as will be explained using Figure 4.2.

An imbalance between hydrostatic and oncotic transcapillary pressures in the injured brain with a disrupted BBB will start filtration and slowly increase ICP. The simultaneous increase in R_{out} (due to the increase in $ICP - P_V$) means a similar increase in P_{out}, which will result in an increase in P_c when partly transferred retrogradely to the capillaries (Figure 4.2). This will result in further filtration and a further increase in ICP until a new steady state is established. It has been calculated that the increase in ICP at steady state can be as much as eight times larger than the initial imbalance between transcapillary hydrostatic pressure (P_c) and the transcapillary oncotic pressure (P_{onc}).[16] This is why the increase in ICP caused by a vasogenic brain edema can be much larger than the initial increase in P_c and decrease in P_{onc}.

Consequently, a reduction in P_c by antihypertensive therapy can reduce ICP at most by eight times more than the initial decrease in P_c caused by antihypertensive therapy. This strengthens the justification for using antihypertensive therapy in head-injured patients with raised ICP, as recommended in the LC (see later discussion).

The decrease in extracranial venous pressure from elevation of the head will cause a corresponding increase in R_{out}, preventing the decrease in extradural venous pressure from being transferred in retrograde manner to the brain.[20] This means that there is no increase in venous drainage from the brain through head elevation. The immediate decrease in ICP often seen after head elevation can instead be explained by a passive decrease in arterial intracranial blood volume when arterial pressure to the brain is reduced.[19–21]

The existence of a passive subdural venous collapse and its hemodynamic consequences are important in our daily life. Without this collapse, there would, for example, be a drastic reduction in intracranial venous blood volume—with marked hemodynamic consequences—when changing from supine to upright position or vice versa.

Positive end expiratory pressure (PEEP) is not recommended as an obligatory therapy in alternative guidelines due to the risk of increase in venous blood volume and ICP.[22] The physiological principles presented earlier contradict such a risk, however, as the increase in extracranial venous pressure from PEEP will not be transferred to the brain. This hypothesis found support in clinical studies by Lou et al.[23] and Caricato et al.[24] The latter showed that PEEP increased central venous pressure (CVP) and jugular venous pressure without affecting ICP.[24] Thus, PEEP (normally 6–8 cm H_2O) has been mandatory in the LC to protect the lungs from atelectasis and acute respiratory distress syndrome (ARDS). The results from several studies now support the use of PEEP in TBI patients.[23–25]

The subdural venous collapse also explains why CPP should be calculated as $P_A -$ ICP and not as $P_A - VP$, as in other organs of the body. CPP is P_A minus the pressure just upstream of R_{out}, which is the same as ICP (Figure 4.2). This means that by accepting CPP as $P_A -$ ICP, we also have to accept the existence of a passive variable subdural venous resistance compensating for extradural variations in P_V (Figure 4.2). If P_V is higher than ICP, there is no protecting venous collapse, and perfusion pressure should be calculated as $P_A - P_V$.[19]

Based on these principles, the LC aims to minimize vasogenic brain edema by reducing the hydrostatic capillary pressure with antihypertensive drugs and preservation of the oncotic pressure with albumin infusion (see later discussion). The antihypertensive drugs used are β_1-blockade and an α_2 agonist and, if necessary, an angiotensin II antagonist. All these drugs reduce arterial pressure without inducing cerebral vasodilation, which had increased ICP. It has been shown that β-blockade and α_2 agonists have no or just minor local effect on cerebral blood flow.[26] Head elevation (maximum of 20 degrees) can also be used, with the purpose of reducing arterial inflow blood pressure to the brain.[2,21]

When introduced, LC was strongly criticized by advocates of the BTF guidelines for the use of antihypertensive treatments such as β-blockade. Several recent studies have shown a significantly improved outcome in s-TBI patients with β-blockade.[27–29] The LC is still the only guideline recommending β-blockade for head-injured patients.

While a disrupted BBB is essential for the development of a vasogenic extracellular brain edema, cytotoxic brain edema is mainly intracellular, caused by damage to cell membranes; for example, from hypoxia and various toxic substances.[30,31] Hypoxia is presumed to be an important triggering mechanism for a secondary injury to the brain.[32,33] The LC makes use of the hypothesis that improvement of perfusion and oxygenation of the most injured hypoxic parts of the brain should help to reduce the cytotoxic brain edema, as will be discussed later.

Perfusion with the Lund Concept

One important purpose of the LC is to maintain or improve microcirculation and oxygenation of the hypoxic parts of the penumbra zone. According to the law of Poisseuille (resistance = constant/radius),[4] the constrictor effect of a vasoconstrictor stimulus is dependent on the initial radius. A vasoconstrictor stimulus in the most injured parts of the penumbra zone, with the radius of the vessels being already reduced by the trauma, may therefore result in a reduction in blood flow, even though there is a simultaneous increase in arterial blood pressure.[3]

Vasoconstrictors may also contribute to hypovolemia as they will increase hydrostatic capillary pressure and transcapillary filtration in the whole body. This is an effect of both an increase in arterial pressure and of postcapillary vasoconstriction. Such an effect has been confirmed both experimentally[34] and clinically.[35] As shown in a study on pigs with head trauma, preservation of normovolemia is important for optimization of microcirculation in the penumbra zone as hypovolemia compromises the circulation through activation of the baroreceptor reflex.[36]

According to these principles, preservation of normovolemia and avoidance of vasoconstrictors may help to preserve microcirculation and oxygenation of the penumbra zone, as also adapted in the LC.

Basal Treatments

Neurosurgical Intervention

An important component in the LC is surgical intervention against intracranial expansivities, suggesting that hematomas and also relatively small contusions (20–30 cm³), if surgically available, should be evacuated in order to reduce ICP and also to reduce the inflammatory burden.

Preservation of Normovolemia

Preservation of normovolemia to optimize microcirculation and oxygenation of the penumbra zone is important in the LC. This is achieved by adequate fluid substitution and measures which reduce transcapillary fluid loss. Such measures are avoidance of high CPP, avoidance of vasopressor treatment, avoidance of low Hb concentrations, and physiotherapy.[2,3,5]

Albumin is kept at greater than 34 g/L using infusion of 20% albumin (at an infusion rate of 100 mL/4 hr). In one randomized study, the SAFE-TBI study,[37] a post hoc analysis of a subgroup from the primary intensive care cohort does not recommend the use of albumin in s-TBI patients. On the strength of the unexpected results of the SAFE-TBI study, many neurointensivists have ceased using albumin, instead using only crystalloids as plasma volume expanders. The SAFE-TBI study has, however, been strongly criticized[38-40] because it is a subgroup analysis with imbalance between the groups regarding initial ICP and age, both disadvantages to the albumin group, but also especially that the 4% albumin solution used was hypotonic (155 mmol/L compared to the normal 190 mmol/L in plasma). Therefore, the SAFE-TBI study has not changed the recommendations on the use of albumin in the LC.

It was also concluded by Ioannidis, analyzing the reliability of randomized studies, that evidence from trials, no matter how impressive, should be interpreted with caution when only one trial is available.[41] This statement is applicable to the SAFE-TBI study.

Glucose (mainly 5%), with addition of sodium and potassium together with saline, is also used in the LC to keep the sodium concentration above 135 mmol/L for nutritional purposes and to maintain an adequate urine production. The amount of crystalloids should be limited to 1–1.5 L/day because of the risk of developing brain edema when the BBB is disrupted.

In the LC, blood transfusions, always using leukocyte-depleted blood, may be used to avoid hypovolemia and to improve oxygenation of the penumbra zone.[2,3] The goal is a hemoglobin concentration of 105–110 g/L. The BTF guidelines do not give any detailed information about fluid therapy.[1,4,6]

Stress Reduction

Head-injured patients benefit from being unstressed because of a lower release of catecholamines and should therefore be sedated to reduce stress-induced increases in ICP and stress-induced release of catecholamines. The heavy sedation also reduces the need for seizure prophylaxis, as shown in a previous study.[42] The degree of sedation should not, however, be deeper than necessary to effectively reduce stress. Midazolam in combination with fentanyl as an analgesic is convenient, but other forms of sedation may be used. The doses can be reduced in relation to the decrease in ICP. Propofol is recommended during the weaning phase.[2]

The antihypertensive drugs recommended in the LC may also reduce stress. Specifically, both β-blockade and α₂ agonists have a stress-reducing effect.[43]

Long-term treatment with barbiturates, and in relatively high doses, is accepted in the BTF guidelines to reduce ICP.[1] Due to severe side effects such as ARDS, pneumonia, high fever, and uncontrolled hypotension, high-dose barbiturate treatment is not a component of the LC. Still, the LC has accepted low doses of barbiturates (0.5–2 mg/kg/hr) for up to 2 days if ICP is critically high in spite of basal LC therapy.

Ventilation

All s-TBI patients (GCS ≤8) should be intubated for adequate control of oxygenation and ventilation, aiming at a Pao_2 of around 12 kPa and a $Paco_2$ of 4.5–5.3 kPa. Hyperventilation should be avoided due to the risk of impaired oxygenation of the penumbra zone.[44,45] Volume-controlled ventilation gives a more stable $Paco_2$. Based on the physiological arguments presented earlier, PEEP (6–8 cm H_2O) is mandatory in the LC to prevent the development of ARDS. It has been observed that ARDS and pneumonia rarely develop when using the LC. This can most likely be explained by a combination of the use of PEEP, the avoidance of vasoconstrictor therapy and barbiturates, and restriction of parenteral fat nutrition in combination with adequate inhalation and fluid therapy.

Monitoring of Intracranial Pressure

Monitoring of ICP is mandatory with the LC, either with an intraparenchymatous or an intraventricular device, with the latter also allowing drainage of CSF.

Monitoring of Cerebral Perfusion Pressure

Monitoring of CPP is important with the LC. CPP should be measured with the arterial 0 level at the same level as the ICP. Thus, if the patient is lying in supine position, the blood pressure has its 0 level at heart level and the ICP has its 0 level at the external auditory canal, the CPP will be measured accurately. If the person is treated with head elevation (e.g., 20 degrees) and the blood pressure 0 level is at heart level, a correction must be made for the difference between the heart and ICP 0 levels. With the LC, CPP stays between 60 and 70 mm Hg in most adult cases, but as low as 50 mm Hg can be accepted in certain cases.[46] A CPP higher than 70 mm Hg should be reduced with more effective antihypertensive treatment or head elevation. Lower CPP values should be used in children, with values depending on the age of the child.

Osmotherapy

The synthetic drug mannitol is the most common osmotic drug used to reduce a raised ICP. Hypertonic saline has become more common during the past two decades. In spite of its use for more than 50 years and its documented ICP-reducing effect, there have still been no studies showing improved outcome with osmotherapy. Mannitol has severe side effects in terms of electrolyte disturbances, rebound effects, and renal insufficiency.[47] Osmotherapy is therefore not a component of the LC, apart from its use for acute prevention of brainstem herniation in a critical situation.

Nutrition

Overnutrition should be avoided as it may induce fever, and parenteral fat in high doses may trigger hemophagocytosis.[48] An initial caloric supply of 15–20 kcal/kg/day through enteral nutrition is recommended from day 2.

Ventricular Drainage and Decompressive Craniectomy

Ventricular drainage via an intraventricular catheter may be used to control a significantly raised ICP. If continuous drainage is used, the drainage level should not be too far below the actual ICP (2–4 mm Hg) to avoid collapse of the ventricular system when the CSF is tapped. For details, see Grande (2006).[3]

If ICP remains elevated (>25–30 mm Hg) in spite of the ICP-reducing measures reviewed in this chapter, a unilateral or bilateral craniectomy can be performed.[49] A cranioplasty or replacement of the bone flap should be done as soon as possible after normalization of the ICP. Side effects of craniectomy in terms brain swelling, especially in the cranial opening, are counteracted by the ICP-reducing (antihypertensive and oncotic) therapy used in the LC.[3]

Active Cooling

The literature lacks support for active cooling in s-TBI patients, and active cooling has never been a component in the LC.[2,3,50]

References

1. Carney N, Totten AM, O'Reilly C, et al. Guidelines for the Management of Severe Traumatic Brain Injury, Fourth Edition. *Neurosurgery.* 2017;80:6–15.

2. Grände PO. The "Lund Concept" for the treatment of severe head trauma-physiological principles and clinical application. *Intensive Care Med.* 2006;32:1475–1484.

3. Grande PO. Critical evaluation of the Lund Concept for treatment of severe traumatic head injury, 25 years after its introduction front. *Neurol.* 2017. https://doi.org/10.3389/fneur.2017.00315

4. Bullock R, Chesnut RM, Clifton C, et al.; Brain Trauma Foundation, American Association of Neurological Surgeons, Joint Section on Neurotrauma and Critical Care. Guidelines for the management of severe head injury. *J Neurotrauma.* 1996;13:641–734.

5. Koskinen LO, Olivecrona M, Grände PO. Severe traumatic brain injury management and clinical outcome using the Lund concept. *Neuroscience.* 2014;283:245–255.

6. Brain Trauma Foundation. Guidelines for the management of severe traumatic brain injury, 3rd ed. *J Neurotrauma.* 2007; 24(suppl 1):1–106.

7. Eker C, Asgeirsson B, Grände PO, Schalén W, Nordström CH. Improved outcome after severe head injury with a new therapy based on principles for brain volume regulation and preserved microcirculation. *Crit Care Med.* 1998;26:1881–1886.

8. Naredi S, Edén E, Zäll S, Stephensen H, Rydenhag B. A standardized neurosurgical neurointensive therapy directed toward vasogenic edema after severe traumatic brain injury: clinical results. *Intensive Care Med.* 1998;24:446–451.

9. Naredi S, Olivecrona M, Lindgren C, Östlund AL, Grände PO, Koskinen LO. An outcome study of severe traumatic head injury using the "Lund therapy" with low-dose prostacyclin. *Acta Anaesthesiol Scand.* 2001;45:402–406.

10. Olivecrona M, Rodling-Wahlström M, Naredi S, Koskinen LO. Prostacyclin treatment in severe traumatic brain injury: a microdialysis and outcome study. *J Neurotrauma.* 2009;26:1251–1262.

11. Gerber LM, Chiu YL, Carney N, Härtl R, Ghajar J. Marked reduction in mortality in patients with severe traumatic brain injury. *J Neurosurg.* 2013;119:1583–1590.

12. Grände PO, Myhre EB, Nordström CH, Schliamser S. Treatment of intracranial hypertension and aspects on lumbar dural puncture in severe bacterial meningitis. *Acta Anaesthesiol Scand.* 2002;46:264–270.

13. Lindvall P, Ahlm C, Ericsson M, Gothefors L, Naredi S, Koskinen LO. Reducing intracranial pressure may increase survival among patients with bacterial meningitis. *Clin Infect Dis.* 2004;38:384–390.

14. Fenstermacher JD. Volume regulation of the central nervous system. In: Staub NC, Taylor AE, eds. *Edema.* New York: Raven Press; 1984: 383–404.

15. Guyton AC, Hall JE. *Textbook of medical physiology*, 10th ed. Philadelphia: Saunders; 2000.

16. Grände PO, Asgeirsson B, Nordström CH. Physiological principles for volume regulation of a tissue enclosed in a rigid shell with application to the injured brain. *J Trauma.* 1997;42:S23–S31.

17. Kongstad L, Grände PO. The role of arterial and venous pressure for volume regulation of an organ enclosed in a rigid compartment with application to the injured brain. *Acta Anaesthesiol Scand.* 1999;43:501–508.

18. Wolf HG, Forbes HS. The cerebral circulation. V. Observations of the pial circulation during changes in intracranial pressure. *Arch Neurol Psychiatr.* 1928;20:1035–1047.

19. Asgeirsson B, Grände PO. Effects of arterial and venous pressure alterations on transcapillary fluid exchange during raised tissue pressure. *Intensive Care Med.* 1994;20:567–572.

20. Kongstad L, Grände PO. Arterial hypertension increases intracranial pressure in cat after opening of the blood-brain barrier. *J Trauma.* 2001;51:490–496

21. Asgeirsson B, Grände PO. Local vascular responses to elevation of an organ above the heart. *Acta Physiol Scand.* 1996;156:9–18.

22. McGuire G1, Crossley D, Richards J, Wong D. Effects of varying levels of positive end-expiratory pressure on intracranial pressure and cerebral perfusion pressure. *Crit Care Med.* 1997;25:1059–1062.

23. Lou M, Xue F, Chen L, Xue Y, Wang K. Is high PEEP ventilation strategy safe for acute respiratory distress syndrome after severe traumatic brain injury? *Brain Inj.* 2012;26:887–890.

24. Caricato A, Conti G, Della Corte F, et al. Effects of PEEP on the intracranial system of patients with head injury and subarachnoid hemorrhage: the role of respiratory system compliance. *J Trauma.* 2005;58:571–576.

25. Cooper KR, Boswell PA, Choi SC. Safe use of PEEP in patients with severe head injury. *J Neurosurg.* 1985;63:552–555.

26. Asgeirsson B, Grände PO, Nordström CH, Berntman L, Messeter K, Ryding E. Effects of hypotensive treatment with alpha 2-agonist and beta 1-antagonist on cerebral haemodynamics in severely head injured patients. *Acta Anaesthesiol Scand.* 1995;39:347–351.

27. Cotton BA, Snodgrass KB, Fleming SB, et al. Beta-blocker exposure is associated with improved survival after severe traumatic brain injury. *J Trauma.* 2007;62:26–33.

28. Arbabi S, Campion EM, Hemmila MR, et al. Beta-blocker use is associated with improved outcomes in adult trauma patients. *J Trauma.* 2007;62:56–61.

29. Inaba K, Teixeira PGR, David JS, et al. Beta-blockers in isolated blunt head injury. *J Am Coll Surg.* 2008;206:432–438.

30. Helmy A, Carpenter KL, Menon DK, Pickard JD, Hutchinson PJ. The cytokine response to human traumatic brain injury: temporal profiles and evidence for cerebral parenchymal production. *J Cereb Blood Flow Metab.* 2011;3:658–670.

31. Werner C, Engelhard K. Pathophysiology of traumatic brain injury. *Br J Anaesth.* 2007;99:4–9.

32. Valadka AB, Gopinath SP, Contant CF, Uzura M, Robertson CS. Relationship of brain tissue PO2 to outcome after severe head injury. *Crit Care Med.* 1998;26:1576–1581.

33. Oddo M, Levine JM, Kumar M, Iglesias K, Frangos S, Maloney-Wilensky E et al. Anemia and brain oxygen after severe traumatic brain injury. *Intensive Care Med.* 2012;38:1497–1504.

34. Dubniks M, Persson J, Grände PO. Effect of blood pressure on plasma volume loss in the rat under increased permeability. *Intensive Care Med.* 2007;33:2192–2198.

35. Nygren A, Redfors B, Thorén A, Ricksten SE. Norepinephrine causes a pressure-dependent plasma volume decrease in clinical vasodilatory shock. *Acta Anaesthesiol Scand.* 2010;54:814–820.

36. Rise IR, Risöe C, Kirkeby OJ. Cerebrovascular effects of high intracranial pressure after moderate hemorrhage. *J Neurosurg Anesthesiol.* 1998;10:224–230.

37. SAFE Study Investigators; Australian and New Zealand Intensive Care Society Clinical Trials Group; Australian Red Cross Blood Service; George Institute for International Health, Myburgh J, Cooper DJ, Finfer S, et al. Saline or albumin for fluid resuscitation in patients with traumatic brain injury. *N Engl J Med.* 2007;30(357): 874–884.

38. Drummond JC, Patel PM, Cole DJ, Kelly PJ. The effect of the reduction of colloid oncotic pressure with and without reduction of osmolality, on post-traumatic cerebral edema. *Anesthesiology.* 1998;88:993–1002.

39. Van Aken HK, Kampmeier TG, Ertmer C, Westphal M. Fluid resuscitation in patients with traumatic brain injury: what is a SAFE approach? *Curr Opin Anaesthesiol.* 2012;25:563–565.

40. Ertmer C, Van Aken H. Fluid therapy in patients with brain injury: what does physiology tell us? *Crit Care.* 2014;18:119.

41. Ioannidis JP. Contradicted and initially stronger effects in highly cited clinical research. *JAMA.* 2005;294:218–28. doi:10.1001/jama.294.2.218

42. Olivecrona M, Zetterlund B, Rodling-Wahlström M, Naredi S, Koskinen LO. Absence of electroencephalographic seizure activity in patients treated for head injury with an intracranial pressure-targeted therapy. *J Neurosurg.* 2009;110:300–305.

43. Cruickshank JM, Neil-Dwyer G, Degaute JP, et al. Reduction of stress/catecholamine-induced cardiac necrosis by beta 1-selective blockade. *Lancet.* 1987;2:585–589.

44. Muizelaar JP, Marmarou A, Ward JD, et al. Adverse effects of prolonged hyperventilation in patients with severe head injury: a randomized clinical trial. *J Neurosurg.* 1991;75:731–739.

45. Stocchetti N, Maas AI, Chieregato A, van der Plas AA. Hyperventilation in head injury: a review. *Chest.* 2005;127: 1812–1827.

46. Nordström CH, Reinstrup P, Xu W, Gärdenfors A, Ungerstedt U. Assessment of the lower limit for cerebral perfusion pressure in severe head injuries by bedside monitoring of regional energy metabolism. *Anesthesiology.* 2003;98:809–814.

47. Grände PO, Romner B. Osmotherapy in brain edema: a questionable therapy. *J Neurosurg Anesthesiol.* 2012;24:407–412. doi:10.1097/01.ana.0000419730.29492.8b.

48. Roth B, Grände PO, Nilsson-Ehle P, Eliasson. Possible role of short-term parenteral nutrition with fat emulsions for development of haemophagocytosis with multiple organ failure in a patient with traumatic brain injury. *Intensive Care Med.* 1993;19:111–114.

49. Olivecrona M, Rodling-Wahlström M, Naredi S, Koskinen LO. Effective ICP reduction by decompressive craniectomy in patients with severe traumatic brain injury treated with an ICP-targeted therapy. *J Neurotrauma.* 2007;24:927–935.

50. Sandestig A, Romner B, Grände PO. Therapeutic hypothermia in children and adults with severe traumatic brain injury. *Ther Hypothermia Temp Manag.* 2014;4:10–20.

Abusive Head Trauma

Rachel Pardes Berger, Jennifer Clarke, and Christine Leeper

5

Epidemiology

Abusive head trauma (AHT) is the leading cause of death from child physical abuse and a source of significant morbidity in those who survive. The most common age at which AHT occurs is 2 months, corresponding with the normal peak developmental period of crying, which is the most commonly identified event preceding AHT.[1] While the majority of AHT cases occur in infants, about 25% occur in older children.[2,3] The incidence is estimated to be 17–34 cases per 100,000 infants less than 12 months of age per year in the United States,[4-7] a rate that is remarkably similar to rates in other developed countries.[3,8-10] By comparison, the incidence of all childhood cancers in the United States is 18 cases per 100,000 children.[11]

The reported incidence of AHT is likely an underestimate due to underdiagnosis. Diagnosis of mild AHT is particularly challenging because children often present with nonspecific clinical signs such as vomiting or fussiness, and healthcare providers may attribute the findings to benign conditions[12,13] or an accidental injury.[14,15] Clinicians may also be reluctant to diagnose AHT due to its legal and social implications.[15-17]

Given the high morbidity and mortality of AHT, there have been significant efforts made at primary prevention. Several studies suggested decreases in AHT rates with parent education,[18,19] but more recent studies have not demonstrated decreases in incidence despite improvement in parental knowledge.[20,21]

Risk Factors

Child, caregiver, and societal factors have been described as risk factors for AHT (Table 5.1). While the presence or absence of risk factors cannot be used for diagnostic purposes, recognizing risk factors is important for programs looking to target prevention programs and so appropriate interventions can be provided after an identified incident of abuse to ensure ongoing safety (e.g. substance abuse treatment, intervention for intimate partner violence).

Presentation

Depending on the severity and type of brain injury (e.g., primarily blunt TBI vs. primarily hypoxic ischemic injury), children with AHT can present with a wide range of symptoms from nonspecific complaints of irritability, poor feeding, or vomiting to life-threatening signs of cardiac arrest or unresponsiveness. There is often a paucity of external findings of trauma, increasing the challenge of accurate diagnosis. Clear documentation of any external findings—including subconjunctival hemorrhages, petechiae,

Table 5.1:
Child, parental, and societal factors associated with an increased risk for abusive head trauma

Child risk factors:
Male gender[4,106–108]
Multiple gestation[4,109]
History of chronic medical problems or developmental delay[107]
Premature birth[108,109]

Parental risk factors:
Young maternal age[4,109]
Lower socioeconomic status[4,107,110]
Caregiver substance abuse[111]
Intimate partner violence[106]

Societal factor:
Economic downturn/recession[112,113]

frenulum tears, palatal or lip injuries, and bruises, particularly in pre-mobile children—by the first medical professional who evaluates the child is imperative. It is often very minor injuries which are most helpful in assessing whether the history provided matches the constellation of injuries the child has. These injuries can heal completely within days and often before extubation. If not clearly documented in the emergency department (ED) and/or prior to any neurosurgical intervention, they may be incorrectly attributed to iatrogenic trauma rather than abuse.

Medical Evaluation

Brain and Spine Injuries

Head computed tomography (CT) remains the imaging modality of choice due to its availability, speed, and high sensitivity for acute hemorrhage, midline shift, and fractures (Table 5.2). Magnetic resonance imaging (MRI) is more sensitive to parenchymal injuries but is less widely available and often requires sedation or general anesthesia.[22] Except in the mildest cases of AHT, brain MRI should be obtained 3–5 days after the injury to better evaluate subtle parenchymal injury and demonstrate injury evolution.[23,24] Simultaneous MRI of the spine is becoming standard of care due to several studies documenting the specificity of spinal subdural hemorrhage and/or ligamentous injuries for AHT.[25–28] In a study of 183 children with brain injuries, cervical spine ligamentous injuries were present in 78% of the AHT group, 46% of the accidental trauma group, and 1% of the nontraumatic group.[25] There remains significant variability in the use of spine imaging, which suggests potential missed opportunities to improve AHT diagnosis.[29]

Subdural hemorrhages (SDHs) are the most common abnormality in AHT. These SDHs are often paradoxically thin despite severe symptoms (Figure 5.1). The reason is likely due to the mechanism by which the SDHs occur in AHT; an acceleration-deceleration injury to the brain is thought to result in tearing of the bridging veins and blood accumulating in the subdural space. The presence of multiple SDHs over the convexities and interhemispheric SDH are also characteristic of AHT.[30]

Table 5.2:
Recommended evaluation for a child with an intracranial injury concerning for abusive head trauma

Test	Reason	Specialist Recommended to Evaluate Results	Other
Brain and spine MRI without contrast	Brain MRI can provide improved information about injury to the brain parenchyma & hypoxia. Spine MRI can identify injuries to the spine, ligaments, and/or soft tissue swelling which are not visible on CT and can assist in determining the mechanism and etiology of injury.	Pediatric neuroradiologist	Some institutions image the entire spine, while others image the cervical spine and extend to thoracic and lumbar spine if abnormalities are noted on cervical spine (vs C-spine) in order to limit sedation time
Dilated ophthalmologic exam[a]	To evaluate for retinal hemorrhages	Pediatric ophthalmologist	Strongly recommend photodocumentation
Skeletal survey including oblique views of ribs[b]	To evaluate for noncranial fractures	Pediatric radiologist	This should not be done as portable films. If there are concerns about acute fractures which may need orthopedic intervention, portable films can be used initially and followed-up with a full skeletal survey.
Follow-up skeletal survey	To evaluate for fractures (especially metaphyseal and rib fractures) which were acute at the time of the initial skeletal survey and could not yet be visualized	Pediatric radiologist	To be done 2–3 weeks after the initial skeletal survey[c]
Screening for possible hematologic etiology of intracranial hemorrhage[d]	PT/PTT, platelets, INR, Factor VIII, Factor IX, d-dimer, fibrinogen	Pediatric hematology consultation recommended if any abnormalities on screening evaluation	A report to CPS should not be delayed until the results of the tests are known.
Serum amino acids and urine organic acids	To rule out glutaric aciduria type I as an etiology in children with isolated intracranial hemorrhage		Glutaric aciduria type I is very rare and its presentation does not overlap entirely with AHT, but should be ruled out as a mimic and considered in cases in which there is isolated intracranial hemorrhage with or without retinal hemorrhages. A report to CPS should not be delayed until the results of the tests are known.
Screen for occult abdominal injury	Liver function tests, pancreatic enzymes		If AST or ALT >80 IU/L, recommend definitive testing (e.g., abdominal CT with contrast)

[a]In children who are too unstable to have their eyes dilated, recommend initial evaluation without dilation and/or sequential dilation of eyes.

[b]In children who die prior to being able to complete a skeletal survey, the skeletal survey should be done postmortem. Any abnormalities need to be relayed to the coroner or medical examiner performing the autopsy.

[c]In children who are too unstable to undergo a skeletal survey until 1 week or more after admission, it is possible to perform a single skeletal survey 2–3 weeks after admission instead of both an initial and follow-up.

[d]Measurement of Factors VII and IX, fibrinogen and d-dimer are not necessary in children who have other, nonhematologic manifestations of abuse (e.g., fractures).

AHT, abusive head trauma; ALT, alanine transaminase; AST, aspartate transaminase; CPS, child protective services; CT, computed tomography; INR, international normalized ratio; MRI, magnetic resonance imaging; PT/PTT, prothrombin time and activated partial thromboplastin.

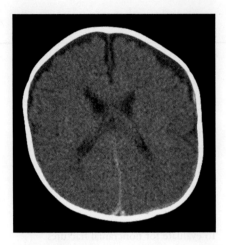

Figure 5.1 Head computed tomography (CT) from a 3-month-old boy who presented with decreased responsiveness without a history of trauma. Glasgow Coma Scale score of 4.

Neuroimaging may help provide information about timing of injury in cases of AHT.[31] However, extreme caution is needed when timing a traumatic event based solely on the signal intensity of the intracranial hemorrhage.[22,32]

Retinal Hemorrhages

The dilated eye examination is a critical part of the evaluation of a child with suspected AHT. The presence or absence of retinal hemorrhage (RH) as well as the number, type, and distribution all help to differentiate RH related to AHT to those from other causes. Large numbers of bilateral RH, RH in all layers of the retina, and extension of the RH into the periphery are all highly associated with AHT.[33] Coagulopathy,[34,35] cardiopulmonary resuscitation,[35,36] and/or increased intracranial pressure (ICP),[34,37] all of which are common in children with severe TBI, do not result in the pattern of RH are seen in AHT. The RH seen in about 10% of cases of severe accidental TBI; they do not have the same characteristics as the RH seen in AHT.

The timing of the dilated eye examination is important. In a study by Binenbaum and colleagues, intraretinal hemorrhages completely resolved within several days in 68% (62/91) of the retinas examined. Due the importance of RH in diagnosing AHT and the speed with which the RH can resolve, dilated indirect ophthalmoscopy by a pediatric ophthalmologist should be performed as early as possible and always within 48 hours of presentation.[38] The need to use the pupillary exam to assess increased ICP during this same time period is an important consideration; serial eye dilation and/or dilation using a mydriatic with a short half-life such as phenylephrine 2.5% are ways to address this issue.[34]

Orthopedic Injuries

A skeletal survey is needed in any child younger than 2 years with concerns for physical abuse including AHT and in most older children (age 2–5) with suspected AHT. A repeat skeletal survey should be obtained approximately 2 weeks after the first[39] since certain fractures (e.g., rib and metaphyseal) that are highly associated with abuse may be difficult to see acutely.

Laboratory Evaluation

Initial laboratory evaluation in cases of suspected AHT should include many of the same lab tests done in children with TBI of any etiology: electrolytes, a complete blood count with platelets, prothrombin time and activated partial thromboplastin (PT/PTT), urine analysis, and liver function tests. The American Academy of Pediatrics section on Hematology/Oncology and the Committee on Child Abuse and Neglect also recommend Factor VIII and Factor IX levels, and a DIC panel (d-dimer and fibrinogen).[40] If any of the initial labs are abnormal, consultation with a pediatric hematologist should be strongly considered. Importantly, patients with severe TBI of any etiology may have a transient coagulopathy that does not reflect an underlying congenital disorder.[41] There may also be additional lab testing which can be driven by the differential diagnosis on a case-by-case basis.[40,42–44]

Differential Diagnosis

AHT is diagnosed after a thorough history and physical examination and supported by laboratory and radiographic findings. Other conditions which should be included in the differential diagnosis of a child with suspected AHT including accidental TBI, metabolic diseases, infection, and coagulation disorders. Taking a detailed history, performing a complete physical examination, and carefully reviewing radiologic and laboratory information almost always distinguishes these other entities from AHT. Additional testing should be able to rule out most other differential diagnoses. There are times when the medical data are insufficient to make a diagnosis of AHT and the diagnosis is, instead, made in combination with data obtained by police and/or child protective services (CPS) including emergency medical services records, social media posts, and other sources of nonmedical data. The importance of the collaborative process among providers within and beyond the medical field cannot be overemphasized.

Being able to provide an assessment of *when* the AHT may have occurred is critical because identification of the perpetrator, while not a medical issue, is needed for child protection. If AHT is diagnosed but the timing of the event is unknown, the infant may be returned to the care of the perpetrator and all the best medical care in the world may be for naught. In order to be better able to pinpoint the time of injury, the physician has a critical role in obtaining a detailed history of the events leading to the presenting symptom(s), determining who was with the infant throughout the timeline, and documenting this clearly in the medical record. There are times, however, when the timing cannot be pinpointed due to limitations of the history, the specific type of injuries, and/or the prolonged symptomatology.

Mechanism of Injury

The exact mechanism of injury that results in the constellation of injuries which define AHT is unknown and likely to be highly variable. AHT, almost by definition, occurs in a child who is too young to talk and by a perpetrator who is unlikely to provide an accurate history of the event. As a result, our understanding of the mechanism and pathophysiology of AHT has been obtained using multiple data sources including descriptive studies,[25,27,28,45–49] postmortem studies,[50–55] biochemical/biomarker analyses,[56,57] confession data,[58,59] animal models,[60–62,63] and computer simulation data.[63] These data suggest that AHT is a variable combination of blunt force trauma, shaking, hypoxic-ischemic injury, and spinal cord injury. Whether shaking in isolation is sufficient to cause severe or fatal head injury in the absence of blunt force trauma has been the topic of a significant amount of research. While a study conducted by Duhaime and colleagues almost 30 years ago suggested that shaking alone was unlikely to cause the pathology seen in their cohort of abused children,[64] contemporary studies using more complex and biofidelic models as well as computer modeling demonstrate that shaking alone is sufficient to cause AHT.[58–61,63,65–69] Evidence of hypoxia-ischemia is common. A study comparing serum biomarkers of neuronal injury in patients with AHT, noninflicted TBI, and hypoxic-ischemic injury found that the biochemical profile seen in AHT was more similar to that of patients with hypoxic-ischemic injury than to that of patients with noninflicted TBI, demonstrating late peak biomarker concentrations that would be consistent with ongoing cell death.[56,57] It has been theorized that hypoxia may result from a delay in seeking medical attention, injury to the respiratory centers in the cervicomedullary junction, and/or cervical spinal cord injury resulting in apnea.[26,47–49,54,55,70] This theory is supported by the clinical observation that children with AHT often have prehospital apnea and/or respiratory compromise[49,71] and by postmortem neuropathologic evaluation of brain tissue that demonstrates findings of hypoxic-ischemic encephalopathy as well as brainstem-specific damage.[52,54,55] As described earlier in the chapter, increased use of spine MRI has improved our ability to discriminate accidental TBI from AHT. It also has offered insight into the mechanism of the injury in AHT and supports the previously unexplained clinical finding of apnea as a prominent symptom, the high incidence of hypoxic-ischemic injuries, and the importance of shaking as a mechanism.[28] In a comparative study of patients with AHT and accidental injury, 81% of children with bilateral hypoxic-ischemic injuries had cervical injuries.[27]

The challenges in understanding the mechanism by which the brain injury in AHT occurs extend to understanding the pathophysiology of RH. Clinical studies, autopsy reports, and simulation studies all suggest that when the body and, consequently, the vitreous is shaken, shearing forces are applied to the retina, particularly at points of attachment, including the macula, retinal vessels, and peripheral retina.[34,50,58,72–75]

The ability to use animal models to improve our understanding of the pathophysiology of the AHT is an evolving field. Early animal models provided suboptimal comparison to humans due to differing anatomy, age-related development, and complex human biomechanics.[60,61] More sophisticated in vivo models are more similar to humans in terms of gyrencephalic structure and maturation.[60,62] Data obtained from these more biofidelic models as well as finite element models[63] are consistent with clinical observations that acceleration-deceleration–type movement of the brain can cause axonal injury and extra axial hemorrhage and that certain types of RH are associated with these specific injury mechanisms.[34,76,77]

Management

Clinical management of AHT is similar to the management of all pediatric TBI. Initial evaluation should be guided by Advanced Trauma Life Support Guidelines and evidence-based guidelines for infants, children, and adolescents with TBI,[78,79] which do not distinguish between accidental TBI and AHT. The same basic principles of care for accidental TBI can be applied with special considerations described later for the specific risks in patients with AHT. While these guidelines do not distinguish injuries based on etiology, appropriate use of them depends on the recognition of trauma as the etiology of a child's symptoms, which can be a challenge in AHT, particularly in its more mild forms.

When AHT is suspected, providers should maintain a low threshold for admission to an intensive care unit for close monitoring. Patients with AHT have significantly higher mortality rates (three- to tenfold in various studies) compared to accidental TBI cohorts,[80,81] even for those with "moderate" injury (9.5% for a Glasgow Coma Scale [GCS] score of 9–11).[82] The mortality at each GCS score is strikingly high in children with AHT[82] and is likely related to the issues discussed earlier. As a result, a higher level of care may be appropriate for this cohort of children at risk of clinical deterioration and poor outcome.

There are several considerations and specific recommendations for patients with AHT. First, more aggressive ICP goals and maintenance of adequate cerebral perfusion pressure (CPP) is indicated. Most studies target ICP at less than 20 mm Hg; however, there are data suggesting that a slightly lower ICP target is better for young children.[83] Two pediatric studies demonstrated that the presence of AHT and a threshold of CPP below 45 mm Hg are associated with poor outcome.[84,85] Aggressive ICP monitoring and prompt intervention is indicated in AHT patients to ensure adequate cerebral blood flow.

Early identification of subclinical seizures is also critical. In two cohorts of patients with TBI who underwent continuous electroencephalographic (EEG) monitoring, AHT was a risk factor for both status epilepticus and subclinical status epilepticus.[86,87] In a cohort of children with AHT admitted to the PICU, the majority had nonconvulsive seizures on EEG or electrographic status epilepticus.[88] Prophylactic use of anticonvulsants and continuous EEG monitoring should, therefore, be considered for all patients with severe AHT.

Finally, early neurosurgical involvement should be considered. In a study of 184 children admitted to the ICU with SDH due to suspected AHT, more than 60% required neurosurgical intervention, although there was little standardization in the index surgical procedure of choice. Subdural puncture and external subdural drainage offered only transient stabilization; many patients required subsequent subdural-peritoneal or subdural-subgaleal shunt to address intracranial hypertension.[89] There is currently no standardized protocol for the neurosurgical treatment of SDH in AHT, though proposed indications include signs of intracranial hypertension, large hematoma size (e.g., >10 mm), and low GCS.[90] While an early study by Cho and colleagues in 1995 suggested that external decompression was associated with a lower mortality rate in AHT,[91] a more recent study by Oluigbo and colleagues comparing outcome after external decompression in both AHT and accidental TBI found increased mortality in AHT patients despite surgical intervention.[80] It is unclear from this study whether decompression is simply unlikely to alter a poor outcome in some victims of AHT or whether decompression may need to be initiated earlier in the clinical course in patients with suspected AHT. More research is clearly needed to define best practices for treatment of AHT.

Interactions Between the Legal and Medical Systems in Suspected AHT

A discussion of AHT is not complete without mention of the legal system. As discussed previously, collaboration among medical professionals, CPS, and police is important both for making the diagnosis and determining if it is possible to time the injury in order to accurately identify a perpetrator and thereby allow nonperpetrating adults to continue their roles as caretakers. Another time when this collaboration is essential is during criminal proceedings. The role of the physician in these proceedings is to provide medical expertise to a jury so that jury members have enough medical knowledge to make the right decision. Although the court system can be a difficult one to interact with, and is a part of the child protection system with which physicians report negative experiences,[92] this part of the process is essential for the safety for children in our community. The child who has already been injured is safer due to involvement in the CPS system, but other children who the perpetrator has access to remain vulnerable unless the criminal system can limit their access to other children.

Another reason why testimony from treating physicians is so important is due to the large number of professional expert defense witnesses.[93] There are extensive peer-reviewed publications characterizing the detailed findings, presentation, and clinical outcome of AHT. There is no legitimate debate regarding the validity of AHT as a diagnosis, neither in the medical literature nor among pediatricians, neurosurgeons, ophthalmologists, neurologists, critical care physicians, emergency medicine physicians, or pediatric rehabilitation physicians.[94] However, theories espoused in the literature and in court by expert defense witnesses[95–97] and published in popular media[98–100] and by the court[101,102] continue to suggest there is debate. Alternative theories of how the constellation of injuries seen in AHT might otherwise occur include coughing, choking, and isolated hypoxia without trauma.[96,103–105] Information from the treating physician is critical in criminal trials to explain why these alternative theories are inadequate and not scientifically sound. As the data presented in this chapter suggest, our scientific understanding of the epidemiology, risks, pathophysiology, and mechanism of AHT has improved greatly over the past 10 years. The next important step will be translating this knowledge into better treatment that can improve the poor outcome from this injury.

References

1. Lee C, Barr RG, Catherine N, Wicks A. Age-related incidence of publicly reported shaken baby syndrome cases: is crying a trigger for shaking? *J Dev Behav Pediatr.* 2007;28(4):288–293.

2. Scribano PV, Makoroff KL, Feldman KW, Berger RP. Association of perpetrator relationship to abusive head trauma clinical outcomes. *Child Abuse Negl.* 2013;37(10):771–777.

3. Bennett S, Ward M, Moreau K, et al. Head injury secondary to suspected child maltreatment: results of a prospective Canadian national surveillance program. *Child Abuse Negl.* 2011;35(11):930–936.

4. Keenan HT, Runyan DK, Marshall SW, Nocera MA, Merten DF, Sinal SH. A population-based study of inflicted traumatic brain injury in young children. *JAMA.* 2003;290(5):621–626.

5. Parrish J, Baldwin-Johnson C, Volz M, Goldsmith Y. Abusive head trauma among children in Alaska: a population-based assessment. *Int J Circumpolar Health*. 2013;72:1. doi:10.3402/ijch. v72i0.21216

6. Gumbs GR, Keenan HT, Sevick CJ, et al. Infant abusive head trauma in a military cohort. *Pediatrics*. 2013;132(4):668–676.

7. Leventhal JM, Martin KD, Asnes AG. Fractures and traumatic brain injuries: abuse versus accidents in a US database of hospitalized children. *Pediatrics*. 2010;126(1):e104–115.

8. Hobbs C, Childs AM, Wynne J, Livingston J, Seal A. Subdural haematoma and effusion in infancy: an epidemiological study. *Arch Dis Child*. 2005;90(9):952–955.

9. Kelly P, Farrant B. Shaken baby syndrome in New Zealand, 2000–2002. *J Paediatr Child Health*. 2008;44(3):99–107.

10. Fanconi M, Lips U. Shaken baby syndrome in Switzerland: results of a prospective follow-up study, 2002–2007. *Eur J Pediatr*. 2010;169(8):1023–1028.

11. National Cancer Institute. Surveillance, Epidemiology, and End Results Program. https://seer.cancer.gov/. 8/12/16.

12. Jenny C, Hymel KP, Ritzen A, Reinert SE, Hay TC. Analysis of missed cases of abusive head trauma. *JAMA*. 1999;281(7):621–626.

13. Letson M, Cooper J, Deans K, et al. Prior opportunities to diagnose abuse in children with abusive head trauma. *Child Abuse Neglect*. 2016;in revision.

14. Jackson AM, Deye KP, Halley T, et al. Curiosity and critical thinking: identifying child abuse before it is too late. *Clin Pediatr (Phila)*. 2015;54(1):54–61.

15. Flaherty EG, Sege RD, Griffith J, et al. From suspicion of physical child abuse to reporting: primary care clinician decision-making. *Pediatrics*. 2008;122(3):611–619.

16. Sege R, Flaherty E, Jones R, et al. To report or not to report: examination of the initial primary care management of suspicious childhood injuries. *Acad Pediatr*. 2011;11(6):460–466.

17. Talsma M, Bengtsson Bostrom K, Ostberg AL. Facing suspected child abuse—what keeps Swedish general practitioners from reporting to child protective services? *Scand J Prim Health Care*. 2015;33(1):21–26.

18. Dias MS, Smith K, DeGuehery K, Mazur P, Li V, Shaffer ML. Preventing abusive head trauma among infants and young children: a hospital-based, parent education program. *Pediatrics*. 2005;115(4):e470–477.

19. Altman RL, Canter J, Patrick PA, Daley N, Butt NK, Brand DA. Parent education by maternity nurses and prevention of abusive head trauma. *Pediatrics*. 2011;128(5):e1164–1172.

20. Zolotor AJ, Runyan DK, Shanahan M, et al. Effectiveness of a statewide abusive head trauma prevention program in North Carolina. *JAMA Pediatr*. 2015;169(12):1126–1131.

21. Dias MS, Rottmund CM, Cappos KM, Reed ME, Wang M, Stetter C, Shaffer ML, Hollenbeak CS, Paul IM, Christian CW, Berger RP, Klevens J. Association of a Postnatal Parent Education Program for Abusive Head Trauma With Subsequent Pediatric Abusive Head Trauma Hospitalization Rates. *JAMA Pediatr*. 2017;171(3):223–229.

22. van Rijn RR, Spevak MR. Imaging of neonatal child abuse with an emphasis on abusive head trauma. *Magn Reson Imaging Clin N Am*. 2011;19(4):791–812;viii.

23. Vazquez E, Delgado I, Sanchez-Montanez A, Fabrega A, Cano P, Martin N. Imaging abusive head trauma: why use both computed tomography and magnetic resonance imaging? *Pediatr Radiol*. 2014;44(suppl 4):S589–603.

24. Hedlund GL, Frasier LD. Neuroimaging of abusive head trauma. *Forensic Sci Med Pathol*. 2009;5(4):280–290.

25. Choudhary AK, Ishak R, Zacharia TT, Dias MS. Imaging of spinal injury in abusive head trauma: a retrospective study. *Pediatr Radiol.* 2014;44(9):1130–1140.

26. Choudhary AK, Bradford RK, Dias MS, Moore GJ, Boal DK. Spinal subdural hemorrhage in abusive head trauma: a retrospective study. *Radiology.* 2012;262(1):216–223.

27. Kadom N, Khademian Z, Vezina G, Shalaby-Rana E, Rice A, Hinds T. Usefulness of MRI detection of cervical spine and brain injuries in the evaluation of abusive head trauma. *Pediatr Radiol.* 2014;44(7):839–848.

28. Kemp A, Cowley L, Maguire S. Spinal injuries in abusive head trauma: patterns and recommendations. *Pediatr Radiol.* 2014 Dec; 44 Suppl 4:S604–12.

29. French B, Song L, Feudtner C, Wood JN. Hospital variation in cervical spine imaging of young children with traumatic brain injury. *Acad Pediatr.* 2016;16(7):684–691.

30. Kemp AM, Jaspan T, Griffiths J, et al. Neuroimaging: what neuroradiological features distinguish abusive from non-abusive head trauma? A systematic review. *Arch Dis Child.* 2011;96(12):1103–1112.

31. Sieswerda-Hoogendoorn T, Postema FA, Verbaan D, Majoie CB, van Rijn RR. Age determination of subdural hematomas with CT and MRI: a systematic review. *Eur J Radiol.* 2014;83(7):1257–1268.

32. Vinchon M, Noule N, Tchofo PJ, Soto-Ares G, Fourier C, Dhellemmes P. Imaging of head injuries in infants: temporal correlates and forensic implications for the diagnosis of child abuse. *J Neurosurg.* 2004;101(1 suppl):44–52.

33. Maguire SA, Watts PO, Shaw AD, et al. Retinal haemorrhages and related findings in abusive and non-abusive head trauma: a systematic review. *Eye (Lond).* 2013;27(1):28–36.

34. Levin AV. Retinal hemorrhage in abusive head trauma. *Pediatrics.* 2010;126(5):961–970.

35. Longmuir SQ, McConnell L, Oral R, Dumitrescu A, Kamath S, Erkonen G. Retinal hemorrhages in intubated pediatric intensive care patients. *J AAPOS.* 2014;18(2):129–133.

36. Odom A, Christ E, Kerr N, et al. Prevalence of retinal hemorrhages in pediatric patients after in-hospital cardiopulmonary resuscitation: a prospective study. *Pediatrics.* 1997;99(6):E3.

37. Morad Y, Kim YM, Armstrong DC, Huyer D, Mian M, Levin AV. Correlation between retinal abnormalities and intracranial abnormalities in the shaken baby syndrome. *Am J Ophthalmol.* 2002;134(3):354–359.

38. Binenbaum G, Chen W, Huang J, Ying GS, Forbes BJ. The natural history of retinal hemorrhage in pediatric head trauma. *J AAPOS.* 2016;20(2):131–135.

39. American College of Radiology. ACR–SPR practice parameter for the performance and interpretation of skeletal surveys in children. https://www.acr.org/-/media/ACR/Files/Practice-Parameters/Rad-Extremity.pdf. Updated 2016.

40. Anderst JD, Carpenter SL, Abshire TC. Evaluation for bleeding disorders in suspected child abuse. *Pediatrics.* 2013;131(4):e1314–1322.

41. Hymel KP, Abshire TC, Luckey DW, Jenny C. Coagulopathy in pediatric abusive head trauma. *Pediatrics.* 1997;99(3):371–375.

42. Bishop FS, Liu JK, McCall TD, Brockmeyer DL. Glutaric aciduria type 1 presenting as bilateral subdural hematomas mimicking nonaccidental trauma. Case report and review of the literature. *J Neurosurg.* 2007;106(3 suppl):222–226.

43. Hartley LM, Khwaja OS, Verity CM. Glutaric aciduria type 1 and nonaccidental head injury. *Pediatrics.* 2001;107(1):174–175.

44. Rooks VJ, Eaton JP, Ruess L, Petermann GW, Keck-Wherley J, Pedersen RC. Prevalence and evolution of intracranial hemorrhage in asymptomatic term infants. *AJNR Am J Neuroradiol*. 2008;29(6):1082–1089.

45. Barber I, Perez-Rossello JM, Wilson CR, Silvera MV, Kleinman PK. Prevalence and relevance of pediatric spinal fractures in suspected child abuse. *Pediatr Radiol*. 2013;43(11):1507–1515.

46. Koumellis P, McConachie NS, Jaspan T. Spinal subdural haematomas in children with non-accidental head injury. *Arch Dis Child*. 2009;94(3):216–219.

47. Feldman KW, Avellino AM, Sugar NF, Ellenbogen RG. Cervical spinal cord injury in abused children. *Pediatr Emerg Care*. 2008;24(4):222–227.

48. King WJ, MacKay M, Sirnick A. Shaken baby syndrome in Canada: clinical characteristics and outcomes of hospital cases. *CMAJ*. 2003;168(2):155–159.

49. Johnson DL, Boal D, Baule R. Role of apnea in nonaccidental head injury. *Pediatr Neurosurg*. 1995;23(6):305–310.

50. Breazzano MP, Unkrich KH, Barker-Griffith AE. Clinicopathological findings in abusive head trauma: analysis of 110 infant autopsy eyes. *Am J Ophthalmol*. 2014;158(6):1146–1154. e1142.

51. Case ME. Distinguishing accidental from inflicted head trauma at autopsy. *Pediatr Radiol*. 2014;44(suppl 4):632–640.

52. Shannon P, Smith CR, Deck J, Ang LC, Ho M, Becker L. Axonal injury and the neuropathology of shaken baby syndrome. *Acta Neuropathol*. 1998;95(6):625–631.

53. Wygnanski-Jaffe T, Levin AV, Shafiq A, et al. Postmortem orbital findings in shaken baby syndrome. *Am J Ophthalmol*. 2006;142(2):233–240.

54. Matschke J, Buttner A, Bergmann M, Hagel C, Puschel K, Glatzel M. Encephalopathy and death in infants with abusive head trauma is due to hypoxic-ischemic injury following local brain trauma to vital brainstem centers. *Int J Legal Med*. 2015;129(1):105–114.

55. Geddes JF, Hackshaw AK, Vowles GH, Nickols CD, Whitwell HL. Neuropathology of inflicted head injury in children. I. Patterns of brain damage. *Brain*. 2001;124(Pt 7):1290–1298.

56. Beers SR, Berger RP, Adelson PD. Neurocognitive outcome and serum biomarkers in inflicted versus non-inflicted traumatic brain injury in young children. *J Neurotrauma*. 2007;24(1):97–105.

57. Berger RP, Adelson PD, Richichi R, Kochanek PM. Serum biomarkers after traumatic and hypoxemic brain injuries: insight into the biochemical response of the pediatric brain to inflicted brain injury. *Dev Neurosci*. 2006;28(4-5):327–335.

58. Bell E, Shouldice M, Levin AV. Abusive head trauma: a perpetrator confesses. *Child Abuse Negl*. 2011;35(1):74–77.

59. Adamsbaum C, Grabar S, Mejean N, Rey-Salmon C. Abusive head trauma: judicial admissions highlight violent and repetitive shaking. *Pediatrics*. 2010;126(3):546–555.

60. Coats B, Binenbaum G, Smith C, et al. Cyclic head rotations produce modest brain injury in infant piglets. *J Neurotrauma*. 2017;34(1):235–247.

61. Ibrahim NG, Ralston J, Smith C, Margulies SS. Physiological and pathological responses to head rotations in toddler piglets. *J Neurotrauma*. 2010;27(6):1021–1035.

62. Lintern TO, Puhulwelle Gamage NT, Bloomfield FH, et al. Head kinematics during shaking associated with abusive head trauma. *J Biomech*. 2015;48(12):3123–3127.

63. Roth S, Raul JS, Ludes B, Willinger R. Finite element analysis of impact and shaking inflicted to a child. *Int J Legal Med*. 2007;121(3):223–228.

64. Duhaime AC, Gennarelli TA, Thibault LE, Bruce DA, Margulies SS, Wiser R. The shaken baby syndrome. A clinical, pathological, and biomechanical study. *J Neurosurg*. 1987;66(3):409–415.

65. Starling SP, Patel S, Burke BL, Sirotnak AP, Stronks S, Rosquist P. Analysis of perpetrator admissions to inflicted traumatic brain injury in children. *Arch Pediatr Adolesc Med*. 2004;158(5):454–458.

66. Biron D, Shelton D. Perpetrator accounts in infant abusive head trauma brought about by a shaking event. *Child Abuse Negl*. 2005;29(12):1347–1358.

67. Case ME. Abusive head injuries in infants and young children. *Leg Med (Tokyo)*. 2007;9(2):83–87.

68. Case ME, Graham MA, Handy TC, Jentzen JM, Monteleone JA. Position paper on fatal abusive head injuries in infants and young children. *Am J Forensic Med Pathol*. 2001;22(2):112–122.

69. Rambaud C. Bridging veins and autopsy findings in abusive head trauma. *Pediatr Radiol*. 2015;45(8):1126–1131.

70. Hadley MN, Sonntag VK, Rekate HL, Murphy A. The infant whiplash-shake injury syndrome: a clinical and pathological study. *Neurosurgery*. 1989;24(4):536–540.

71. Falcone RA Jr, Brown RL, Garcia VF. Disparities in child abuse mortality are not explained by injury severity. *J Pediatr Surg*. 2007;42(6):1031–1036; discussion 1036–1037.

72. Sturm V, Landau K, Menke MN. Optical coherence tomography findings in Shaken Baby syndrome. *Am J Ophthalmol*. 2008;146(3):363–368.

73. Yamazaki J, Yoshida M, Mizunuma H. Experimental analyses of the retinal and subretinal haemorrhages accompanied by shaken baby syndrome/abusive head trauma using a dummy doll. *Injury*. 2014;45(8):1196–1206.

74. Gardner HB. Optical coherence tomography findings in shaken baby syndrome: Forbes editorial. *Am J Ophthalmol*. 2009;147(3):559–60; author reply 560–1.

75. Muni RH, Kohly RP, Sohn EH, Lee TC. Hand-held spectral domain optical coherence tomography finding in shaken-baby syndrome. *Retina ()*. 2010;30(4 suppl):S45–50.

76. Coats B, Binenbaum G, Peiffer RL, Forbes BJ, Margulies SS. Ocular hemorrhages in neonatal porcine eyes from single, rapid rotational events. *Invest Ophthalmol Vis Sci*. 2010;51(9):4792–4797.

77. Morad Y, Wygnansky-Jaffe T, Levin AV. Retinal haemorrhage in abusive head trauma. *Clin Exp Ophthalmol*. 2010;38(5):514–520.

78. American College of Surgeons. *Advanced trauma life support*. Chicago, IL: American College of Surgeons; 2015.

79. Kochanek PM, Carney N, Adelson PD, et al. Guidelines for the acute medical management of severe traumatic brain injury in infants, children, and adolescents—second edition. *Pediatr Crit Care Med*. 2012;13(suppl 1):S1–82.

80. Oluigbo CO, Wilkinson CC, Stence NV, Fenton LZ, McNatt SA, Handler MH. Comparison of outcomes following decompressive craniectomy in children with accidental and nonaccidental blunt cranial trauma. *J Neurosurg Pediatr*. 2012;9(2):125–132.

81. Davies FC, Coats TJ, Fisher R, Lawrence T, Lecky FE. A profile of suspected child abuse as a subgroup of major trauma patients. *Emerg Med J*. 2015;32(12):921–925.

82. Shein SL, Bell MJ, Kochanek PM, et al. Risk factors for mortality in children with abusive head trauma. *J Pediatr*. 2012;161(4):716–722 e711.

83. Chambers IR, Stobbart L, Jones PA, et al. Age-related differences in intracranial pressure and cerebral perfusion pressure in the first 6 hours of monitoring after children's head injury: association with outcome. *Childs Nerv Syst*. 2005;21(3):195–199.

84. Miller Ferguson N, Shein SL, Kochanek PM, et al. Intracranial hypertension and cerebral hypoperfusion in children with severe traumatic brain injury: thresholds and burden in accidental and abusive insults. *Pediatr Crit Care Med*. 2016;17(5):444–450.

85. Mehta A, Kochanek PM, Tyler-Kabara E, et al. Relationship of intracranial pressure and cerebral perfusion pressure with outcome in young children after severe traumatic brain injury. *Dev Neurosci*. 2010;32(5-6):413–419.

86. Arndt DH, Lerner JT, Matsumoto JH, et al. Subclinical early posttraumatic seizures detected by continuous EEG monitoring in a consecutive pediatric cohort. *Epilepsia*. 2013;54(10):1780–1788.

87. O'Neill BR, Handler MH, Tong S, Chapman KE. Incidence of seizures on continuous EEG monitoring following traumatic brain injury in children. *J Neurosurg Pediatr*. 2015;16(2):167–176.

88. Hasbani DM, Topjian AA, Friess SH, et al. Nonconvulsive electrographic seizures are common in children with abusive head trauma. *Pediatr Crit Care Med*. 2013;14(7):709–715.

89. Melo JR, Di Rocco F, Bourgeois M, et al. Surgical options for treatment of traumatic subdural hematomas in children younger than 2 years of age. *J Neurosurg Pediatr*. 2014;13(4):456–461.

90. Nishimoto H. Recent progress and future issues in the management of abusive head trauma. *Neurol Med Chir (Tokyo)*. 2015;55(4):296–304.

91. Cho DY, Wang YC, Chi CS. Decompressive craniotomy for acute shaken/impact baby syndrome. *Pediatr Neurosurg*. 1995;23(4):192–198.

92. Flaherty EG, Sege R. Barriers to physician identification and reporting of child abuse. *Pediatr Ann*. 2005;34(5):349–356.

93. National District Attorneys Association 2016; http://www.ndaa.org/ncpca_prosecution_defense.html.

94. Narang SK, Estrada C, Greenberg S, Lindberg D. Acceptance of shaken baby syndrome and abusive head trauma as medical diagnoses. *J Pediatr*. 2016;177:273–278.

95. Squier W. Shaken baby syndrome: the quest for evidence. *Dev Med Child Neurol*. 2008;50(1):10–14.

96. Barnes PD, Galaznik J, Gardner H, Shuman M. Infant acute life-threatening event—dysphagic choking versus nonaccidental injury. *Semin Pediatr Neurol*. 2010;17(1):7–11.

97. Miller R, Miller M. Overrepresentation of males in traumatic brain injury of infancy and in infants with macrocephaly: further evidence that questions the existence of shaken baby syndrome. *Am J Forensic Med Pathol*. 2010;31(2):165–173.

98. Tuerkheimer D. Anatomy of a misdiagnosis. *New York Times*. September 20, 2010;opinion pages.

99. Goldsmith M. *The Syndrome* [documentary]. 2016. https://www.imdb.com/title/tt3183936/

100. Bazelon E. Shaken-baby syndrome faces new questions in court. *New York Times Magazine*. February 2, 2011. https://www.nytimes.com/2011/02/06/magazine/06baby-t.html

101. *State of Wisconsin v. Edmunds*. No. 2007AP933. (WI Ct. App., 2008).

102. *Del Prete v. Thompson*. No. 1:2010cv05070. (N.D. Ill., 2014).

103. Donohoe M. Evidence-based medicine and shaken baby syndrome: part I: literature review, 1966–1998. *Am J Forensic Med Pathol*. 2003;24(3):239–242.

104. Geddes JF, Talbert DG. Paroxysmal coughing, subdural and retinal bleeding: a computer modelling approach. *Neuropathol Appl Neurobiol*. 2006;32(6):625–634.

105. Geddes JF, Tasker RC, Hackshaw AK, et al. Dural haemorrhage in non-traumatic infant deaths: does it explain the bleeding in 'shaken baby syndrome'? *Neuropathol Appl Neurobiol.* 2003;29(1):14–22.

106. Ricci L, Giantris A, Merriam P, Hodge S, Doyle T. Abusive head trauma in Maine infants: medical, child protective, and law enforcement analysis. *Child Abuse Negl.* 2003;27(3):271–283.

107. Niederkrotenthaler T, Xu L, Parks SE, Sugerman DE. Descriptive factors of abusive head trauma in young children—United States, 2000–2009. *Child Abuse Negl.* 2013;37(7):446–455.

108. Tursz A, Cook JM. Epidemiological data on shaken baby syndrome in France using judicial sources. *Pediatr Radiol.* 2014;44(suppl 4):641–646.

109. Sieswerda-Hoogendoorn T, Bilo RA, van Duurling LL, et al. Abusive head trauma in young children in the Netherlands: evidence for multiple incidents of abuse. *Acta Paediatr.* 2013;102(11):e497–501.

110. Kesler H, Dias MS, Shaffer M, Rottmund C, Cappos K, Thomas NJ. Demographics of abusive head trauma in the Commonwealth of Pennsylvania. *J Neurosurg Pediatr.* 2008;1(5):351–356.

111. Diaz-Olavarrieta C, Garcia-Pina CA, Loredo-Abdala A, Paz F, Garcia SG, Schilmann A. Abusive head trauma at a tertiary care children's hospital in Mexico City. A preliminary study. *Child Abuse Negl.* 2011;35(11):915–923.

112. Huang MI, O'Riordan MA, Fitzenrider E, McDavid L, Cohen AR, Robinson S. Increased incidence of nonaccidental head trauma in infants associated with the economic recession. *J Neurosurg Pediatr.* 2011;8(2):171–176.

113. Berger RP, Fromkin JB, Stutz H, et al. Abusive head trauma during a time of increased unemployment: a multicenter analysis. *Pediatrics.* 2011;128(4):637–643.

Traumatic Cerebral Vascular Injury

Kimbra Kenney, Margalit Haber, and Ramon Diaz-Arrastia

6

Introduction

While the complex molecular and cellular mechanisms responsible for traumatic brain injury (TBI)-associated deficits are incompletely understood, substantial data suggest that traumatic cerebral vascular injury (TCVI), at least partially, underlies TBI-related disability. Because the cerebral vasculature is highly plastic, TCVI also represents an attractive target for therapies. There are well-established pharmacologic and nonpharmacologic approaches that promote vascular health, such as exercise, phosphodiesterase-5 (PDE-5) inhibitors, hydroxymethylglutaryl-CoA (HMG-CoA) reductase inhibitors, high-density lipoprotein (HDL) mimetics, and peroxisome proliferator-activated receptor-γ (PPAR-γ) agonists, among others, and several have shown efficacy in both chronic neurovascular and neurodegenerative conditions.[1] This chapter will focus on TCVI preclinical and clinical data that support TCVI as a unique pathophysiologic TBI endophenotype and novel imaging techniques that can be used to assess its association with TBI-related symptoms and disability, as well as predictive and pharmacodynamic biomarkers of vascular-targeted TCVI therapy.

The Neurovascular Unit

The micro-network regulating cerebral blood flow (CBF), vascular permeability, and angiogenesis was recognized more than 130 years ago at the end of the nineteenth century by Paul Ehrlich[2] and has been coined the neurovascular unit (NVU).[3–5] The NVU comprises endothelial cells, astrocytes, microglia, pericytes, neurons, and the extracellular matrix that are physiologically linked in normal brain function. But it also actively participates in the pathogenesis of many brain disorders, including common conditions such as hypertension, diabetes, and neurodegenerative disorders (e.g., Alzheimer's disease).[5,6] The NVU has been an intense focus of research in a myriad of acute and chronic neurologic disorders.[7]

Pathophysiology of Neurovascular Unit Injury After TBI

TCVI can result from both primary and secondary injuries (e.g., blood–brain barrier [BBB] disruption, increased intracellular calcium, mitochondrial dysfunction, neuroinflammation).[7] After TBI, the changes seen in the BBB are biphasic—immediate changes caused by direct physical damage to endothelial cells followed by changes from secondary metabolic injuries in other elements of the NVU (neurons, astrocytes, pericytes, microglia, and the extracellular matrix).[8] Diminished CBF and focal tissue hypoxia is a common precipitant of NVU pathophysiology and is mediated through multiple pathophysiologic cascades (e.g. BBB disruption, edema, focal ischemia).[3,9,10] In animal TBI models, focal cortical impact has been shown to result in BBB break-down.[11–14] The onset of the early first phase is rapid, with the BBB permeability max-imal within a few hours of injury. Nearly immediately, BBB dysfunction is associated with microvascular changes, including an increase in endothelial caveolae with increased transcytosis of plasma proteins[15,16] and decreases in expression of junctional adhesion and tight junction proteins.[17,18] An increase in pericytes[19] and a proliferation of blood vessels in response to vascular endothelial growth factor (VEGF)[20] at the neurovascular junction have also been observed. The onset of the second phase is delayed, starting from 3–7 days following TBI. When injured, the NVU rapidly increases blood flow in order to restore normal oxygen supply and induces factors that promote angiogen-esis.[8,21] However, the NVU also attempts self-repair through mechanisms with potential deleterious consequences that enhance secondary injury if homeostasis is not quickly restored.[8] These changes often occur remote from the TBI impact and represent sec-ondary NVU changes.

Pathology of Microvascular Injury in Acute TBI: Primary Injury

Preclinical Studies of Acute Changes

Microvascular injury is a near universal finding in experimental TBI and has been re-ported in nearly all animal models, including impact acceleration,[22,23] fluid percussion injury,[24] and controlled cortical impact (CCI).[25] Early studies with fluid percussion injury showed peri-contusion petechial hemorrhages around small venules, pyknotic neurons, and swollen astrocytes. Ultrastructural analysis revealed early vessel wall damage in areas with irreversible neuronal injury.[26] Another fluid percussion injury study showed reduced microvascular density (57% loss) within cortical contusions.[27] After CCI, acute migration of pericytes was observed from microvascular locations to thinning areas of the basal lamina.[28] Electron microscopy in primates showed endothelial changes at 3 hours that persisted 1 week post-injury.[29] Sangiorgi et al.[30] described microvascular in-jury changes similar to those found in humans the first 3 weeks after injury.[21] Casts of the cerebra microvasculature taken 3 hours after CCI showed extravasation consistent with subarachnoid, subdural, and intraparenchymal haemorrhage, a result of primary injury. By 12 hours, the major finding was microvascular constriction and distal caliber reduction, potentially reflecting cytotoxic edema.[30] A study of microvascular pathology in the CCI model at both acute and chronic time points shows microvascular injury associated with inflammation, BBB disruption, and progressive white matter injury.[31]

Human Neuropathological Observations in Acute/Subacute TBI

TCVI is a near universal feature of severe TBI.[23,32] There are abundant pathological reports describing TCVI after fatal TBI[33] and, although less frequently, also in individuals who died from non–TBI related complications after mild TBI.[21,34] Microscopic perivascular hemorrhages are seen even when macroscopic hemorrhage is absent. Microscopically, there are abundant intravascular microthrombi in the microvasculature. In samples from noncontused or contused sections after fatal TBI cases, intravascular microthrombi are seen in both, only varying in density and correlated with focal areas of neuronal necrosis[34] suggesting a possible link between microthrombi and neuronal death.[26] Rodriquez-Baeza and colleagues studied the cerebral microvasculature ultrastructurally in 10 TBI patients who died between 1 and 20 days after injury.[21] Corrosion casts of the microvasculature revealed three changes in the arterioles and capillaries of the middle and deep cortical vascular zones in TBI brains: (1) longitudinal folds, (2) sunken vascular surfaces with craters at endothelial junctions, and (3) reduction of the vessel lumen (Figure 6.1).[21] Recent electron microscopy studies after severe TBI describe the following capillary and pericyte changes: thickening of the basement membrane 3–8 times normal; rarefaction, vacuolization, and splitting of the capillary basement membrane; pericyte hypertrophy; pericyte rarefaction and necrosis; and lipofuscin and lipid deposits in pericyte cytoplasm,[35,36] indicating widespread microvascular injury after TBI.[21,35,36]

For most patients, clinical data indicate that BBB permeability returns to normal within days to weeks following TBI,[37–39] In some patients, BBB disruption has been documented months or years after mild injuries.[40,41] As a result of forces from the initial injury, microvascular endothelia often sustain a shear injury,[21] resulting in BBB, CBF, and metabolic derangements. Additionally, BBB damage can arise from nonvascular causes including astrocytic dysfunction, inflammation-related mechanisms, and metabolic disturbances. BBB disruption results in an increase in endothelial permeability and, in turn, can result in brain edema from the entry of a protein-rich exudate through the widened endothelial tight junctions. The inflammatory response in patients with TBI begins within hours after injury and lasts up to several weeks.[42] Following infiltration, leukocytes release proinflammatory cytokines, cytotoxic proteases, and reactive oxygen species, which activates local microglia, and these further expand BBB opening.[43] BBB dysfunction is associated with increased levels of Aβ in the cerebrospinal fluid after TBI.[44]

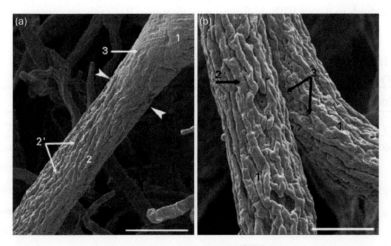

Figure 6.1 Scanning electron micrographs showing electron microscope microvascular changes in two arteriolar vessels from the frontal lobe after traumatic brain injury.[21] (A) Arteriole with longitudinal folds (2′) with transition from smooth to folds (*arrowheads*). 1 = subpial zone; 2 = superficial zone; 3 = cortical zone. Scale bar = 86 μm. (B) Arteriolar vessels (1) with longitudinal folds (2) and nuclear imprints of endothelial cells (3) at higher power. Scale bar = 23 μm.

Pathology of Microvascular Injury in Chronic TBI: Microvascular Repair

Injured blood vessels respond to TBI through local repair (Table 6.1). The cerebral microvasculature effects this through increased protein synthesis along with cell hypertrophy and hyperplasia.[7] These time-dependent responses are not seen until 3 hours to 7 weeks after TBI and can be used in forensic injury dating.[32] In animal models, therapies that promote vascular repair and/or angiogenesis, such as statins[53] or sildenafil,[54,55] promote neurologic recovery.

Pathology of Cerebral Microvascular Injury in Chronic Traumatic Encephalopathy

Prominent microvasculopathy is also described in chronic traumatic encephalopathy (CTE).[56,57] Cortical vascular changes, such as thickened perforating arteries, absence of nuclei in vascular cells, and diffuse hyaline, were described in the initial CTE cases.[58] Among CTE cases in the Corsellis collection, diffuse perivascular hemosiderin collections in macrophages, neuroglia, or extracellular space were described.[59] In sports-related CTE cases, striking vascular changes such as perivascular microgliosis and astrocytosis, neurofibrillary tangles, and spindle-shaped neurites in the sulcal depths of cortical gyri and hemosiderin-laden perivascular macrophages have been described.[60] In a series of blast-associated CTE cases, McKee similarly noted perivascular lymphocytic cuffing, hemosiderin-laden macrophages within cerebral vessel walls, and focal calcifications of penetrating small thalamic and deep white matter vessels[61] similar to that seen in mouse models of TCVI.[32,56]

Noninvasive Assessment of the Blood–Brain Barrier

There are currently both computed tomography (CT) and magnetic resonance imaging (MRI) methods to detect BBB dysfunction qualitatively. Both rely on contrast-enhanced

Table 6.1:
Summary of major components of traumatic vascular injury (TVI)

Major Components of Acute Traumatic Vascular Injury (TVI)		
Category of Injury	Site/Function	Effect[Ref]
Morphologic injury	Endothelial lesion	Increased[45]
	Endothelial barrier antigen	Decreased[46]
Physiologic injury	Vascular reactivity	Decreased[47]
	Vasoconstriction	Increased[48]
	Vasodilation	Decreased[48]
	BBB damage	Increased[49]
	O consumption2	Decreased[45]
Biochemical/Molecular injury	iNOS/eNOS expression	Increased[50]
	Endothelial cell activation	Increased[51]
	von Willebrand factor activation	Increased[52]

imaging techniques using iohexol and gadolinium-labeled diethylenetriamine penta-acetic acid, respectively. A new class of MRI contrast agents—the superparamagnetic iron oxide nanoparticle compounds—is increasingly being used to image brain infiltration of macrophages and indirectly quantify BBB disruption.[62] There are also semi-quantitative methods to assess BBB integrity that compare pre- and postcontrast images[40,63] as well as dynamic contrast-enhanced imaging (DCE-MRI).[64,65] Friedman et al. examined 15 amateur football players and 13 athlete controls with DCE-MRI and created BBB permeability maps for each subject. They found BBB pathology in 40% of the football players versus 8.3% of the athlete controls but no association between BBB pathology and concussion history.[66]

Noninvasive Assessment of Traumatic Cerebral Vascular Injury

There are two methods to assess cerebral microvascular function: functional neuroimaging and cerebrovascular reactivity (CVR) measurements. Novel neuroimaging sequences have been coupled with dynamic procedures that increase physiologic demand to measure the cerebral microvasculature's ability to respond to the increased demand and, indirectly, demonstrate TCVI.

Neuroimaging and Cerebrovascular Reactivity in Experimental Animals

Neuroimaging studies consistently show reduced CBF acutely after experimental TBI by fMRI[67] and laser Doppler flowometry.[68] In fluid percussion injury, CBF measured via continuous arterial spin label (ASL) imaging showed reductions the first 2 weeks after injury, corresponding with decreases in cortical small vessel density.[67]

CVR can be assessed in experimental models through cranial windows that allow direct visualization of the pial microvasculature. The anesthetized animals undergo a hypercapnia challenge with 3–5% carbon dioxide while the pial microvasculature is assessed. One week after injury, there is a significant decrease in CVR compared to sham injured controls.[22] Other studies report that TBI causes a loss of the normal vasodilatory response to potent vasodilators (acetylcholine, adenosine, and sodium nitroprusside).[24]

Neuroimaging Studies in Humans

CBF has been extensively studied after TBI in humans, especially in the acute period, when CBF deficits are common and generally show focal or multifocal CBF reduction.[68] Bonne et al.[69] used single-photon emission computed tomography (SPECT) to measure regional CBF in symptomatic, chronic TBI patients and found areas of cerebral hypoperfusion. However, it is unclear whether decreased CBF reflects a primary vascular injury or a compensatory response to a primary neuronal injury with reduced metabolic demand. With SPECT, Lewine et al.[70] described CBF abnormalities in 40% of 30 chronic symptomatic mild TBI patients and found SPECT to be significantly more sensitive than MRI. A recent meta-review concluded that SPECT outperformed CT and MRI in both acute and chronic TBI diagnosis.[71] In all 10 studies that compared SPECT to CT or MRI, SPECT identified CBF deficits that were not seen by conventional imaging.

Other advanced MRI techniques have been helpful in evaluating TCVI. ASL provides a direct measurement of arterial perfusion in absolute units of CBF. Kim et al. showed that chronic moderate or severe TBI patients have reduced global CBF in the resting state, as well as decreased regional perfusion in the thalamus, posterior cingulate cortex, and frontal cortex.[72] Regional CBF can also be calculated by perfusion-weighted imaging (PWI). In 15 symptomatic sports-related concussion patients studied 6 months postconcussion, PWI showed reduced CBF in the thalami bilaterally and reduced cerebral blood volume in the left thalamus compared to controls.[9] Susceptibility-weighted imaging (SWI) detects microbleeds better than gradient recalled echo MRI in traumatic axonal injury, and the total number and volume of microbleeds correlate with TBI-associated functional outcomes.[73] Traumatic microbleeds are seen in 23% of mild TBI patients scanned between 8 and 60 days after injury, and their presence inversely correlates with neurocognitive testing.[74] However, one of the limitations of CBF measurements is that these methods cannot distinguish decreased CBF as a result of diminished neuronal activity versus vascular dysfunction.

Assessment of Cerebrovascular Reactivity in Humans

Several methods exist to study CVR noninvasively in humans, including hypercapnia challenge, breath-holding, or acetazolamide administration[75] via transcranial Doppler (TCD), fMRI, or near infra-red spectroscopy (NIRS). While TCD and NIRS offer the advantage of high temporal resolution, MRI offers superb spatial resolution. A prospective study of 299 moderate to severe TBI patients assessed cerebral vasospasm with TCD.[76] Nearly half (45.2%) of the patients had vasospasm with the highest risk at day 3 after injury. CVR, measured by both TCD and NIRS, was decreased in 12 professional boxers[77] 72 hours after a bout. Compared to controls, the boxers also had chronically impaired CVR by both modalities and lower CVR measurements correlated with increased neurocognitive dysfunction and inversely correlated with TBI exposure. A meta-analysis reported reduced CVR via TCD in 42 athletes examined between 2 and 5 days after sports-related concussion.[78]

Functional NIRS (fNIRS), another noninvasive measure of CVR, is currently also being used to assess microvascular function in TBI. fNIRS allows CVR measurements during dynamic challenges that are independent of hemoglobin concentration, skull thickness, and extracranial circulation.[79] Using a NIRS-based CVR index in 40 acute TBI patients, a total hemoglobin reactivity index measured by NIRS correlated with the intracranial pressure–derived cerebrovascular pressure reactivity index.[80] A study of 37 critically ill TBI patients showed a good correlation between hemoglobin reactivity index measured via NIRS and intracranial pressure.

Hypercapnia-BOLD MRI Reliably Measures CVR Deficits in Chronic Stage After TBI

Direct measures of microvascular injury require assessment of CVR using manipulations that directly affect endothelial function without altering neuronal metabolism. One method combines MRI with the blood oxygen dependent (BOLD) signal in response to hypercapnia challenge and provides excellent spatial resolution.[81–89] The hypercapnia challenge is administered during the MRI by the inhalation of room air alternating with room air admixed with 5% CO_2. The CVR is the ratio of change in BOLD signal to the change in end-tidal CO_2; with voxel-by-voxel measurements, a CVR map can be drawn.

Mutch et al. examined CVR in adolescents with chronic postconcussive syndrome (PCS) after sports concussion and age-matched healthy controls with fMRI-BOLD and found decreased mean CVR in the PCS group.[86] Our group recently reported a study of CVR by MRI-BOLD with hypercapnia challenge in 27 chronic stage TBI patients at least 6 months after injury compared to 15 age- and gender-matched controls.[88] At baseline, CBF and CVR were measured both before and after administration of a single dose of sildenafil, a specific phosphodiesterase-5 inhibitor (PDE5) and a candidate therapy for traumatic vascular injury based on its vascular reparative mechanisms of action. Chronic TBI subjects showed a significant reduction in mean global, gray matter (GM), and white matter (WM) CVR compared to healthy volunteers ($p < 0.001$). Mean GM CVR had the greatest effect size (Cohen's d = 0.9). CVR maps in chronic TBI subjects show patchy, multifocal CVR deficits. By contrast, CBF discriminated poorly between TBI subjects and healthy volunteers and did not correlate with CVR (Figure 6.2, images A2, B2, C2).[89] After a single dose of sildenafil, TBI subjects showed a significant increase in global CVR compared to healthy controls ($p < 0.001$, d = 0.9). Post-sildenafil CVR maps showed near-normalization of CVR in many regions where baseline CVR was low, predominantly within areas without structural abnormalities (Figure 6.2, images A4–5, B4–5, C4–5).[88] Within this cohort of TBI subjects, we compared microstructural tissue integrity (via mean diffusivity [MD] and fractional anisotropy [FA]) and altered vascular function (via CBF and CVR) within regions of visible encephalomalacia on fluid-attenuated inversion recovery (FLAIR) sequences compared to areas without visible encephalomalacia on FLAIR. There was a significant reduction in FA, CBF, and CVR with a complementary increase in MD within regions of FLAIR-visible encephalomalacia ($p < 0.05$ for all comparisons). By contrast, in normal-appearing brain regions, only CVR was significantly reduced relative to controls ($p < 0.05$). These findings indicate that vascular dysfunction represents a TBI endophenotype that is distinct from structural injury detected using conventional MRI and may be present even in the absence of visible structural injury.[90]

We adapted the hypercapnia challenge to NIRS testing and found similar CVR reductions in chronic TBI and a strong correlation with the MRI-BOLD results. Focal CVR deficits seen on CVR maps by fMRI are also observed in the same areas by fNIRS in the frontal regions (Franck Amyot, personal communication). Global CVR is significantly lower in chronic TBI patients and is reliably measured by both fMRI and fNIRS, Both methods show promise as noninvasive measures of CVR function after TBI. CVR may prove to be a useful predictive and pharmacodynamic biomarker in therapeutic trials of TCVI.

Advances in noninvasive imaging techniques that examine cerebral vascular integrity and physiology show potential in TCVI research. Recently, Lu et al. reported a novel multiparametric imaging scheme that simultaneously measures baseline venous cerebral blood volume (vCBV), CVR, bolus arrival time (BAT), and resting-state function connectivity (fcMRI) using concomitant oxygen and carbon dioxide gas inhalation and a rapid (<10 minute) BOLD sequence.[91] FcMRI networks were identified from the gas-inhalation MRI data and correlated highly with conventional fcMRI acquisition,

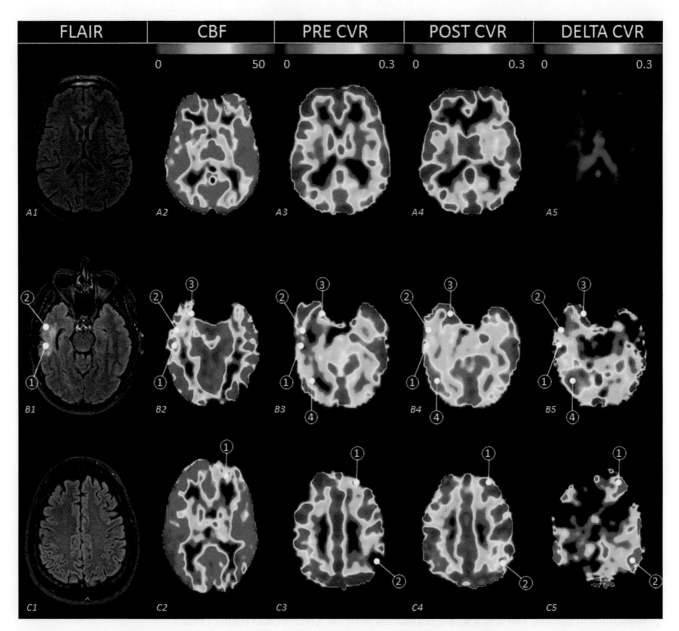

FLAIR	CBF	PRE CVR	POST CVR	DELTA CVR
	0 — 50	0 — 0.3	0 — 0.3	0 — 0.3

Figure 6.2 Structural (fluid-attenuated inversion recovery [FLAIR] magnetic resonance image), cerebral blood flow (CBF), and cerebrovascular reactivity (CVR) maps of one healthy control (A1 to A5), one TBI subject with focal gliosis (B1 to B5), and one traumatic brain injury subject with no structural abnormality (C1 to C5). CBF and pre-sildenafil CVR maps were acquired before sildenafil administration. Post-sildenafil CVR maps were acquired 1 hour after single dose of sildenafil 50 mg. ΔCVR is the difference between the post-sildenafil and the pre-sildenafil CVR maps. All images were co-registered and resliced with the structural image (FLAIR). Regions of visible encephalomalacia (region B2) typically showed low CBF, low CVR, and low ΔCVR. We interpret these findings as indicating that in regions with extensive microvasculature damage, there is not enough nitrous oxide (NO) produced to allow potentiation by sildenafil. More commonly in regions where there is no visible encephalomalacia noted on FLAIR (such as in regions B4, C1, and C2) CBF may be normal or low, but CVR is low, and a robust ΔCVR is noted. We interpret these findings as indicating that, in these areas without structural abnormality, some NO is produced by damaged endothelial cells, insufficient to produce normal vasodilation to the hypercapnia stimulus but enough to produce normal or near-normal vasodilation with the addition of NO enhancement by PDE5 inhibition.

including the default mode network and the primary visual network. Lu et al. examined healthy controls and subjects with Moyamoya syndrome and showed focal reductions of CVR in stenosis-affected arteries in the Moyamoya patients.

A recent report of single-dose sildenafil in Alzheimer disease patients, documented the vascular reparative effects of PDE-5 with improvements in cerebral hemodynamic function and increased cerebral oxygen metabolism.[92] We recently reported a safety and tolerance phase II clinical trial of sildenafil in chronic moderate-severe TBI and showed that single-dose sildenafil improved CVR and was safe and well-tolerated.[88]

Conclusion

TCVI has been an underrecognized TBI endophenotype despite a robust theoretical construct and a large body of empirical evidence. The studies reviewed here support the hypothesis that TCVI is near ubiquitous after TBI. TCVI plays a potentially important role in chronic postconcussive symptoms and even in TBI-associated neurodegenerative disorders. Further neuropathological studies are required to characterize the extent and time course of TCVI. As novel vascular technologies are developed, we will achieve a better understanding of TCVI's role in clinical symptoms both acutely and remotely after TBI. Understanding the pathophysiology of TCVI will aid in developing effective treatments targeting the underlying pathology.

Acknowledgments

Work in the authors' laboratory was supported by the Center for Neuroscience and Regenerative Medicine (CNRM) and by the Chronic Effects of Neurotrauma Consortium (CENC). The contents of this chapter are solely the responsibility of the authors and do not represent the official views of the Department of Defense, CRNM, or CENC.

References

1. Nicolakakis N, Hamel E. Neurovascular function in Alzheimer's disease patients and experimental models. *J Cereb Blood Flow Metab.* 2011;31(6):1354–1370.

2. Ehrlich P. Oxygen need by the organism: analytical study using color [German]. *Hirschwald.* 1885;8:167.

3. Lecrux C, Hamel E. The neurovascular unit in brain function and disease. *Acta Physiol (Oxf).* 2011;203(1):47–59.

4. Kenney K, Amyot F, Haber M, et al. Cerebral vascular injury in traumatic brain injury. *Exp Neurol.* 2016;275(Pt 3):353–366.

5. Zlokovic BV. Neurovascular pathways to neurodegeneration in Alzheimer's disease and other disorders. *Nat Rev Neurosci.* 2011;12(12):723–738.

6. Zlokovic BV. The blood-brain barrier in health and chronic neurodegenerative disorders. *Neuron.* 2008;57(2):178–201.

7. Golding EM. Sequelae following traumatic brain injury. The cerebrovascular perspective. *Brain Res Brain Res Rev.* 2002;38(3):377–388.

8. Shlosberg D, Benifla M, Kaufer D, Friedman A. Blood-brain barrier breakdown as a therapeutic target in traumatic brain injury. *Nat Rev Neurol.* 2010;6(7):393–403.

9. Bartnik-Olson BL, Holshouser B, Wang H, et al. Impaired neurovascular unit function contributes to persistent symptoms after concussion: a pilot study. *J Neurotrauma.* 2014;31(17):1497–1506.

10. Xing C, Hayakawa K, Lok J, Arai K, Lo EH. Injury and repair in the neurovascular unit. *Neurol Res.* 2012;34(4):325–330.

11. Barzó P, Marmarou A, Fatouros P, Corwin F, Dunbar J. Magnetic resonance imaging-monitored acute blood–brain barrier changes in experimental traumatic brain injury. *J Neurosurg.* 1996;85:1113–1121.

12. Csuka E, Morganti-Kossmann MC, Lenzlinger PM, Joller H, Tretz O, Kossmann T. IL-10 levels in cerebrospinal fluid and serum of patients with severe traumatic brain injury: relationship to IL-6, TNF-α, TGF-β1 and blood–brain barrier function. *J Neuroimmunol.* 1999;101:211–221.

13. Morganti-Kossmann MC, Hans VH, Lenzlinger PM, et al. TGF-β is elevated in the CSF of patients with severe traumatic brain injuries and parallels blood–brain barrier function. *J Neurotrauma.* 1999;16:617–628.

14. Shapira Y, Setton D, Artru AA, Shohami E. Blood–brain barrier permeability, cerebral edema, and neurologic function after closed head injury in rats. *Anesth Analg.* 1993;77:141–148.

15. Nag S, Venugopalan R, Stewart DJ. Increased caveolin-1 expression precedes decreased expression of occludin and claudin-5 during blood–brain barrier breakdown. *Acta Neuropathol.* 2007;114:459–469.

16. Nag S, Manias JL, Stewart DJ. Expression of endothelial phosphorylated caveolin-1 is increased in brain injury. *Neuropathol Appl Neurobiol.* 2009;35:417–426.

17. Zhao J, Moore AN, Redell JB, Dash PK. Enhancing expression of Nrf2-driven genes protects the blood brain barrier after brain injury. *J Neurosci.* 2007;27:10240–10248.

18. Yeung D, Manias JL, Stewart DJ, Nag S. Decreased junctional adhesion molecule-A expression during blood–brain barrier breakdown. *Acta Neuropathol.* 2008;115:635–642.

19. Dore-Duffy P, Owen C, Balabanov R, Murphy S, Beaumont T, Rafols JA. Pericyte migration from the vascular wall in response to traumatic brain injury. *Microvasc Res.* 2000;60:55–69.

20. Nag S, Takahashi JL, Kilty D. Role of vascular endothelial growth factor in blood–brain barrier breakdown and angiogenesis in brain trauma. *J Neuropathol Exp Neurol.* 1997;56:912–921.

21. Rodriguez-Baeza A, Reina-de la Torre F, Poca A, Marti M, Garnacho A. Morphological features in human cortical brain microvessels after head injury: a three-dimensional and immunocytochemical study. *Anat Rec A Discov Mol Cell Evol Biol.* 2003;273(1):583–593.

22. Baranova AI, Wei EP, Ueda Y, Sholley MM, Kontos HA, Povlishock JT. Cerebral vascular responsiveness after experimental traumatic brain injury: the beneficial effects of delayed hypothermia combined with superoxide dismutase administration. *J Neurosurg.* 2008;109(3):502–509.

23. Gao G, Oda Y, Wei EP, Povlishock JT. The adverse pial arteriolar and axonal consequences of traumatic brain injury complicated by hypoxia and their therapeutic modulation with hypothermia in rat. *J Cereb Blood Flow Metab.* 2010;30(3):628–637.

24. Wei EP, Hamm RJ, Baranova AI, Povlishock JT. The long-term microvascular and behavioral consequences of experimental traumatic brain injury after hypothermic intervention. *J Neurotrauma.* 2009;26(4):527–537.

25. Cherian L, Goodman JC, Robertson C. Improved cerebrovascular function and reduced histological damage with darbepoietin alfa administration after cortical impact injury in rats. *J Pharmacol Exp Ther.* 2011;337(2):451–456.

26. Dietrich WD, Alonso O, Halley M. Early microvascular and neuronal consequences of traumatic brain injury: a light and electron microscopic study in rats. *J Neurotrauma.* 1994;11(3):289–301.

27. Corsellis JA, Brierley JB. Observations on the pathology of insidious dementia following head injury. *J Ment Sci.* 1959;105:714–720.

28. Dore-Duffy P, Owen C, Balabanov R, Murphy S, Beaumont T, Rafols JA. Pericyte migration from the vascular wall in response to traumatic brain injury. *Microvasc Res.* 2000;60(1):55–69.

29. Maxwell RJ, Martinez-Perez I, Cerdan S, et al. Pattern recognition analysis of 1H NMR spectra from perchloric acid extracts of human brain tumor biopsies. *Magn Reson Med.* 1998;39(6):869–877.

30. Sangiorgi S, DeBenedictis A, Protasoni M, et al. Early-stage microvascular alterations of a new model of controlled cortical traumatic brain injury: 3D morphological analysis using scanning electron microscopy and corrosion casting. *J Neurosurg.* 2013;118(4):763–774.

31. Glushakova OY, Johnson D, Hayes RL. Delayed increases in microvascular pathology after experimental traumatic brain injury are associated with prolonged inflammation, blood-brain barrier disruption, and progressive white matter damage. *J Neurotrauma.* 2014;31(13):1180–1193.

32. Hausmann R, Betz P. The time course of the vascular response to human brain injury—an immunohistochemical study. *Int J Legal Med.* 2000;113(5):288–292.

33. Tomlinson BE. Brain-stem lesions after head injury. *J Clin Pathol Suppl (R Coll Pathol).* 1970;4:154–165.

34. Stein SC, Graham DI, Chen XH, Smith DH. Association between intravascular microthrombosis and cerebral ischemia in traumatic brain injury. *Neurosurgery.* 2004;54(3):687–691.

35. Castejon OJ. Ultrastructural pathology of cortical capillary pericytes in human traumatic brain oedema. *Folia Neuropathol.* 2011;49(3):162–173.

36. Castejon OJ. Ultrastructural alterations of human cortical capillary basement membrane in human brain oedema. *Folia Neuropathol.* 2014;52(1):10–21.

37. Kirchhoff C, Stegmaier J, Bogner V, et al. Intrathecal and systemic concentration of NT-proBNP in patients with severe traumatic brain injury. *J Neurotrauma.* 2006;23:943–949.

38. Lenzlinger PM, Marx A, Trentz O, Kossmann T, Morganti-Kossmann MC. Prolonged intrathecal release of soluble Fas following severe traumatic brain injury in humans. *J Neuroimmunol.* 2002;122:167–174.

39. Stahel PF, Morganti-Kossmann MC, Perez D, et al. Intrathecal levels of complement-derived soluble membrane attack complex (sC5b-9) correlate with blood–brain barrier dysfunction in patients with traumatic brain injury. *J Neurotrauma.* 2001;18:773–781.

40. Tomkins O, Shelef I, Kaizerman I, et al. Blood–brain barrier disruption in post-traumatic epilepsy. *J Neurol Neurosurg Psych.* 2008;79:774–777.

41. Korn A, Golan H, Melamed I, Pascual-Marqui R, Friedman A. Focal cortical dysfunction and blood–brain barrier disruption in patients with postconcussion syndrome. *J Clin Neurophysiol.* 2005;22:1–9.

42. Morganti-Kossmann MC, Satgunaseelan L, Bye N, Kossmann T. Modulation of immune response by head injury. *Injury.* 2007;38:1392–1400.

43. Stamatovic SM, Dimitrijevic OB, Keep RF, Andjelkovic AV. Inflammation and brain edema: new insights into the role of chemokines and their receptors. *Acta Neurochir Suppl.* 2006;96:444–450.

44. Emmerling MR, Morgannti-Kossmann MC, Kkossmann T, et al. Traumatic brain injury elevates the Alzheimer's amyloid peptide Aβ42 in human CSF. A possible role for nerve cell injury. *Ann NY Acad Sci.* 2000;903:118–122.

45. Wei EP, Dietrich WD, Povlishock JT, Navari RM, Kontos HA. Functional, morphological, and metabolic abnormalities of the cerebral microcirculation after concussive brain injury in cats. *Circ Res.* 1980;46:37–47.

46. Lin B, Ginsberg MD, Zhao W, et al. Quantitative analysis of microvascular alterations in traumatic brain injury by endothelial barrier antigen immunohistochemistry. *J Neurotrauma.* 2001;18(4):389–397.

47. Martin NA, Patwardhan RV, Alexander MJ, et al. Characterization of cerebral hemodynamic phases following severe head trauma: hypoperfusion, hyperemia, and vasospasm. *J Neurosurg.* 1997;87:9–19.

48. Golding EM, Robertson CS, Bryan RM. The consequences of traumatic brain injury on cerebral blood flow and autoregulation: a review. *Clin Exp Hypertens.* 1999;21:299–332.

49. Tanno H, Nockels RP, Pitts LH, et al. Breakdown of the blood-brain barrier after fluid percussive brain injury in the rat. Part 1: Distribution and time course of protein extravasation. *J Neurotrauma.* 1992;9:335–347.

50. Gahm C, Holmin S, Mathiesen T. Temporal profiles and cellular sources of three nitric oxide synthase isoforms in the brain after experimental contusion. *Neurosurgery.* 2000;46:1319–1326.

51. Balabanov R, Goldman H, Murphy S, et al. Endothelial cell activation following moderate traumatic brain injury. *Neurol Res.* 2001;23:175–182.

52. Yokota H, Naoe Y, Nakabayashi M, et al. Cerebral endothelial injury in severe head injury: the significance of measurements of serum thrombomodulin and the von Willebrand factor. *J Neurotrauma.* 2002;19:1007–1015.

53. Wu H, Jiang H, Lu D, et al. Induction of angiogenesis and modulation of vascular endothelial growth factor receptor-2 by simvastatin after traumatic brain injury. *Neurosurgery.* 2011;68(5):1363–1371.

54. Zhang R, Wang Y, Zhang L, et al. Sildenafil (Viagra) induces neurogenesis and promotes functional recovery after stroke in rats. *Stroke.* 2002;33(11):2675–2680.

55. Pifarre P, Prado J, Giralt M, Molinero A, Hidalgo J, Garcia A. Cyclic GMP phosphodiesterase inhibition alters the glial inflammatory response, reduces oxidative stress and cell death and increases angiogenesis following focal brain injury. *J Neurochem.* 2010;112(3):807–817.

56. Goldstein LE, Fisher AM, Tagge CA, et al. Chronic traumatic encephalopathy in blast-exposed military veterans and a blast neurotrauma mouse model. *Sci Transl Med.* 2012;4(134):134ra160.

57. McKee AC, Stern RA, Nowinski CJ, et al. The spectrum of disease in chronic traumatic encephalopathy. *Brain.* 2013;136(Pt 1):43–64.

58. Corsellis JA, Bruton CJ, Freeman-Browne D. The aftermath of boxing. *Psychol Med.* 1973;3(3):270–303.

59. Adams CW, Bruton CJ. The cerebral vasculature in dementia pugilistica. *J Neurol Neurosurg Psychiatry.* 1989;52(5):600–604.

60. McKee AC, Daneshvar DH, Alvarez VE, Stein TD. The neuropathology of sport. *Acta Neuropathol.* 2014;127(1):29–51.

61. McKee AC, Robinson ME. Military-related traumatic brain injury and neurodegeneration. *Alzheimers Dement.* 2014;10(3 suppl):S242–253.

62. Jander S, Schroeter M, Saleh A. Imaging inflammation in acute brain ischemia. *Stroke.* 2007;38:642–645.

63. Tomkins O, Kaufer D, Korn A, et al. Frequent blood–brain barrier disruption in the human cerebral cortex. *Cell Mol Neurobiol.* 2001;21:675–691.

64. Tofts PS, Kermode AG. Measurement of the blood–brain barrier permeability and leakage space using dynamic Mr imaging. 1 Fundamental concepts. *Magn Reson Med.* 1991;17:357–367.

65. Zaharchuk G. Theoretical basis of hemodynamic Mr imaging techniques to measure cerebral blood volume, cerebral blood flow, and permeability. *AJNR Am J Neuroradiol.* 2007;28:1850–1858.

66. Weissberg I, Veksler R, Kamintsky L, et al. Imaging blood-brain barrier dysfunction in football players. *JAMA Neurol.* 2014;71(11):1453–1455.

67. Hayward NM, Tuunanen PI, Immonen R, Ndode-Ekane XE, Pitkanen A, Grohn O. Magnetic resonance imaging of regional hemodynamic and cerebrovascular recovery after lateral fluid-percussion brain injury in rats. *J Cereb Blood Flow Metab.* 2011;31(1):166–177.

68. Thomale UW, Kroppenstedt SN, Beyer TF, Schaser KD, Unterberg AW, Stover JF. Temporal profile of cortical perfusion and microcirculation after controlled cortical impact injury in rats. *J Neurotrauma.* 2002;19(4):403–413.

69. Bonne O, Gilboa A, Louzoun Y, et al. Cerebral blood flow in chronic symptomatic mild traumatic brain injury. *Psychiatry Res.* 2003;124(3):141–152.

70. Lewine JD, Davis JT, Bigler ED, et al. Objective documentation of traumatic brain injury subsequent to mild head trauma: multimodal brain imaging with MEG, SPECT, and MRI. *J Head Trauma Rehabil.* 2007;22(3):141–155.

71. Raji CA, Tarzwell R, Pavel D, et al. Clinical utility of SPECT neuroimaging in the diagnosis and treatment of traumatic brain injury: a systematic review. *PLoS One.* 2014;9(3):e91088.

72. Kim J, Whyte J, Patel S, et al. Resting cerebral blood flow alterations in chronic traumatic brain injury: an arterial spin labeling perfusion FMRI study. *J Neurotrauma.* 2010;27(8):1399–1411.

73. Tong KA, Ashwal S, Holshouser BA, et al. Diffuse axonal injury in children: clinical correlation with hemorrhagic lesions. *Ann Neurol.* 2004;56(1):36–50.

74. Huang YL, Kuo YS, Tseng YC, Chen DY, Chiu WT, Chen CJ. Susceptibility- weighted MRI in mild traumatic brain injury. *Neurology.* 2015;84(6):580–585.

75. Kassner A, Roberts TP. Beyond perfusion: cerebral vascular reactivity and assessment of microvascular permeability. *Top Magn Reson Imaging.* 2004;15(1):58–65.

76. Oertel M, Boscardin WJ, Obrist WD, et al. Posttraumatic vasospasm: the epidemiology, severity, and time course of an underestimated phenomenon: a prospective study performed in 299 patients. *J Neurosurg.* 2005;103(5):812–824.

77. Bailey DM, Jones DW, Sinnott A, et al. Impaired cerebral haemodynamic function associated with chronic traumatic brain injury in professional boxers. *Clin Sci (Lond).* 2013;124(3):177–189.

78. Gardner AJ, Tan CO, Ainslie PN, et al. Cerebrovascular reactivity assessed by transcranial Doppler ultrasound in sport-related concussion: a systematic review. *Br J Sports Med.* 2015;49(16):1050–1055.

79. Kainerstorfer JM, Sassaroli A, Hallacoglu B, Pierro ML, Fantini S. Practical steps for applying a new dynamic model to near-infrared spectroscopy measurements of hemodynamic oscillations and transient changes: implications for cerebrovascular and functional brain studies. *Acad Radiol.* 2014;21(2):185–196.

80. Zweifel C, Castellani G, Czosnyka M, et al. Noninvasive monitoring of cerebrovascular reactivity with near infrared spectroscopy in head- injured patients. *J Neurotrauma.* 2010;27(11):1951–1958.

81. Lu H, Liu P, Yezhuvath U, Cheng Y, Marshall O, Ge Y. MRI mapping of cerebrovascular reactivity via gas inhalation challenges. *J Vis Exp.* 2014;94:52306.

82. Mutch WA, Ellis MJ, Graham MR, et al. Brain MRI CO2 stress testing: a pilot study in patients with concussion. *PLoS One.* 2014;9:e102181.

83. Ellis MJ, Ryner LN, Sobczyk O, et al. Neuroimaging assessment of cerebrovascular reactivity in concussion: current concepts, methodological considerations, and review of the literature. *Front Neurol.* 2016;7:61.

84. Mutch WA, Ellis MJ, Ryner LN, et al. Longitudinal brain magnetic resonance imaging CO2 stress testing in individual adolescent sports-related concussion patients: a pilot study. *Front Neurol.* 2016;7:107.

85. Yezhuvath US, Lewis-Amezcua K, Varghese R, Xiao G, Lu H. On the assessment of cerebrovascular reactivity using hypercapnia BOLD MRI. *NMR Biomed.* 2009;22:779–786.

86. Yezhuvath US, Uh J, Cheng Y, et al. Forebrain-dominant deficit in cerebrovascular reactivity in Alzheimer's disease. *Neurobiol Aging.* 2012;33:75–82.

87. Mutch WA, Ellis MJ, Ryner LN, et al. Brain magnetic resonance imaging CO2 stress testing in adolescent postconcussion syndrome. *J Neurosurg.* 2016;125:648–660.

88. Kenney K, Amyot F, Moore C, et al. Phosphodiesterase-5 inhibition potentiates cerebrovascular reactivity in chronic traumatic brain injury. *Ann Clin Trans Neur.* 2018; 5(4):418–428.

89. Amyot F, Kenney K, Moore C, et al. Imaging of cerebrovascular function in chronic traumatic brain injury [published online ahead of print October 25, 2017]. *J Neurotrauma* 2018.

90. Haber M, Amyot F, Kenney K, et al. Vascular abnormalities within normal appearing tissue in chronic traumatic brain injury. [published online ahead of print June 7, 2018]. *J Neurotrauma.* 2018.

91. Liu P, Welch BG, Li Y, et al. Multiparametric imaging of brain hemodynamics and function using gas-inhalation MIR. *NeuroImage.* 2017;146:715–723.

92. Sheng M, Lu H, Liu P, et al. Sildenafil improves vascular and metabolic function in patients with Alzheimer's disease. *J Alzheimers Dis.* 2017;60(4):1351–1364.

Disorders of Consciousness: Common Findings in Brain Injury

Calixto Machado, Mario Estévez, Rafael Rodríguez, Mauricio Chinchilla, and Jesús Pérez-Nellar

Introduction

The Terri Schiavo case raised new controversies about the diagnosis and management of the persistent vegetative state (PVS) and the minimally conscious state (MCS). This debate has dominated national US discourse, reaching from the media, the courts, the Florida legislature, the Governor of Florida, Congress, all the way to the President of United States.[1–4] The Schiavo case and other famous patients,[1–4] including Karen Ann Quinlan[5] and Nancy Cruzan in United States[6] and Tony Bland in United Kingdom,[7] have made it necessary for neurologists and neuroscientists to propose reliable diagnostic guidelines for testing brain function in altered states of consciousness.

The term "persistent vegetative state" was coined by Jennett and Plum in 1972 to describe the condition of patients with severe brain damage in whom coma has progressed to a state of wakefulness without detectable awareness. Such patients have sleep–wake cycles but no ascertainable cerebral cortical function. Jennett and Plum thought that patients in a PVS could be distinguished clinically from those with other conditions associated with disturbances of consciousness. These authors described a specific syndrome of reflex reactions without any meaningful response to the environment in patients who have a sleep–awake pattern. They introduced the term because they were dissatisfied with other terms used at the time. These terms referred to states that were not true coma (e.g., prolonged coma or coma vigil) because the patients, by definition, were not in coma, or described specific syndromes (e.g., decerebrate dementia, parasomnia, or akinetic mutism).[8] The term *apallic syndrome*, still used in some European countries, implies lack of the cortex (pallium), but this is not the only pathologic pattern found in these cases.[9]

Controversies exist in the use of present-day clinical terminology, including terms that may be pejorative in describing patients. Terms that are utilized to describe disorders of consciousness (DOC) may also be pejorative and have the potential to complicate patient care.[10] The term "persistent vegetative state" was originally used to describe patients with severe brain damage in whom coma had progressed to a state of wakefulness without detectable awareness by bedside clinical examination.[10,11]

Kretschmer in 1940 had originally used the term "apallic syndrome" to describe patients who were open-eyed, uncommunicative, and unresponsive due to a diversity of brain injuries such as cerebral arteriosclerosis, lues, and gunshot wounds.[12] This term was scarcely used until Viennese neurologists and neuropathologists began to apply to describe survivors after anoxic insults or poisoning.[13] Ingvar described the complete apallic syndrome or less severe forms that he termed "dyspallic" or "incomplete apallic." For this author, the main characteristics of the complete apallic syndrome were a complete loss of higher (telencephalic) function with an isoelectric electroencephalogram (EEG) and much-reduced cerebral blood flow and metabolism in supratentorial structures, and the syndrome was caused by the destruction of the "pallium, the cortical gray matter that covers the thelencephalon."[14] Although term implies lack of the cortex (pallium), diffuse damage of intra- and subcortical connections in the cerebral hemispheres white matter, and necrosis of the thalamus may also lead to this syndrome.[10,11,15]

PVS refers to the only circumstance in which an apparent dissociation of both components of consciousness is found characterized by preservation of wakefulness with an apparent loss of awareness.[11,15] The term minimally conscious state (MCS) was introduced to portray some patients as in a transitional phase toward the partial recovery of self-awareness or environmental awareness while emerging from the PVS.[16]

We now understand that PVS patients may show unequivocal signs of awareness and command-following, rendering the concept of vegetative state inappropriate and demanding new and representative terms.[10] Several functional neuroimaging and neurophysiological studies have demonstrated that a small subset of unresponsive "vegetative" patients may show unambiguous signs of consciousness and command-following that is inaccessible to clinical examination at the bedside.[17] Gosseries et al. have pointed out negative associations intrinsic to the term "vegetative state" and resultant diagnostic errors and their potential effect on the treatment and care for these patients.[18] The clinical examination of patients who suffer from altered states of consciousness is conducted at the bedside and remains largely unchanged from the times of Jennett and Plum.[10,11,15]

The tools we use are susceptible to environmental and physiological factors and often depend on the patient's ability to communicate through speech or movement. In order to address these problems, various functional brain imaging paradigms, which do not rely on the patient's ability to move or speak, have demonstrated the potential to inform the diagnostic decision-making process.[11,17] Jennett and Plum argued that the *Oxford English Dictionary* defined the word *vegetative* as "to live a merely physical life, devoid of intellectual activity or social intercourse" and also to describe "an organic body capable of growth and development but devoid of sensation and thought."[18]

Most of our patients use Spanish as their native language. The term *estado vegetativo* used in Spanish by physicians to describe PVS came from a literal English–Spanish translation. According to the *Real Academia Española*, the Spanish term "*vegetativo*" is related to unconscious vital functions, and "*vegetal*" is relative to plants. According to our experience, when a physician informs a patient's relatives that their family member's diagnosis is a *estado vegetativo*, they understand that he or she is no longer a human being, that there is no hope of recovery. Hence, many neurologists, including our group, feel uncomfortable when referring to human beings as being vegetative or as a "vegetable." We find it difficult to embrace the humanism of a patient who is in an altered state of consciousness when he or she is labeled with a term that has a pejorative connotation. As physicians, we find that it is very difficult to tell any person that someone they love or respect is in a vegetative state. We must strive to maintain these people's rights as human beings and treat them with respect in all things, including the language of our discipline.[10,11,15,17]

Fortunately, we are not alone in our desire for a better classification of syndromes of MCSs. After 35 years, the European Task Force on Disorders of Consciousness has proposed a new term, *unresponsive wakefulness syndrome* (*UWS*), to assist society in avoiding the deprecatory term "vegetative state."[19]

We submitted a response to the paper by Giacino et al., proposing the use of the term "minimally aware state" instead of "minimally conscious state."[20] Our group has embraced the use of the new term "UWS" and might suggest that we change our concept and use of the term MCS to *minimally responsive wakefulness state* (MRWS) or minimally aware wakefulness state (MAWS).[10]

Therefore, physicians must constantly strive to serve humankind, not only with our skills and training but also with the use of language that demonstrates the respect we have for humankind. We embrace, applaud, and agree on the importance of finding new terms to describe those patients with DOC. We also are aware of the need for change in the terminology of non–English speaking societies. Medical terms must be current and avoid any pejorative description of patients, which will promote our abilities to serve humankind and challenge neuroscientists to offer society new and realistic hopes for neurorehabilitation.[10,11,15,17,20]

Clinical Findings in Patients in a Persistent Vegetative State

The main finding in PVS is preservation of wakefulness with apparent loss of awareness.[19–22] The diagnosis of PVS has been made more difficult by recognition of the MCS as a transitional phase in the partial recovery of self-awareness or environmental awareness while emerging from the PVS, leading to a relatively high proportion of errors.[15,16,20]

Diagnostic criteria for PVS include lack of evidence of awareness of self or environment, lack of interaction with others, and lack of comprehension or expression of language. By implication, external stimuli do not evoke purposeful or sustained and reproducible voluntary behavioral responses.[11,15,16,20]

The accurate diagnosis of PVS requires the skills of a multidisciplinary team experienced in the management of people with complex disabilities and consciousness disorders. Accurate clinical assessments of patients in these conditions must be obtained before they undergo neuroimaging. Moreover, in reports of neuroimaging studies, all relevant clinical details must be available for comparisons between studies.[15,16,20,23–25]

According to the Multi-Society Task Force on PVS,[26,27] the vegetative state can be diagnosed considering certain criteria, including a lack of awareness of self or environment and the inability to interact with others; a lack of sustained, reproducible, purposeful, or voluntary behavioral responses to visual, auditory, tactile, or noxious stimuli; and a lack of evidence of language comprehension or expression. There is intermittent wakefulness manifested by the presence of sleep–wake cycles; sufficient hypothalamic and brainstem autonomic function for survival with medical and nursing care; bowel and bladder incontinence; and, finally, there are variably preserved cranial nerve reflexes and spinal reflexes. The crux of the problem lies in determining a person's internal mental state using external proof.[26–28]

Eye tracking and emotional responses are the most common ways of determining whether a patient is responding and therefore is no longer in a vegetative state. The first sign of a patient emerging from PVS is the localizing of the eyes on a visual stimulus.

This can be observed because persons in a vegetative state are unable to track moving objects or fixate their vision on an object, and, as a patient recovers, he regains this ability.[11] Several authors have reported that recovery of visual pursuit may presage recuperation of other signs of consciousness.[28] However, Andrews et al. have emphasized that many patients who are misdiagnosed as being in a vegetative state are blind or have severe visual handicap, and thus lack of eye blink to threat or absence of visual tracking might be not reliable signs for diagnosing a vegetative state.[29]

Giacino et al. have developed the JFK Coma Recovery Scale (CRS-R) to follow-up the clinical evolution in these patients and their potential recovery. If the CRS-R is applied by trained examiners and in repeated measurements, it could yield stable estimates of patient status. This scale contains six subscale scores: auditory function, visual function, motor function, oromotor/verbal function, communication, and arousal scales.[30]

Misdiagnoses of the vegetative state, MCS, and *locked-in syndrome* are common. Unexpected and well-documented recoveries of cognitive functions have been described in patients diagnosed by neurologists experienced and skilled in the diagnosis of this condition.[31–33] Childs et al. reported that 37% of 49 cases admitted to a special unit for rehabilitation were incorrectly diagnosed according to the American Medical Association guidelines on PVS and the decision process on withdrawing support.[31]

Although imaging techniques have the potential to improve both diagnostic and prognostic accuracy, careful and repeated neurological assessment by a trained examiner remains best practice.[11]

Nonetheless, emotional and self-relevant stimuli are able to automatically attract attention, and their use in patients suffering from DOC might help detect otherwise hidden signs of cognition. We reported a patient clinically diagnosed as being in vegetative state or UWS who showed emotional content responses to his mother's voice as assessed by EEG and heart rate variability (HRV).[17,34]

Comparison of Coma, Vegetative State, MCS, and Locked-In Syndrome

Coma

Coma is a sleep-like state characterized by the absence of arousal and awareness. The patient lies with the eyes closed, cannot be aroused, and has no awareness of self and surroundings. Stimulation cannot produce spontaneous periods of wakefulness and eye-opening in patients in a coma, unlike patients in a vegetative state. In order to make a clear distinction from other states of transient loss of consciousness, such as syncope, concussion, and the like, coma must endure for at least 1 hour. Coma can result from diffuse bihemispheric cortical or white-matter damage after neuronal or axonal injury, or from focal brainstem lesions that affect the pontomesencephalic tegmentum or paramedian thalami bilaterally.[11,35,36]

Locked-In Syndrome

Locked-in syndrome is defined as state characterized by sustained eye opening (bilateral ptosis should be ruled out as a complicating factor), aphonia or hypophonia, quadriplegia or quadriparesis, and vertical or lateral eye movement or blinking of the upper eyelid to signal yes–no responses; these patients preserve awareness of their environment.

Eye or eyelid movements are the main method of communication. This state entails a serious issue for physicians, nurses, and the whole staff because patients can hear and understand commentaries about their critical health state. The term "locked-in syndrome" was coined by Plum and Posner to describe the quadriplegia and anarthria consequential from the disruption of corticospinal and corticobulbar pathways, correspondingly.[36,37]

Minimally Conscious State

MCS patients show limited but clear evidence of awareness of themselves or their environments on a reproducible or sustained basis by at least one of several behaviors: gestural or verbal yes–no response (regardless of accuracy), following simple commands, intelligible speech, and purposeful behavior (including movements or affective behaviors that happen in response to stimuli in the environment and are not due to reflexive activity). MCS in some patients is a transitional phase toward the partial recovery of self- or environmental awareness while emerging from the vegetative state.

Giacino proposed a group of diagnostic criteria for MCS to demonstrate a clear and discernible evidence of self- or environmental awareness on a reproducible or sustained basis:[32]

Akinetic mutism was first described in a Cairn in a girl with a craniopharyngiomatous cyst that compressed the walls of the third ventricle.[38] Akinetic mutism is a rare state that has been described as a subcategory of the MCS because, although the syndrome has fairly identifiable characteristics, it is on a continuum with and overlaps the MCS.[39]

The main clinical features are an abulic emotionless state, unresponsiveness, and eye-tracking of object or person movement in the hospital room or intensive care unit. According to Wijdicks, the description of this syndrome is debatable because most patients with akinetic mutism are not fully akinetic, and many may respond with movements. (However, a few patients are really mute; many are able to utter only a single word.) Wijdicks also remarked that the ability of a patient to follow the examiner moving about the room or to be abruptly prompted to response by a person coming into the room is comparable to the observation of hypermetamorphosis in monkeys that have had their temporal lobes removed: these animals apparently respond to movement rather than objects.[40]

It has been suggested that this syndrome is caused by bilateral lesions of the cingulate gyri. The anterior cingulate cortex lesions affect executive functions and vocalization and, as this area is highly connected with the supplementary motor area, impair initiation of movement.[41] Nonetheless, other brain lesions have been reported to explain this syndrome, such as lesions affecting the diencephalic structures such as the thalamus or basal ganglia, or even mesencephalic structures involving the reticular activating system.[41,42] Akinetic mutism has been described associated with hypothalamic lesions and in obstructive hydrocephalus, aneurysmal subarachnoid hemorrhage producing bifrontal lesions, and an infiltrative astrocytoma in the fornix.[11]

Brain Connectivity in Disorders of Consciousness

The assessment of brain connectivity is essential to explain the pathophysiology of DOC. Brain connectivity estimators represent patterns of links in the brain. Connectivity can be considered at different levels of the brain's organization, from neurons to neural assemblies and brain structures. Brain connectivity involves different concepts, such as *neuroanatomical* or *structural connectivity* (pattern of anatomical links), *functional connectivity* (usually understood as statistical dependencies), and *effective connectivity* (referring to causal interactions).[43–45]

Although there exists an association between structural or anatomic connectivity (AC) and functional connectivity (FC), AC may be dissociated from FC.[43] Other authors have defined a new type of FC, *effective connectivity*.[43,46]

The development of diffusion-weighted magnetic resonance imaging (DW-MRI) techniques in the past several decade makes possible the noninvasive study of the anatomical circuitry of the living human brain. DW-MRI techniques have being widely used to estimate the nervous fiber pathways connecting brain regions of interest.[43–45] Recently, a novel DW-MRI and graph theory methodology were introduced with the principal purpose of summarizing patterns of anatomical connections between brain gray matter areas.[44]

Some brain connectivity estimators evaluate FC from brain activity time series such as EEG, local field potential (LFP), or spike trains, which have an effect on directed connectivity. These estimators can be applied to functional MRI (fMRI) data if the required image sequences are available. Among estimators of connectivity are linear and nonlinear, bivariate, and multivariate measures. Certain estimators also indicate directionality. Different methods of connectivity estimation vary in their effectiveness.[43,44]

To our knowledge, our group has introduced for the first time the use of graph theoretical approaches and DTI to differentiate the topological organization of white matter networks in patients in a vegetative state and with locked-in syndrome. In order to identify the characteristic properties of injured networks in comparison with healthy architectures, we used network-based statistics. In this study, we therefore sought to suggest essential differences in reduced global network efficiency and altered nodal efficiency between these DOC.[43]

Conclusion

The study of DOC is a challenge for present and future neurologists and neuroscientists. An accurate and reliable assessment of the level and content of consciousness in DOC is critical for subsequent patient management and rehabilitation, as well as for legal and ethical decision-making. To date, the gold standard for diagnosis of the level of consciousness is behavioral. However, clinical diagnosis is limited by the scope and reliability of available scales, examiner experience, and overlapping of impairments in consciousness. These concerns may lead examiners to misdiagnose patients with locked-in syndrome in whom cortical functions are preserved but who lack the ability to produce voluntary motor behavior and may resemble patients in a vegetative state.[11,43–46]

Our group showed that DTI is a potent tool for dissecting the complex neuroanatomic substrate of different DOC. Although the results of brain fiber tracking were not necessarily parallel to clinical symptoms, essential differences between patients in a vegetative state and those with locked-in syndrome are evidenced in Figure 7.1.

Viewed as a network disorder, the vegetative state shows widespread impairment in cortico-cortical connectivity in addition to impairments in brainstem connections. This result suggests that the loss of awareness in patients with brainstem lesions might be

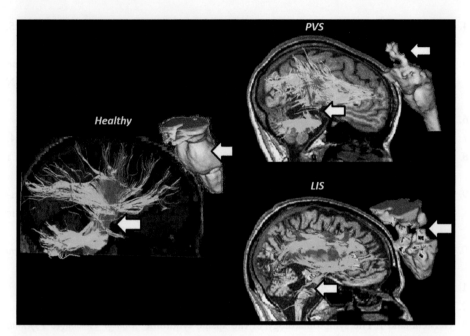

Figure 7.1 Anatomical damage (magnetic resonance image, T1), streamLine fiber tractography, and spatial correlation of impairments in patients. Healthy subject (control), persistent vegetative state (PVS), and locked-in-syndrome (LIS). PVS patient shows a widespread disruption in cortical and subcortical connectivity. Patient with LIS demonstrates an injury in pontine crossing tracts and preserved cortical networking. The healthy subject shows preservation of both anatomy and network.

associated with aberrant neuronal connectivity among widely distributed brain regions and provide structural evidence for the notion of the vegetative state as a disconnection syndrome. Significant reduction of all structural network attributes in this pathological condition might be interpreted as a considerable decline in the amount of possible nervous information that can be exchanged throughout the brain and how efficiently it can be managed at local and global levels.

On the contrary, patient with locked-in syndrome showed a cortical connectivity pattern comparable to that observed in healthy controls. Disruption of connections between brainstem, basal ganglia, and frontal motor regions is consistent with quadriplegia, aphonia, quadriplegia, and paralysis of the cranial nerves, while cortical networks supporting consciousness remain intact. Those results are highly consistent with the remarkable functional and cognitive differences between these pathological states, as extensively reported in previous studies.[11,43]

References

1. McHugh P. Annihilating Terri Schiavo. *Hum Life Rev.* 2005;31:67–77.

2. Silverman HJ. Withdrawal of feeding-tubes from incompetent patients: the Terri Schiavo case raises new issues regarding who decides in end-of-life decision making. *Intensive Care Med.* 2005;31:480–481.

3. Wolfson J. Defined by her dying, not her death: the guardian ad litem's view of Schiavo. *Death Stud.* 2006;30:113–120.

4. Newman M. Gov. Bush's role is ended in feeding tube dispute. *NY Times (Print).* January 25, 2005:A21.

5. Kinney HC, Korein J, Panigrahy A, Dikkes P, Goode R. Neuropathological findings in the brain of Karen Ann Quinlan. The role of the thalamus in the persistent vegetative state. *N Engl J Med.* 1994;330:1469–1475.

6. McCormick RA. The Nancy Cruzan case. *Midwest Med Ethics.* 1989;5:2–31.

7. Dyer C. Law lords rule that Tony Bland does not create precedent. *BMJ.* 1993;306:413–414.

8. Jennett B, Plum F. Persistent vegetative state after brain damage. A syndrome in search of a name. *Lancet.* 1972;1:734–737.

9. Hassler R, Ore GD, Dieckmann G, Bricolo A, Dolce G. Behavioural and EEG arousal induced by stimulation of unspecific projection systems in a patient with post-traumatic apallic syndrome. *Electroencephalogr Clin Neurophysiol.* 1969;27:306–310.

10. Machado C, Estévez M, Carrick FR, et al. Vegetative state is a pejorative term. *Neuro Rehabilitation.* 2012;31(4):345–347.

11. Machado C. *Brain Death: A Reappraisal.* New York: Springer; 2007.

12. Kretschmer E. Das apallische syndrom. *Z Ges Neurol Psychiat.* 1940;169:576–579.

13. Gerstenbrand F. The symptomatology of the apallic syndrome. *Monogr Gesamtgeb Psychiatr Psychiatry Ser.* 1977;14:14–21.

14. Ingvar DH, Brun A. [The complete apallic syndrome]. *Arch Psychiatr Nervenkr.* 1972;215:219–239.

15. Machado C, Korein J. Persistent vegetative and minimally conscious states. *Rev Neurosci.* 2009;20:203–220.

16. Giacino, JT, Ashwal, S, Childs, N, et al. The minimally conscious state: definition and diagnostic criteria. *Neurology.* 2002;58:349–353.

17. Machado C, Korein J, Aubert E, et al. Recognizing a mother's voice in the persistent vegetative state. *Clin EEG Neurosci.* 2007;38(3):124–126.

18. Gosseries O, Bruno MA, Chatelle C, et al. Disorders of consciousness: what's in a name? *Neuro Rehabilitation.* 2011;28:3–14.

19. Laureys, S, Celesia, GG, Cohadon, F, et al. Unresponsive wakefulness syndrome: a new name for the vegetative state or apallic syndrome. *BMC Med.* 2010;8:68.

20. Machado, C. The minimally conscious state: definition and diagnostic criteria. *Neurology.* 2002;59:1473–1474.

21. Machado C, Estévez M, Rodríguez R, et al. Are persistent vegetative state patients isolated from the outer world? *J Functional Neurol Rehab Ergonomics.* 2011;1:357–378.

22. Laureys S. The neural correlate of (un)awareness: lessons from the vegetative state. *Trends Cogn Sci.* 2005;9:556–559.

23. Fins JJ. neuroethics and disorders of consciousness: discerning brain states in clinical practice and research. *J Ethics.* 2016;18:1182–1191.

24. Noel JP, Blanke O, Serino A, Salomon R. Interplay between narrative and bodily self in access to consciousness: no difference between self- and non-self attributes. *Front Psychol.* 2017;8:72.

25. Wannez S, Gosseries O, Azzolini D, et al. Prevalence of coma-recovery scale-revised signs of consciousness in patients in minimally conscious state. *Neuropsychol Rehabil.* 2017;11:1–10.

26. Multi-Society Task Force on PVS. Medical aspects of the persistent vegetative state (1). *N Engl J Med.* 1994;330:1499–1508.

27. Multi-Society Task Force on PVS. Medical aspects of the persistent vegetative state (2). *N Engl J Med*. 1994;330:1572–1579.

28. Shiel A, Horn SA, Wilson BA, Watson MJ, Campbell MJ, McLellan DL. The Wessex Head Injury Matrix (WHIM) main scale: a preliminary report on a scale to assess and monitor patient recovery after severe head injury. *Clin Rehabil*. 2000;14:408–416.

29. Andrews K. Recovery of patients after four months or more in the persistent vegetative state. *BMJ*. 1993;306:1597–1600.

30. Giacino JT, Kalmar K, Whyte J. The JFK Coma Recovery Scale-revised: measurement characteristics and diagnostic utility. *Arch Phys Med Rehabil*. 2004;85:2020–2029.

31. Childs NL, Mercer WN. Misdiagnosing the persistent vegetative state. Misdiagnosis certainly occurs. *BMJ*. 1996;313:944.

32. Giacino JT, Kalmar K. Diagnostic and prognostic guidelines for the vegetative and minimally conscious states. *Neuropsychol Rehabil*. 2005;15:166–174.

33. Del Giudice R, Blume C, Wislowska M, et al. Can self-relevant stimuli help assessing patients with disorders of consciousness? *Conscious Cogn*. 2016;44:51–60.

34. Machado C, Estévez M, Gutiérrez J, et al. Recognition of the mom's voice with an emotional content in a PVS patient. *Clin Neurophysiol*. 2011;122:1059–1060.

35. Laureys S, Owen AM, Schiff ND. Brain function in coma, vegetative state, and related disorders. *Lancet Neurol*. 2004;3:537–546.

36. Plum F, Posner JB. *The Diagnosis of Stupor and Coma*. Philadelphia, PA: FA Davis; 1980.

37. Warabi Y, Hayashi K, Nagao M, Shimizu T. Marked widespread atrophy of the cerebral cortex and brainstem in sporadic amyotrophic lateral sclerosis in a totally locked-in state. *BMJ Case Rep*. 2017. pii: bcr2016218952.

38. Cairns H, Oldfield RC, Pennybacker JB, Whitteridge D. Akinetic mutism with epidermoid cyst of the third ventricle (with a report on associated disturbance of brain potentials). *Brain*. 1941;64:273–290.

39. Jang SH, Kwon HG. Akinetic mutism in a patient with mild traumatic brain injury: a diffusion tensor tractography study. *Brain Inj*. 2017;13:1–5.

40. Wijdicks EF, Cranford RE. Clinical diagnosis of prolonged states of impaired consciousness in adults. *Mayo Clin Proc*. 2005;80:1037–1046.

41. Buge A, Escourolle R, Rancurel G, Poisson M. [Akinetic mutism and bicingular softening. 3 anatomo-clinical cases]. *Rev Neurol (Paris)*. 1975;131:121–131.

42. Castaigne P, Lhermitte F, Buge A, Escourolle R, Hauw JJ, Lyon-Caen O. Paramedian thalamic and midbrain infarct: clinical and neuropathological study. *Ann Neurol*. 1981;10:127–148.

43. Machado C, Estevez M, Rodriguez R, et al. Anatomic and functional connectivity relationship in autistic children during three different experimental conditions. *Brain Connect*. 2015;5(8):487–496.

44. Iturria-Medina Y, Canales-Rodríguez EJ, Melie-García L, et al. Characterizing brain anatomical connections using diffusion weighted MRI and graph theory. *Neuroimage*. 2007;36:645–660.

45. Fan J, Zhong M, Zhu X, et al. Resting-state functional connectivity between right anterior insula and right orbital frontal cortex correlate with insight level in obsessive-compulsive disorder. *Neuroimage Clin*. 2017;15:1–7.

46. Harding JH, Yucel M, Harrison BJ, Pantelis C, Breakspear M. Effective connectivity within the frontoparietal control network differentiates cognitive control and working memory. *Neuroimage*. 2014;106C:144–153.

Section II

Mild Traumatic Brain Injury and Concussions

The TRACK-TBI Approach: Redefining Severity and Outcome Assessments

John K. Yue, Ethan A. Winkler, Hansen Deng,
Amy J. Markowitz, Kevin K. W. Wang, and Geoffrey T. Manley

Introduction

Traumatic brain injury (TBI) is highly heterogeneous in cause, severity, pathology, and clinical course.[1] Severity classifications and the availability of sensitive outcome measures for detecting deficits have remained static for the past three decades. Patients continue to be classified into mild, moderate, and severe TBI using the initial Glasgow Coma Scale (GCS; mild 13–15; moderate 9–12; severe 3–8) based upon three behavioral responses: eye opening (1–4 scale), verbal response (1–5), and motor response (1–6).[2] While the simplicity of the GCS allows for rapid assessment of level of consciousness/ obtundation and neurological decline, it lacks nuance that may be important for appropriate TBI diagnosis, prognosis, and treatment planning. Although low GCS (≤8) has high diagnostic specificity for severe TBI (~82%)[3] and is predictive (80–84%)[4] of in-hospital mortality[5] and favorable versus unfavorable outcome (Glasgow Outcome Scale (GOS); good recovery/moderate disability versus severe disability/death) at multiple time points postinjury,[4,6,7] the diagnostic sensitivity of GCS is low and it cannot readily distinguish between types of intracranial pathologies.[3] Furthermore, the GCS has a ceiling effect in the upper range, and its predictive utility at the milder end of the TBI spectrum is equivocal. Elderly patients also demonstrate differential responses to GCS, with less incidence of observable neurologic deficit[8] but higher odds of mortality compared to younger patients with identical GCS.[9] In practice, the GCS may vary depending on rater experience and time of rating—further complicating its objectivity. While the shortcomings of the GCS are well understood, few recommendations exist on how to improve on the diagnostic structure of TBI.

The Glasgow Outcome Scale-Extended (GOSE)[10] is an 8-point scale of functional recovery (1, "death"; 8, "back to baseline") and has been in use for the past four decades as the consensus measure for TBI.[11] However, the GOSE remains relatively insensitive to domain-specific impairment, limiting the study design of trials for targeted therapies for any one of the many subdomains encompassed in this global outcome metric.

In addition to the limitations of a precise disease classification model based on pathoanatomic and molecular features and consensus outcome measures sensitive to subdomains of deficits, TBI research has been further limited by lack of standards for data collection, curation, and multidisciplinary sharing and/or collaboration. Historically, this has hampered the rate of progress to advance clinical care and to address these and other limitations.

IMPACT Trials

Over the past 40 years, multicenter trials in TBI therapeutics have encountered significant challenges, in part due to inconsistent inclusion criteria, center effects, lack of surrogate biomarkers, variations in management, and lack of standardization to enable data pooling and robust analyses.[12] To address this, in the first coordinated effort within the field of TBI, the International Mission for Prognosis and Analysis of Clinical Trials in TBI (IMPACT) project merged clinical data from a summative number of randomized controlled trials (RCTs) and observational studies in TBI from 1984 to 1997. Clinical data from time of injury and postresuscitation to 6-month outcome were collated in 9,205 total patients, from which three validated prognostic models for severe and moderate TBI were developed and remain currently in use.[13,14] From IMPACT, a set of data variables deemed critically important to collect across all TBI clinical research emerged, termed *common data elements* (CDEs). The rationale for CDEs was to establish standard data definitions and collection methods in order to standardize data collection across future TBI clinical studies and thus ensure that the most relevant variables were collected in all trials, as well as to ensure data fidelity and data pooling to achieve statistical power in forming clinical conclusions.

NINDS Common Data Elements, Version 1

Informed by the IMPACT trials, the National Institutes of Health (NIH) and National Institute of Neurological Disorders and Stroke (NINDS) led the initiative to establish TBI CDEs, co-sponsored by the Department of Veterans Affairs, National Institute on Disability and Rehabilitation Research, industry stakeholders, and others.[15] Consensus interagency working groups consisting of experts from 49 institutes were formed for four major domains of data collection: demographics and clinical assessment, biospecimens and biomarkers, neuroimaging, and outcome measures. These groups were responsible for determining three levels of data granularity per domain: "core" (minimal set of measures to characterize the broad spectrum of subjects), "supplemental" (intended for greater depth/breadth of exploration for more specialized populations), and "emerging" (require further validation but may fill gaps in currently valid measures and/or substitute for recommended measures).[16–20] These working groups aimed to restructure the definition of TBI severity stratified across demographic/clinical risk factors, diagnostic and prognostic serum proteins and baseline genome susceptibility, objective neuroimaging pathology, and, of course, the multidimensional assessment of TBI outcomes in each and every patient rather than specialty measures from any single study.

The rationales behind each of the four domains are as follows:

- *Demographics and clinical assessment.* Participant/subject characteristics, clinical history, injury-/disease-related events, and injury assessments and examinations constitute a wide range of data variables with disparate definitions across studies. These were cohered into a set of CDEs with standard definitions.[17]
- *Biospecimens and biomarkers.* A sensitive and specific biomarker may be utilized earlier during the injury course during a routine blood draw, in lieu of delaying optimal treatment until neuroimaging is obtained, and/or in some cases replacing the need for computed tomography (CT) imaging and thus reducing radiation exposure.

Although a biomarker has yet to be validated for TBI diagnosis, over the past three decades, there is increasing evidence for the role of serum glial fibrillary acidic protein (GFAP) and ubiquitin c-terminal hydrolase-L1 (UCH-L1).[21,22] Considerable variability in biofluid type (whole blood, plasma, serum, others), collection, processing, and storage methods exists and should be standardized with best practices to reduce costs and accelerate genomic, proteomic, and metabolomic research in TBI.[23]

• *Neuroimaging.* This workgroup focused on five major components: (1) defining lesions strictly and objectively to maximize interrater reliability, with precise terms following exact definitions; (2) using specific radiologic protocols including CT, magnetic resonance imaging (MRI), magnetic resonance perfusion, diffusion tensor imaging (DTI), positron emission tomography (PET), functional MRI (fMRI), and others, with flexibility to accommodate evolving techniques; (3) determining levels of granularity encompassing presence/absence, quantification, and/or responses to intervention appropriate for the lesion type; (4) designing an electronic database with dropdown menus instead of hard-copy forms; and (5) designing a flexible dataset to allow for a range of specific population studies (rather than the traditional "comatose adults with CT").[20]

• *Outcome measures.* Measures targeting primary clinical research objectives and documenting the natural course of recovery from TBI and that were suitable for comparison across studies were selected to include "core" measures of functional recovery, neuropsychological impairment, psychological status, TBI-related symptoms, executive function, cognitive and physical limitations, social role participation, and health-related quality of life to be assessed at the standard follow-up timepoint of 6 months postinjury.[19] "Core" measures were the GOSE, Rey Auditory Verbal Learning Test (RAVLT), Trail Making Test (TMT), WAIS-IV Processing Speed Index (WAIS-PSI), Brief Symptom Inventory 18 (BSI18), Rivermead Post Concussional Symptoms Questionnaire (RPQ), Functional Independence Measure (FIM) Cognition Subscale, Craig Handicap Assessment and Reporting Technique Short Form (CHART-SF), and Satisfaction with Life Scale (SWLS).[19]

TRACK-TBI Pilot: Implementation

Under the American Reinvestment and Recovery Act, in 2009, NINDS funded the prospective, multicenter Transforming Research and Clinical Knowledge Pilot (TRACK-TBI Pilot) study to validate the feasibility of implementing the CDEs and to assess their utility across the four CDEs domains: (1) demographic, social, clinical, and injury history data; (2) biospecimens and biomarkers for genetic and proteomic analyses; (3) neuroimaging studies using CT and MRI; and (4) multidimensional outcome measures at 3 and 6 months postinjury.[24] Infrastructure for building data repositories across clinical data, plasma and whole blood biospecimens, neuroimaging, and outcome measures was implemented successfully to create a high-quality, accessible information commons for future TBI research.

The TRACK-TBI Pilot was conducted at three Level 1 trauma centers (San Francisco General Hospital, University of Pittsburgh Medical Center, and University of Medical Center Brackenridge in Austin, Texas) and one rehabilitation center (Mount Sinai Rehabilitation Center in New York City) and enrolled patients from April 2010 to June 2011. Patients aged 0–100 presenting to the emergency department (ED) with external force trauma to the head sufficient to triage to a clinical brain CT scan within 24 hours of injury were eligible for enrollment. Exclusion criteria were pregnancy, incarceration, involuntary psychiatric hold, concurrent life-threatening disease, and non-English speaking status due to certain outcome measures being normed only in English. No exclusion criteria were set for TBI severity. Data were transferred into electronic case report forms (eCRFs) on the secure, Health Insurance Portability and Accountability Act (HIPAA)-compliant online clinical database with built-in relational inconsistency checks. Upon completion of data collection and checks for NIH CDE compliance, TRACK-TBI Pilot data were submitted to the Federal Interagency Traumatic Brain Injury Research (FITBIR) repository.

The TRACK-TBI Pilot aimed to replicate the goals of the TBI CDEs: to create a comprehensive, relevant framework with sufficient breadth and depth of data capture in which refinements to TBI severity classification and stratification can be performed. "Emerging-level" demographic and clinical history data were collected to encompass subject characteristics, subject and family history, disease-/injury-related events, and injury assessments and examinations as previously stated. Each patient admitted to the hospital had an additional standard set of variables collected per day for medications, laboratory tests, vital signs, surgeries, and injury severity classifications. Biospecimens were collected within 24 hours of injury via venipuncture and prepared separately in 250 μL plasma aliquots for proteomic analysis and whole-blood samples for DNA analysis, and frozen at −80°C within 1 hour of collection.[18]

All patients received standard clinical brain CT scans, and, in addition, a 3 Tesla outpatient brain MRI at 2 weeks postinjury was obtained in patients able to return for a scan. TRACK-TBI neuroradiologists implemented equivalent imaging protocols at all sites and reviewed each imaging sequence with knowledge of only patient gender and age. Imaging findings were coded according to the "core" consensus CDEs developed by the neuroimaging working group. The de-identified images were securely shared via a radiology picture archiving system (rPACS) in Digital Imaging and Communications in Medicine (DICOM) format for consensus remote visualization by multiple authorized users.

All CDE "core" and two "supplemental" outcome measures were collected at 6 months postinjury, including a measure of posttraumatic stress disorder (PTSD) due to its high incidence and coexistence with TBI and especially mild TBI. While not part of standard follow-up, a 3-month postinjury outcomes assessment was added to include the GOSE, 22 symptoms from the Acute Concussion Evaluation, and standard information on postdischarge outpatient care and return to work status, which were repeated as part of the 6-month outcomes battery.

TRACK-TBI Pilot: Findings and Lessons Learned

The TRACK-TBI Pilot reported successful implementation of the TBI CDEs version 1 via 599 enrolled patients with acute TBI presenting to Level 1 trauma centers and 51 patients with chronic TBI presenting to TBI rehabilitation centers. In the setting of intact data warehouses and infrastructure prior to enrollment, biospecimens were obtained from 75% of patients, 2-week MRI in 40%, and 3- and 6-month outcomes in 77% and 69% respectively. The estimated time for full study completion per patient was approximately 20 hours. Across the spectrum of TBI, per GCS definition, 83% of participants had "mild" TBI, 4% had "moderate," and 13% had "severe," which are consistent with prior reports. Capturing the TBI CDEs enabled the refinement of TBI severity classifications, which were reported to the NINDS at regular intervals between 2010 and 2014. Reports to date from TRACK-TBI Pilot are displayed in Table 8.1.

The term "mild" TBI continues to be a misnomer and underscores the critical need to develop classification strategies for targeted therapy, especially when a large subpopulation of patients report persistent functional impairment up to 12 months postinjury, with certain subdomains of symptoms (e.g., sleep, emotional) no different at 12 months versus 3 months.[25] From the TRACK-TBI Pilot data to date, the strongest predictors of outcome include older age, pre-injury psychiatric disorders, lower education, injury via assault, extracranial injuries, lower GCS, and prior TBI.[26–28] Yuh et al. demonstrated that 27% of TRACK-TBI Pilot patients with GCS of 13–15 and a normal initial brain CT had abnormalities on 2-week brain MRI that were strongly associated with poorer 3-month outcome, thus emphasizing the addition of early CT and MRI as part of a prognostic model.[29] In the same analysis, the specific lesion type of subarachnoid hemorrhage on CT was found to be predictive of lower 3-month GOSE, but was outperformed by MRI evidence of cerebral contusions and/or foci of axonal shear injury. In a separate analysis, MR DTI surpassed all other predictors for both 3- and 6-month outcome prediction, in particular for mild TBI patients without prior neuropsychiatric and substance abuse history.[30] As for patients without detectable CT/MRI abnormalities, Palacios et al. recently reported that spatial maps of the resting state networks (RSNs) may be sensitive biomarkers for neurocognitive outcome.[31]

Regarding biomarkers, day-of-injury values for circulating plasma GFAP (marker of glial injury) and UCH-L1 (marker of neuronal injury) were analyzed; when combined, superior sensitivity and specificity for diagnosing TBI was obtained.[32] GFAP demonstrated an area under the receiver-operating characteristic curves (AUCs) of 0.88 for differentiating between positive and negative brain CTs, and 0.91 for differentiating TBI from healthy controls; for UCH-L1, AUCs were 0.87 and 0.71, respectively.[33,34] Allelic association analyses are currently under way as well, including the role of single-nucleotide polymorphisms (SNPs) on post-injury recovery. SNPs of cellular responses to stress and DNA damage (poly [ADP-ribose] polymerase 1; PARP1) and in striatal dopamine processing (ankyrin repeat and kinase domain containing 1[ANKK1], catechol-o-methyltransferase [COMT], dopamine receptor type D2 [DRD2]) were found to be associated with 6-month neurocognitive outcomes.[35–39] The upregulation of the autoimmune response to specific brain antigens (e.g., circulating autoantibodies to GFAP) may be detectable as a marker of repeated brain injury.[40] Furthermore, day-of-injury serum brain-derived neurotrophic factor (BDNF), a marker of neuronal outgrowth, may be associated with improved 6-month outcomes post-injury.[41]

The multidimensional CDE "core" outcomes battery has proved to be specific, necessary, and invaluable in characterizing differential profiles of recovery following the spectrum of TBI, elucidating risk factors for certain subdomains, and enabling predictive models for subpopulations. Due to the more pressing nature of validating a diagnostic biomarker for TBI, biomarker studies to date have focused peripherally on predicting outcome using primarily the GOSE. However, in the realm of more specialized genetic

Table 8.1:
TRACK-TBI pilot results to date

Title	Author, Journal, and Year	Domain 1 = Clinical/Demographic 2 = Biomarker 3 = Neuroimaging 4 = Outcomes	Results, Conclusions, and Lessons Learned
Resting-State Functional Connectivity Alterations Associated with Six-Month Outcomes in Mild Traumatic Brain Injury	Palacios et al., *J Neurotrauma*, 2017	3, 4	Alterations were found in spatial maps of resting-state networks (RSNs) between 75 mTBI patients versus healthy controls and were predictive of mTBI outcomes at 6 months postinjury. These resting-state functional MRI results demonstrate that even mTBI patients without brain lesions on conventional CT/MRI scans can have alterations of functional connectivity at the semi-acute stage that help explain their outcomes. RsfMRI may be a sensitive biomarker for early diagnosis and prediction of cognitive and behavioral performance.
Development of a Prediction Model for Post-Concussive Symptoms following Mild Traumatic Brain Injury: A TRACK-TBI Pilot Study	Cnossen et al., *J Neurotrauma*, 2017	1, 4	In 277 mTBI patients, education, pre-injury psychiatric disorders, and prior TBI were the strongest predictors of 6-month postconcussive symptoms (PCS). The total set of predictors explained 21% of the variance, which decreased to 14% after bootstrap validation. These variables explain less than one-fifth of the total variance in outcome. Model refinement with larger datasets, more granular variables, and objective biomarkers are needed before implementation in clinical practice.
Uncovering Precision Phenotype-Biomarker Associations in Traumatic Brain Injury Using Topological Data Analysis	Nielson et al., *PLoS One*, 2017	1, 2, 3, 4	Topological data analysis (TDA) algorithms organized and mapped the data of 586 TBI patients to identify a subset of mTBI patients with a specific multivariate phenotype associated with unfavorable outcome at 3 and 6 months post-injury. This patient subset had high rates of posttraumatic stress disorder (PTSD) and enrichment in several distinct genetic polymorphisms associated with cellular responses to stress and DNA damage (PARP1) and in striatal dopamine processing (ANKK1, COMT, DRD2).

COMT Val158Met Polymorphism is Associated with Post-Traumatic Stress Disorder and Functional Outcome Following Mild Traumatic Brain Injury	Winkler et al., *J Clin Neurosci*, 2017	2, 4	In 83 mTBI patients, COMT Val158Met is associated with lower incidence of PTSD after controlling for race and psychiatric disorders/substance abuse. PTSD is a strong predictor of poorer outcome on GOSE (OR 0.09 [0.03–0.26]), which persists after controlling for age, GCS, and race. When accounting for PTSD in multivariable analysis, the association of COMT genotype and GOSE did not remain significant. Whether COMT genotype indirectly influences global functional outcome through PTSD remains to be determined, and larger studies in more diverse populations are needed to confirm these findings.
Screening for Post-Traumatic Stress Disorder in a Civilian Emergency Department Population with Traumatic Brain Injury	Haarbauer-Krupa et al., *J Neurotrauma*, 2017	1, 4	In 280 mTBI patients, incidence of screening positive for PTSD was conducted using the PTSD Checklist-Civilian Version (PCL-C) at 6 months postinjury; 26.8% screened positive for PTSD. Screening positive was significantly associated with concurrent functional disability, postconcussive and psychiatric symptomatology, decreased satisfaction with life, and decreased visual processing and mental flexibility. Assault mechanism (OR 3.59 [1.69–7.63]) and psychiatric history (OR 2.56 [1.42–4.61]) remained significant predictors of screening positive for PTSD, while education (per-year OR 0.88 [0.79–0.98]) was associated with decreased odds of PTSD. Standardized data collection and review of pre-injury education, psychiatric history, and injury mechanism during initial hospital presentation can aid in identifying patients with mTBI at risk for developing PTSD symptoms who may benefit from closer follow-up.
DRD2 C957T Polymorphism is Associated with Improved 6-Month Verbal Learning Following Traumatic Brain Injury	Yue et al., *Neurogenetics*, 2017	2, 4	In 128 Caucasian subjects, DRD2 C957T polymorphism (rs6277) and 6-month CVLT-II, WAIS-PSI, and TMT were assessed. The rs6277 T-allele associates with better verbal learning and recall on CVLT-II Trials 1–5 (T-allele carrier 52.8 ± 1.3 points, C/C 47.9 ± 1.7 points; mean increase 4.9 points [0.9 to 8.8]), Short-Delay Free Recall (T-carrier 10.9 ± 0.4, C/C 9.7 ± 0.5; mean increase 1.2 [0.1 to 2.5]), and Long-Delay Free Recall (T-carrier 11.5 ± 0.4, C/C 10.2 ± 0.5; mean increase 1.3 [0.1 to 2.5]) after adjusting for age, education years, GCS, acute intracranial pathology on acute brain CT, and ANKK1 SNP rs1800497. No association was found between DRD2 and nonverbal processing speed (WAIS-PSI) or mental flexibility (TMT) at 6 months. DRD2 C947T (rs6277) may be associated with better performance on select cognitive domains independent of ANKK1 following TBI.

(continued)

Table 8.1: Continued

Title	Author, Journal, and Year	Domain 1 = Clinical/Demographic 2 = Biomarker 3 = Neuroimaging 4 = Outcomes	Results, Conclusions, and Lessons Learned
Plasma Anti-Glial Fibrillary Acidic Protein Autoantibody Levels during the Acute and Chronic Phases of Traumatic Brain Injury: A Transforming Research and Clinical Knowledge in Traumatic Brain Injury Pilot Study	Wang et al., *J Neurotrauma*, 2016	2, 4	In 196 TBI patients, history of prior TBI with LOC had higher day 1 glial fibrillary acidic protein autoantibody (AutoAb[GFAP]) levels (9.11 ± 1.42) versus healthy controls (2.90 ± 0.92; $p = 0.032$) and patients reporting no prior TBI (2.97 ± 0.37; $p < 0.001$), but not patients reporting prior TBI without LOC (8.01 ± 1.80; $p = 0.906$). AutoAb[GFAP] levels for chronic TBI (average post-TBI time 176 days or 6.21 months) were significantly higher (15.08 ± 2.82) than in healthy controls ($p < 0.001$). These data suggest a persistent upregulation of the autoimmune response to specific brain antigen in the subacute to chronic phase after TBI and after repeated TBI insults. Hence, AutoAb[GFAP] may be a sensitive assay to study the dynamic interactions between post-injury brain and patient-specific autoimmune responses across acute and chronic settings after TBI.
Collaborative Targeted Maximum Likelihood Estimation for Variable Importance Measure: Illustration for Functional Outcome Prediction in Mild Traumatic Brain Injuries	Pirracchio et al., *Stat Methods Med Res*, 2016	1, 2, 3, 4	In 365 mTBI patients, clinically important predictors among a set of risk factors were identified using a variable importance analysis based on targeted maximum likelihood estimators (TMLE) and collaborative TMLE (cTMLE). cTMLE estimator demonstrated substantially less positivity bias compared to TMLE. Automated cTMLE can target model selection in TBI clinical studies via machine learning to estimate VIMs in complicated, high-dimensional data.
Circulating Brain–Derived Neurotrophic Factor Has Diagnostic and Prognostic Value in Traumatic Brain Injury	Korley et al., *J Neurotrauma*, 2016	2, 4	The associations among BDNF, GFAP, UCH-L1 and recovery from TBI at 6 months were investigated in 159 patients. Median BDNF concentrations (ng/mL) were higher in mild (8.3) than in moderate (4.3) or severe TBI (4.0; $p = 0.004$). The 75 (71.4%) subjects with very low BDNF values (<the 1st percentile; <14.2 ng/mL) had higher odds of incomplete recovery than those who did not have very low values (OR 4.0 [1.5–11.0]). The AUC for discriminating complete and incomplete recovery was 0.65 [0.52–0.78] for BDNF, 0.61 [0.49–0.73] for GFAP, and 0.55 [0.43–0.66] for UCH-L1. The addition of GFAP/UCH-L1 to BDNF did not improve outcome prediction significantly. Day-of-injury serum BDNF is associated with TBI diagnosis, provides 6-month prognostic information for recovery and may aid in TBI risk stratification.

COMT Val158Met Polymorphism is Associated with Nonverbal Cognition Following Mild Traumatic Brain Injury	Winkler et al., *Neurogenetics*, 2016	2, 4	In 100 uncomplicated mTBI patients, the COMT Met158 allele associated with higher nonverbal processing speed on the WAIS-PSI (101.6±SE 2.1) when compared to Val158/Val158 (93.8±SE 3.0) after controlling for demographics and injury severity (mean increase 7.9 points, [1.4 to 14.3], *p* = 0.017). The COMT Val158Met polymorphism did not associate with mental flexibility on the TMT or with verbal learning on the CVLT-II.
Association of a Common Genetic Variant within ANKK1 with Six-month Cognitive Performance after Traumatic Brain Injury	Yue et al., *Neurogenetics*, 2015	2, 4	In a combined 492 TBI patients from two prospective multicenter studies, Citicoline Brain Injury Treatment (COBRIT) and TRACK-TBI Pilot, a dose-dependent effect for the T allele was found for 6-month verbal learning, with T/T homozygotes scoring lowest on the CVLT-II (T/T 45.1, C/T 51.1, C/C 52.1, ANOVA, *p*=0.008). Post hoc testing with multiple comparison–correction indicated that T/T patients performed significantly worse than C/T and C/C patients. Similar effects were observed in a test of nonverbal processing (WAIS-PSI). These results extend those of previous studies reporting a negative relationship of the ANKK1 T allele with cognitive performance after TBI. The authors demonstrate the value of pooling shared clinical, biomarker, and outcome variables from two large datasets applying the NIH TBI CDEs.
Measurement of the Glial Fibrillary Acidic Protein and its Breakdown Products GFAP-BDP Biomarker for the Detection of Traumatic Brain Injury Compared to Computed Tomography and Magnetic Resonance Imaging	McMahon et al., *J Neurotrauma*, 2015	2, 3, 4	In 215 subjects, GFAP-BDP demonstrated very good predictive ability (AUC = 0.87) and discrimination of injury severity (OR 1.45 [1.29–1.64]). Use of GFAP-BDP yielded a net benefit above clinical screening alone and a net reduction in unnecessary scans by 12–30%. Used in conjunction with other clinical information, rapid measurement of GFAP-BDP is useful in establishing or excluding the diagnosis of radiographically apparent intracranial injury. As an adjunct to current screening practices, GFAP-BDP may help avoid unnecessary CT scans without sacrificing sensitivity.
Outcome Prediction After Mild and Complicated Mild Traumatic Brain Injury: External Validation of Existing Models and Identification of New Predictors Using the TRACK-TBI Pilot Study	Lingsma et al., *J Neurotrauma*, 2015	1, 4	Multivariable analyses of 386 mTBI subjects showed that strongest predictors of decreased 3- and 6-month GOSE were older age, pre-existing psychiatric conditions, and lower education. Assault injury, extracranial injuries, and lower GCS were also predictive of lower GOSE. Existing models for mTBI performed unsatisfactorily. For mTBI, different predictors are relevant as for moderate and severe TBI. These include age, preexisting psychiatric conditions, and lower education. Development of a valid prediction model for mTBI patients requires further research efforts.

(continued)

Table 8.1: Continued

Title	Author, Journal, and Year	Domain 1 = Clinical/Demographic 2 = Biomarker 3 = Neuroimaging 4 = Outcomes	Results, Conclusions, and Lessons Learned
Genetic Data Sharing and Privacy	Sorani et al., *Neuroinformatics*, 2015	2	TRACK–TBI research group experiences illustrate that data privacy and sharing can be accomplished simultaneously, and highlight an approach in the context of an ambitious basic and clinical research collaboration.
Diffusion Tensor Imaging for Outcome Prediction in Mild Traumatic Brain Injury: A TRACK–TBI Study	Yuh et al., *J Neurotrauma*, 2014	3, 4	Significant predictors in 76 mTBI patients for 6-month GOSE included ≥1 region-of-interest with severely reduced fractional anisotropy (OR 2.7; p = 0.048), neuropsychiatric history (OR 3.7; p = 0.01), and years of education (OR 0.82/year; p = 0.03). For 37 patients without neuropsychiatric and substance abuse history, MRI surpassed all other predictors for both 3- and 6-month outcome prediction. This is the first study to compare diffusion tensor imaging (DTI) in individual mTBI patients to conventional imaging and demographic/clinical characteristics for outcome prediction. DTI demonstrated utility in a group of TBI patients with heterogeneous backgrounds and in a subset of patients without neuropsychiatric or substance abuse history.
ED Disposition of the Glasgow Coma Scale 13 to 15 Traumatic Brain Injury Patient: Analysis of the Transforming Research and Clinical Knowledge in TBI Study	Ratcliff et al., *Am J Emerg Med*, 2014	1, 4	In 304 mTBI patients, admission to the ICU compared with floor admission varied by: study site; antiplatelet/anticoagulation therapy (OR 7.46 [1.79–31.13]); skull fracture (OR 7.60 [2.44–23.73]); and lower GCS (OR 2.36 [1.05–5.30]). No difference in outcome was observed among the three levels of care (ED discharge, floor admission, ICU admission). Clinical characteristics and local practice patterns contribute to mTBI disposition decisions. Level of care was not associated with outcomes. Intracranial hemorrhage, GCS 13 to 14, skull fracture, and current antiplatelet/anticoagulant therapy influenced disposition decisions.
Symptomatology and Functional Outcome in Mild Traumatic Brain Injury: Results from the Prospective TRACK–TBI Study	McMahon et al., *J Neurotrauma*, 2014	1, 4	At 6 and 12 months after mTBI, 82% (n = 250; n = 163) of patients reported at least one postconcussional symptom (PCS); 44.5% and 40.3% of patients had significantly reduced SWLS scores. At 3 months post-injury, 33% were functionally impaired (GOSE ≤6); 22.4% remained below full functional recovery at 12 months. The term "mild" continues to be a misnomer for this patient population and underscores the need for evolving classification strategies for TBI for targeted therapy.

Acute Biomarkers of Traumatic Brain Injury: Relationship Between Plasma Levels of Ubiquitin C–Terminal Hydrolase–L1 and Glial Fibrillary Acidic Protein	Diaz–Arrastia et al., *J Neurotrauma*, 2014	2, 4	UCH–L1 and GFAP are among of the most widely studied biomarkers for TBI. When biomarkers were combined, superior sensitivity and specificity for diagnosing TBI was obtained (AUC 0.94) in 206 patients. Both biomarkers discriminated between TBI patients with intracranial lesions on CT scan. GFAP was significantly more sensitive and specific (AUC 0.88 vs. 0.71 for UCH–L1). For association with 3–month outcome (GOSE), neither biomarker had adequate sensitivity and specificity (GFAP AUC 0.65–0.74, UCH–L1 AUC 0.59–0.80). The study supports a role for multiple biomarker measurements in TBI research.
The Impact of Previous Traumatic Brain Injury on Health and Functioning: A TRACK–TBI Study	Dams–O'Connor et al., *J Neurotrauma*, 2013	1, 4	In 586 subjects, those with a prior TBI had less-severe acute injuries but experienced worse outcomes at 6 months. Multivariable regressions controlling for demographics and acute injury severity indicated that individuals with prior TBI reported more mood symptoms, more postconcussive symptoms, lower life satisfaction, and had slower processing speed and poorer verbal learning compared to those with no prior TBI. These findings suggest that history of TBI with LOC may have important implications for health and psychological functioning after TBI in community-based samples.
Transforming Research and Clinical Knowledge in Traumatic Brain Injury Pilot: Multicenter Implementation of the Common Data Elements for Traumatic Brain Injury	Yue et al., *J Neurotrauma*, 2013	1, 2, 3, 4	Demonstrated the feasibility of implementing the NINDS TBI CDEs through successful recruitment and multidimensional data collection of 650 patients. Curated the TRACK–TBI Pilot dataset to enable collaborative opportunities to more precisely characterize TBI and improve the design of future therapeutic trials in TBI.

(*continued*)

Table 8.1: Continued

Title	Author, Journal, and Year	Domain 1 = Clinical/Demographic 2 = Biomarker 3 = Neuroimaging 4 = Outcomes	Results, Conclusions, and Lessons Learned
GFAP-BDP as an Acute Diagnostic Marker in Traumatic Brain Injury: Results from the Prospective Transforming Research and Clinical Knowledge in Traumatic Brain Injury Study	Okonkwo et al., *J Neurotrauma*, 2013	2, 4	GFAP-BDP ability to discriminate patients with traumatic lesions on CT shown by AUC 0.88 [0.84–0.93] in 215 TBI patients. The optimal cutoff of 0.68 ng/mL for plasma GFAP-BDP level was associated with a 21.61 OR for traumatic findings on head CT. Six-month outcome (GOSE) AUC 0.65 [0.55–0.74] with OR 2.07 for unfavorable outcome (GOSE 1–4). Larger prospective validation trial needed for GFAP-BDP as routine diagnostic biomarker.
Magnetic Resonance Imaging Improves 3-Month Outcome Prediction in Mild Traumatic Brain Injury	Yuh et al., *Ann Neurol*, 2013	1, 3, 4	In 135 mTBI patients, 27% of those with normal admission brain CT had abnormal early brain MRI. CT evidence of subarachnoid hemorrhage was associated with a multivariate OR of 3.5 ($p = 0.01$) for poorer 3–month outcome on GOSE, after adjusting for demographic/clinical factors. One or more brain contusions on MRI and ≥4 foci of hemorrhagic axonal injury on MRI independently associated with poorer 3–month outcome, with OR 4.5 ($p = 0.01$) and 3.2 ($p = 0.03$), respectively. The addition of early CT and MRI to a prognostic model based on known demographic, clinical, and socioeconomic predictors resulted in a greater than twofold increase in the explained variance in 3–month GOSE.

studies, individual outcome measures have been targeted with encouraging results. For example, ANKK1 and DRD2 SNPs were associated with subscales of verbal learning/memory,[35,39] while COMT Val158Met was associated with nonverbal memory measures and PTSD.[36,38] Prediction models have been constructed for GOSE using supervised and unsupervised approaches,[27,42] and preliminary models for 6-month postconcussive symptoms (PCS) and PTSD await validation in larger cohorts.[26,43] Importantly, due to the inclusive design of the CDE "core" outcome battery, performance on specialized outcome measures can be compared against the GOSE, which has enabled analysis of GOSE score substrata and/or questions that may relate to poorer performance on individual measures.

Evolution of the TBI CDEs, Current Status, and Future Directions

The successful implementation of the TBI CDEs in the TRACK-TBI Pilot and feedback to NINDS CDE working groups spurred the development of the NINDS TBI CDEs, version 2. In practice, version 1 was deemed appropriate for acute hospitalized patients; version 2 aimed to update with recommendations relevant to all ages, levels of injury severity, and phases of recovery, as well as multiple types of research studies (epidemiological, acute hospitalized, rehabilitation).[44] In comparison to the original CDE strata of "core," "supplemental," and "emerging," version 2 working groups deemed a small set of refined "core" CDEs to be "fully relevant" for all study types, a much broader set of "highly relevant" variables applicable across study types termed the "basic" CDEs, and an expanded set of "supplemental" CDEs recommended for use depending on study goals and culminating in a descriptive data dictionary of 900 total CDEs. As described previously, determining analytic results from the TRACK-TBI Pilot regarding development and refinement of severity stratification continues to make progress. In 2013, the NINDS working groups formally recognized that different sets of CDEs, including relevant demographic/clinical variables and outcome measures, may be applicable to mild TBI (GCS 13–15) versus moderate/severe TBI (GCS 3–12) and acute TBI versus TBI rehabilitation.[44] This follows the evolving views on TBI over the past decade—the vastly heterogeneous subgroup of "mild TBI" is no longer sufficient due to varying intracranial pathologies, contusions, and shearing injuries that appear on MRI but not CT, and the range of persistent deficits that exist even in patients negative for intracranial pathology on imaging. Accordingly, outcome measures should no longer be confined to the unidimensional nature of the GOSE, but instead incorporate a time-efficient battery inclusive of the necessary subdomains to fully characterize TBI heterogeneity.

The TRACK-TBI Pilot distinguished the need for a flexible outcomes battery to be sensitive to the deficits suffered across broad classifications of TBI patients. Certain outcome assessments focusing on the subtle sequelae of TBI were more appropriate for patients suffering milder injuries, while other "core" outcome measures remain better suited for those with severe functional disabilities (GOSE 2–4). This finding aligns with the current version 2 of the CDEs, which has designated mild TBI and moderate/severe TBI as subgroups requiring distinct sets of CDEs.[44] The TRACK-TBI Pilot also demonstrated the importance of utilizing the full battery at all study time points for improved prognostic value and for monitoring comparative trajectories of recovery—including the ability to delineate risk factors for those who improve versus those who decline over time. Furthermore, TRACK-TBI identified gaps in documenting the recovery process, particularly in mental health and health economics, that version 1 of the "core" CDE outcome measures did not capture in patients at the upper end of recovery (e.g., GOSE 7–8), constituting ongoing discussion in the field.[45]

To address the limitations and lessons learned from the TRACK-TBI Pilot, the ongoing, 12-center prospective Transforming Research and Clinical Knowledge in Traumatic Brain Injury (TRACK-TBI; tracktbi.ucsf.edu; currently enrolling; 2014–2018 [projected]) was funded by NINDS and other agencies as a cooperative agreement (U01), with expanded granularity of CDEs to include the "supplemental" tier of the TBI CDEs version 2 for demographic/clinical assessment; biospecimen draws for whole blood, serum, and RNA at day 1, 3, and 5 and at 2 weeks, and 6 months; 3 Tesla MRI at 2 weeks and 6 months; and outcome assessments at 2 weeks and at 3, 6, and 12 months. In an effort to delineate outcome severity, the current outcome assessments have formally been stratified into two tiers (*battery* and *comprehensive battery*) using the Galveston Orientation and Amnesia Test (GOAT), a measure of attention and orientation. The abbreviated battery was tailored to patients with more severe injuries lacking orientation (GOAT <75) to include assessments of consciousness/basic cognition (Coma Recovery Scale [CRS], Cognitive Assessment Protocol [CAP]) rather than more advanced cognitive tests, PCS, and psychological health and quality-of-life surveys for those who are oriented at follow-up time points (Figure 8.1). Patients who improve can be moved from the abbreviated battery to the comprehensive battery at outcome assessment time points if they improve sufficiently in neurologic orientation. Through the flexibility of this battery and multiple assessment time points, deep data analytics can be utilized to effectively assess trajectories of recovery over the first year.

One major success of the TRACK-TBI Pilot was the creation of a comprehensive data repository—biospecimen and neuroimaging banking—as one of the first studies submitted to FITBIR to enable legacy analyses. Pursuant of the aims of the TBI CDEs, the TRACK-TBI Pilot, along with recent large drug trials utilizing CDEs version 1 (Citicoline Brain Injury Treatment Trial [COBRIT],[46] Progesterone for the Treatment of Traumatic Brain Injury III [ProTECT][47]), concurrent acute TBI trials utilizing CDEs version 2 (TRACK-TBI U01; Collaborative European NeuroTrauma Effectiveness Research in Traumatic Brain Injury [CENTER-TBI; www.center-tbi.eu][48]), and trials in chronic (Chronic Effects of Neurotrauma Consortium [CENC])[49] and sports TBI (Concussion Assessment, Research and Education Consortium [CARE])[50] will be harmonized and continually curated as part of the collaborative, multidisciplinary US Department of Defense (DoD)-funded Traumatic Brain Injury Endpoints (TED) Initiative.[51] The goals of the TED Initiative, comprising clinician scientists working collaboratively with industry leaders, patient advocacy organizations, and regulatory authorities from the US Food and Drug Administration (FDA), are to create a comprehensive meta-dataset and to validate a range of refined clinical outcome assessments and sensitive biomarkers that the FDA could consider for use in stratification of patients in TBI clinical trials.

Conclusion

Advances in TBI research have been limited over the past four decades, in part due to imprecise classification approaches lacking pathoanatomic and molecular features and

Domain	Outcome Measure	Estimated Completion Time	Comprehensive Assessment (CA) Cohort	Brief Assessment (BA) Cohort
Screening Protocol (5-9 minutes)				
Screening	• Assessment of speech intelligibility • Galveston Orientation and Amnesia Test (Standard, Written, and Modified GOAT) • Post-traumatic amnesia (PTA) assessment	2m 5m 2m	2W, then as needed	N/A
Abbreviated Battery (60-85 minutes- includes screening)				

Participant/ Surrogate Interviews	• Sections:
	  • Demographic Variables
	  • Vocational History
	  • Pre-morbid medical history
	  • Prior TBI screen
	  • Alcohol Use Disorders Identification Test (AUDIT-C)
	  • 3-Item Drug Use Interview
		15 min	2W, 3M (T), 6M, 12M	N/A

Consciousness and Basic Cognition	• Confusion Assessment Protocol (CAP) • Coma Recovery Scale Revised (CRS-R)	15m 15-30m	2W, 6M, 12M	N/A
Global Outcome	• Glasgow Outcome Scale Extended (GOSE) • Expanded Disability Rating Scale Post-Acute Interview (E-DRS-PI)	8m 5-15m	2W, 3M (T), 6M, 12M	GOSE: 2W (T), 3M (T), 6M (T), 12M (T)
Comprehensive Assessment Battery (136-148 minutes- includes screening; excludes BTACT)				
Global Outcome	• Glasgow Outcome Scale Extended (GOSE) • Expanded Disability Rating Scale Post-Acute Interview (E-DRS-PI)	8m 5-15m	2W, 3M (T), 6M, 12M	N/A

Participant/ Surrogate Interviews	• Sections:
	  • Demographic Variables
	  • Vocational History
	  • Pre-morbid medical history
	  • Prior TBI screen
	  • Alcohol Use Disorders Identification Test (AUDIT-C)
	  • 3-Item Drug Use Interview
		15 min	2W, 3M (T), 6M, 12M	N/A

Cognition	• Rey Auditory Verbal Learning Test II (RAVLT) • Trail Making Test (TMT) • Wechsler Adult Intelligence Scale IV Processing Speed Index (WAIS-IV PSI) • NIH Toolbox Cognitive Battery • Brief Test of Adult Cognition by Telephone (BTACT)	15m 5m 4m 30m 20m	2W, 6M, 12M ------------------------ 6M (T)	N/A
Post-Concussive/TBI-Related Symptoms	• Rivermead Post-Concussion Questionnaire (RPQ) • Participant Reported Outcome Measurement Information System Pain Intensity and Interference Instruments (PROMIS-PAIN) • Insomnia Severity Index	6m 5m 3m	2W, 3M (T), 6M, 12M	N/A
Participation and Quality of Life (QoL)	• Quality of Life After Brain Injury- Overall Scale (Qolibri-OS) • Mayo-Portland Adaptability Inventory- (MPAI4-PART) • Satisfaction With Life Scale (SWLS) • SF-12 Version 2	5m 2m 3m 3m	2W, 3M (T), 6M, 12M	N/A
Psychological Health	• PTSD Checklist (PCL-5) • Brief Symptom Inventory 18 (BSI18) • Participant Health Questionnaire- 9 (PHQ-9) • Columbia Suicide Severity Rating Scale (C-SSRS)* (*Only required if ≥1 on the PHQ-9 or the BSI-18)	6m 6m 5m 5m	2W, 3M (T), 6M, 12M	N/A

Figure 8.1 Flexible outcomes assessment framework for ongoing, prospective 12–center Transforming Research and Clinical Knowledge in Traumatic Brain Injury (TRACK-TBI U01) study.

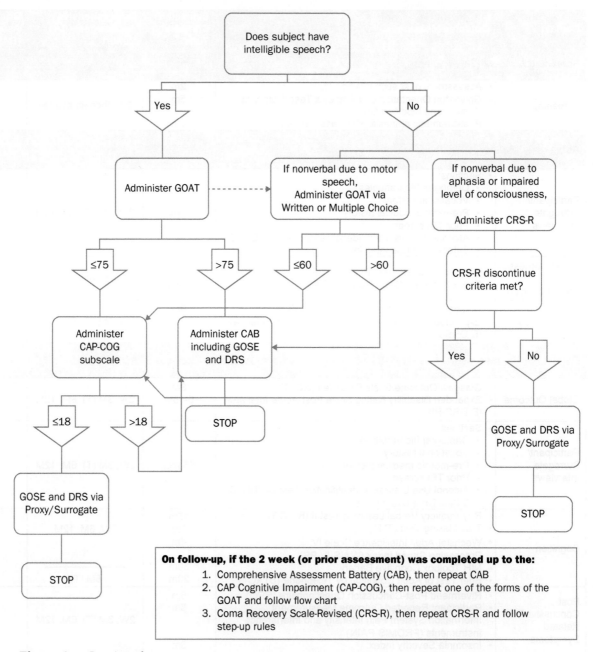

Figure 8.1 Continued

insensitive outcome measures to subdomains of recovery from a vastly heterogeneous disease. The NINDS TBI CDE project aimed to standardize data collection, discover new diagnostic tools (e.g., proteomic, genetic, and imaging biomarkers), and develop a multidimensional outcomes endpoint sensitive to differential profiles of recovery. The prospective, multicenter TRACK–TBI Pilot study (2010–2012) demonstrated the feasibility of implementing the TBI CDEs version 1 and the utility of uniform data standards to enable creation of high-quality data repositories comprising deeply granular data from a comprehensive range of critical TBI clinical data domains. Feedback and lessons learned from the TRACK–TBI Pilot have assisted in the formation of the NIH TBI

CDEs version 2, currently employed across numerous large-scale TBI clinical studies. Harmonized, curated data from these studies will be deposited into a TED Initiative meta-dataset to enable the discovery and validation of refined severity markers and outcome endpoints.

References

1. Lingsma HF, Roozenbeek B, Steyerberg EW, Murray GD, Maas AIR. Early prognosis in traumatic brain injury: from prophecies to predictions. *Lancet Neurol.* 2010;9(5):543–554.

2. Teasdale G, Jennett B. Assessment of coma and impaired consciousness. A practical scale. *Lancet.* 1974;2(7872):81–84.

3. Grote S, Böcker W, Mutschler W, Bouillon B, Lefering R. Diagnostic value of the Glasgow Coma Scale for traumatic brain injury in 18,002 patients with severe multiple injuries. *J Neurotrauma.* 2011;28(4):527–534.

4. McNett M. A review of the predictive ability of Glasgow Coma Scale scores in head-injured patients. *J Neurosci Nurs.* 2007;39(2):68–75.

5. Cho DY, Wang YC. Comparison of the APACHE III, APACHE II and Glasgow Coma Scale in acute head injury for prediction of mortality and functional outcome. *Intensive Care Med.* 1997;23(1):77–84.

6. Timmons SD, Bee T, Webb S, Diaz-Arrastia RR, Hesdorffer D. Using the abbreviated injury severity and Glasgow Coma Scale scores to predict 2-week mortality after traumatic brain injury. *J Trauma.* 2011;71(5):1172–1178.

7. Majdan M, Steyerberg EW, Nieboer D, Mauritz W, Rusnak M, Lingsma HF. Glasgow coma scale motor score and pupillary reaction to predict six-month mortality in patients with traumatic brain injury: comparison of field and admission assessment. *J Neurotrauma.* 2015;32(2):101–108.

8. Salottolo K, Levy AS, Slone DS, Mains CW, Bar-Or D. The effect of age on Glasgow Coma Scale score in patients with traumatic brain injury. *JAMA Surg.* 2014;149(7):727–734.

9. Caterino JM, Raubenolt A, Cudnik MT. Modification of Glasgow Coma Scale criteria for injured elders. *Acad Emerg Med.* 2011;18(10):1014–1021.

10. Teasdale GM, Pettigrew LE, Wilson JT, Murray G, Jennett B. Analyzing outcome of treatment of severe head injury: a review and update on advancing the use of the Glasgow Outcome Scale. *J Neurotrauma.* 1998;15(8):587–597.

11. McMillan T, Wilson L, Ponsford J, Levin H, Teasdale G, Bond M. The Glasgow Outcome Scale—40 years of application and refinement. *Nat Rev Neurol.* 2016;12(8):477–485.

12. Maas AIR, Roozenbeek B, Manley GT. Clinical trials in traumatic brain injury: past experience and current developments. *Neurotherapeutics.* 2010;7(1):115–126.

13. Maas AIR, Steyerberg EW, Marmarou A, et al. IMPACT recommendations for improving the design and analysis of clinical trials in moderate to severe traumatic brain injury. *Neurotherapeutics.* 2010;7(1):127–134.

14. Marmarou A, Lu J, Butcher I, et al. IMPACT database of traumatic brain injury: design and description. *J Neurotrauma.* 2007;24(2):239–250.

15. Saatman KE, Duhaime A-C, Bullock R, et al. Classification of traumatic brain injury for targeted therapies. *J Neurotrauma.* 2008;25(7):719–738.

16. Whyte J, Vasterling J, Manley GT. Common data elements for research on traumatic brain injury and psychological health: current status and future development. *Arch Phys Med Rehabil.* 2010;91(11):1692–1696.

17. Maas AI, Harrison-Felix CL, Menon D, et al. Common data elements for traumatic brain injury: recommendations from the interagency working group on demographics and clinical assessment. *Arch Phys Med Rehabil.* 2010;91(11):1641–1649.

18. Manley GT, Diaz-Arrastia R, Brophy M, et al. Common data elements for traumatic brain injury: recommendations from the biospecimens and biomarkers working group. *Archives of Physical Medicine and Rehabilitation.* 2010;91(11):1667–1672.

19. Wilde EA, Whiteneck GG, Bogner J, et al. Recommendations for the use of common outcome measures in traumatic brain injury research. *Arch Phys Med Rehabil.* 2010;91(11):1650–1660.e17.

20. Duhaime A-C, Gean AD, Haacke EM, et al. Common data elements in radiologic imaging of traumatic brain injury. *Arch Phys Med Rehabil.* 2010;91(11):1661–1666.

21. Vos PE, Lamers KJB, Hendriks JCM, et al. Glial and neuronal proteins in serum predict outcome after severe traumatic brain injury. *Neurology.* 2004;62(8):1303–1310.

22. Vos PE, Jacobs B, Andriessen TMJC, et al. GFAP and S100B are biomarkers of traumatic brain injury: an observational cohort study. *Neurology.* 2010;75(20):1786–1793.

23. Manley GT, Diaz–Arrastia R, Brophy M, et al. Common data elements for traumatic brain injury: recommendation from the biospecimens and biomarkers working group. *Arch Phys Med Rehabil.* 2010;91:1667–1672.

24. Yue JK, Vassar MJ, Lingsma HF, et al. Transforming research and clinical knowledge in traumatic brain injury pilot: multicenter implementation of the common data elements for traumatic brain injury. *J Neurotrauma.* 2013;30(22):1831–1844.

25. McMahon P, Hricik A, Yue JK, et al. Symptomatology and functional outcome in mild traumatic brain injury: results from the prospective TRACK-TBI study. *J Neurotrauma.* 2014;31(1):26–33.

26. Cnossen MC, Winkler EA, Yue JK, et al. Development of a prediction model for postconcussive symptoms following mild traumatic brain injury: a TRACK-TBI pilot study. *J Neurotrauma.* Mar 2017. doi:10.1089/neu.2016.4819.

27. Lingsma HF, Yue JK, Maas AIR, Steyerberg EW, Manley GT, TRACK-TBI Investigators. Outcome prediction after mild and complicated mild traumatic brain injury: external validation of existing models and identification of new predictors using the TRACK-TBI pilot study. *J Neurotrauma.* 2015;32(2):83–94.

28. Ratcliff JJ, Adeoye O, Lindsell CJ, et al. ED disposition of the Glasgow Coma Scale 13 to 15 traumatic brain injury patient: analysis of the Transforming Research and Clinical Knowledge in TBI study. *Am J Emerg Med.* 2014;32(8):844–850.

29. Yuh EL, Mukherjee P, Lingsma HF, et al. Magnetic resonance imaging improves 3-month outcome prediction in mild traumatic brain injury. *Ann Neurol.* 2013;73(2):224–235.

30. Yuh EL, Cooper SR, Mukherjee P, et al. Diffusion tensor imaging for outcome prediction in mild traumatic brain injury: a TRACK-TBI study. *J Neurotrauma.* 2014;31(17):1457–1477.

31. Palacios EM, Yuh EL, Chang Y-S, et al. Resting-state functional connectivity alterations associated with six-month outcomes in mild traumatic brain injury. *J Neurotrauma.* 2017;34(8):1546–1557.

32. Diaz-Arrastia R, Wang KKW, Papa L, et al. Acute biomarkers of traumatic brain injury: relationship between plasma levels of ubiquitin C-terminal hydrolase-L1 and glial fibrillary acidic protein. *J Neurotrauma.* 2014;31(1):19–25.

33. Okonkwo DO, Yue JK, Puccio AM, et al. GFAP-BDP as an acute diagnostic marker in traumatic brain injury: results from the prospective transforming research and clinical knowledge in traumatic brain injury study. *J Neurotrauma*. 2013;30(17):1490–1497.

34. McMahon PJ, Panczykowski DM, Yue JK, et al. Measurement of the glial fibrillary acidic protein and its breakdown products GFAP-BDP biomarker for the detection of traumatic brain injury compared to computed tomography and magnetic resonance imaging. *J Neurotrauma*. 2015;32(8):527–533.

35. Yue JK, Winkler EA, Rick JW, et al. DRD2 C957T polymorphism is associated with improved 6-month verbal learning following traumatic brain injury. *Neurogenetics*. 2017;18(1):29–38.

36. Winkler EA, Yue JK, Ferguson AR, et al. COMT Val(158)Met polymorphism is associated with post-traumatic stress disorder and functional outcome following mild traumatic brain injury. *J Clin Neurosci*. 2017;35:109–116.

37. Nielson JL, Cooper SR, Yue JK, et al. Uncovering precision phenotype-biomarker associations in traumatic brain injury using topological data analysis. *PLoS One*. 2017;12(3):e0169490.

38. Winkler EA, Yue JK, McAllister TW, et al. COMT Val 158 Met polymorphism is associated with nonverbal cognition following mild traumatic brain injury. *Neurogenetics*. 2016;17(1):31–41.

39. Yue JK, Pronger AM, Ferguson AR, et al. Association of a common genetic variant within ANKK1 with six-month cognitive performance after traumatic brain injury. *Neurogenetics*. 2015;16(3):169–180.

40. Wang KKW, Yang Z, Yue JK, et al. Plasma anti-glial fibrillary acidic protein autoantibody levels during the acute and chronic phases of traumatic brain injury: a Transforming Research and Clinical Knowledge in Traumatic Brain Injury pilot study. *J Neurotrauma*. 2016;33(13):1270–1277.

41. Korley FK, Diaz-Arrastia R, Wu AHB, et al. Circulating brain-derived neurotrophic factor has diagnostic and prognostic value in traumatic brain injury. *J Neurotrauma*. 2016;33(2):215–225.

42. Pirracchio R, Yue JK, Manley GT, van der Laan MJ, Hubbard AE; TRACK-TBI Investigators. Collaborative targeted maximum likelihood estimation for variable importance measure: illustration for functional outcome prediction in mild traumatic brain injuries. *Stat Methods Med Res*. Jun 2016. doi:10.1177/0962280215627335.

43. Haarbauer-Krupa J, Taylor CA, Yue JK, et al. Screening for post-traumatic stress disorder in a civilian emergency department population with traumatic brain injury. *J Neurotrauma*. 2017;34(1):50–58.

44. Hicks R, Giacino J, Harrison-Felix C, Manley G, Valadka A, Wilde EA. Progress in developing common data elements for traumatic brain injury research: version two: the end of the beginning. *J Neurotrauma*. 2013;30(22):1852–1861.

45. Silverberg ND, Crane PK, Dams-O'Connor K, et al. Developing a cognition endpoint for traumatic brain injury clinical trials. *J Neurotrauma*. 2017;34(2):363–371.

46. Zafonte RD, Bagiella E, Ansel BM, et al. Effect of citicoline on functional and cognitive status among patients with traumatic brain injury: Citicoline Brain Injury Treatment Trial (COBRIT). *JAMA*. 2012;308(19):1993–2000.

47. Wright DW, Yeatts SD, Silbergleit R, et al. Very early administration of progesterone for acute traumatic brain injury. *N Engl J Med*. 2014;371(26):2457–2466.

48. Maas AIR, Menon DK, Steyerberg EW, et al. Collaborative European NeuroTrauma Effectiveness Research in Traumatic Brain Injury (CENTER-TBI): a prospective longitudinal observational study. *Neurosurgery*. 2015;76(1):67–80.

49. Walker WC, Carne W, Franke LM, et al. The Chronic Effects of Neurotrauma Consortium (CENC) multi-centre observational study: description of study and characteristics of early participants. *Brain Inj.* 2016;30(12):1469–1480.

50. Broglio SP, McCrea M, McAllister T, et al. A national study on the effects of concussion in collegiate athletes and US military service academy members: the NCAA-DoD Concussion Assessment, Research and Education (CARE) consortium structure and methods. *Sports Med.* March 2017. doi:10.1007/s40279-017-0707-1.

51. Manley GT, MacDonald CL, Markowitz A, et al. The Traumatic Brain Injury Endpoints Development (TED) initiative: progress on a public-private regulatory collaboration to accelerate diagnosis and treatment of traumatic brain injury. *J Neurotrauma*. March 2017. doi:10.1089/neu.2016.4729.

Acute Assessment of Mild Traumatic Brain Injury

Linda Papa

9

Prevalence and Definition of Traumatic Brain Injury

According to Center of Disease Control (CDC) estimates, there were about 2.8 million traumatic brain injury (TBI)-related emergency department (ED) visits, hospitalizations, and deaths in the United States in 2013. That is close to 2% of the total injury- and non–injury-related ED visits, hospitalizations, and deaths.[1] In 2012, an estimated 329,290 children (age 19 or younger) were treated in US EDs for sports and recreation-related injuries that included a diagnosis of concussion or TBI. From 2001 to 2012, the rate of ED visits for sports and recreation-related injuries with a diagnosis of concussion or TBI, alone or in combination with other injuries, more than doubled among children younger than 20 years.[2]

The CDC defines a traumatic brain injury as a disruption in the normal function of the brain that can be caused by a bump, blow, or jolt to the head or by penetrating head injury. Among clinicians and researchers, there is variability in the nomenclature and definition of a mild TBI (mTBI). Many terms have been used to describe the severity of this injury including minor, minimal, grade I, class I, and low-risk.[3] Moreover, the terms "head trauma," "head injury," and "brain injury" are used in similar contexts but are distinct. *Head trauma* is a broad term describing an external trauma to the craniofacial area of the body from either blunt, penetrating, blast, rotational, or acceleration/deceleration forces; *head injury* refers to a clinically evident injury on physical exam; and *brain injury* indicates an injury to the brain itself.[3,4] *Concussion* is within the spectrum of mTBI and is a term commonly used to describe mTBI in sports. Traditionally, TBI has been classified into three very broad categories: mild, moderate, and severe. The severity of TBI is initially based on the Glasgow Coma Scale (GCS) score which uses ocular, verbal, and motor responses to determine central nervous system impairment. "Mild" injuries result in a brief change in mental status or consciousness with a GCS score between 13 and 15. "Severe" injuries lead to an extended period of unconsciousness after the injury and have a GCS score between 3 to 8, and "moderate" injuries typically have a GCS score of 9–12. However, the vast majority of all reported TBI cases are "mild."[5] The GCS score was originally developed during a time when computed tomography (CT) scanning was not available to communicate changes in neurologic status in comatose patients with TBI.[6] Due to its ease of use, CT has been adopted in the routine assessment of all trauma patients, including those with mTBI who are not in coma.[7]

The diagnosis of brain injury can be elusive because it is not always evident on physical exam, particularly mTBI. According to the American Congress of Rehabilitation Medicine, a patient with mTBI is a person with a GCS of 13–15 who has had a traumatically induced physiological disruption of brain function as manifested by at least one of the following: (1) any period of loss of consciousness less than 30 minutes, (2) any loss of memory for events immediately before or after the accident (posttraumatic amnesia should last less than 24 hours), (3) any alteration in mental state at the time of the accident (e.g., feeling, dazed, disoriented, or confused), and (4) focal neurological deficits that may or may not be transient.[8,9] Those who evaluate TBI acutely do not have the luxury of waiting to make the diagnosis days or weeks after injury and must rely on acute indices of "disruption of brain function" such as loss of consciousness, amnesia, feeling dazed, feeling disoriented, being confused, or having neurologic deficits following head trauma. However, the GCS score can reflect impairment from conditions other than brain injury such as intoxication from drugs and alcohol, hypoxemia, distracting injuries, and sedative medications.[10] Furthermore, about 13% of patients who become comatose start with a GCS 15.[11,12] Patients can deteriorate from an expanding intracranial hematoma after what appears clinically to be a mild TBI. Therefore, it is very important to observe upward and downward trends in GCS score by performing serial assessments.[3,13,14]

Initial Management of Mild Traumatic Brain Injury

Initial management of suspected mTBI in the ED starts with the principles of Advanced Trauma Life Support and protecting the cervical spine.[7] In an individual with multisystem trauma, clinicians must keep a high index of suspicion for mTBI since concomitant injuries can serve to distract from a potential brain injury. Clinicians should take a comprehensive history and gather information about the mechanism of injury, consumption of alcohol or drugs, comorbidities, and symptoms of other potential injuries. At this time, the diagnosis of mTBI is largely clinical, and it is essential to obtain a history of symptoms of confusion, loss of consciousness, and amnesia. Patients may also report headache, dizziness, balance problems, nausea and vomiting, and sensitivity to light and noise, as well as impaired cognition, memory, and communication. All patients should undergo a comprehensive physical exam including a detailed neurologic examination and repeated GCS scores. The motor component of the GCS is the strongest predictor of outcome following TBI.[15]

The term "mild" does not reflect the true nature of this type of injury. Individuals with mTBI are acutely at risk for serious intracranial injuries.[16,17–19] Approximately 5–17% of patients with suspected mTBI in the ED have abnormal CT scans.[16–19] These patients have a small but important risk of subsequent deterioration because of intracranial bleeding. Therefore, it is critical to identify these high-risk patients.

Currently, CT of the head is the diagnostic standard for identifying intracranial injury in the ED. It is widely availability, rapid, and compatible with life support devices. However, CT is associated with exposure to ionizing radiation and higher healthcare costs.[20] Therefore, a number of clinical decision rules have been prospectively derived and validated to identify those at risk for neurosurgical intervention and intracranial lesions on CT scan among adult patients with suspected mTBI in the ED.[17–19] Structural magnetic resonance imaging (MRI) may improve sensitivity for detecting abnormalities,[21] but limitations to MRI use include availability and contraindications.

Novel structural and functional neuroimaging techniques are emerging that are identifying undetected brain abnormalities in mTBI. More subtle structural abnormalities in mTBI are best seen with MRI sequences, such as gradient-recalled echo (GRE) and fluid-attenuated inversion recovery (FLAIR).[21] A significant advancement in the imaging of mTBI is susceptibility-weighted imaging (SWI), which uses differences in magnetic susceptibility between tissues and is particularly helpful for the evaluation of axonal injury.[22] Diffusion tensor imaging (DTI) also uses MRI technology to perform tractography (i.e., visualization of major white matter pathways) to assess damaged nerve fiber tracts.[23] DTI has been shown to detect white matter abnormalities and underlying cognitive deficits following mTBI when conventional imaging is normal.[24,25]

Biomarkers for Mild Traumatic Brain Injury

Discovery of biomarkers that are specific for TBI is a quest that has been ongoing for several decades.[26] The pursuit of these elusive markers has been most intense over the past 20 years.[27–31] Commercialization of these biomarkers is ongoing, and a number of companies are seeking FDA approval to market their tests for clinical applications. In 2018, the FDA US Food and Drug Administration approved the use of a blood test combining UCH-L1 and GFAP for detecting lesions on computed tomography CT scan in adults with mTBI within 12 hours of injury. Recent systematic reviews of biomarkers in sports concussion and children showed that there are at least 11 different biomarkers assessed in athletes[30] and 99 biomarkers in children.[29] These include calcium binding protein B S100β, glial fibrillary acidic protein (GFAP), neuron-specific enolase (NSE), tau, neurofilament (NF), ubiquitin c-terminal hydrolase (UCH-L1), brain-derived neurotrophic factor (BDNF), and myelin basic protein (MBP). Some of these markers are discussed next.

S100β

S100β is the best-studied biomarker in mTBI for potentially screening patients for head CT. S100β is found in astrocytes and helps to regulate intracellular levels of calcium. A number of studies have found significant correlations between elevated serum levels of S100β and CT abnormalities in adults[32–34] and weak correlations in children.[35,36] It has been suggested that adding the measurement of S100β concentration to clinical decision tools for mTBI patients could potentially reduce the number of CT scans by 30%.[34] However, other investigators have failed to detect associations between S100β with CT abnormalities in both adults and children.[37–41] Its utility in the setting of multiple trauma remains controversial because it is also elevated in trauma patients without direct head trauma[42–45] and can be found in adipocytes, chondrocytes, and melanocytes.[46,47]

Glial Fibrillary Acidic Protein

A number of recent studies have shown GFAP to be a promising brain-specific biomarker for mTBI in adults and children.[45,48–53] GFAP is a protein found in the astroglial skeleton of white and gray matter[54] and is released into serum following an mTBI within an hour of injury.[45,48,53] Unlike S100β, GFAP is elevated in mTBI patients with axonal injury as evidenced by MRI at 3 months post-injury.[49]

Serum GFAP levels distinguish mTBI patients from trauma patients without TBI and detect intracranial lesions on CT with a sensitivity of 94–100% in children and 97–100% in adults.[45,48,51,53,55] Moreover, GFAP outperforms S100β in detecting CT lesions in the setting of multiple trauma when extracranial fractures are present,[45,51] and it also predicts the need for neurosurgical intervention in patients presenting with a GCS of 15.[48,53] Most recently, the temporal profile of GFAP was evaluated in a large cohort of 584 trauma patients seen at the ED. GFAP performed consistently over 7 days in identifying concussion and mild to moderate TBI, detecting traumatic intracranial lesions on head CT and predicting neurosurgical intervention.[53] This study of the pathophysiological kinetics of GFAP renders it a promising contender for clinical use for mTBI and concussion diagnosis within a week of injury.[53] GFAP is released into serum following a mTBI within an hour of injury and remains elevated for several days after.[45,48,53]

Ubiquitin C-terminal Hydrolase

Another promising candidate biomarker for TBI currently under investigation is UCH-L1. This protein is involved in the addition and removal of ubiquitin from proteins that are destined for metabolism.[56,57] UCH-L1 was previously used as a histological marker for neurons because it is so copious.[58] Clinical studies performed in humans with severe TBI have established that the UCH-L1 protein is significantly elevated in human cerebrospinal fluid (CSF) and is detectable very early after injury.[59–61] Concentrations of UCH-L1 remain significantly elevated for at least 7 days post-injury,[53,60,61] and there is very good correlation between CSF and serum levels.[62] Serum UCH-L1 is also elevated in children with moderate and severe TBI.[63] Most recently, UCH-L1 was detected in the serum of mTBI adults[52,53,64] and children within an hour of injury.[65] Serum levels of UCH-L1 discriminated mTBI patients of all ages from uninjured and non–head injured trauma control patients who had orthopedic injuries or motor vehicle trauma without head injury.[53,64,65] A handful of studies have shown serum UCH-L1 levels to be significantly higher in those with intracranial lesions on CT than those without lesions[50,52,53,64,65] and to be much higher in those eventually requiring a neurosurgical intervention.[53,64] The temporal profile of UCH-L1 was evaluated in a large cohort of ED trauma patients; UCH-L1 rose rapidly and peaked at 8 hours after injury and declined rapidly over 48 hours.[53]

Tau

Total tau (t-tau) has been found to be correlated with severity of injury in severe TBI.[66–69] Recently, a study of professional hockey players showed that serum t-tau outperformed S-100β and NSE in detecting concussion at 1 hour after injury and that levels were significantly higher in postconcussion samples at all times compared with preseason levels.[70] T-tau at 1 hour after concussion also correlated with the number of days it took for concussion symptoms to resolve. Accordingly, t-tau remained significantly elevated at 144 hours in players with postconcussive symptoms (PCS) lasting more than 6 days versus players with PCS for less than 6 days.[70] Phosphorylated-tau (p-tau) is also being examined following head trauma and may have some association with chronic encephalopathy.[71] It appears that enhanced tau protein phosphorylation occurs with more severe injuries.[72,73]

Conclusion

Most patients with mTBI can be discharged from the ED with a normal examination and after a reasonable period of observation and/or following a negative head CT.[74] Any athlete suspected of having a concussion should be immediately removed from play.[75] Studies of ED patients have indicated that as many as 30% of patients with a discharge diagnosis of mTBI will have symptoms at 3 months post-injury, and up to 15% will continue to be symptomatic at 1 year post-injury.[76,77] Appropriate referrals should be made based on symptoms before discharging patients from the ED. Serum markers have the potential to better manage patients with mTBI and reduce the need for head CT scans. Unlike clinical variables, serum marker measurements offer a more objective measure of injury and could complement clinical decision-making in the management of mTBI acutely after injury. Although there are an abundance of papers being published, many lack the rigorous methods and reporting required to adequately evaluate these markers for clinical use. Well-designed studies with adequate sample sizes, appropriate control groups and outcome measures, clear definition, proper timing of sample collection, and well-described performance characteristics of the assays will be needed to introduce biomarkers into clinical practice.[26]

References

1. Taylor CA, Bell JM, Breiding MJ, Xu L. Traumatic brain injury-related emergency department visits, hospitalizations, and deaths—United States, 2007 and 2013. *MMWR Surveill Summ.* 2017;66:1–16.

2. Coronado VG, Haileyesus T, Cheng TA, et al. Trends in sports- and recreation-related traumatic brain injuries treated in US emergency departments: the National Electronic Injury Surveillance System-All Injury Program (NEISS-AIP) 2001–2012. *J Head Trauma Rehabil.* 2015;30:185–197.

3. Jagoda AS, Bazarian JJ, Bruns JJ Jr, et al. Clinical policy: neuroimaging and decision making in adult mild traumatic brain injury in the acute setting. *Ann Emerg Med* 2008;52:714–748.

4. Menon DK, Schwab K, Wright DW, Maas AI. Position statement: definition of traumatic brain injury. *Arch Phys Med Rehabil.* 2010;91:1637–1640.

5. Faul M, Xu L, Wald MM, Coronado VG. Traumatic brain injury in the United States. Emergency department visits, hospitalizations and deaths 2002–2006. https://www.cdc.gov/traumaticbraininjury/pdf/blue_book.pdf. Published March, 2010.

6. Teasdale G, Jennett B. Assessment of coma and impaired consciousness. A practical scale. *Lancet.* 1974;2:81–84.

7. ATLS Subcommittee; American College of Surgeons' Committee on Trauma; Internationa ATLS Working Group. Advanced trauma life support (ATLS®): the ninth edition. *J Trauma Acute Care Surg.* 2013;74:1363–1366.

8. Kay T, Harrington DE, Adams R, et al. Definition of mild traumatic brain injury. *J Head Trauma Rehabil.* 1993;8:86–87.

9. Ruff RM, Iverson GL, Barth JT, Bush SS, Broshek DK. Recommendations for diagnosing a mild traumatic brain injury: a National Academy of Neuropsychology education paper. *Arch Clin Neuropsychol.* 2009;24:3–10.

10. Cook LS, Levitt MA, Simon B, Williams VL. Identification of ethanol-intoxicated patients with minor head trauma requiring computed tomography scans. *Acad Emerg Med.* 1994;1:227–234.

11. Marshall LF, Toole BM, Bowers SA. The National Traumatic Coma Data Bank. Part 2: Patients who talk and deteriorate: implications for treatment. *J Neurosurg.* 1983;59:285–288.

12. Jennett B, Teasdale G, Galbraith S, et al. Severe head injuries in three countries. *J Neurol Neurosurg Psychiatry.* 1977;40:291–298.

13. Almenawer SA, Bogza I, Yarascavitch B, et al. The value of scheduled repeat cranial computed tomography after mild head injury: single-center series and meta-analysis. *Neurosurgery.* 2013;72:56–62

14. Stippler M, Smith C, McLean AR, et al. Utility of routine follow-up head CT scanning after mild traumatic brain injury: a systematic review of the literature. *Emerg Med J.* 2012;29:528–532.

15. Hoffmann M, Lefering R, Rueger JM, et al. Pupil evaluation in addition to Glasgow Coma Scale components in prediction of traumatic brain injury and mortality. *Br J Surg.* 2012 Jan; 99 Suppl 1:122–30.

16. Stein SC, Ross SE. Mild head injury: a plea for routine early CT scanning. *J Trauma.* 1992;33:11–13.

17. Stiell IG, Wells GA, Vandemheen K, et al. The Canadian CT Head Rule for patients with minor head injury. *Lancet.* 2001;357:1391–1396.

18. Haydel MJ, Preston CA, Mills TJ, Luber S, Blaudeau E. DeBlieux PM Indications for computed tomography in patients with minor head injury. *N Engl J Med.* 2000;343:100–105.

19. Mower WR, Hoffman JR, Herbert M, Wolfson AB, Pollack CV Jr, Zucker MI. Developing a decision instrument to guide computed tomographic imaging of blunt head injury patients. *J Trauma.* 2005;59:954–959.

20. Melnick ER, Szlezak CM, Bentley SK, Dziura JD, Kotlyar S, Post LA. CT overuse for mild traumatic brain injury. *Jt Comm J Qual Patient Saf.* 2012;38:483–489.

21. Mechtler LL, Shastri KK, Crutchfield KE. Advanced neuroimaging of mild traumatic brain injury. *Neurol Clin.* 2014;32:31–58.

22. Mittal S, Wu Z, Neelavalli J, Haacke EM. Susceptibility-weighted imaging: technical aspects and clinical applications, part 2. *AJNR Am J Neuroradiol.* 2009;30:232–252.

23. Cubon VA, Putukian M, Boyer C, Dettwiler A. A diffusion tensor imaging study on the white matter skeleton in individuals with sports-related concussion. *J Neurotrauma.* 2011;28:189–201.

24. Wilde EA, McCauley SR, Hunter JV, et al. Diffusion tensor imaging of acute mild traumatic brain injury in adolescents. *Neurology.* 2008;70:948–955.

25. Hellyer PJ, Leech R, Ham TE, Bonnelle V, Sharp DJ. Individual prediction of white matter injury following traumatic brain injury. *Ann Neurol.* 2013;73:489–499.

26. Papa L, Wang KK. Raising the bar on traumatic brain injury biomarker research—methods make a difference. *J Neurotrauma.* 2017;34(13):2187–2189.

27. Papa L. Exploring the role of biomarkers for the diagnosis and management of traumatic brain injury patients. In: Man TK, Flores RJ, eds. *Proteomics—Human Diseases and Protein Functions.* London: IntechOpen; 2012.

28. Zetterberg H, Smith DH, Blennow K. Biomarkers of mild traumatic brain injury in cerebrospinal fluid and blood. *Nat Rev Neurol.* 2013;9:201–210.

29. Papa L, Ramia MM, Kelly JM, Burks SS, Pawlowicz A, Berger RP. Systematic review of clinical research on biomarkers for pediatric traumatic brain injury. *J Neurotrauma.* 2013;30:324–338.

30. Papa L, Ramia MM, Edwards D, Johnson BD, Slobounov SM. Systematic review of clinical studies examining biomarkers of brain injury in athletes after sports-related concussion. *J Neurotrauma.* 2015;32:661–673.

31. Papa L. (2016) Potential blood-based biomarkers for concussion. *Sports Med Arthrosc.* 2016;24:108–115.

32. Ingebrigtsen T, Romner B, Marup-Jensen S, et al. The clinical value of serum S-100 protein measurements in minor head injury: a Scandinavian multicentre study. *Brain Inj.* 2000;14:1047–1055.

33. Muller K, Townend W, Biasca N, et al. S100B serum level predicts computed tomography findings after minor head injury. *J Trauma.* 2007;62:1452–1456.

34. Biberthaler P, Linsenmeier U, Pfeifer KJ, et al. Serum S-100B concentration provides additional information fot [sic] the indication of computed tomography in patients after minor head injury: a prospective multicenter study. *Shock.* 2006;25:446–453.

35. Bechtel K, Frasure S, Marshall C, Dziura J, Simpson C. Relationship of serum S100B levels and intracranial injury in children with closed head trauma. *Pediatrics.* 2009;124:e697–704.

36. Castellani C, Bimbashi P, Ruttenstock E, Sacherer P, Stojakovic T, Weinberg AM. Neuroprotein S-100B—a useful parameter in paediatric patients with mild traumatic brain injury? *Acta Paediatr.* 2009;98:1607–1612.

37. Phillips JP, Jones HM, Hitchcock R, Adama N, Thompson RJ. Radioimmunoassay of serum creatine kinase BB as index of brain damage after head injury. *Br Med J.* 1980;281:777–779.

38. Rothoerl RD, Woertgen C, Holzschuh M, Metz C, Brawanski A. S-100 serum levels after minor and major head injury. *J Trauma.* 1998;45:765–767.

39. Piazza O, Storti MP, Cotena S, et al. S100B is not a reliable prognostic index in paediatric TBI. *Pediatr Neurosurg.* 2007;43:258–264.

40. Berger RP, Pierce MC, Wisniewski SR, Adelson PD, Kochanek PM. Serum S100B concentrations are increased after closed head injury in children: a preliminary study. *J Neurotrauma.* 2002;19:1405–1409.

41. Swanson CA, Burns JC, Peterson BM. Low plasma D-dimer concentration predicts the absence of traumatic brain injury in children. *J Trauma.* 2010;68(5):1072–1077.

42. Anderson RE, Hansson LO, Nilsson O, Dijlai-Merzoug R, Settergren G: High serum S100B levels for trauma patients without head injuries. *Neurosurgery* 2001;48(6):1255–1258; discussion 1258–1260.

43. Pelinka LE, Kroepfl A, Schmidhammer R, et al. Glial fibrillary acidic protein in serum after traumatic brain injury and multiple trauma. *J Trauma.* 2004;57:1006–1012.

44. Unden J, Bellner J, Eneroth M, Alling C, Ingebrigtsen T, Romner B. Raised serum S100B levels after acute bone fractures without cerebral injury. *J Trauma.* 2005;58:59–61.

45. Papa L, Silvestri S, Brophy GM, et al. GFAP out-performs S100beta in detecting traumatic intracranial lesions on computed tomography in trauma patients with mild traumatic brain injury and those with extracranial lesions. *J Neurotrauma.* 2014;31:1815–1822.

46. Zimmer DB, Cornwall EH, Landar A, Song W. The S100 protein family: history, function, and expression. *Brain Res Bull.* 1995;37:417–429.

47. Olsson B, Zetterberg H, Hampel H, Blennow K. Biomarker-based dissection of neurodegenerative diseases. *Prog Neurobiol.* 2011;95:520–534.

48. Papa L, Lewis LM, Falk JL, et al. Elevated levels of serum glial fibrillary acidic protein breakdown products in mild and moderate traumatic brain injury are associated with intracranial lesions and neurosurgical intervention. *Ann Emerg Med.* 2012;59:471–483.

49. Metting Z, Wilczak N, Rodiger LA, Schaaf JM, van der Naalt J. GFAP and S100B in the acute phase of mild traumatic brain injury. *Neurology.* 2012;78:1428–1433.

50. Diaz-Arrastia R, Wang KK, Papa L, et al. Acute biomarkers of traumatic brain injury: relationship between plasma levels of ubiquitin C-terminal hydrolase-L1 and glial fibrillary acidic protein. *J Neurotrauma.* 2014;31:19–25.

51. Papa L, Zonfrillo MR, Ramirez J, Silvestri S, et al. Performance of glial fibrillary acidic protein in detecting traumatic intracranial lesions on computed tomography in children and youth with mild head trauma. *Acad Emerg Med.* 2015;22:1274–1282.

52. Welch RD, Ayaz SI, Lewis LM, et al. Ability of serum glial fibrillary acidic protein, ubiquitin c-terminal hydrolase-L1, and S100B to differentiate normal and abnormal head computed tomography findings in patients with suspected mild or moderate traumatic brain injury. *J Neurotrauma.* 2016;33:203–214.

53. Papa L, Brophy GM, Welch RD, et al. Time course and diagnostic accuracy of glial and neuronal blood biomarkers GFAP and UCH-L1 in a large cohort of trauma patients with and without mild traumatic brain injury. *JAMA Neurol.* 2016;73:551–560.

54. Eng LF, Vanderhaeghen JJ, Bignami A, Gerstl B. An acidic protein isolated from fibrous astrocytes. *Brain Res.* 1971;28:351–354.

55. Papa L, Mittal MK, Ramirez J, et al. In children and youth with mild and moderate traumatic brain injury, glial fibrillary acidic protein out-performs S100beta in detecting traumatic intracranial lesions on computed tomography. *J Neurotrauma.* 2016;33:58–64.

56. Tongaonkar P, Chen L, Lambertson D, Ko B, Madura K. Evidence for an interaction between ubiquitin-conjugating enzymes and the 26S proteasome. *Mol Cell Biol.* 2000;20:4691–4698.

57. Gong B, Leznik E. The role of ubiquitin C-terminal hydrolase L1 in neurodegenerative disorders. *Drug News Perspect.* 2007;20:365–370.

58. Jackson P, Thompson RJ. The demonstration of new human brain-specific proteins by high-resolution two-dimensional polyacrylamide gel electrophoresis. *J Neurol Sci.* 1981;49:429–438.

59. Siman R, Toraskar N, Dang A, et al. A panel of neuron-enriched proteins as markers for traumatic brain injury in humans. *J Neurotrauma.* 2009;26:1867–1877.

60. Papa L, Akinyi L, Liu MC, et al. Ubiquitin C-terminal hydrolase is a novel biomarker in humans for severe traumatic brain injury. *Crit Care Med.* 2010;38:138–144.

61. Papa L, Robertson CS, Wang KK, et al. Biomarkers improve clinical outcome predictors of mortality following non-penetrating severe traumatic brain injury. *Neurocrit Care.* 2015;22:52–64.

62. Brophy G, Mondello S, Papa L, et al. Biokinetic analysis of Ubiquitin C-Terminal Hydrolase-L1 (UCHL1) in severe traumatic brain injury patient biofluids. *J Neurotrauma.* 2011;28(6):861–870.

63. Berger RP, Beers SR, Papa L, Bell M. Common data elements for pediatric traumatic brain injury: recommendations from the biospecimens and biomarkers workgroup. *J Neurotrauma.* 2012;29:672–677.

64. Papa L, Lewis LM, Silvestri S, et al. Serum levels of ubiquitin C-terminal hydrolase distinguish mild traumatic brain injury from trauma controls and are elevated in mild and moderate traumatic brain injury patients with intracranial lesions and neurosurgical intervention. *J Trauma Acute Care Surg.* 2012;72:1335–1344.

65. Papa L, Mittal MK, Ramirez J, et al. Neuronal biomarker Ubiquitin C-Terminal Hydrolase (UCH-L1) detects traumatic intracranial lesions on CT in children and youth with mild traumatic brain injury. *J Neurotrauma.* 2017;34(13):2132–2140.

66. Franz G, Beer R, Kampfl A, et al. Amyloid beta 1-42 and tau in cerebrospinal fluid after severe traumatic brain injury. *Neurology.* 2003;60:1457–1461.

67. Marklund N, Blennow K, Zetterberg H, Ronne-Engstrom E, Enblad P, Hillered L. Monitoring of brain interstitial total tau and beta amyloid proteins by microdialysis in patients with traumatic brain injury. *J Neurosurg.* 2009;110:1227–1237.

68. Ost M, Nylen K, Csajbok L, et al. Initial CSF total tau correlates with 1-year outcome in patients with traumatic brain injury. *Neurology.* 2006;67:1600–1604.

69. Sjogren M, Blomberg M, Jonsson M, et al. Neurofilament protein in cerebrospinal fluid: a marker of white matter changes. *J Neurosci Res.* 2001;66:510–516.

70. Shahim P, Tegner Y, Wilson DH, et al. Blood biomarkers for brain injury in concussed professional ice hockey players. *JAMA Neurol.* 2014:71:684–692.

71. Puvenna V, Engeler M, Banjara M, et al. Is phosphorylated tau unique to chronic traumatic encephalopathy? Phosphorylated tau in epileptic brain and chronic traumatic encephalopathy. *Brain Res.* 2016;1630:225–240.

72. Rubenstein R, Chang B, Davies P, Wagner AK, Robertson CS, Wang KK. A novel, ultrasensitive assay for tau: potential for assessing traumatic brain injury in tissues and biofluids. *J Neurotrauma.* 2015;32:342–352.

73. Yang WJ, Chen W, Chen L, et al. Involvement of tau phosphorylation in traumatic brain injury patients. *Acta Neurol Scand.* 2016;135(6):622–627.

74. Geijerstam JL, Oredsson S, Britton M. Medical outcome after immediate computed tomography or admission for observation in patients with mild head injury: randomised controlled trial. *BMJ.* 2006;333:465.

75. Zimmer A, Marcinak J, Hibyan S, Webbe F. Normative values of major SCAT2 and SCAT3 components for a college athlete population. *Appl Neuropsychol Adult.* 2015;22:132–140.

76. Langlois JA, Rutland-Brown W, Wald MM. The epidemiology and impact of traumatic brain injury: a brief overview. *J Head Trauma Rehabil.* 2006;21:375–378.

77. Lannsjo M, af Geijerstam JL, Johansson U, Bring J, Borg J. Prevalence and structure of symptoms at 3 months after mild traumatic brain injury in a national cohort. *Brain Inj.* 2009;23:213–219.

Blast Traumatic Brain Injury Mechanisms

*Elizabeth McNeil, Zachary Bailey, Allison Guettler,
and Pamela VandeVord*

10

Introduction

More than 25% of the veterans returning from Operation Enduring Freedom (OEF), Operation Iraqi Freedom (OIF), and Operation New Dawn (OND) are suffering from closed head injuries due to blast exposure.[1] Blast traumatic brain injury (bTBI) is the second most common cause of injuries from blast. In 2016, there were 13,634 servicemen and -women diagnosed with a TBI, with 86% categorized as mild TBI (mTBI).[2] To further complicate the injury, combat personnel can be exposed to multiple low-level blasts, which could lead to long-term sequelae.[3] A study by Wilk et al. surveyed 587 US Army soldiers returning from Iraq with a self-reported concussion.[4] Of these mild head injuries, 72.2% reported a blast mechanism as the cause of injury, highlighting the importance of understanding the mechanism of bTBI.

Introduction to Blast Physics

An explosive free-field blast has four distinct flow regions: explosive, near-field, mid-field, and far-field. These are associated with the explosion itself, the fireball, a nonuniform flow containing shrapnel, and a uniform flow, respectively. The far-field region is well-characterized from a physics perspective; therefore, the majority of experimental research on bTBI has been focused within this region.

Two general parameters that characterize a free-field blast are static and dynamic pressure. *Static pressure* (i.e., hydrostatic pressure, side-on pressure, or overpressure) is the pressure experienced on a surface parallel to the direction of fluid flow and acting as a principle stress on the surface. *Dynamic pressure* is a measure of the specific kinetic energy of the flow and has a lower magnitude than static pressure. The sum of static and dynamic pressure is the *stagnation*, or *total pressure*. A third pressure type, *reflected pressure*, has the largest magnitude and describes the force experienced by a surface normal to the blast wave. Reflected pressure is not a parameter of a free-field blast but a description of how the wave interacts with objects or structures in its path. The magnitude of the reflected pressure is dependent on the object shape and size, its angle with respect to the shock front, and location on the object's surface. The relative speed of the shock wave can be used to determine the conditions of the shock front using *Rankine-Hugoniot relations*.

At any observation point in the far-field region, an area will experience an abrupt increase in static pressure as the shock wave passes, followed by a blast wind. The amount

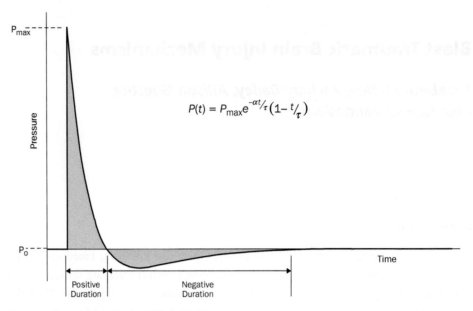

$$P(t) = P_{max}e^{-\alpha t/\tau}\left(1 - t/\tau\right)$$

Figure 10.1 Friedlander waveform showing the pressure profile of an ideal blast wave where P is the overpressure, P_{max} is the maximum overpressure, τ is the positive duration, and α is a decay constant.

of time to reach peak positive pressure is called the *rise time* and is in the nanosecond range. Then, the wind reverses and travels toward the origin, which now has a pressure below ambient conditions, and causes a negative pressure at the observation point, eventually returning to ambient. The negative phase has a much smaller magnitude than the positive phase and typically has a longer duration. The *Friedlander equation* is a simplified approximation of the pressure profile of the blast event at a given point in the far-field region (Figure 10.1).

Injury Categories

There are four main modes of blast injury. *Primary injury*, or *barotrauma*, is an injury due to blast pressure. *Secondary injuries* are due to shrapnel or objects thrown by the blast wave. *Tertiary injuries* are caused by acceleration of the body, including impact with structures after being thrown by the blast. *Quaternary injuries* focus on direct effects of the explosion and may include thermal burns or chemical exposures. Individuals may be exposed to one or more of these injury modes, which contributes to the unique pathology of bTBI.

Theories of Blast Brain Injury Mechanisms

How does exposure to a blast wave cause brain injury? This is a question that has yet to be answered. There are theories speculating how the brain becomes injured yet little evidence to support one as a major contender. As shown in Figure 10.2, there are four main theories of primary bTBI mechanisms that will be examined here: blast wave transmission through skull orifices, direct cranial transmission, thoracic surge, and skull

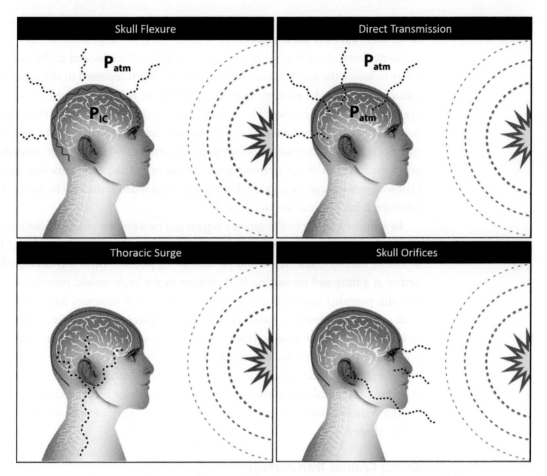

Figure 10.2 Summary of current theories of primary blast transmission to the brain. Dotted lines represent the proposed route of transmission. The skull flexure and direct transmission theories differ on the transfer of blast wave across the skull. In the direct transmission theory, the blast wave transverses the skull leading to an intracranial pressure (ICP) similar to that of the atmosphere (P_{atm}). In the skull flexure theory, the blast causes flexure of the skull, which disturbs ICP but may not directly relate to P_{atm}.

flexure dynamics. Other mechanisms of primary bTBI have been proposed and will be summarized.

Skull Orifices

The skull has several orifices that provide potential entrance to the intracranial space. In the skull orifice theory, the blast wave enters the cranium through the nasal canal, auditory canal, and/or the ocular orbits leading to intracranial pressure (ICP) disturbances that can injure the brain. Studies have reported injury to these sensory systems following blast exposure, such as tympanic membrane rupture and intraocular foreign bodies.[5–10] An evaluation of 120 Marines in Iraq revealed prevalent upper extremity and head injuries (70%).[5] They found ear injuries to be common and speculated they could be reduced by wearing earplugs. Eye injuries were uncommon (0.5%), likely due to ballistic eye protection. If head injuries are prevalent even though eye injuries are low, then it may be reasonable to assume that bTBI mechanisms cannot be solely based on entrance of the blast wave via the orbits.

Some finite element modeling and *in vivo* studies have looked at this mechanism as a way to injure the brain. Neurodegeneration has been reported in the retina and brain visual centers due to primary blast overpressure in rodents exposed to blast without eye protection.[11-15] Another *in vivo* study showed that changes in ICP occurred independently from the presence of eye protection during a primary blast wave exposure suggesting another mechanism of blast energy transfer.[16] However, other orifices were not investigated. A finite element investigation of human blast exposure showed that blast overpressure can be amplified in the ear canal when it directly faces the blast wave; however, it has minimal impact on ICP.[17]

In summary, injury to the sensory organs can be a consequence of blast exposure but there is little evidence supporting this theory as a mechanism of primary bTBI. More *in vivo* or cadaveric research could be used to support the theory. Blocking all but one orifice at a time and measuring ICP changes in the brain would provide useful insight into this potential mechanism. Even if there are no ICP increases due to entry into the skull orifices, this does not rule out focal injury adjacent to the orifices possibly leading to secondary injury responses. Injury to the axon bundles running through the orifices could lead to downstream effects such as neurodegeneration in the retina and brain visual centers.[11-15] Additional *in vivo* research studying each orifice, the involved neurons, evaluating the signaling pathway, and identifying relevant behavioral deficits could also provide valuable insight. In conclusion, there is a scarcity of data supporting the skull orifice theory.

Direct Cranial Transmission

A second mechanism of injury debated in literature is blast energy directly transmitted to the brain through the skull. Direct wave transmission, also called *transosteal wave propagation*, concerns the processes by which an air-borne shock wave interacts with the material interface of the skull and transmits a "through-thickness" stress by direct compression of the skull material. The energy transmitted through the skull is thought to be governed by the acoustic impedances of the two media. When the blast wave is transmitted between two media of similar acoustic impedances, the wave is assumed to travel with little energy dissipation. However, when traveling between two media with different acoustic impedances the blast wave will be transmitted and reflected. The rate of transmission of the blast wave is dependent on the acoustic impedance mismatch at the boundary. Following direct transmission, the pressure waves within the cranium are capable of creating patterns of diffuse damage in brain tissue through shear stress and other various physical phenomenon including spallation, implosion, and inertia.

The effects of acoustic impedance mismatch may be particularly relevant when considering the blast wave interaction with the skull. The wave transmission from air to bone is accompanied by a large impedance mismatch, which may suggest large rarefaction from the skull. Still, several computational models have demonstrated the effects of direct transmission.[18-20] However, these models have yet to be validated with physiologically relevant experimental data.

Changes in ICP have been observed in several studies of blast exposure.[16,21–23] Chandra and Sundaramurthy (2015) demonstrated changes in ICP following blast exposure to postmortem human surrogate heads.[22] The ICP pressure trace showed similar trends to the incident pressure wave and increased accordingly with incident pressure. The maximum ICP recorded was behind the forehead (following frontal blast exposure) and exceeded the peak overpressure of the incident blast wave. The authors suggest a role for direct transmission of the blast wave into the cranium. However, by this theory, wave attenuation through the skull would be expected. Other mechanisms are possibly involved, which leads to the observed wave amplification within the cranium.

Thoracic Surge Mechanism

Blast exposure in theater and in most experimental models subjects the whole body to the blast wave. Therefore, the mechanism of blast transmission to the brain may not involve an isolated interaction with the skull. Instead, the thoracic surge mechanism postulates that the blast wave causes compression of the thorax and abdomen, which can propagate through soft tissue and vasculature. A pressure surge within the vasculature may travel to the more sensitive vessels of the brain and create a diffuse injury pattern. In both clinical and preclinical studies of blast exposure, thorax and abdomen compression have been observed that results in a diverse array of soft tissue damage.[24,25] These injuries include lacerations, perforations, and hematomas to organs including the lung, liver, spleen, and small intestine.[24] Damage to cerebral vasculature has been characterized following blast exposure, although it has not been sufficiently attributed to vascular surge.[26–30]

Despite evidence of thorax trauma, the thoracic surge mechanism as a method of blast transmission to the brain is met with little experimental or biomechanical support. Studies have attempted to isolate thoracic mechanisms in various preclinical models of blast neurotrauma.[31–34] Simard et al. reported an inflammatory response occurring within the brain following a thorax-only blast exposure.[33] The inflammatory response was mitigated by jugular vein ligation and was reproduced by an intravenous pressure pulse. Cernak et al. also reported localized chest exposure to blast that resulted in ultrastructural and biochemical alterations, along with cognitive deficits in rodents.[32] Similar results were found by Long et al., who showed that the presence of a Kevlar protective vest reduced mortality and mitigated fiber degeneration in the brain following low-level blast exposure.[34] However, at a higher magnitude of blast overpressure, the vest was not able to mitigate fiber degeneration. While these studies have demonstrated differences in injury patterns dependent on the presence of thorax or head protection, the injury metrics used do not provide direct mechanistic evidence of primary blast transmission. Rather, the presence of cellular and molecular pathology in the brain may result from a systemic response to distal organ/tissue injury.[35]

Other studies have observed little to no role of a thoracic mechanism in blast transmission to the brain. Romba and Martin noticed that changes in ICP were only observed when the head of a rhesus monkey was exposed to the blast.[36] Chest-only exposure led to minimal pressure changes in both the thorax and head. Goldstein et al. exposed a mouse and an isolated mouse head to a blast and measured ICP dynamics.[37] In both tests, ICP closely mirrored the blast wave, questioning the contribution of a thoracic surge mechanism. However, the duration of ICP change appeared to decrease in the isolated head.[37] This may imply a contributory role for a thoracic mechanism, but also could result from the absence of cerebral perfusion in the isolated head.

To properly assess the role of a thoracic mechanism, previous studies rely on the ability to isolate thorax exposure from blast wave exposure to the head. However, this is experimentally difficult to achieve as simple incorporation of head protection may not sufficiently prevent blast wave–skull interaction. In fact, studies have demonstrated that the mechanics of blast wave interaction with a helmet involve pressure intensification between the skull and helmet.[22,38] Therefore, it is possible that "chest-only" exposures include confounding exposure of the blast wave with the skull.

Proper investigation of the thoracic mechanism has proved to be experimentally difficult. As such, bTBI pathology cannot be confidently attributed to a thoracic mechanism. However, the experimental and computational studies discussed previously provide support for a potential contributory role in the injury pathology. To better understand the effects of this mechanism, future experiments should seek to better isolate thoracic mechanisms from skull interactions and secondary injury cascades.

Skull Flexure Dynamics

The skull flexure dynamics theory is based on the principle that the blast wave cannot directly transmit through the skull into the brain. Instead, the blast wave energy interacts with the skull causing deformation or vibration.[21,39–42] This phenomenon can be explained by the high impedance mismatch between the air and the skull, causing the majority of the blast pressure to be reflected off the surface of the skull. The stress wave in the skull may travel much faster than the blast wave in the air and lead to complex strain profiles over the entire skull as the blast wave propagates. These skull dynamics cause ICP disturbances and gradients. The brain, being incompressible but viscoelastic, is susceptible to shear forces and deformation caused by these changes. With this theory, diffuse injury patterns of the brain are expected, which has been observed in several preclinical blast models.[43–49]

Measured oscillatory ICP responses provide support for this theory. To determine the source of these ICP oscillations, Romba and Martin placed pressure sensors in a sacrificed primate's brain and reported ICP profiles.[37] They found distinct pressure pulses in the brain did not mirror the ambient pressure profile, contradicting the direct cranial transmission theory. Additionally, they investigated the effect of shielding the thorax of the animal while subjecting the head to blast exposure. Their results indicated ICP oscillations were found despite the presence of thorax protection, contradicting the thoracic surge hypothesis. Recently, similar results demonstrated that strong blast-induced ICP was inflicted in swine despite being fitted with thoracic protection.[50] Sophisticated computational models have been developed to investigate skull flexure. Moss et al. created a computational model of the human head interacting with the shock wave from a blast.[41] The main conclusion from this work is that the blast wave will cause the skull to dynamically flex inward; this will create a ripple effect on the skull surface that propagates outward. This rippling will result in variable pressure regions that produce pressure gradients in the brain. It was also reported that the deflections caused by the shock front will lead to magnified levels of pressure within the brain, potentially leading to significant neurotrauma. Research of blast mechanics in simplified physical models has also been undertaken. Alley et al. investigated the effects of spherical shells with and without apertures, and with two different types of brain simulant of varying viscosities to determine the effects of impedance mismatches in the human head when exposed to a blast wave.[51] Their results showed noticeable pressure oscillations within the simulant, and those regions of compression and tension could possibly lead to neurotrauma in an organism. Bolander et al. went a step further and measured skull deformation during blast with strain gauges.[39] They found oscillations in the strain data from the skull and in the ICP measurements in the brain. The delay in rise time of the ICP response in the brain compared to the incident shock wave was attributed to the skull acting as a medium between the external environment and the intracranial contents. This study supports skull flexure and provides evidence against the direct cranial transmission theory (strain and ICP oscillations).[39] Chandra and Sundaramurthy also reported strain profiles on the skull, which may play an important role in the injury pathology.[22] Based on these studies, transference of shock wave energy into the brain by means of skull flexure may likely contribute to the mechanism of primary blast neurotrauma.

Other Mechanisms

In addition to the main theories just explained, other theories warrant mention. One hypothesis for bTBI is that there is a combination of rotational and translational accelerations of the head caused during the blast event. While some consider acceleration to be the primary blast injury mechanism,[37] others have shown head acceleration may be a confounding factor by studying pure-rotation versus blast neurotrauma[52] and the effects of head restraint during primary blast wave exposure.[53] Experiments and simulations using a sphere and simulations with the ALE3D head model provide time-course evidence to support that acceleration may not be the primary injury mechanism and is better classified as a tertiary injury mode.[41,51]

Another hypothesis for causing bTBI is through cavitation. This theory works in conjunction with the direct skull transmission or the skull flexure theory, where there is an increase of ICP due to either direct transmission of the blast wave or skull flexure dynamics. The increase in coup pressure creates a contre coup negative pressure, which can form cavitation bubbles. The collapse of these bubbles can cause damage to the adjacent brain tissue. Many modeling and surrogate studies have shown the development of negative ICP contre coup to the blast wave during an exposure.[54-56] However, experimental evidence does not exist to support negative pressure and cavitation being injurious to the surrounding brain tissue. Cavitation during a blunt impact in monkeys was reported but did not appear to produce injury up to a negative peak ICP of 1 atm.[57] Similar experiments would help discern the importance of cavitation as a mechanism of blast brain injury.

In summary, there are still many unknowns surrounding blast brain injury mechanisms. It is possible that these theories do not occur exclusively from each other, but rather that several of these mechanisms lead to brain injury following blast exposure. Biomechanical investigation with *in vivo*, cadaver, and finite element models would greatly increase our knowledge of blast brain injury mechanisms.

References

1. MacGregor AJ, Dougherty AL, Galarneau MR. Injury-specific correlates of combat-related traumatic brain injury in Operation Iraqi Freedom. *J Head Trauma Rehabil.* 2011;26(4):312–318.

2. Defense and Veterans Brain Injury Center (DVBIC). Department of Defense numbers for traumatic brain injury worldwide. http://dvbic.dcoe.mil/files/tbi-numbers/DoD-TBI-Worldwide-Totals_2016_Q1-Q3_Nov-10-2016_v1.0_508_2016-12-27.pdf. Published 2016.

3. Elder GA, Gama Sosa MA, De Gasperi R, et al. Vascular and inflammatory factors in the pathophysiology of blast-induced brain injury. *Front Neurol.* 2015;6:48.

4. Wilk JE, Thomas JL, McGurk DM, Riviere LA, Castro CA, Hoge CW. Mild traumatic brain injury (concussion) during combat: lack of association of blast mechanism with persistent postconcussive symptoms. *J Head Trauma Rehabil.* 2010;25(1):9–14.

5. Gondusky JS, Reiter MP. Protecting military convoys in Iraq: an examination of battle injuries sustained by a mechanized battalion during Operation Iraqi Freedom II. *Mil Med.* 2005;170(6):546.

6. Eskridge SL, Macera CA, Galarneau MR, et al. Injuries from combat explosions in Iraq: injury type, location, and severity. *Injury.* 2012;43(10):1678–1682.

7. Peters P. Primary blast injury: an intact tympanic membrane does not indicate the lack of a pulmonary blast injury. *Mil Med.* 2011;176(1):110.

8. Harrison CD, Bebarta VS, Grant GA. Tympanic membrane perforation after combat blast exposure in Iraq: a poor biomarker of primary blast injury. *J Trauma Acute Care Surg.* 2009;67(1):210–211.

9. Xydakis MS, Mulligan LP, Smith AB, Olsen CH, Lyon DM, Belluscio L. Olfactory impairment and traumatic brain injury in blast-injured combat troops A cohort study. *J Neurol.* 2015;84(15):1559–1567.

10. Morley MG, Nguyen JK, Heier JS, Shingleton BJ, Pasternak JF, Bower KS. Blast eye injuries: a review for first responders. *Disaster Med Public Health Prep.* 2010;4(2):154–160.

11. DeMar J, Sharrow K, Hill M, Berman J, Oliver T, Long J. Effects of primary blast overpressure on retina and optic tract in rats. *Front Neurol.* 2016;7:59.

12. Petras J, Bauman RA, Elsayed NM. Visual system degeneration induced by blast overpressure. *J Toxicol.* 1997;121(1):41–49.

13. Koliatsos VE, Cernak I, Xu L, et al. A mouse model of blast injury to brain: initial pathological, neuropathological, and behavioral characterization. *J Neuropathol Exp Neurol.* 2011;70(5):399–416.

14. Wang H-CH, Choi J-H, Greene WA, et al. Pathophysiology of blast-induced ocular trauma with apoptosis in the retina and optic nerve. *Mil Med.* 2014;179(8S):34–40.

15. Choi JH, Greene WA, Johnson AJ, et al. Pathophysiology of blast-induced ocular trauma in rats after repeated exposure to low-level blast overpressure. *Clin Exp.* 2015;43(3):239–246.

16. Leonardi AD, Bir CA, Ritzel DV, VandeVord PJ. Intracranial pressure increases during exposure to a shock wave. *J Neurotrauma.* 2011;28(1):85–94.

17. Akula P, Hua Y, Gu L. Blast-induced mild traumatic brain injury through ear canal: a finite element study. *Biomed Eng Lett.* 2015;5(4):281–288.

18. Nyein MK, Jason AM, Yu L, et al. In silico investigation of intracranial blast mitigation with relevance to military traumatic brain injury. *Proc Natl Acad Sci.* 2010;107(48):20703–20708.

19. Moore DF, Jerusalem A, Nyein M, Noels L, Jaffee MS, Radovitzky RA. Computational biology—modeling of primary blast effects on the central nervous system. *NeuroImage.* 2009;47(suppl 2):T10–20.

20. Selvan V, Ganpule S, Kleinschmit N, Chandra N. Blast wave loading pathways in heterogeneous material systems-experimental and numerical approaches. *J Biomech Eng.* 2013;135(6):61002–61014.

21. Leonardi AD. *An investigation of the biomechanical response from shock wave loading to the head* [dissertation]. Detroit, MI: Wayne State University; 2011.

22. Chandra N, Sundaramurthy A. Acute pathophysiology of blast injury-from biomechanics to experiments and computations: implications on head and polytrauma. In: Kobeissy FH, ed. *Brain Neurotrauma: Molecular, Neuropsychological, and Rehabilitation Aspects.* Boca Raton, FL: CRC Press/Taylor & Francis; 2015:199–258.

23. Chavko M, Koller WA, Prusaczyk WK, McCarron RM. Measurement of blast wave by a miniature fiber optic pressure transducer in the rat brain. *J Neurosci Methods.* 2007;159(2):277–281.

24. Wani I, Parray FQ, Sheikh T, et al. Spectrum of abdominal organ injury in a primary blast type. *World J Emerg Surg.* 2009;4(1):46.

25. Clemedson CJ. Blast injury. *Physiol Rev.* 1956;36(3):336–354.

26. Pun PB, Kan EM, Salim A, et al. Low level primary blast injury in rodent brain. *Front Neurol.* 2011;2:19.

27. Gama Sosa MA, De Gasperi R, Janssen PL, et al. Selective vulnerability of the cerebral vasculature to blast injury in a rat model of mild traumatic brain injury. *Acta Neuropathol Commun.* 2014;2:67.

28. Gama Sosa MA, De Gasperi R, Paulino AJ, et al. Blast overpressure induces shear-related injuries in the brain of rats exposed to a mild traumatic brain injury. *Acta Neuropathol Commun.* 2013;1(1):51.

29. Bir C, Vandevord P, Shen Y, Raza W, Haacke EM. Effects of variable blast pressures on blood flow and oxygen saturation in rat brain as evidenced using MRI. *J Magn Reson Imaging.* 2012;30(4):527–534.

30. Kamnaksh A, Kwon SK, Kovesdi E, et al. Neurobehavioral, cellular, and molecular consequences of single and multiple mild blast exposure. *Electrophoresis.* 2012;33(24):3680–3692.

31. Cernak I, Savic J, Malicevic Z, Zunic G, Radosevic P, Ivanovic I. Leukotrienes in the pathogenesis of pulmonary blast injury. *J Trauma.* 1996;40(3 suppl):S148–151.

32. Cernak I, Wang Z, Jiang J, Bian X, Savic J. Ultrastructural and functional characteristics of blast injury-induced neurotrauma. *J Trauma.* 2001;50(4):695–706.

33. Simard JM, Pampori A, Keledjian K, et al. Exposure of the thorax to a sublethal blast wave causes a hydrodynamic pulse that leads to perivenular inflammation in the brain. *J Neurotrauma.* 2014;31(14):1292–1304.

34. Long JB, Bentley TL, Wessner KA, Cerone C, Sweeney S, Bauman RA. Blast overpressure in rats: recreating a battlefield injury in the laboratory. *J Neurotrauma.* 2009;26(6):827–840.

35. Committee on Gulf War and Health: Long-Term Effects of Blast Exposures, Board on the Health of Select Populations, Institute of Medicine. *Gulf War and Health: Long-Term Effects of Blast Exposures.* Vol 9. Washington, DC: National Academy Press; 2014.

36. Romba J, Martin P. *The propagation of air shock waves on a biophysical model.* (Report No. AD0264932). Human Engineering Lab Aberdeen Proving Ground, MD; 1961.

37. Goldstein LE, Fisher AM, Tagge CA, et al. Chronic traumatic encephalopathy in blast-exposed military veterans and a blast neurotrauma mouse model. *Sci Transl Med.* 2012;4(134):134ra160.

38. Ganpule S, Gu L, Alai A, Chandra N. Role of helmet in the mechanics of shock wave propagation under blast loading conditions. *Comput Methods Biomech Biomed Engin.* 2012;15(11):1233–1244.

39. Bolander R, Mathie B, Bir C, Ritzel D, VandeVord P. Skull flexure as a contributing factor in the mechanism of injury in the rat when exposed to a shock wave. *Ann Biomed Eng.* 2011;39(10):2550–2559.

40. Dal Cengio Leonardi A, Keane NJ, Bir CA, Ryan AG, Xu L, Vandevord PJ. Head orientation affects the intracranial pressure response resulting from shock wave loading in the rat. *J Biomech.* 2012;45(15):2595–2602.

41. Moss WC, King MJ, Blackman EG. Skull flexure from blast waves: a mechanism for brain injury with implications for helmet design. *Phys Rev Lett.* 2009;103(10):108702.

42. Zhu F, Wagner C, Dal Cengio Leonardi A, et al. Using a gel/plastic surrogate to study the biomechanical response of the head under air shock loading: a combined experimental and numerical investigation. *Biomech Model Mechanobiol.* 2012;11(3-4):341–353.

43. Sajja VS, Ereifej ES, VandeVord PJ. Hippocampal vulnerability and subacute response following varied blast magnitudes. *Neurosci Lett.* 2014;570:33–37.

44. Sajja VS, Galloway M, Ghoddoussi F, Kepsel A, VandeVord P. Effects of blast-induced neurotrauma on the nucleus accumbens. *J Neurosci Res.* 2013;91(4):593–601.

45. Sajja VSSS, Hubbard WB, Hall CS, Ghoddoussi F, Galloway MP, VandeVord PJ. Enduring deficits in memory and neuronal pathology after blast-induced traumatic brain injury. *Sci Rep.* 2015;5:15075.

46. Vandevord PJ, Bolander R, Sajja VS, Hay K, Bir CA. Mild neurotrauma indicates a range-specific pressure response to low level shock wave exposure. *Ann Biomed Eng.* 2012;40(1):227–236.

47. Saljo A, Arrhen F, Bolouri H, Mayorga M, Hamberger A. Neuropathology and pressure in the pig brain resulting from low-impulse noise exposure. *J Neurotrauma.* 2008;25(12):1397–1406.

48. Kamnaksh A, Kovesdi E, Kwon SK, et al. Factors affecting blast traumatic brain injury. *J Neurotrauma.* 2011;28(10):2145–2153.

49. Garman RH, Jenkins LW, Switzer RC III, et al. Blast exposure in rats with body shielding is characterized primarily by diffuse axonal injury. *J Neurotrauma.* 2011;28(6):947–959.

50. Bauman RA, Ling G, Tong L, et al. An introductory characterization of a combat-casualty-care relevant swine model of closed head injury resulting from exposure to explosive blast. *J Neurotrauma.* 2009;26(6):841–860.

51. Alley MD, Schimizze BR, Son SF. Experimental modeling of explosive blast-related traumatic brain injuries. *NeuroImage.* 2011 Jan;54 Suppl 1:S45–54.

52. Stemper BD, Shah AS, Budde MD, et al. Behavioral outcomes differ between rotational acceleration and blast mechanisms of mild traumatic brain injury. *Front Neurol.* 2016;7(31):1–13.

53. Gullotti DM, Beamer M, Panzer MB, et al. Significant head accelerations can influence immediate neurological impairments in a murine model of blast-induced traumatic brain injury. *J Biomech Eng.* 2014;136(9):091004.

54. Goeller J, Wardlaw A, Treichler D, O'Bruba J, Weiss G. Investigation of cavitation as a possible damage mechanism in blast-induced traumatic brain injury. *J Neurotrauma.* 2012;29(10):1970–1981.

55. Salzar RS, Treichler D, Wardlaw A, Weiss G, Goeller J. Experimental investigation of cavitation as a possible damage mechanism in blast-induced traumatic brain injury in post-mortem human subject heads. *J Neurotrauma*. 2017;34(8):1589–1602.

56. Wardlaw A, Goeller J. Cavitation as a possible traumatic brain injury (TBI) damage mechanism. Paper presented at: 26th Southern Biomedical Engineering Conference (SBEC) 2010; April 30–May 2, 2010, College Park, MD.

57. Nusholtz GS, Lux P, Kaiker P, Janicki MA. Head impact response—Skull deformation and angular accelerations. SAE Technical Paper 841657. In: *Proceedings of the 28th Stapp Car Crash Conference*. Warrenton, PA: Society of Automotive Engineers; 1984.

Adult and Pediatric Mild and Moderate Head Injury Management in Scandinavian Countries

Zandra Olivecrona and Johan Undén

11

Introduction

Denmark, Norway, and Sweden constitute the Scandinavian countries. At 3,425,804 square kilometers, the combined area of the Nordic countries would form the seventh-largest country in the world. In 2017, the region had a population of around 27 million people.[1] The countries have similar healthcare and political systems. In general, there is a public, three-level hospital structure, with local hospitals serving small areas, central hospitals serving a larger area (county), and university hospitals serving these other hospitals in a regionalized manner.[2] The university hospitals are Level 1 trauma centers with neurosurgical departments. There are six neurosurgical departments in Sweden (and a consultatory neurosurgical service at the youngest university hospital in Örebro) and five in Denmark, Finland, and Norway, respectively. All neurosurgical departments treat patients with traumatic head injury, except one of the two departments in Oslo, Norway.

The Scandinavian Neurotrauma Committee (SNC) was founded in 1998 to strengthen the care of neurotrauma patients in the Nordic countries. The committee consists of dedicated neurosurgeons, neuroanesthesiologists, and neurointensivists from Sweden, Norway, Denmark, Finland, and Iceland.[3]

In 2000, the SNC presented evidence-based guidelines for initial management of minimal, mild, and moderate head injuries in adults.[4] In 2016, the corresponding pediatric guidelines were published[5]. These guidelines are continuously updated.[6]

The aim of the guidelines is to guide physicians in the emergency department (ED) during initial (the first 24 hours) management of adult and pediatric patients with minimal, mild, and moderate head injuries; specifically, to decide which patients are to receive computed tomography (CT) scanning, admission, or discharge (or combinations of these) from the ED. In 2007, S100β was adapted into the existing Scandinavian management guidelines for adults to reduce CT usage and costs. There is an ongoing multicenter study running to investigate if S100β also can be implemented in the pediatric guidelines for mild head injuries.

Scandinavian Guidelines for Initial Management of Minimal, Mild, and Moderate Head Injuries in Adults

The guidelines apply to all adults (>18 years of age) who have sustained a head trauma within the past 24 hours.

Minimal represents patients with a Glasgow Coma Scale (GCS) score of 15 and no risk factors, mild is a GCS score of 14 or 15 with risk factors (such as amnesia or loss of consciousness [LOC]), and moderate is a GCS score of 9–13. The brain injury marker S100β is now included in the guidelines, aiming at reducing unnecessary CT scanning.

Minimal

These patients are GCS 15 with no risk factors. These patients are considered as having a very low risk of developing a serious intracranial complication and can therefore be discharged from the hospital without a CT scan.

Mild, Low-Risk

These patients are GCS 14 with no risk factors, or they are GCS 15 and have confirmed or suspected LOC (i.e., the patient cannot clearly deny LOC) or at least to episodes of vomiting. If less than 6 hours have passed since the trauma and S100β analysis is readily available, serum should be sample. If S100β is less than 0.10 μg/L, the patient has a very low risk of serious intracranial complication and can be discharged. A CT scan should be done if:

- S100β is 0.10 μg/L or greater
- More than 6 hours have passed since trauma
- The patient has significant extracranial injuries (e.g., large bone fractures may result in elevated S100β levels)
- S100β analysis is unavailable

If the CT is normal, the patient can be discharged.

Mild, Medium-Risk

These patients are GCS 14–15, 65 years or older, and are also on antiplatelet medication (such as aspirin, clopidogrel, ticlopidine, or dipyridamole). These patients have a moderate risk of intracranial complication and should have a CT scan; if normal, they can be discharged.

Mild, High-Risk

These patients are GCS 14–15 and have either one or more of the following risk factors:

- Intraventricular shunt
- Posttraumatic seizures
- Clinical signs of depressed skull fracture (palpable depression or abnormal discontinuity of skull) or basal skull fracture (raccoon eyes, Battle's sign, hemotympanum, cerebrospinal fluid [CSF] rhinorrhea)
- Focal neurological deficits
- Anticoagulation medication (low-molecular-weight heparins Coumadin/warfarin, dabigatran, or other pharmacologic anticoagulation)
- Coagulation disorders (such as hemophilia, thrombocytopenia, or liver cirrhosis with pathological INR [>1.5]).

These patients have a relatively high risk of intracranial complication. They should have a CT and also be admitted for close neurological observation for at least 24 hours, irrespective of CT findings.

Moderate

These patients are GCS 9–13. They should have a CT and also be admitted for close neurological observation for at least 24 hours, irrespective of CT findings.

Admission

CT is recommended as the primary management routine. If CT is logistically difficult or unavailable, some patients may be admitted for close neurological observation for at least 12 hours after injury.

Patients with high-risk mild and moderate head injury should be admitted, irrespective of CT findings, for at least 24 hours. Observation includes GCS, a simplified neurological exam, pupil size/reactivity, blood pressure, pulse rate, oxygen saturation and respiration rate, and these should be performed every 15 minutes for the first 4 hours after injury, every 30 minutes for the following 4 hours, and at least every hour hereafter.

Some patients with minimal head injury or normal CT/serum S100β following mild head injury, where discharge is recommended, may need admission for other reasons than head injury (such as patients with other injuries, intoxicated patients, or elderly patients without sufficient help at home). Since these patients have a very low risk of intracranial injury, they do not need the observation routine just mentioned.

Computed Tomography

A non–contrast-enhanced CT should be done as soon as possible, with a greater urgency for more severe head injuries according to the preceding guidelines. The patient should be adequately observed while waiting for the CT scan. If CT is abnormal, consider contacting a neurosurgeon or neurotrauma center for advice concerning further management.

Repeat Computed Tomography

Routine repeat CT is not recommended. However, a repeat CT should be done immediately in patients deteriorating in GCS ($\geq$2 points) or with new or progressive neurological deficits.

Discharge

All patients with head injury should receive oral and written information (general advice concerning their head injury) at discharge.

Scandinavian Guidelines for Initial Management of Minimal, Mild, and Moderate Head Trauma in Children

The guidelines apply to all children (<18 years of age) who have sustained a head trauma within the past 24 hours. The pediatric GCS can be used for nonverbal children younger than 5 years of age.[7]

Children younger than 1 year of age may be difficult to assess clinically, thus admitting the child for in-hospital observation after a head trauma may be an option regardless of the child being asymptomatic. A bulging fontanel in an infant (examined when the child is not crying) can be a sign of increased intracranial pressure, which is usually also accompanied with a decreased level of consciousness or other neurological deficits. These patients should be admitted to the hospital and CT scanned.

Minimal

These patients have a GCS score of 15 and have no risk factors. These patients have a very low risk of serious intracranial complication and can be discharged from the emergency department without a CT scan.

Mild, Low-Risk

These children have a GCS score of 15 and have one or more of the following risk factors:

- Suspected or confirmed brief LOC (i.e., exclusion of loss of consciousness is not possible),
- Confirmed posttraumatic amnesia,
- At least two episodes of vomiting
- Severe or progressive headache
- A ventricular shunt
- Behaving abnormally according to their guardians

Children younger than 2 years with a GCS score of 15 and presenting with a large scalp hematoma or a hematoma in the temporal or parietal region, or if the child seems irritable to normal touch or stimulus, is also classified as mild, low-risk. These children should be clinically observed for at least 6 hours (from the time of trauma) until the symptoms have resolved (e.g., headache or vomiting) and the child is fully awake and stable without signs of deterioration. If multiple risk factors are present, consider doing a CT scan instead.

Mild, Medium-Risk

These children have are GCS 14 or 15 and have at least one of the following risk factors:

- LOC for 1 minute or more
- Coagulation disorder (such as hemophilia, thrombocytopenia, or liver disorders with pathological INR [>1.4])
- Taking anticoagulation medication (Coumadin/warfarin, low-molecular-weight heparins, or other pharmacologic anticoagulation)

These patients have a moderate risk of intracranial complication and should be admitted for observation for at least 12 hours (from time of trauma). Alternatively, the child could have a CT scan and, if normal, can be discharged with close follow-up.

Mild, High-Risk

These children are GCS 14–15 and have at least one of the following risk factors:

- Clinical signs of depressed skull fracture (palpable depression or abnormal discontinuity of skull) or basal skull fracture (raccoon eyes, Battle's sign, hemotympanum, CSF rhinorrhea or otorrhea)
- Focal neurological deficits
- Have had a posttraumatic seizure

These patients have a relatively high risk of intracranial complications. They should have a CT and also be admitted for close neurological observation for at least 24 hours, even if the CT is normal.

Moderate

These children are GCS 9–13. They should have a CT and also be admitted for close observation for at least 24 hours, even if the CT is normal.

Admission and Observation

CT is recommended as the primary management routine. Patients with mild, high-risk and moderate head trauma should be admitted irrespective of CT findings for at least 24 hours. Observation should include the level of consciousness (GCS score), a simplified neurological examination (strength testing in extremities, language, and speech), and pulse rate check, and these may be further extended to assessment of headache intensity and pupil size and reactivity especially in children with decreased level of consciousness. The assessment should be performed every 15 minutes for the first 4 hours *after injury*, every 30 minutes for the following 4 hours, and at least every hour hereafter.

Some with minimal head trauma or normal CT following mild head trauma may need admission for reasons other than the head trauma (e.g., children with insufficient guardian supervision, children with other injuries, or heavily intoxicated adolescents). Since these patients have a very low risk of intracranial injury, they need to be checked at least every 4 hours, but do not need the extensive observation routine just mentioned.

Computed Tomography

A non–contrast-enhanced CT should be done as soon as possible, with a greater urgency for mild, high-risk, and moderate head trauma. The child should be adequately monitored when waiting for the CT scan. When CT is abnormal, consider contacting a neurosurgeon for advice concerning further management. Repeat CT should be done immediately in patients deteriorating in GCS ($\geq$2 points) or new/progressive neurological deficits.

Discharge

Guardians to all children with head trauma should receive oral and written instructions at discharge as well as general information about head injuries and contact information.

References

1. "Definition of Scandinavia in English." Oxford Dictionaries. https://en.oxforddictionaries.com/definition/us/scandinavia. Retrieved December 23, 2016.

2. Socialstyrelsen. About the Swedish healthcare system. http://www.socialstyrelsen.se/healthcare-visitors-sweden/about-swedish-healthcare-system/public-private-healthcare-sweden. Sept 25, 2013.

3. Scandinavian Neurotrauma Committee. http://www.neurotrauma.nu/.

4. Ingebrigtsen T, Romner B, Kock-Jensen C; Scandinavian Neurotrauma Committee. Scandinavian guidelines for initial management of minimal, mild, and moderate head injuries. *J Trauma*. 2000;48(4):760–766.

5. Astrand R, Rosenlund C, Unden J; Scandinavian Neurotrauma Committee. Scandinavian guidelines for initial management of minor and moderate head trauma in children. *BMC Med*. 2016;14:33.

6. Unden J, Ingebrigtsen T, Romner B; Scandinavian Neurotrauma Committee. Scandinavian guidelines for initial management of minimal, mild and moderate head injuries in adults: an evidence- and consensus-based update. *BMC Med*. 2013;11:50.

7. Holmes JF, Palchak MJ, MacFarlane T, Kuppermann N. Performance of the pediatric Glasgow Coma Scale in children with blunt head trauma. *Acad Emerg Med*. 2005;12(9):814–819.

Challenges in Neurotrauma Management in India and Rapidly Growing Developing Countries

Virendra Deo Sinha, G. K. Prusty, and Amit Chakrabarty

12

The global burden of disease (GBD) related to all injuries or "trauma" is the leading cause of loss of human potential around the world, especially in low- and middle-income countries (LMICs)[1]. Among all trauma-related injuries, traumatic brain injuries (TBI) and spinal cord injuries (SCI) are the largest causes of death and disability.

Most countries in Asia are experiencing a rapid growth in economic liberalization leading to increased risk factors for TBI in the region. The increased exposure to risk factors coupled with health systems that are often not able to provide adequate treatment and rehabilitation services to TBI patients creates a "double risk." The lack of national epidemiological data on TBI and the use of dated global data from the 1990s both reflect a serious gap in health information systems in Asia. The economic consequences of TBI are reported to be enormous, and yet estimates of the cost of TBI within Asia could not be found in the literature. Given the preventable nature of TBI, it is important to elucidate the true burden of disease in Asia in order to tailor specific prevention programs aimed at alleviating this increasing epidemic.

TBI is a significant public health problem worldwide and is predicted to surpass many diseases as a major cause of death and disability by 2020. The majority of TBI cases (60%) are a result of road traffic injuries, followed by falls (20–30%) and violence (10%). In comparison to all other global regions, Asia has the highest percentage of TBI-related outcomes as a result of falls (77%) and other unintentional injuries (57%).[1]

Magnitude of the Problem

Globally, injuries account for 10% of total deaths and 15% of disability adjusted life years (DALYs). India and other developing countries face major challenges in prevention, prehospital care, and rehabilitation in their rapidly changing environments to reduce the burden of TBI.

Minor head injuries form the bulk of head injuries, ranging from 80% to 90%.

Presently, comprehensive studies of TBI in India are lacking. In India 60–70% of TBI results from road traffic accidents (RTAs), and RTAs in India have increased dramatically in recent years due to widespread motor vehicle access and inadequate safety protocols. India has the highest mortality rates from RTAs in the world, with 161,736 RTA deaths in 2010 (according to the National Crime Records Bureau, India). For each RTA-related death, at least 20 serious injuries occur in India. This equates to 3.2 million serious RTA-related injuries in 2010.

Again, there is lack of population-based data on how many RTAs result in TBI. Because RTAs contribute to 60–70% of all TBIs (http://indianheadinjuryfoundation. org/affect-tbi.html), this would lead to 3–3.5 million TBI (from all cases) in 2010 in India. So, given the long-term disability rate of approximately 50% after TBI, India is generating about 1.5–1.7 million neurologically disabled people every year due to TBI alone.[2]

Causes

Trauma care in India is in its infancy, the budget for primary and secondary trauma care is grossly inadequate, health functionaries are unskilled, and disparities exist between states in developing countries.

Low literacy rates, ignorance, road age and poor road conditions, carefree attitudes while driving, improper implementation of traffic rules, driving under the influence of alcohol, and inadequate signage are a few of the causes of RTAs in India.

Teaching, nonteaching, and corporate hospitals are the major providers of secondary and tertiary healthcare in Indian cities, but little attempt has been made to include them in the trauma care system. A strategy for integrated, coordinated trauma care and injury prevention activities needs to be developed in developing countries.

Paediatric Neurotrauma

TBIs among children are an important cause of concern in all countries. A study from Nepal retrospectively examined pediatric head trauma, and all children with head injury who were younger than 16 years from April 2005 to March 2006 were included. Fall from height was the most common cause (65.1%), followed by RTA (25.6%). Mild head injury, defined as a Glasgow Coma Scale (GCS) score of 13–15, was most common. In urban areas in Nepal, RTA is the most common cause of TBI, and in rural areas, fall from height is the more common cause. A study from Taiwan examined pediatric neurotrauma over an 8-year period and showed that traffic injury is the most common cause of neurotrauma (47.3%), followed by falls (40.3%). Cricket is a popular game in several southeast Asian countries and in Africa. A prospective study undertaken in Srinagar, India, shows that pediatric TBI due to cricket ball impact is quite serious even if a plastic ball is used instead of a standard cricket ball. Public awareness and appropriate safety precautions would prevent such incidents.[3]

Challenges in Epidemiology

Unlike in developed countries, there is no well-established system for collecting and managing information on various diseases in India. Thus it is a daunting task to obtain reliable information about acquired brain injury. In the course of conducting a systematic review on the epidemiology of TBI in India, we recognized several challenges which hampered our effort. Inadequate case definition, lack of centralized reporting mechanisms, lack of population-based studies, absence of standardized survey protocols, and inadequate mortality statistics are some of the major obstacles. Following a standard case definition; linking multiple hospital-based registries; initiating a state- or nationwide population-based registry; conducting population-based studies that are methodologically robust; and introducing centralized, standard reporting mechanisms for TBI are some of the strategies that could help facilitate a thorough investigation into the epidemiology and understanding of TBI. This may help improve policies on the prevention and management of acquired brain injury in India.[1]

Challenges in Prevention

There are many ways in which society, government, and nongovernmental organizations (NGOs) can contribute to preventing head injury. The approach should be holistic.

Some important aspects of injury control are motor vehicle safety programs that target youth in information campaigns on alcohol usage, restraints and helmets, driving habits, road conditions, and speed limits. In addition, every new car launched onto the market should go through strict safety checks and crash tests. Because this invariably increases the cost of vehicle, manufacturers try to evade safety norms to stay in this competitive market.

Young drivers are at highest risk for RTAs. The combination of lack of driving experience and liability to impulsive behavior appears to be the cause. Graduated licensing programs and requiring an adult escort appear to be effective. Alcohol appears to be disproportionately risky for young drivers, and higher minimum drinking ages and laws that prescribe lower legal blood alcohol levels for young drivers are effective in reducing injury.

Legislation is very effective in promoting seat belt and helmet use. Educational status does effect the use of helmets or restraints, although many of the violators in cities are college students. Resistance to the use of helmets comes from youth under various pretexts (being uncomfortable, hot weather, partial cutoff of auditory input, etc.).

Segregation of slow-moving and fast-moving vehicles and cyclists is very important. In smaller cities where the number of cyclists is very high, there are currently no ways to segregate them from the rest of traffic.

Pedestrians usually either do not use designated footpaths or else there are no walkable footpaths. Also, to cross busy roads, subways and overhead bridges are rarely used. The provision of escalators at the entrance to subways may encourage their use[4].

Road safety and the prevention of accidents should be a part of the curriculum for schoolchildren because they form a very large group.[4,5]

The World Health Organization in its report *World Report on Road Traffic Injury Prevention*[6] recommends:

- Making road safety a political priority
- Appointing a lead agency for road safety, giving it adequate resources, and making it publicly accountable
- Developing a multidisciplinary approach to road safety
- Setting appropriate road safety targets and establishing national road safety plans to achieve them
- Creating budgets for road safety and increasing investment in demonstrably effective road safety activities

Challenges in Prehospital Care

Despite understanding the need of prehospital emergency care, the quality of pre-hospital emergency care is far from satisfactory in developing countries, including India. Considering economic-, educational-, infrastructural-, communication-, and transportation-related issues and the deficiency of trained manpower, the initial focus should be on first-responder care and basic prehospital care. An advanced level of care is more practical in urban areas, provided that skilled professional help and ambulance support are readily available. The goal of the prehospital emergency care system should be to match the needs of patients to the available resources so that optimal, prompt, and cost-effective care can be offered. To bridge the wide gap between the actual and ex-pected levels of care, this urgent need must be appreciated by the community, govern-ment administration, and medical professionals, and very positive steps should be taken to meet future challenges.

A prehospital trauma care service remains a dynamic field of medicine for the care of trauma patients. Therefore, improvements in the field of trauma services are required to ensure that "golden-hour" compliance for all trauma victims is an achiev-able goal by coordinating activities between prehospital care and specialized hospital care services.

Improving accessibility and establishing a uniform emergency access telephone number are basic challenges to overcome. A specific and unique model system should be developed to address the needs of the trauma patient. The goal should be to get "the right patient, to the right place, at the right time, to receive the right care" following trauma.[7]

Challenges in Rehabilitation

For the family of a person living with a brain injury, the treatment and psychosocial re-habilitation process is a semi-rational sequence of demands, challenges, disappointment, and rewards. An important question to consider is where, when, and how families are going to get the support, resources, knowledge, encouragement, role models, and skills they need to negotiate the emotional and physical perils of a changing healthcare system and demanding psychosocial rehabilitation process.

TBI is the leading cause of disability in people younger than 40 years of age, and dis-ability can be classified in a simple fashion using the Glasgow Outcome Scale. Disability after moderate or severe TBI may take various forms:

- Mental sequelae with personality change, memory disorder, and apathy (a defective recent memory may be particularly incapacitating)
- Disturbed motor function of an arm or a leg
- Speech disturbance
- Epilepsy (in 1–5% of patients)

Brain injury rehabilitation occurs as inpatient rehabilitation, outpatient rehabilita-tion, and/or community rehabilitation. There are many rehabilitation services across India run by government and private firms. Choosing which rehabilitation unit to refer someone with a brain injury should involve the clinical team, the patient, and his or her family. Once a referral has been made, the rehabilitation unit will usually carry out an assessment to make sure their service is suitable to that patient.

Lack of patient follow-up that provides more information in terms of the patient's ability to perform activities of daily living at home and the barriers (both environmental and due to disability and handicap) the patient faces needs to be overcome/modified.

Other limitations to adequate rehabilitation are financial constraints (many families spend most of their saving in treating the head injury, leaving little in the way of funds for rehabilitation), lack of trained physiotherapists and psychologists in suburban and rural areas, and ignorance of the importance of rehabilitation after head injury among lower socioeconomic groups [8].

Auditing Process and Outcome

As clinical innovation has matured into respectable clinical practice, the emphasis has begun to shift toward auditing processes and outcomes. It may be that the aim is to reassure ourselves and others that we are doing our best, but an audit can also demonstrate local variability in the quality of trauma care. Greater governmental and public scrutiny of hospital services in the coming years is likely to yield interesting findings about variations in the organization and quality of trauma care.[9,10]

Conclusion

The organization of a trauma system has four impact pillars: organization of prehospital care facilities, hospital networking, communication systems, and organization of in-hospital care (acute care and definitive care). An integrated approach is required at all levels: human resources (staffing and training), physical resources (infrastructure, equipment, and supplies), and process (organization and administration). Compared to the Western world, trauma care services in India lack each of these elements. Most of the physical resources for in-hospital care in terms of infrastructure and equipment are already available at secondary and tertiary care hospitals and need only moderate upgrades.[7] Therefore, the areas where greatest focus is needed in the field of trauma services are as follows:

1. Provide physical resources for prehospital care and communication systems.
2. Provide well-trained staff at all levels of care, from prehospital to definitive trauma care and rehabilitation. Providers should be well-trained and should understand the critical needs of a trauma victim. Skill-based training programs for doctors as well as paramedical staff in acute life support (ALS) procedures are needed.
3. Organize and integrate prehospital services with definitive care facilities (hospital) so that a patient is shifted to an appropriate facility in the shortest possible time.

References

1. Puvanachandra P, Hyder AA. The burden of traumatic brain injury in Asia: a call for research. *Pak J Neurol Sci.* 2009;4(1):27–32.
2. Abhijit Das, Botticello AL, Wylie GR, Radhakrishnan K. Neurologic disability: a hidden epidemic for India. *Neurology.* 2013;81(1):97.

3. Wani AA, Ramzan AU, Tariq R, Kirmani AR, Bhat AR. Head injury in children due to cricket ball scenario in developing countries. *Pediatr Neurosurg.* 2008;44(3):204–207.

4. Bhatoe HS. Preventing head injury: a project tiger for neurosciences. *Ind J Neurotrauma.* 2005;2(2):63–65.

5. Mohan D, Tiwari G, Bhalla K. *Road Safety in India Status Report.* Transportation Research and Injury Prevention Programme. 2016 accessed July 18, 2018. tripp.iitd.ernet.in/assets/publication/road_safety_in_India_StatusReport1.pdf

6. Peden M, Scurfield R, Sleet D, Mohan D, Hyder AA, Jarawan E, Mathers C. World Report on Road Traffic Injury Prevention. *World Health Organization,* 2004. ISBN 92-4-156260-9. www.who.int/violence_injury_prevention/publications/road_traffic/world_report/en/ pp 1-201.

7. Lakesh Kumar Anand, Manpreet Singh, Dheeraj Kapoor. Prehospital trauma care services in developing countries. *Anaesth Pain Intensive Care.* 2013;17(1) 65–70.

8. Gentleman D. Improving outcome after traumatic brain injury—progress and challenges. *Br Med Bull.* 1999;55(4):910–926.

9. Gupta A, Gupta E. Challenges in organizing trauma care systems in India. *Ind J Comm Med.* 2009;34(1):75–76.

10. Prusty GK, Gururaj G, Dey KK. Neurotrauma: an emerging epidemic in low- and middle-income countries. In: Morganti-Kossman C, Raghupathi R, Mass A, eds. *Traumatic Brain and Spinal Cord Injury.* Cambridge University Press; 2012:17–29. Cambridge, UK.

Chronic TBI in Veterans and Service Members: Clinical Assessment, Interventions, and Differentiation from PTSD

Harvey S. Levin, Randall S. Scheibel, Maya Troyanskaya, Karin Thompson, and Helene Henson

13

Traumatic brain injury (TBI) is one of the most frequent types of injury sustained by active duty service members during Operation Enduring Freedom (OEF), Operation Iraqi Freedom (OIF), and Operation New Dawn (OND). Since 2000, 12–23% of OEF/OIF/OND service members sustained a TBI[1]; the Armed Forces Health Surveillance Branch has recorded 379,519 cases of TBI in service members worldwide over this time period, including 312,495 cases of mild TBI which constitute 82.3% of the total number (Defense and Veterans Brain Injury Center, February14, 20168).[2] In deployment-related TBI during OEF/OIF and OND, an explosive device causing blast-related injury was involved in 79% of the TBI cases.[3] However, most TBIs sustained by service members are not combat-related; training and off-duty injuries such as motor vehicle crashes and falls account for most of the TBIs sustained by service members. Moreover, blast-related TBI typically involves concomitant non-blast mechanisms. This chapter provides an overview of the chronic effects of TBI in service members and veterans, including clinical assessment, brain imaging, and treatment strategies currently employed by the Veterans Health Administration (VHA). We also discuss the overlapping and distinctive features of TBI as compared with posttraumatic stress disorder (PTSD).

Subacute Versus Chronic Effects of mTBI

Clinical management of acute mTBI in active duty service members has evolved to emphasize rest followed by progressive return to activities, a regimen which ensures return to duty in the majority of cases.[1] In contrast to the typical trajectory of resolving symptoms and improving cognitive performance during the initial days to months after mTBI in civilians, comorbidities such as PTSD and depression often develop and intensify over time following combat-related mTBI. Comorbid PTSD was diagnosed by self-report measures in 43.9% of service members who indicated at 3 to 4 months post-deployment that they had sustained mTBI associated with loss of consciousness.[4] One of the few prospective longitudinal studies found no differences in the percent of disability at 6–12 months between blast + impact (77%) and non-blast TBI (79%) cohorts who were medically evacuated ostensibly for polytrauma.[5] Comorbid PTSD at follow-up was present in 41.5% and 48.3% of these cohorts, respectively.

Large prospective studies and critical reviews of the literature on chronic, post-deployment morbidity have concluded that the chronic effects of deployment-related mTBI on persistent symptoms and poor cognitive performance in veterans are mitigated after statistically adjusting for comorbid PTSD, depression, and other comorbidities.[1,6] In contrast, the effects of PTSD on persistent symptoms and poor cognitive performance in veterans are robust even after statistically adjusting for mTBI.

Assessing the Chronic Effects of mTBI in Veterans

Evaluating the chronic effects of TBI in returning veterans presents unique challenges: (1) the assessment typically takes place months, sometimes years, after injury; (2) due to the predominantly mild character of injuries, medical records completed right after the incident may be unavailable, necessitating reliance on self-report; (3) repetitive mTBIs, which are frequent in blast-related injuries, might have cumulative effects but could be difficult for the veteran to accurately recall, and repetitive injuries might also be associated with repetitive subconcussive head impacts, prolonged exposure to combat, and other stressful events that contribute to the development of PTSD; (4) multiple deployments; (5) ongoing comorbid psychiatric conditions; and (6) financial incentives for reporting symptoms and deficits. In summary, it is often difficult for the veteran and the clinician to pinpoint a specific concussive event as the cause of chronic sequelae.

To improve diagnosis and provide adequate services, in 2007, the VHA implemented a policy requiring TBI screening for all individuals who were deployed as part of OEF/OIF/OND, and a clinical reminder was added to the VA computerized medical record system.[7] Since that time, the TBI clinical reminder used the Brief Traumatic Brain Injury Screen[8] which consists of four questions; answering "yes" to all four questions triggered a second-level evaluation with a TBI specialist such as a physiatrist or neurologist and included deployment history (e.g., blast and non-blast incidents), lifetime history of any injuries, and physical examination. In addition, veterans seen for the second-level evaluation are asked to fill out the Neurobehavioral Symptom Inventory (NSI),[9] PTSD Checklist—Civilian Version (PCL-C),[10] and the Participation Index (M2PI) of the Mayo-Portland Adaptability Inventory (MPAI).[11] The outcome of the evaluation determines future steps in the patient's care. Despite concerns[4,12] and challenges[13] regarding its validity and reliability, the post-deployment TBI assessment system has proved to be a valuable tool in veterans' care. Persistence of postconcussive symptoms (PCS) in the somatic (e.g., headache, dizziness), cognitive (e.g., poor memory, reduced concentration), and emotional (e.g., depression, anxiety) domains for months following an mTBI is often referred to as "postconcussion syndrome." However, the usefulness of this diagnosis (ICD-10) has been questioned because the symptoms are subjective, nonspecific, and often not causally linked to functional deficits or objective findings such as imaging or other diagnostic tests.

Validity of Clinical Assessment Data

The use of performance validity tests (PVT) and symptom validity tests (SVT)[14] is common practice in the assessment of recently deployed service personnel and veterans, especially those with a history of mTBI and comorbid conditions. Since clinicians and researchers have to rely on self-report years after an injury, it is imperative to use both the PVT and SVT measures.

In general, the PVT and SVT failure rates in this population are much higher compared to civilians with a history of mTBI[15] with some groups reporting PVT failure rates as high as 58%[16] and others as low as 4–9%.[17] These differences are most likely due to research setting and enrollment of participants who are not actively seeking treatment or compensation. In addition, individuals with mTBI and comorbid PTSD were more likely to fail the measures of PVT and SVT.[18]

Role of Neuroimaging

Neuroimaging with computerized tomography (CT) and clinical magnetic resonance imaging (MRI) does not currently contribute to the differential diagnosis of PTSD and the chronic effects of mTBI (including posttraumatic syndrome) in the VHA. According to the VA/DoD clinical practice guideline,[19] the criteria for mTBI require normal structural imaging while the diagnosis of PTSD depends on exposure to psychologically traumatic events or stressors[20] that are often associated with combat. Functional neuroimaging and other advanced research methods have characterized neurobiological mechanisms that may underlie TBI and PTSD and have provided insights into why their clinical presentation is often similar.[21,22] However, these advances in research have not yet been applied to clinical management in the VHA or in civilian practice.

Neurobiological Model of PTSD

As noted in an earlier section, PTSD is a frequent comorbidity of deployment related mTBI. Consequently, the neurobiology of PTSD and its relation to TBI is relevant to clinicians and researchers. Preclinical research and functional neuroimaging studies using trauma- or fear-related stimuli support a neurobiological model of PTSD that includes dysfunction within the brain's fear circuitry, including structures such as the amygdala, ventromedial prefrontal cortex, insula, and hippocampus.[23,24] The amygdala has often been reported to be overactive or hyperreactive in response to fear-invoking stimuli in individuals with PTSD, while the ventromedial prefrontal cortex is hypoactive.[25] When considered in combination, these findings are major contributors to a model of PTSD in which the medial prefrontal cortex is unable to exert sufficient top-down inhibitory control over a hyperactive amygdala, leading to exaggerated fear responses and chronic stress.[24,25]

Pathophysiology of TBI

The structures and connections of the frontal and limbic regions are also among the tissues that have been said to be most vulnerable to TBI due to impact and inertial forces.[22,26,27] Findings from numerous studies, most of which have been conducted in civilian samples with moderate to severe TBI due to blunt head trauma, are consistent with a mixed and highly heterogeneous neuropathology that may include multifocal or diffuse axonal injury, as well as focal lesions such as contusions and lacerations.[28] Secondary injury may also occur as a result of edema, herniation, hemorrhage, ischemia, inflammation, and excitotoxic processes.[26,28] The distribution of focal lesions has been reported to favor anterior brain structures within the frontal and temporal lobes, while axonal injury often occurs within the frontal white matter and long fiber tracts.[26–28] Neuroimaging research with mTBI, again mostly with blunt impact injury and acceleration-deceleration injury in civilians, has been less consistent in revealing signs of diffuse axonal injury and other structural neuropathology.[27,29] However, there is evidence that tissue volume loss and white matter hyperintensities can occur with mTBI, and, as with more severe injuries, these pathological changes may also follow a rostrocaudal gradient that favors the frontal lobes and limbic structures such as the hippocampus.[27,30,31]

Brain Imaging Findings in Combat-Related TBI

Whether similar types of neuropathology occur regularly with combat-related mTBI, including that associated with blast, is currently an area of intense investigation (see Wilde et al. for a review[31]). Anecdotally, small white matter hyperintensities and hemosiderin deposits have been observed in veterans and service members who had sustained combat-related injuries.[31] If research confirms the presence of such pathology with an anatomical pattern similar to that found with civilian TBI, then this may explain some of the symptom overlap between PTSD and persistent PCS.[22] So far, no formal studies have specifically addressed this aspect of combat-related mTBI, and those using various forms of diffusion imaging have provided mixed findings, including some negative results[32,33] and others which are generally consistent with diffuse white matter injury,[34,35] heterogeneous and spatially dispersed focal areas of decreased white matter integrity,[33,36] or injury to vulnerable areas such as the orbitofrontal white matter, cingulum bundle, and cerebellar peduncles.[37] These inconsistent results likely reflect heterogeneity in the neuropathology produced by combat-related mTBI, as well as different post-deployment subject samples and methodology.

There is still the possibility that advanced neuroimaging techniques may be able to describe the neuropathological mechanisms associated with PTSD and persistent PCS, and, ultimately, this research may contribute to the development of tools for differential diagnosis.[21] Using high field strength (i.e., 7 Tesla) magnetic resonance spectroscopy in military personnel after mTBI, Hetherington and colleagues[38] found a decrease in hippocampal N-acetyl aspartate (NAA) to creatine and NAA to choline ratios similar to those previously reported in civilian TBI. These differences appear to be specific for the brain injury since they were not related to the presence of PTSD, anxiety, depression, or alcohol dependence.

Functional neuroimaging studies using cognitive tasks have also started to report differences between PTSD and TBI.[39,40] A common finding in civilian TBI is greater and more extensive activation during task conditions placing demands upon working memory, cognitive control, and other executive functions.[41–43] Veterans and service members with a history of blast-related mTBI have been found to exhibit a similar hyperactivation pattern during cognitive control (e.g., tasks involving stimulus–response conflict, cognitive interference, or inhibition), including increases within the anterior cingulate gyrus, medial frontal cortex, and posterior cerebral areas (Figures 13.1A and 13.1B).[39] However, those who had not experienced TBI or blast exposure during deployment but had elevated posttraumatic stress symptoms (PTSS) at the time of the study were found to have extensive deactivation while engaging cognitive control, and there was also a negative correlation between PTSS and activation within several cortical association areas, including the dorsolateral prefrontal cortex.[40] In

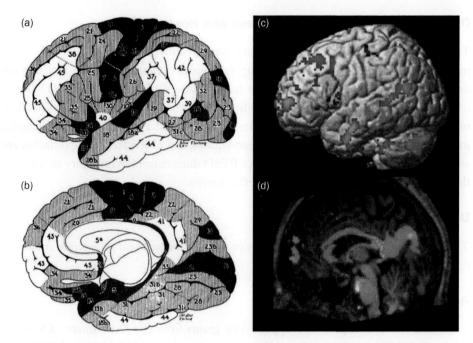

Figure 13.1 During cognitive control, increasing posttraumatic stress symptoms (PTSS) are associated with an activation shift away from complex, late-maturing cortical areas to those that develop earlier. (A) Lateral view of the brain showing the developmental order of myelination (i.e., myelinogenesis) with cortical areas that undergo late maturation indicated in white. (B) Medial view depicting the cortical myelination pattern. (C) Lateral view of a surface-rendered image showing the correlation pattern for Arrows Task cognitive control activation with PTSS. Areas with a positive correlation are displayed using a red–yellow scale, while those with a negative correlation are in blue–green. (D) The correlation of Arrows Task activation with PTSS in medial view.

A is from G. Bonin, *Essay on the Cerebral Cortex*, 1950, Charles C. Thomas Publisher, Springfield, IL; B is from Scheibel et al., *Brain Imaging and Behavior*, 2015. Reproduced with permission from the publisher.

contrast, more severe PTSS was associated with increased activation within a number of different structures, including the somatomotor cortex, insula, and basal ganglia (Figures 13.1C and 13.1D). Other studies of PTSD and PTSS have also found altered activation during cognitive tasks, including decreased activation within brain structures involved in executive functions,[44–46] and some investigators have suggested that such changes may reflect a bias favoring bottom-up over top-down processing that is related to increased noradrenergic activity.[40,44,47] Results from additional functional neuroimaging research of this type may support a modified model of PTSD neurobiology that includes more extensive cortical dysfunction, provides a better description of differences in the neuropathology associated with PTSD and persistent PCS due to mTBI, and contributes to the development of new tools for differential diagnosis and to monitor treatment effects.

Directions for Clinical Management and Research

The trend in the VHA is toward symptomatic treatment of the chronic effects of mTBI and comorbid PTSD, emphasizing functional outcomes without focusing on differentiating the contributions of these mechanisms. With evidence that PTSD and depression contribute more toward disability and morbidity than the chronic effects of mTBI, therapies to treat these comorbidities are emphasized. However, advanced imaging studies, preclinical research, behavioral interventions, and pharmacologic approaches are continuing to elucidate the mechanisms of PTSD distinct from brain injury to improve the accuracy of diagnosis and treatment effectiveness.

Disclaimer

The contents do not represent the views of the US Department of Veterans Affairs or the United States Government.

Acknowledgments

Preparation of this chapter was supported by grants from the Department of Veterans Affairs, Rehabilitation Research and Development Service (B1320-I), "An fMRI Study of Deployment-Related TBI in Veterans and Service Members and a Longitudinal Study of Chronic TBI in OEF/OIF/OND Veterans and Service Members." We are grateful to English Pratts and to Rhonda O'Donovan for editorial assistance.

References

1. O'Neil ME, Carlson KF, Storzbach D, et al. Factors associated with mild traumatic brain injury in veterans and military personnel: a systematic review. *J Int Neuropsychol Soc.* 2014;(20):249–261.

2. (Defense and Veterans Brain Injury Center, February 14, 2018).

3. Owens BD, Kragh JF, Wenke JC, Macaitis J, Wade CE, Holcomb JB. Combat wounds in operation Iraqi Freedom and Operation Enduring Freedom. *J Trauma.* 2008;(64):295–299.

4. Hoge CW, McGurk D, Thomas JL, Cox AL, Engel CC, Castro CA. Mild traumatic brain injury in US soldiers returning from Iraq. *N Engl J Med.* 2008;358(5):453–463.

5. MacDonald CL, Johnson AM, Wierzechowski L, et al. Prospectively assessment clinical outcomes in concussive blast vs nonblast traumatic brain injury among evacuated US military personnel. *JAMA Neurology.* 2014;(71)8:994–1002.

6. Vasterling JJ, Brailey K, Proctor SP, Kane R, Heeren T, Franz M. Neuropsychological outcomes of mild traumatic brain injury, post-traumatic stress disorder and depression in Iraq-deployed US Army soldiers. *Br J Psychiatry.* 2012;(201):186–192. doi:10.1192/bjp.bp.111.096461.

7. Department of Veterans Affairs and Department of Defense. VA/DOD clinical practice guideline for the management of concussion/mild traumatic brain injury. http://www.healthquality.va.gov/mtbi/concussion.

8. Schwab KA, Ivins B, Cramer G, et al. Screening for traumatic brain injury in troops returning from deployment in Afghanistan and Iraq: initial investigation of the usefulness of a short screening tool for traumatic brain injury. *J Head Trauma Rehabil.* 2007;22(6):377–389. PMID:18025970.

9. Cicerone K, Kalmar K. Persistent post-concussive syndrome: structure of subjective complaints after mild traumatic brain injury. *J Head Trauma Rehabil.* 1995;10:1–17.

10. Dobie DJ, Kivlahan DR, Maynard C, et al. Screening for post-traumatic stress disorder in female Veteran's Affairs patients: validation of the PTSD checklist. *Gen Hosp Psychiatry*. 2002;24(6): 367–374.

11. Malec J. The Mayo-Portland adaptability inventory. The Center for Outcome Measurement in Brain Injury. http://www.tbims.org/combi/mpai Published 2005. Accessed December 10, 2016.

12. Belanger HG, Uomoto JM, Vanderploeg RD. The Veterans Health Administration's (VHA's) Polytrauma System of Care for mild traumatic brain injury: costs, benefits, and controversies. *J Head Trauma Rehabil*. 2009;24(1):4–13.

13. Iverson GL, Langlois JA, McCrea MA, Kelly JP. Challenges associated with post-deployment screening for mild traumatic brain injury in military personnel. *Clin Neuropsychol*. 2009;23(8):1299–1314.

14. Larrabee GJ. Performance validity and symptom validity in neuropsychological assessment. *J Int Neuropsychol Soc*. 2012;18:625.

15. Gfeller JD, Roskos PT. A comparison of insufficient effort rates, neuropsychological functioning, and neuropsychiatric symptom reporting in military veterans and civilians with chronic traumatic brain injury. *Behav Sci Law*. 2013;31:833–849.

16. Armistead-Jehle P. Symptom validity test performance in US veterans referred for evaluation of mild TBI. *Appl Neuropsychol*. 2010;17: 52–59.

17. Clark AL, Amick MM, Fortier C, Milberg WP, McGlinchey RE. Poor performance validity predicts clinical characteristics and cognitive test performance of OEF/OIF/OND veterans in a research setting. *Clin Neuropsychol*. 2014;28:802–825.

18. Greiffenstein MF, Baker WJ. Validity testing in dually diagnosed post-traumatic stress disorder and mild closed head injury. *Clin Neuropsychol*. 2008;22:565–582.

19. Management of Concussion-Mild Traumatic Brain Injury Working Group. *VA/DoD Clinical Practice Guideline for the Management of Concussion-Mild Traumatic Brain Injury*. Version 2.0. Washington, DC: Veterans Health Administration and Department of Defense; 2016.

20. American Psychiatric Association. *Diagnostic and Statistical Manual of Mental Disorders*. 5th ed. Washington, DC: American Psychiatric Association.

21. Brenner LA. Neuropsychological and neuroimaging findings in traumatic brain injury and post-traumatic stress disorder. *Dial Clin Neurosci*. 2011;12(3):311–323.

22. Stein MB, McAllister TW. Exploring the convergence of posttraumatic stress disorder and mild traumatic brain injury. *Am J Psychiatry*. 2009;166:768–776.

23. Bremner JD. Neuroimaging in posttraumatic stress disorder and other stress-related disorders. *Neuroimaging Clin N Am*. 2007;17(4):523–538.

24. Shin LM, Handwerger K. Is posttraumatic stress disorder a stress-induced fear circuitry disorder? *J Trauma Stress*. 2009;22(5):409–415.

25. Francati V, Vermetten E, Bremner JD. Functional neuroimaging studies in posttraumatic stress disorder: review of current methods and findings. *Depress Anxiety*. 2007;24:202–218.

26. Bigler ED. Traumatic brain injury, neuroimaging, and neurodegeneration. *Front Human Neurosci*. 2013;7:395. doi:10.3389/fnhum.2013.00395.

27. Levine B, Kovacevic N, Nica EI, et al. The Toronto traumatic brain injury study: injury severity and quantified MRI. *Neurology*. 2008;70:771–778.

28. Povlishock JT, Katz DI. Update of neuropathology and neurological recovery after traumatic brain injury. *J Head Trauma Rehabil*. 2005;20(1):76–94.

29. Tate DF, Wade BSC, Velez CS, et al. Volumetric and shape analyses of subcortical structures in United States service members with mild traumatic brain injury. *J Neurol.* 2016;263:2065–2079.

30. Levin HS, Williams DH, Eisenberg HM, High WM, Guinto FC. Serial MRI and neurobehavioral findings after mild to moderate closed head injury. *J Neurol Neurosurg Psychiatry.* 1992;55:255–262.

31. Wilde EA, Bouix S, Tate DF, et al. Advanced neuroimaging applied to veterans and service personnel with traumatic brain injury: state of the art and potential benefits. *Brain Imaging Behav.* 2015;9:367–402.

32. Levin HS, Wilde E, Troyanskaya M, et al. Diffusion tensor imaging of mild to moderate blast-related traumatic brain injury and its sequelae. *J Neurotrauma.* 2010;27(4):683–694. doi:10.1089/neu.2009.1073.

33. Jorge RE, Acion L, White T, et al. White matter abnormalities in veterans with mild traumatic brain injury. *Am J Psychiatry.* 2012;169(12):1284–1291. doi:10.1176/appi.ajp.2012.12050600.

34. Davenport ND, Lim KO, Armstrong MT, Sponheim SR. Diffuse and spatially variable white matter disruptions are associated with blast-related mild traumatic brain injury. *NeuroImage.* 2012;59(3):2017–2024. doi:10.1016/j.neuroimage.2011.10.050.

35. Morey RA, Haswell CC, Selgrade ES, et al. Effects of chronic mild traumatic brain injury on white matter integrity in Iraq and Afghanistan war veterans. *Hum Brain Mapp.* 2013;34(11):2986–2999. doi:10.1002/hbm.22117.

36. Taber KH, Hurley RA, Haswell CC, et al. White matter compromise in veterans exposed to primary blast forces. *J Head Trauma Rehabil.* 2015;30(1):E15–E25. doi:10.1097/HTR.0000000000000030.

37. MacDonald CL, Johnson AM, Cooper D, et al. Detection of blast-related traumatic brain injury in US military personnel. *N Engl J Med.* 2011;364(22):2091–2100. doi:10.1056/NEJMoa1008069.

38. Hetherington HP, Hamid H, Kulas J, et al. MRSI of the medial temporal lobe at 7 T in explosive blast mild traumatic brain injury. *Magn Reson Med.* 2014;71(4):1358–1367. doi:10.1002/mrm.24814.

39. Scheibel RS, Newsome MR, Troyanskaya M, et al. Altered brain activation in military personnel with one or more traumatic brain injuries following blast. *J Int Neuropscyhol Soc.* 2012;18(1):89–100.

40. Scheibel RS, Pastorek NJ, Troyanskaya M, et al. The suppression of brain activation in post-deployment military personnel with posttraumatic stress symptoms. *Brain Imaging Behav.* 2015;9:513–526.

41. Scheibel RS, Newsome MR, Troyanskaya M, et al. Effects of severity of traumatic brain injury and brain reserve on cognitive-control related brain activation. *J Neurotrauma.* 2009;26:1447–1461.

42. Hillary FG. Neuroimaging of working memory dysfunction and the dilemma with brain reorganization hypotheses. *J Int Neuropsychol Soc.* 2008;14:526–534.

43. Maruishi M, Miyatani M, Nakao T, Muranaka H. Compensatory cortical activation during performance of an attention task by patients with diffuse axonal injury: a functional magnetic resonance imaging study. *J Neurol Neurosurg Psychiatry.* 2007;78:168–173.

44. Falconer E, Bryant R, Felmingham KL, et al. The neural networks of inhibitory control in posttraumatic stress disorder. *J Psychiatr Neurosci.* 2008;33(5):413–422.

45. Hayes PH, LaBar KS, Petty CM, McCarthy G, Morey RA. Alterations in the neural circuitry for emotion and attention associated with posttraumatic stress symptomatology. *Psychiatr Res Neuroimag*. 2009;172:7–15.

46. Morey RA, Petty CM, Cooper DA, LaBar KS, McCarthy G. Neural systems for executive and emotional processing are modulated by symptoms of posttraumatic stress disorder in Iraq War veterans. *Psychiatry Res*. 2008;162:59–72.

47. Heilman KM, Nadeau SE, Beversdorf DO. Creative innovation: possible brain mechanisms. *Neurocase*. 2003;9(5):369–379.

Chemosensory Impairment After Traumatic Brain Injury

Shanna Williams and Nathan Zasler

14

Introduction

Posttraumatic olfactory and gustatory impairments following traumatic brain injury (TBI) are more common than many clinicians appreciate and have a variety of different causes. It is important to fully assess this class of posttraumatic impairments due to the implications of such sensory loss on daily life functions that we otherwise take for granted. Additionally, smell loss in and of itself may be an indicator of dysexecutive impairments and/or a risk marker for anterior parenchymal contusional injury. Such impairments may impede vocational pursuits, produce work and home safety risks, and impede hedonistic appreciation of various normal life experiences.[1] There are assessment and management strategies for chemosensory impairments in both the acute and long-term care settings that all clinicians treating persons with TBI should be aware of. Proper early education, including prognosis information, is critical to provide to the patient affected by these types of sensory losses. Medicolegal aspects of assessing impairment and disability secondary to chemosensory impairment are often an issue in litigated cases involving TBI, and it is therefore important for clinicians to understand the nuances of these issues.

Olfaction

Overview

Posttraumatic sensory system impairment has the potential to adversely impact our sense of safety, ability to perform an assortment of routine daily tasks, and one's perception of normalcy. In 2013, the National Institute on Deafness and Other Communication Disorders (NIDCD) cited that more than 200,000 people report chemosensory problems every year, with 1–2% of the North American population reporting smell difficulties.[2]

Approximately 1.7 million individuals suffer a TBI each year, with an estimated 20% presenting with olfactory dysfunction.[3,4] Schofield, Moore, and Gardner (2014) found that the incidence of olfactory dysfunction ranged from 20% to 61% depending on the severity of brain injury, with other studies noting a higher incidence following injuries to the occipital lobe.[5,6] Fortin, Lefebvre, and Ptito (2010) noted that 40–44% of TBI survivors had olfactory dysfunction that they were unaware of.[7] In a recent systematic review, it was noted that patients with mild TBI had a relatively high prevalence of olfactory dysfunction; however, it was frequently underdiagnosed.[8]

Olfactory impairment after TBI may be quantitative or qualitative in nature. Absence of smell is referred to as anosmia, whereas decreased smell is referred to as hyposmia, and altered perception is known as dysosmia. Phantosmias are the perception of smell in the absence of an odor stimulus, parosmia is a distorted perception of an actual odor, and cacosmia is an unpleasant, sometimes foul-smelling odor.[6]

Anatomy

Although olfactory dysfunction after TBI may occur due to injury to frontotemporal smell centers, it can also occur due to injuries involving the sinonasal tract or destruction of olfactory nerve filaments via tearing or shearing.[9] The neural process of olfaction is initiated with a multitude of smell receptors located within the mucous membranes of the nasal passages detecting the odor stimulant and signaling to the olfactory bulb for processing. From the olfactory bulb, physiological signals are then delivered to the different olfactory areas of the brain for odor identification and memorization, emotional processing, and determination of response to the stimulus.[10] The olfactory neuromatrix is complex and can be affected on multiple levels by TBI-related injury (Table 14.1).

Examination

Although chemosensory impairment is a common sequelae of TBI, its functional consequences are often not adequately appreciated by practitioners, patients, and/or caregivers. Establishment of consistent procedures for evaluation could facilitate identification of impairment sooner and promote earlier treatment and adequate differential

Table 14.1:
Olfactory neuromatrix[9]

Olfactory Function	Area(s) of Brain
Primary olfactory center	Pyriform, amygdalar, periamygdalar and enterorhinal cortices
Secondary olfactory center	Orbitofrontal cortex (via the mediodorsal nucleus of the thalamus)
Identification of odor intensity, responsiveness to aversive stimuli, controls feeding behaviors through integration of olfactory and neuroendocrine stimuli, emotional memories, unconscious emotional signal recognition	Amygdala (with secondary connections to the hypothalamus)
Controls long-term memory, responses to stress, and contextualizes emotional experiences	Hippocampus
Activated with pleasant and unpleasant odor stimuli, integrates body sensations for emotional status of person, houses primary taste centers	Insula
Activated by olfactory stimulations, underlies emotional proportions of pain	Anterior cingulate cortex (aka limbic lobe)
Odor identification	Anterior insular cortex

diagnosis of the condition, as well as better adjustment and quality of life for those affected. The presence of anosmia has historically been associated as a marker of dysexecutive impairment,[11,12] although recent research has brought this relationship into question.[13] Regardless, olfactory testing should always be formally assessed as part of the neurological exam after any TBI due to its potential functional and injury pathology implications. Ideally, standardized olfactory assessments should be used to determine the presence of olfactory impairment even in the absence of olfactory complaints. Olfactory screening should include basic questions to alert the professional to warning signs of olfactory dysfunction and the need for more in-depth testing. Questions should not only target any perceived changes in one's sense of smell, but also in the sense of taste (as loss of smell often subjectively presents as perceived loss of taste), changes in food preferences and appetite, changes in libido, and impact on quality of life including safety. The patient's ability to cope with his or her impairment and any associated secondary affective responses should also be explored. The patient should be asked to elaborate on whether the loss is complete or partial, constant or intermittent, for all odors or only some, experienced by a sudden or gradual onset, and/or associated with cacosmia (i.e., smelling burning or fecal odors) among other questions (Note that the reporting of cacosmias may also indicate an underlying temporolimbic epileptic focus.) Generally, persons with posttraumatic anosmia retain the ability to detect trigeminal odor stimulants, but this should also be assessed.[14]

Determining the presence of other symptoms or conditions that may impact olfaction is also important. Assess any history of nasal stuffiness or obstruction, facial pain and headaches, allergies, substance abuse, neurodegenerative disorders (including family history), occupational and/or environmental exposures (including smoking), prior radiation therapy, previous operations, and medication use. Practitioners should be aware of olfactory side effects of medications such as adrenal corticosteroids, antithyroids, opiates, and cardiovascular or antihypertensive medications.[14–16] If smell dysfunction is a result of medication use, discontinuation of the medication does not necessarily guarantee improvements in the condition. Such information is important in guiding the examiner to identify warning signs of olfactory impairment and the need for further testing and imaging procedures in the pursuit of a diagnosis.

Once olfactory dysfunction is identified, further evaluations may be warranted. The medical professional treating the individual should conduct a thorough exam including the nose, ears, upper respiratory tract, head, and neck. Referral to an otolaryngologist may be warranted for a thorough examination of the olfactory neuroepithelium, nasal mucous membrane, and oral cavity. A thorough neurological examination should also be conducted on all cranial nerves and frontotemporal functions.[16]

Neuroradiological Assessment

To localize the site of injury responsible for olfactory loss, high-resolution imaging has been shown to be most revealing. Computed tomography (CT) showing the best resolution for structures in the sinonasal cavity, including both soft tissue and bony structures, with 1 mm or less cuts should be utilized to optimize results. If there is a desire to image small parenchymal lesions at the bone parenchyma interface, then magnetic resonance imaging (MRI) is the preferred test of choice as imaging of such areas as the olfactory bulb will otherwise be compromised by artifact and volume averaging if CT is used. Recent work has also shown that diffusion tensor imaging may be helpful in evidencing posttraumatic fiber pathway abnormalities consistent with injury and possibly shed light on recovery mechanisms.[17]

Clinical tests of chemosensory function are used to confirm patient complaints, quantify sensory deficits, and track changes in function over time. Such testing may be particularly helpful in impairment and disability evaluation and/or forensic assessments. Table 14.2 lists the better-known clinical chemosensory evaluation centers.[18–21]

There are various assessments used to test olfactory impairment, focusing primarily on odor identification and detection thresholds. Many of these assessments are available commercially, although only a small number of them have any research examining their utility in patients with TBI (Table 14.3).[7,22–24]

Management

As olfactory impairment is often a permanent change in chemosensory function following TBI, a comprehensive approach to treatment should include strategies to improve quality of life, safety, and coping. Practitioners should be aware of the impact smell impairment has on function and be able to provide basic compensatory strategies or make referrals to other professionals to assist the patient in managing his or her smell impairment. This approach should include strategies to alleviate the patient's concerns through education while assisting and promoting health, quality of life, and safety. Options for treating posttraumatic olfactory impairment should focus on management of symptomatology related to the injury. These may include the use of topical or oral corticosteroids, a combination of the two, or surgical interventions to correct structural damage to the nasal passages as a result of trauma depending on the etiology of the smell loss.[22,25,26] There is some early evidence that short-term (4 month) "olfactory training" increases identification abilities more so than discrimination abilities[27] and that such training may be effective in improving phenyl ethyl alcohol (PEA) thresholds in persons with traumatic anosmia.[28] There is also preclinical work suggesting that restoration of smell may be feasible through olfactory neuroepithelial transplantation surgery.[29]

Patients and caregivers may wish to consider therapy options for coping with the loss of smell as well as rehabilitative compensatory strategies. Consultations with a nutritionist should be considered for menu planning, healthy seasoning alternatives, and use of additional flavors and textures to compensate for diminished quality of taste that is normally perceived with anosmia.[9] A referral to an occupational therapist (OT) would be beneficial in identifying the impact olfactory dysfunction can have on the patient's daily activities, with treatment emphasizing compensatory strategies to encourage optimal performance within the patient's environment or occupational role.[30] OT focus should include but not be limited to activities of daily living (ADLs) with regards to hygiene, body odor, sexual activity, and consumption of nutritional and safe food options. Additional areas of intervention should address instrumental activities of daily living (IADLs) such as vigilance with food preparation and expiration dates, home management responsibilities, infant/child or family caregiving, and pet maintenance relative to hygiene. Specific interventions may involve changing clothes regularly and even on a schedule if memory impaired, use of "measured" cologne or perfume applications, and regular use of deodorants, as well as dietary measures such as using different spices,

Table 14.2:
Chemosensory evaluation centers

National Centers: Monell Chemical Senses Center 3500 Market St. Philadelphia, PA 19104-3308 Phone: 267-519-4700 General Information: mcsc@monell.org Website: www.monell.org Taste and Smell Disorder Clinic 1200 Lakeway Dr., Suite 8 Austin, TX 78734 Phone: 512-261-7909 and Fax: 512-402-9241 Website: http://www.tastesmell.com/

The Smell and Taste Treatment and Research Foundation, Ltd. 233 East Erie, Suite 712 Chicago, IL 60611 Phone: 888-381-8040 OR 847-274-2267 Foundation e-mail: dr.hirsch@smellandtaste.org Website: http://www.smellandtaste.org

The Taste and Smell Clinic for Molecular Nutrition and Sensory Disorders 5125 MacArthur Blvd., NW#20 Washington, DC 20016 Phone: 202-364-4180, Toll Free: 1-877-MYSMELL Email: Doc@TasteandSmell.com<mailto:Doc@TasteandSmell.com Website: http://www.tasteandsmell.com/

The University of Colorado Rocky Mountain Taste and Smell Center Website: www.uchealth.org/Pages/Services/Ear-Nose-and-Throat-ENT.aspx Locations:

Anschutz Medical Campus- Anschutz Outpatient Pavilion 1635 Aurora Ct. Aurora, CO 80045 Phone: 720-848-2820 Greeley 5881 W 16th Street, Suite F Greeley, CO 80634 Phone: 970-313-2700

Longmont 1925 W Mountain View Ave Longmont, CO 80501 Phone: 720-494-3120 Sterling 620 Iris Dr. Sterling, CO 80751 Phone: 970-313-2740 UC Gardner Neurosensory Disorders Center University of Cincinnati Medical Center 234 Goodman St. Cincinnati, OH 45219 Phone: 866-941-8264 Website: www.uchealth.com/neurosensory

UC San Diego Health Sinus and Nasal Dysfunction 200 W Arbor Dr. San Diego, CA 92103 Phone: 858-657-8590

University of Connecticut Taste and Smell Center 263 Farmington Ave Farmington, CT 06030-5311 Phone: 860-679-2000 (University of Connecticut Health Operator) OR 844-388-2666 (For Appointment) Website: http://uconntasteandsmell.uchc.edu

University of Florida Center for Smell and Taste PO Box 100127 Gainesville, FL 32610-0127 Phone: 352-294-5360 Email: ufcst@ufl.edu Website: www.cst.ufl.edu

University of Pennsylvania Smell and Taste Center 5 Ravdin Pavilion 3400 Spruce St. Philadelphia, PA 19104-4283 Phone: 215-662-2797 and Fax: 215-349-5266 Website: http://www.med.upenn.edu/stc/index.html

Virginia Commonwealth University Smell and Taste Disorders Clinic Phone: 804-628-4ENT (804-628-4368) Website: http://www.vcu.edu/ent/clinical/smelltaste/index.html Locations:

Colonial Heights 2035 Waterside Dr., Suite 100 Prince George, VA 23875 Nelson Clinic 401 N. 11th Street 7th floor, room 7-100 PO Box 980146 Richmond, VA 23298-0146 Phone: 804-628-4368 Stony Point 9109 Stony Point Dr., Suite 1200 Richmond, VA 23235

International Centers:

Canada: St. Paul's Sinus Center St. Paul's Hospital Foundation 178-1081 Burrard St. Vancouver, BCV6Z 1Y6 Phone: 604-682-8206 OR 800-720-2983

Germany: University Hospital Mannheim ENT Clinic Theodor-Kutzer-Ufer 1-3 68167 Mannheim, Germany Website: https://w2.umm.de/index.php?id=5300

University of Dresden Medical School

Interdisciplinary Center for Smelling and Tasting Fetscherstrasse 74 01307 Dresden, Germany Phone: +49 (0) 351 458 4189 Website: www.uniklinikum-dresden.de/hno/riechen

Greece: Smell and Taste Clinic Aristotle University Papageorgiou Ring Rd Thessaloniki, Greece Phone: 00302313323523 Mexico: Smell and Taste Clinic Hospital ABC Campus Santa Fe Consultorio 154 Phone: 1664 7078 OR 1664 7079 Email: gustoyolfayto@gmail.com Website: www.gustoyolacto.org OR www.otorrino.com.mx Switzerland:

University of Geneva Hospitals ENT/Head and Neck Surgery Rue Gabrielle-Perret-Gentil 4 1205 GENEVA, Building C, Level 3 Phone: 41-0-22-382-3423 and Fax: 41-0-22-372-8244 Email: Basile.Landis@hcuge.ch Website: www.hug-ge.ch/Rhinologie

United Kingdom: Rhinology Clinic at Freeman Hospital Freeman Hospital High Heaton Newcastle, NE7 7DW Phone: 0191 2137635

The Sinus Clinic at Royal Surrey County Hospital The Royal Surrey County Hospital Egerton Rd. Guildford, GU2 7XX Phone: 01483 571122

The Smell and Taste Clinic at Birmingham Queen Elizabeth Hospital Queen Elizabeth Medical Centre, Edg Baston Birmingham, B15 2TH Phone: 0121-627-2000 Website: www.uhb.nhs.uk/ent.htm

The Smell and Taste Clinic at James Paget Hospital James Paget University Hospital Gorleston Great Yarmouth, NR31 6LA Phone: 01493-452832 Website: www.uea.ac.uk/rhinology-group/smell-and-taste-disorders

Table 14.3:
Olfactory assessment instruments studied in persons with traumatic brain injury[7,17–19]

Name	Commercially Available (Yes/No)	Administration Time and Procedure	Company and Contact Info	Test–Retest Reliability	Malingering Cutoff
Alberta Smell Test (AST)	Yes. $12	Time: ~20–30 minutes Procedure: Use scented markers with authentic essences. Instruct subject to close eyes, present stimuli monorhinally in 10 trials. Subject is then presented a list of eight options from which to identify the odor. Scoring: Normal olfaction = ≥3 correct responses out of 10 per nostril.	Green's Publishing Dr. Paul Green drpgreen@ telus.net	N/A	2/20 or lower
University of Pennsylvania Smell & Taste Center Smell Test (UPSIT) aka Smell Identification Test (SIT)	Yes. $26.95 × 7 min.= $188.65 Price does not include administration, manual, or additional scoring keys.	Time: 15 minutes. Procedure: 40-item scratch-sniff, forced choice test. Scoring: Normal olfaction = 34–40 correct responses (males) and 35–40 (females), 6 categories of dysfunction: anosmia, severe hyposmia, moderate hyposmia, mild hyposmia, normosmia, and malingering	Sensonics. com- "Smell ID Test" Available in multiple languages and shorter versions	0.981	Score of 5/ 40 or lower

textures, and temperatures to make food more enticing. Safety measures might include assurance of smoke detectors in the home, use of smell detectors for personnel working around toxic substances, and/or restrictions from involvement with certain activities that, due to smell loss, would be unsafe or otherwise compromised in quality performance such as might occur with cooks, firefighters, chemists, nannies, and other professions.[1,31]

Prognosis

Although often considered irreversible, posttraumatic anosmia has been shown to have potential for improvement with time; typically, the prognosis for recovery declines as time post-injury increases. Varying degrees of spontaneous recovery are estimated to occur with one-third of individuals experiencing posttraumatic anosmia.[25] There are likely different mechanisms involved in early versus late recovery, with the former more related to resolution of acute swelling and inflammation and the latter more likely related to neural regenerative changes. Beyond 1 year post-injury, recovery of smell function is deemed to be atypical, although late cases of recovery have been reported.[6] On occasion, patients with anosmia may have aberrant or maladaptive neural regeneration leading to parosmias.[32]

Gustation

Overview

Gustatory impairment after TBI is a relatively rare occurrence on a neurogenic basis. From a functional standpoint, posttraumatic anosmia is the most common etiology of the subjective perception of reporting taste impairment after TBI. Patients will often report that their taste is impaired as a consequence of this phenomena due to the intimate networking of the smell and taste systems. Taste disorders are traditionally classified as either quantitative or qualitative, with the former including ageusia (loss of taste), hypogeusia (decreased taste), and dysgeusia (altered perception), and the latter including parageusia (distorted taste with an actual stimulus), phantogeusia (taste without an actual stimulus), and cacogeusia (unpleasant or foul taste).[6,33,34]

Anatomy

The anatomical pathway responsible for mediation of taste has its start at the level of the taste receptor cells of the tongue, which transmit information to the taste sensory neurons in the brainstem, which then relays information from the gustatory nucleus through cranial nerves VII, IX, and X to the somatosensory and frontal cortices, amygdala, and hypothalamus, as well as the hippocampus. These structures mediate conscious perception of taste, emotional quality of taste, and memories of taste, respectively.[35] Damage to structures in the pons and thalamus have also been shown to have the potential to adversely impact taste perception.[36,37]

Gustatory loss can be either conductive or neurosensory. Saliva serves as the primary vehicle for the taste receptors of the tongue and oropharyngeal mucosa to be activated by gustatory stimuli. Salivary function can be disrupted by trauma but is more commonly adversely affected by medications that may have anticholinergic or other mechanisms that lead to dry mouth and, as a consequence, have the potential to adversely impact gustation. Some of the offending agents that fall into this category include angiotensin converting enzyme (ACE) inhibitors, acetazolamide, certain antidepressants, antipsychotics, anticonvulsants, anticholinergic bladder medications, and opiates, among others.[34]

Neurosensory deficits can be due to cranial nerve injury to one of the three nerves mediating taste function, specifically cranial nerves VII, IX, or X. These types of injuries, aside from peripheral cranial nerve VII injuries, are very uncommon and generally inconsequential to taste function due to the aforementioned redundancy in the taste system innervation that occurs secondary to bilateral innervation to the tongue. The ninth and tenth cranial nerves are deep and less prone to injury than superficial nerves like the seventh cranial nerve, which can be injured in several places along its course and, in particular, is at high risk of traumatization with temporal bone fractures (about half of all cases). Longitudinal fractures result in facial nerve deficits in only a minority of cases.

The pathway for gustation involves a complex, integrated neuromatrix starting from the taste receptor cells on the tongue, where information is then transmitted via taste sensory neurons in the brainstem to the gustatory nucleus (brainstem taste relay cells) and on to the somatosensory and frontal cortex, amygdala, and hypothalamus, as well as the hippocampus. The cortical structures mediate conscious perception of taste, whereas the amygdala and hypothalamus mediate the emotional quality of taste and the hippocampus facilitates taste memories.[38]

Examination

For gustatory complaints in the absence of olfactory dysfunction, the oral cavity should be inspected for trauma to the tongue; findings consistent with impairment of cranial nerves V, VII, IX, or X; and the quantity and quality (viscosity, clarity, color) of saliva. Conditions that may be associated with dysgeusias include caries, infected tonsils, and the like. Facial nerve injury should be suspected with ipsilateral facial weakness and taste loss and/or a history of ear canal laceration or bony step-offs, Battle's sign, cerebrospinal fluid (CSF) otorrhea, or hemotympanum. Diagnostic testing may include use of various techniques including electromyography and nerve conduction studies, evoked and event-related potentials, and/or quantitative testing. Assessment of lacrimation and stapedial reflex response can assist in localizing the site of cranial nerve VII lesions.[4,39]

Quantitative testing of gustation is more challenging in the traditional hospital or outpatient clinic setting. This type of testing utilizes multiple dilutions of stimuli applied to different areas of the mouth and/or tongue (i.e., anterior two-thirds then posterior one-third of the tongue and/or to the whole mouth). The clinician evaluates both stimulant detection and identification to try to localize the area of impairment and the taste sensation that is impaired.[40]

Neuroradiological Assessment

Radiologic testing may be useful in assessing those rare cases that present with subjective complaints of taste loss. Acute CT may demonstrate parenchymal pathology associated with cortical or subcortical gustatory sensation processing. Two-plane high-resolution CT (HRCT) of the temporal bone may identify fractures through the course of the facial nerve (cranial nerve VII) or in the vicinity of cranial nerves IX and X at the jugular foramen. MRI is more sensitive at detecting smaller parenchymal abnormalities, but its role in assessing gustatory loss is probably limited. HRCT is capable of detecting bony abnormalities, obstructive lesions, or sinusitis, which represent the primary treatable causes of posttraumatic chemosensory disturbances, but the additional cost of MRI is seldom justified in this application. Functional imaging studies have mainly demonstrated frontal hypoperfusion in anosmic patients following TBI.[41]

Management

There are no currently accepted treatments for gustatory impairments that occur on a central basis following TBI. Peripheral injuries to the seventh cranial nerve may be amenable to surgical approaches such as decompression surgery or reconstruction in the acute post-injury period (the latter if there is traumatic severing of the nerve).[42] If facial nerve injury involves edema or inflammation, then steroids will typically be employed. Reversible causes for taste impairment should be explored including medications that may adversely affect salivary transmission of taste stimuli and/or medications that produce dysgeusias.[6]

Appropriate patient education is important as gustatory impairment can have substantive ramifications on an individual's quality of life in terms of both health and safety. Patients may compensate for taste loss by increasing the saltiness or spiciness of their food, sometimes to the point of excess or contraindication in terms of other medical comorbid conditions (i.e., hypertension, reflux, gastritis). Taste impairment may also impact choice of foods and may have negative ramifications on food preparation abilities. Based on the these issues, dietary assessment is crucial with any type of chemosensory loss.[43] Appropriate rehabilitative compensatory strategies including careful use of seasonings, salt substitutes, and spices, as well as recommendations for integrating different food textures and temperatures into ones' eating habits to help improve the hedonistic aspects of eating. As far as meal preparation is concerned, patients with dysgeusia or, in extreme cases, ageusia should be instructed to strictly follow recipes and not rely on their own taste functions to prepare meals. Strict use of food labeling to avoid eating spoiled foods should be encouraged, although if smell function is intact this becomes less of a challenge.

Prognosis

Surprisingly, recovery of posttraumatic taste impairment seems to occur more frequently than that associated with posttraumatic olfactory impairment. Posttraumatic taste impairments may have a delayed or immediate onset. Bitter sensation tends to be more affected than the other four (i.e., sweetness, sourness, saltiness, and umami). Aberrant neuronal regeneration may lead to parageusias. The small existing literature on this topic suggests that recovery tends to occur over the first few months post-injury and that different taste modalities recover at steroid rates with seventh cranial nerve sensations (i.e., sweetness) recovering faster than glossopharyngeal mediated taste sensation (i.e., bitterness).

Medicolegal Issues in Chemosensory Impairment

While seemingly minor compared with some other type of post-TBI impairments, chemosensory disturbances can have a considerable impact on a person's quality of life and functional abilities depending on their roles (both vocational and otherwise). The sixth edition of the American Medical Association (AMA) *Guides to Evaluation of Permanent Impairment* (GEPI) rates impairment from 1–5% of the whole person when there is partial or complete bilateral loss of either sense due to peripheral lesions. There is a greater emphasis in the latest edition of the GEPI on objective chemosensory testing when compared with prior versions.[44] There is not adequate discussion, however, of the need to assess symptom and performance validity in regards to any performed chemosensory assessment given the risk for symptom magnification in patients involved in processes that may be associated with secondary gain behaviors such as workers' compensation and personal injury litigation.[45]

The real-world impact of such deficits varies greatly with a patient's pursuits, whether vocational or avocational. Patients who work as cooks, firefighters, plumbers, chemists, nannies, and cosmeticians, among other occupations, may have significant difficulty resuming work after suffering posttraumatic chemosensory loss. Work clearance should also be gauged on the risks to the injured worker as well as to others, given the safety ramifications of such impairment.[1]

Conclusion

Chemosensory impairment is a common sequela of TBI, with olfactory impairment having a higher incidence than gustatory impairment. Therefore, it is important for practitioners to be aware of the incidence of chemosensory impairment within this population and the necessity for thorough assessment. Patients with impairment should be provided with therapeutic interventions to offer guidance and assistance with developing strategies for management and coping to improve life satisfaction and safety.

Chemosensory impairment may result in both anxiety and depression. Even when specific treatment does not exist to restore function, patient assessment may help educate both the patient and his or her family, as well as decrease secondary affective response to this type of loss. Patients and caregivers should be taught appropriate compensatory strategies for chemosensory impairments in all relevant environments in which they will be functioning and be encouraged to contact local resource centers for further treatment, guidance, and support. Organizations such as the Anosmia Foundation (http://www.anosmiafoundation.com/intro.shtml) and Fifth Sense (http://www.fifthsense.org.uk/about-fifth-sense/) can provide patients and families with information and support services.

Further prospective, randomized, and blinded research is needed to define the true incidence of olfactory and gustatory impairment after TBI, the etiology of said impairment, risk factors across the severity spectrum, and the best tests for assessment, as well as to examine the efficacy of management strategies, including both neuromedical and rehabilitative, in an effort to establish a systematic, functionally oriented, holistic approach to this class of impairments.

References

1. Santos DV, Reiter ER, DiNardo LJ, Costanzo RM. Hazardous events associated with impaired olfactory function. *Arch Otolaryngol Head Neck Surg.* 2004;130:317–319.

2. National Institute on Deafness and Other Communication Disorders article title- Smell Disorders Fact Sheet, NIH Pub. No. 09-3231, September 2013, Reprinted October 2014. https://www.nidcd.nih.gov/sites/default/files/Documents/health/smelltaste/NIDCD-Smell-Disorders.pdf. Accessed June 12, 2016.

3. Brain Injury Facts, Brain Injury Statistics, Brain Injury Association of America, http://biamo.org/Portals/0/BIAA%20Brain%20Injury%20Statistics%20Fact%20Sheet.pdf.

4. Reiter ER, Costanzo RM. Chemosensory impairment after traumatic brain injury: assessment and management. *Int Neurotrauma Lett.* 2012;23:3. http://www.ncbi.nlm.nih.gov/pmc/articles/PMC3798071/. Accessed June 20, 2016.

5. Schofield PW, Moore TM, Gardner A. Traumatic brain injury and olfaction: a systematic review. *Front Neurol.* 2014;5:5. doi:10.3389/fneur.2014.00005.

6. Costanzo RM, Reiter RJ, Yelverton JC. Smell and taste. In: Zasler ND, Katz DL, Zafonte RD, eds. *Brain Injury Medicine: Principles and Practice.* 2nd ed. New York: Demos Medical Publishing; 2013:794–808.

7. Fortin A, Lefebvre MB, Ptito M. Traumatic brain injury and olfactory deficits: the tale of two smell tests! *Brain Injury.* 2010;24(1):27–33. doi:10.3109/02699050903446815.

8. Proskynitopoulos PJ, Stippler M, Kasper EM. Posttraumatic anosmia. In patients with mild traumatic brain injury (mTBI): a systematic and illustrated review. *Surg Neurol Int.* 2016;7(suppl 10):S263–S275.

9. Costanzo RM, DiNardo LJ, Zasler ND. Head injury and olfaction. In: Doty RL, ed. *Handbook of Olfaction and Gustation.* New York: Marcel Dekker; 1995:493–502.

10. Soudry Y, Lemogne C, Malinvaud D, Consoli S-M, Bonfils P. Olfactory system and emotion: common substrates. *Eur Ann Otorhinolaryngol Head Neck Dis.* 2011;128(1):18–23. doi:10.1016/j.anorl.2010.09.007.

11. Roberts RJ, Sheehan W. Thurber S, et al. functional neuroimaging in posttraumatic olfactory impairment. *Indian J Psychol Med*. 2010;32(2):93–98.

12. Xydakis MS, Mulligan LP, Smith AB, et al. Olfactory impairment in traumatic brain injury in blast-induced combat troops: a cohort study. *Neurology*. 2015;84 (15)1559–1567.

13. Bakker K, Catroppa C, Anderson V. The relationship between olfactory dysfunction and executive function in children with traumatic brain injury. *J Clin Exp Neuropsychol*. 2017;39(9):876–889.

14. Duncan HJ, Smith DV. Clinical disorders of olfaction. In: Doty RL, ed. *Handbook of Olfaction and Gustation*. New York: Marcel Dekker; 1995:345–365.

15. Snow JB, Doty RL, Bartoshuk LM. Clinical Evaluation of Olfactory and Gustatory Disorders. In: Getchell TV, Doty RL, Bartoshuk LM, Snow JB, eds. *Smell and Taste in Health and Disease*. New York: Raven Press; 1991:463–467.

16. Wrobel BB, Leopold DA. Clinical assessment of patients with smell and taste disorders. *Otolaryngol Clin N Am*. 2004;37(6):1127–1142.

17. Bonanno L, Marino S, DeSalvo S, et al. role of diffusion tensor imaging in diagnosis and management of posttraumatic anosmia. *Brain Inj*. 2017;31(13-14):1964–1968.

18. NIDCD—Directory of Organizations. https://directory.nidcd.nih.gov/area.aspx?areatype=smelltopic. Accessed June 12, 2016.

19. Clinics—Fifth Sense. http://www.fifthsense.org.uk/smell-and-taste-clinics/. Accessed June 12, 2016.

20. OUTSIDE THE US—Barb Stuckey. http://barbstuckey.com/treatment_centers/outside-the-us/. Accessed June 12, 2016.

21. Research/Clinical Centers—Association for Chemoreception Sciences. http://www.achems.org/i4a/pages/Index.cfm?pageID=3342. Accessed June 12, 2016.

22. Kalogjera L, Dzepina D. Management of smell dysfunction. *Curr Allergy Asthma Rep*. 2012;12(2):154–162.

23. Scadding G, Hellings P, Alobid I, et al. Diagnostic tools in rhinology: EAACI position paper. *Clin Transl Allergy*. 2011;1:2. doi:10.1186/2045-7022-1-2.

24. Doty R, Shaman P, Kimmelman C, Dann M. University of Pennsylvania Smell Identification Test: a rapid quantitative olfactory function test for the clinic. *Laryngoscope*. 1984;94(Pt 2):176–178.

25. Coelho DH, Costanzo RM. Post-traumatic olfactory dysfunction. *Auris Nasus Larynx*. 2016;43(2):137–143.

26. Jiang RS, Wu SH, Liang KL, et al. Steroid treatment for posttraumatic anosmia. *Eur Arch Otorhinolaryngol*. 2010;267(10):1563–1567.

27. Konstantinidis I, Tsakiropoulou E, Bekiaridou P, et al. Use of olfactory training in post-traumatic and post-infectious olfactory dysfunction. *Laryngoscope*. 2013;123(12):E85–90.

28. Jiang R, Twu CW, Liang KL. The effect of olfactory training on the odor threshold in patients with traumatic anosmia. *Am J Rhinol Allergy*. 2017;31(5):317–322.

29. Costanzo RM, Yagi S. Olfactory epithelial transplantation: possible mechanism for restoration of smell. *Curr Opin Otolaryngol Head Neck Surg*. 2011;19(1):54–57.

30. Zasler ND, McNeny R, Heywood PG. Rehabilitative management of olfactory and gustatory dysfunction following brain injury. *J Head Trauma Rehabil*. 1992;7(1):66–75.

31. Pence TS, Reiter ER, DiNard LJ, Costanzo RM. Risk factor for hazardous events in olfactory impaired patients. *JAMA Otolaryngol Head Neck Surg*. 2014;140(10):951–955.

32. Sumner D. Post-traumatic ageusia. *Brain*. 1967;90(1):187–202.

33. Costanzo RM, Zasler ND. Epidemiology and pathophysiology of olfactory and gustatory dysfunction in head trauma. *J Head Trauma Rehabil*. 1992;7:15–24.

34. Welge-Lussen A. Re-establishment of olfactory and taste functions. *GMS Curr Top Otorhinolarygol Head Neck Surg*. 2005;4:Doc06. Published online September 28, 2005.

35. De Araujo IE, Simon SA. The gustatory cortex and multisensory integration. *Int J Obes*. 2009;33(suppl 2):S34–S43.

36. Rousseaux M, Muller P, Gahide I, Mottin Y, Romon M. Disorders of smell, taste, and food intake in a patient with a dorsomedial thalamic infarct. *Stroke*. 1996;27:2328–2330.

37. Sunada I, Akano Y, Yamamoto S, Tashiro T. Pontine haemorrhage causing disturbance of taste. *Neuroradiology*. 1995;37:659.

38. Dutta TM, Josiah AF, Cronin CA, et al. Altered taste and stroke: a case report and literature review. *Top Stroke Rehabil*. 2013;20(1):78–86.

39. Hummel T, Landis BN, Huttenbrink KB. Smell and taste disorder [published online ahead of print, April 26, 2012]. *GMS Curr Top Otorhinolarygol Head Neck Surg*. 2011;10:Doc04. doi:10.3205/cto000077.

40. Maheswaran T, Abikshyeet P, Sitra G. Gustatory dysfunction. *J Pharm Bioallied Sci*. 2014;6(suppl 1): S30–S33. doi:10.4103/0975-7406.137257. PMCID: PMC4157276.

41. Roberts RJ, Sheehan W, Thurber S, Roberts MA. Functional neuroimaging and post-traumatic olfactory impairment. *Indian J Psychol Med*. 2010;32(2):93–98.

42. Sofferman PA. Facial nerve injury and decompression. In: Nadol JB, Schuknecht HF, eds. *Surgery of the Ear and Temporal Bone*. New York: Raven Press; 1993:329–344.

43. Mattes RD, Cowart BJ. Dietary assessment of patients with chemosensory disorders. *J Am Diet Assoc*. 1994;94:50–56.

44. American Medical Association. *AMA Guides to the Evaluation of Permanent Impairment*. 6th ed. Chicago, IL: AMA Press; 2012.

45. Green P, Iverson GL. Effects of injury severity and cognitive exaggeration on olfactory deficits in head injury compensation claims. *Neuro Rehabilitation*. 2001;16:237–243.

Return to Play, School, or Work After Concussion

Charles H. Tator

15

Introduction

The management of concussions, including their diagnosis and treatment, have improved greatly in the past 15 years or so. There is much greater public awareness about the importance of concussions and their consequences. More research has been done, and it is now clear that a large number of concussions occur annually in every country and that concussion is the most common brain injury. It is also well known that not everyone recovers from concussions.[1]

The management of athletes returning to play has been facilitated by the International Consensus Conferences of the Concussion in Sport Group (CISG) that have been held among concussion experts since 2001[2] and every 4–5 years since, with the goal of developing evidence-based protocols for management. The management guides in this chapter reflect the information contained in the most recent international conference, held in 2016 in Berlin and subsequently published in 2017.[3]

Management guidelines for return to play (RTP) have always been regarded as an important aspect of concussion management. Indeed, even prior to the international guidelines, there were many national schemes suggested in the United States and Canada that were based on the severity of concussion as determined by various grading schemes that were not evidence-based and are no longer used.[4,5] In Canada, the Canadian Association of Sports Medicine or CASM, as it was called at the time, published a "concussion protocol" specifying removal from the game or practice of any player *suspected of a concussion* followed by examination by a medical doctor for establishment of the *diagnosis of concussion*. This was an important document because it delineated two phases for the initial RTP protocol. The first phase was *recognition* of a possible concussion by non-healthcare personnel such as players themselves, coaches, teachers, and parents. The second phase was *diagnosis* of concussion by a medical doctor. All this was essential for proper management and speedy RTP. The intent was "manage better and return earlier." Appropriate RTP management was considered to be of high importance for primary and secondary injury prevention.

There was also early recognition of the wisdom of the principle that every concussed athlete should be assessed initially by a medical doctor and then subsequently during the RTP process to ensure that the athlete was ready to return to collision drills and game play.[6]

Several years later, after accomplishing useful RTP protocols, the attention of researchers, clinical leaders, educators, and occupational health experts turned to the development and testing of the return to school or return to learn (RTL) processes after concussion in students. These protocols are still evolving and have not been evaluated for as long a time as RTP protocols. Then, a few years later, concussion experts were asked by schools to provide a protocol for return to school or return to learn that would also facilitate earlier and safe return to the classroom. Gradually, the protocols for return to school have become developed and are now more useful for sufferers, their families, and for educators.

The last of the "return" protocols to be developed is the return to work (RTW) protocol, and there has been very little evaluation and experience with them. In general, the RTL and the RTW protocols are much more complex than RTP because of the greater variety of school levels and variety of instruction and learning for each age group. Similarly, the RTW protocols are very complex and must be individualized for type, complexity, and risk factors for an infinite variety of work situations. RTW has always been a major problem for concussion sufferers, their families, and their advocates including their lawyers and insurers. The medical profession has always had to play a role in helping with the rehabilitation of concussed workers and has attempted to provide safe and effective protocols. This has been perhaps the most difficult area for progress.

Return to Play

Prior to 2000, there was very little consensus about which of several protocols to follow, but, after the development of the International Consensus Conferences of the Concussion in Sport Group (CISG), the majority of sports medicine specialists and other medical specialties and non-medical healthcare professionals began to follow the RTP recommendations of the international group. There was early recognition of the merit in following the international guidelines for secondary injury prevention purposes. Secondary injury prevention is designed to lessen the chance for worsening the injury after a concussion has occurred. Thus, readiness to play was interpreted as readiness to risk a second concussion and that RTP should be delayed for as long as it takes for the brain to recover fully from the first concussion. Waiting for the brain to heal after the first concussion is the best biomarker we have to indicate that the effects of the second concussion would be minimized. Unfortunately, there is no fluid biomarker in blood or cerebrospinal fluid (CSF) or imaging biomarker that signifies the extent of brain healing. The best we have is the clinical biomarker and that is determined by the athlete's tolerance and subjective response to graded exercise. There was early recognition that a graduated or staged process was necessary to determine the readiness of the brain for complete return to participation in sports and that the best way for the athlete to assess brain readiness was to subject the recovering, concussed athlete to a series of graduated exercises in terms of progressively more active increases in effort and duration. In general, a five-step graduated process was developed for noncollision sports and a six-step process for collision sports.[7] One of the earliest principles is that there should be at least 1 day between steps and that, if an athlete provokes symptoms at any step, the athlete should return to the previous level at which symptoms were not provoked. Thus, the earliest that an athlete should RTP is 1 week for adults and at least double that for children and adolescents.

There has been a trend toward increasing the interval between steps for children and young adolescents, who have been shown to take longer to recover from concussion than adults. For example, the majority of adults take 7–10 days to recover with about 80–85% recovering fully within that time. In contrast, normal recovery in children and young adolescents is now considered to be about 1 month.[3]

There are a large number of current guidelines for RTP, but virtually all are based on the principles of graduated increase in physical and mental activity, with the recommended threshold determined by the response elicited by going up to the *threshold* for provocation of symptoms. The principle of the threshold was clearly indicated in the 2017 document.[3] This principle of graduated physical and mental exercise was established by the earliest International Consensus Conferences of the Concussion in Sport Group (CISG) and has been confirmed at each subsequent Conference. In general, the five-step regimen for noncontact sports and the six-step regimen for contact sports were confirmed.[7] These graded regimens have been published widely after each conference, and the response from many sports worldwide has been very good. Most guidelines recommend that the RTP process should be monitored by a healthcare professional such as a clinical therapist and does not require step-by-step monitoring by a medical doctor. However, most guidelines recommended a return visit to a medical doctor between steps 4 and 5 for both contact and noncontact sports.

Prior to the Berlin conference, the duration of step 1 involved complete abstinence from physical and mental activity until all symptoms had resolved, but this has now been shortened to no more than 24–48 hours. Thus, it is no longer necessary to remain at rest for longer than 1–2 days. There is no evidence that staying at complete rest for a longer time will enhance recovery. Thus, players recovering from concussion should attempt to perform increasing levels of physical and mental activity up to their personal threshold for onset or aggravation of symptoms. They are advised to "push the envelope a bit."

Some researchers have advocated the use of heart rate as a guide to how much exercise should be taken,[8] and, indeed, there has been a trend toward monitoring heart rate as an index of the amount of exercise to strive for. In my view, there is no compelling evidence for recommending the concept that a specific optimum heart rate at a specific time in the recovery process for a given patient adds precision to the advice for a graduated increase to the threshold of symptom onset or aggravation.

The issue of baseline testing as an adjunct for guiding the RTP process has been a highly controversial topic. There are now a plethora of computerized and noncomputerized methods for obtaining baseline data on neurological, motor, or neuropsychological aspects of brain function. In my view, these are unnecessary for monitoring function during the RTP process, and this is the view of CISG.[3] If a practitioner feels otherwise, the new Sport Concussion Assessment Tool (SCAT5) can be downloaded free from several websites and can be used for baseline and follow-up purposes.

It is recognized that improved athlete compliance requires the provision of sport-specific guidelines during the graduated RTP process. For example, the steps recommended for equestrian sports cannot be the same as for football. Sport-specificity is essential so that athletes can participate in activities related to a specific sport that they are pursuing, such as skating for hockey players and running for football players. In equestrian sports, the activities progress from on the ground activities to horse-mounted activities. In addition to sport-specificity, the ideal RTP guidelines will have to be age-specific. Compliance has been studied with respect to RTP and has been found to be problematic, with a significant number of athletes being noncompliant with graduated exercise regimens.[9]

Elite athletes and professionals have shown poor compliance with these recommendations, and coaches, trainers, and medical doctors are often under pressure to return athletes to play at earlier times after concussion. It is uncertain whether these superbly trained athletes can tolerate earlier return without being more vulnerable to sustaining another concussion because of incomplete brain recovery or sustain long-term consequences such as the second-impact syndrome, postconcussion syndrome (PCS), or chronic traumatic encephalopathy (CTE).

The proliferation of RTP guidelines has also had some negative consequences because parents and athletes can be uncertain about which ones to follow. The Internet now contains a multitude of guidelines initiated by sports organizations or clinicians advertising for patients. In some countries, ministries of education and sports have tried to create a consensus among schools, sports organizations, and practitioners and have published their own guidelines. The most reliable websites for concussion and information guidelines are offered by governments (cdc.gov) or nonprofit organizations (parachutecanada.org). In Canada, we have recently created harmonized guidelines for all sports, and this is a good example for other countries to follow (see parachutecanada.org).

There are situations in which the advice on RTP should be "never return to collision sports," and this is often required in football, hockey, rugby, boxing, and soccer. The author's criteria for offering this advice are shown in Table 15.1. A recommendation for "never return" is based on many criteria; the number of concussions; the interval between concussions; the length of time to recover from each concussion; the presence of clinical neurological or neuropsychological deficits, especially cognitive decline; the presence of imaging lesions, such as intracerebral hemorrhage or contusion; and the riskiness for further concussion in the sport involved. In my view,

Table 15.1:
Concussions: Guidelines for can return to play or never return to play

Criterion	Can Return to Play	Never Return to Play
1. Neurological history and examination	No neurological deficits No persisting symptoms	Presence of any neurological deficits or significant symptoms
2. Number and interval of previous concussions	Small number, dispersed in time (such as several years), with complete recovery	Multiple, over a short time, such as weeks
3. Length of time to achieve recovery after the last or prior concussions	Short duration (days)	Long duration (months)
4. Neuropsychological evaluation	No cognitive deficits	Presence of cognitive deficits
5. MR/CT findings	No abnormalities	Presence of lesions
6. Riskiness of sport	Low risk (e.g., golf)	High risk (e.g., football)

the advice given to amateurs and professionals should be the same, although the decision made by the concussed individual will vary in relation to this issue.

Return to Learn

During the RTL process, teamwork is essential, and it is important for the school to designate the leaders and members of the team who will be responsible for supervising and facilitating the student's return. For example, it is advantageous to have the school principal or delegate as the leader of the team, and the members should include a guidance counselor and perhaps a physical and health education teacher. If there is an athletic trainer and public health nurse attached to a given school, they should also be involved.[10]

The Berlin conference reinforced the concept that RTL takes precedence over RTP for school-aged children and adolescents and that the RTL process should be graduated and commenced prior to RTP. The accommodations required and the overall format of the RTL for a given student must be individualized. In general, the RTL process is much more complex than the RTP process and there is a much greater need for personal attention and supervision. Unfortunately, the process is one of clinical evaluation of each step because of the absence of objective biomarkers to assess the response or to objectively guide the process.

The graduated RTL may consist of 2 hours a day at school at first, and, if tolerated, this can be gradually increased. If a student cannot tolerate 2 hours a day, even with full accommodations, it may be better to commence graduated home schooling. After the initial step of the RTL protocol is accomplished, the RTP protocol can begin. The RTL process occurs on a graduated basis based on the tolerance of the individual student. The emphasis is once again on determining a given student's thresholds for specific activities such as work with a computer, which is often a difficult challenge for a concussed student. Wearing sunglasses, and turning down the screen's brightness and changing the colors are often helpful accommodations.

Some students will need their course loads adjusted, and courses may have to be dropped if not tolerated. The accommodations necessary may also include extension of assignment deadlines and more time for examinations. Accommodations may also need to include a room with low lighting and minimal noise if photophobia and sonophobia are major symptoms.

Obviously, steps must be taken to minimize the possibility of a student sustaining another blow to the head or body during the RTL process. Stray balls at recess, wet floors, and objects left on the floor are some of the potential causes of repeat concussions.

Return to Work

Similar to RTL, RTW also requires communication, individualization, and a graduated process with accommodations. In general, the RTW process is even more complex than RTP because of the myriad of workplace situations, each with its own opportunities and difficulties for providing a graduated return process with the accommodations that may be required. Also, some jobs take place in an environment in which the risks of a further concussion are significant. Similar to RTP is the shortcoming that clinical judgment is all that is available to design and monitor the process for establishing a worker's thresholds since there are no objective biomarkers to guide the process. The process requires good communication, teamwork, and feedback for optimal results.

There are many jobs to which the concussed worker cannot return during the recovery process, such as those requiring repetitive climbing, driving, heavy lifting, and day-long computer work. Computers can be especially symptom-producing for patients with headaches, photophobia, and vertigo.

The precise graduation of time at work needs to be individualized based on thresholds of tolerance for each component of a worker's role, which may include cognitive tasks such as communication with customers and physical work such as heavy lifting. The emotional effects of isolation from the previous team of workers and the necessity of RTW in a new environment with new team members may evoke anxiety. Thus, there is considerable risk for exacerbation of mental health problems during the RTW process. A frequent source of anxiety is pressure from insurers to accelerate or regiment the RTW schedule.

During the RTW process, it is essential to minimize the possibility of a worker sustaining another blow to the head or body. Depending on the risks involved, it is often necessary to conduct most of the initial stages of the graduated RTW process in a specific job different from the one that caused the concussion if it was work-related. Climbing stairs, wet floors, objects falling from shelves, and floors covered with pipes, wires, and other objects are special work-related hazards and potential causes of repeat concussions.

Conclusions

Recovery of the brain shows great variability during recovery from concussions. There is a long list of modifiers that various studies have been found to influence the duration and completeness of recovery. Much of the research has shown disagreement among authors about the precise factors that affect recovery. The pre-injury demographic factors are age and sex of the individual and preexisting conditions such as migraine headaches, depression, attention deficit disorder, attention deficit hyperactivity disorder, and previous concussions. The type of activity in which the concussions occurred does not seem to affect recovery time and RTP.

Unfortunately, there is no specific treatment, such as a pharmaceutical or nutritional supplement, or physical treatment proven to enhance recovery and RTP, RTL, and RTW. However, any treatment that effectively reduces or eliminates symptoms, such as, medication for headaches, physiotherapy for an associated whiplash or other cervical spine injury, antidepressant medication or psychotherapy for concussion-induced depression, or vestibular therapy for dizziness, will hasten return to normal activities. (Management of headaches in concussed athletes is very important for early RTP in my experience.) Similarly, accommodations in the school and work environment are essential for early RTL and RTW.

References

1. Hiploylee C, Dufort PA, Davis HS, et al. Longitudinal study of postconcussion syndrome: not everyone recovers. *J Neurotrauma*. 2017;34(8):1511–1523.

2. Aubry M, Cantu R, Dvorak J, et al. Summary and agreement statement of the First International Conference on Concussion in Sport, Vienna 2001. Recommendations for the improvement of safety and health of athletes who may suffer concussive injuries. *Br J Sports Med*. 2002;36(1):6–10.

3. McCrory P, Meeuwisse W, Dvorak J, et al. Consensus statement on concussion in sport: the 5th International Conference on Concussion in Sport held in Berlin, October 2016. *Br J Sports Med*. 2017;51(11):838–847.

4. Kelly JP, Rosenberg JH. Diagnosis and management of concussion in sports. *Neurology*. 1997;48(3):575–580.

5. Cantu RC. Guidelines for return to contact sports after a cerebral concussion. *Phys Sports Med*. 1986;14:75–83.

6. Canadian Academy of Sport Medicine Concussion Committee. Guidelines for assessment and management of sport-related concussion. *Clin J Sport Med*. 2000;10:209–211.

7. McCrory P, Meeuwisse WH, Aubry M, et al. Consensus statement on concussion in sport: the 4th International Conference on Concussion in Sport held in Zurich, November 2012. *Br J Sports Med*. 2013;47(5):250–258.

8. Leddy JJ, Baker JG, Willer B. Active rehabilitation of concussion and post-concussion syndrome. *Phys Med Rehabil Clin N Am*. 2016;27(2):437–454.

9. Ackery A, Provvidenza C, Tator CH. Concussion in hockey: compliance with return to play advice and follow-up status. *Can J Neurol Sci*. 2009;36(2):207–212.

10. McGrath N. Supporting the student-athlete's return to the classroom after a sport-related concussion. *J Athl Train*. 2010;45(5):492–498.

The Link Between Traumatic Brain Injury and Neurodegenerative Diseases

Richard Rubenstein

16

Traumatic brain injury (TBI) is generally defined as an insult to the brain caused by an external force leading to altered brain functioning, possible unconsciousness, and impaired cognition. Symptoms of a TBI can be mild, moderate, or severe, depending on the extent of the damage to the brain. The majority of people with a mild TBI (mTBI) usually remain conscious or, in some cases, may experience a loss of consciousness for a few seconds or minutes. Other symptoms of mTBI include headache, confusion, lightheadedness, dizziness, blurred vision or tired eyes, ringing in the ears, bad taste in the mouth, fatigue or lethargy, a change in sleep patterns, behavioral or mood changes, and trouble with memory, concentration, attention, or thinking. Approximately 80–90% of all the neurotrauma cases are classified as mTBI[1] but are difficult to diagnose due to the transient and heterogeneous nature of mTBI symptoms. As a result, a large portion of these injuries are undiagnosed. Often referred to as *concussion*, mTBI is classified by a Glasgow Coma Score (GCS) of 13–15. Severe TBI (sTBI) is referred to as head injuries that result in either permanent or an extended period of unconsciousness, amnesia, or death following a head injury and is quantitatively classified by a GCS of 3–8. Moderate TBI (modTBI) consists of a period of unconsciousness or amnesia ranging from 30 minutes to 24 hours with a GCS of 9–12. A person with a modTBI or sTBI may have a headache that gets worse or does not go away, repeated vomiting or nausea, convulsions or seizures, an inability to awaken from sleep, dilation of one or both pupils of the eyes, slurred speech, weakness or numbness in the extremities, loss of coordination, and increased confusion, restlessness, or agitation. Disabilities resulting from a TBI depend on the severity of the injury, the location of the injury, and the age and general health of the individual. Some common disabilities include problems with cognition (thinking, memory, and reasoning), sensory processing (sight, hearing, touch, taste, and smell), communication (expression and understanding), and behavior or mental health (depression, anxiety, personality changes, aggression, acting out, and social inappropriateness). More serious head injuries may result in stupor (a temporary unresponsive state), coma (a state in which an individual is totally unconscious, unresponsive, unaware, and unarousable), vegetative state (an individual is unconscious and unaware of his or her surroundings but continues to have a sleep–wake cycle and periods of alertness), or a persistent vegetative state (an individual stays in a vegetative state for more than a month).

TBI is a worldwide health and socioeconomic problem and a leading cause of death and disability in children and young adults. According to the World Health Organization (WHO), on an annual basis there are approximately 10 million people affected by head trauma mainly as a result of increasing automobile accidents and awareness of sports-related injuries.[2] Furthermore, it is estimated that the annual incidence of mTBI is 100–600 people per 100,000 worldwide. People between the ages of 15 and 24 experience the highest number of TBIs. The next highest risks for TBI are children 5–9 years of age and adults over the age of 80. Males have twice the risk of sustaining a TBI than females and fourfold the chance of resultant death.

In addition to its effect on human health, TBIs present a significant economic liability. Without accounting for neurodegenerative diseases, the Centers for Disease and Control (CDC) reported that mTBIs alone cost the United States $17 billion annually, and that number jumped to $57 billion when all TBIs were included.[3] More recently, the cost for hospitalized cases of TBI in the United States is estimated at $77 billion.[4] This number does not include patients treated only in the emergency department, outpatient facilities, or those who omit medical care all together. When sports-related concussions are taken into consideration, mTBI accounted for 20% (306,000) of the 1.5 million TBIs in the United States.[5] Of those 306,000 patients, 55% received outpatient care and 34% received no medical attention.[5,6] This means that only 12% of these patients were hospitalized and, therefore, only 12% would be accounted for in the CDC's $57 billion estimate for the economic toll for TBIs. The CDC also acknowledges that its incidence figures underestimate the amount of TBIs primarily due to the fact that there is still no standard definition for a concussion and therefore a large number of TBIs are not being reported.[3,7]

TBI results in acceleration–deceleration forces and/or rotational forces acting on the brain. Both linear and angular/rotational acceleration forces contribute to TBIs, and they are classified as either focal or diffuse injuries depending on the mechanism of the injury. They are designated as focal injuries when the acceleration–deceleration forces cause impact between the brain and inner protrusions of the skull. Diffuse injuries, on the other hand, occur when the differential motion of the brain causes shearing and tearing of the axons, which results in diffuse axonal injuries (DAIs).[8] DAIs are considered one of the major causes of morbidity and mortality following head trauma. DAIs cause damage and swelling to the axonal cytoskeleton which results in impaired axoplasmic transport.[9] This impaired axonal transport leads to the abnormal production and accumulation of toxic proteins, peptides, and their aggregates immediately following the trauma.[9,10]

Whole-brain volume is age-dependent, and, over time, even in the healthy individual, declines. TBI can enhance brain volume loss, which initiates numerous disease processes leading to acute and long-term neuroinflammation with chronic neurodegeneration.[11,12] Within the first 6 months after head injury, significant brain atrophy is an initial sign of neurodegeneration.[13] Concomitantly, the TBI-induced neuroinflammatory response in the form of microglial activation develops within the first week, persists for several months, and returns to normal levels after several years. In the case of DAIs, this microglial reaction is particularly pronounced in the white matter. This TBI-induced release of cytokines activates microglia, which then stimulates additional cytokine release in proportion to the severity of the head injury.[14] This progressive process initiates a sustained inflammatory response which can lead to chronic neurodegeneration.

TBI and Alzheimer Disease

TBI is more of a disease process than an event that is associated with immediate and long-term sensomotor, psychological, and cognitive impairments. TBI is the best known established epigenetic risk factor for later development of neurodegenerative diseases and dementia. Single or repetitive injury has been associated with Alzheimer disease (AD), Parkinson disease (PD), amyotrophic lateral sclerosis (ALS), frontotemporal dementia (FTD), and chronic traumatic encephalopathy (CTE). The similar pathophysiologies among all of these disorders, consisting of the gradual degeneration of brain cells and gradual loss of brain functions, suggests a common mechanistic link to TBI. Individuals subjected to a TBI are approximately four times more likely to develop dementia at a later stage. Single brain injury is linked to later development of symptoms resembling AD while repetitive brain injuries are linked to later development of CTE. Furthermore, the existence of multiple factors associated with the neurodegenerative diseases (such as slow disease progression, neuroinflammation, and genetics) makes the definitive identification of etiologies problematic.[11,15–19] The long-term pathological consequences of TBI are a major concern. The varying degrees of injury are associated with progressive atrophy of gray and white matter structures that may persist months to years after injury.

The genetic background of β-amyloid precursor protein, apolipoprotein E (ApoE), presenilin, and neprilysin genes is associated with exacerbation of the neurodegenerative process after TBI. ApoE is a plasma lipoprotein primarily responsible for transporting lipids through the central nervous system (CNS), and it plays a vital role in synaptogenesis along with maintaining, repairing, and remodeling neuronal tissue.[20] Of the various neurodegenerative diseases, there is the strongest evidence suggesting a link between head trauma and AD. Individuals with a history of TBI were 60% more likely to develop AD compared with others.[21] Within a population of AD patients, it has also been reported that a history of TBI accelerates the onset of AD.[22,23] Carriers of the ApoE4 allele with a history of TBI have a 10-fold increased risk of AD whereas noncarriers of this allele with a TBI history had no increased risk of dementia.[24] In comparison, possessing the ApoE4 allele with no history of head trauma indicated a twofold increase risk of AD.[24]

The major pathological hallmarks in the brain of AD patients are neuronal loss, synaptic dysfunction,[25] and plaque deposition, which primarily consists of amyloid-β (Aβ) peptide and neurofibrillary tangles (NFTs) composed of phosphorylated tau (p-tau) protein.[26] Studies in humans[27] and experimental animal models[28] have revealed abnormal accumulations of extracellular senile plaques and intracellular NFTs following TBI.

Aβ aggregation is regarded as a major component in the pathogenesis of AD.[29] Aβ deposition primarily occurs in cortical regions responsible for memory and learning as well as in the small blood vessels of the meninges and cerebral cortex.[26] As a result of head trauma, the presence of DAIs results in NFTs and Aβ accumulation, aggregation, and the deposition of Aβ plaques and NFTs at a rate greater than aging alone.[30,31] A consequence of TBI is altered axonal transport as a result of cytoskeletal changes. The affected axonal transport influences the levels and/or activity of α-synuclein, amyloid precursor protein (APP), β-Secretase 1 (BACE1), tau, ApoE4, presenilin 1 (PS1), and caspase-3, which in turn may be involved in APP processing contributing to AD.[32,33] A recent study[34] investigated amyloid pathology using amyloid tracer 11C-Pittsburgh compound B (11C-PiB) with positron emission tomography (PET; 11C-PiB-PET) combined with diffusion tensor imaging (DTI), which estimates the degree of axonal injury following TBI. Increased 11C-PiB binding was present in long-term survivors of TBI in a distribution overlapping with AD but also involving the cerebellum.[35] A mechanistic link between axonal injury and amyloid pathology was suggested by the relationship between cortical ^{11}C-PiB binding and white matter damage in connected tracts.

Moreover, studies in various animal models indicated that the expression of amyloidogenic β- and γ-secretases and their substrate APP is increased after TBI, suggesting that Aβ peptides are generated de novo after TBI.[36,37] Oxidative stress and mitochondrial dysfunction are also key contributors to the pathological cascade leading to AD.[38]

After TBI, hypoxia and hypertension are common.[39,40] Hypoxia facilitates the pathogenesis of AD by accelerating the accumulation of Aβ and by increasing the hyperphosphorylation of tau, leading to the chronic process of neurodegeneration.[41] Hypoxia markedly increases Aβ deposition and potentiates memory deficits in AD.[42] Accumulating evidence shows that stroke and ischemic attacks significantly increase the risk of AD because of the drive in cerebral Aβ accumulation and related apoptotic events in the brain.[43,44]

TBI and Parkinson Disease

Parkinson disease (PD) is a progressive neurodegenerative disorder characterized by loss of pigmented dopaminergic neurons in the substantia nigra (SN) as well as the presence of abnormal α-synuclein-containing Lewy bodies and Lewy neurites.[45] The mechanisms associated with linking neurotrauma with the PD neurodegenerative processes are unknown.

Recent studies[46] suggested α-synuclein as a pathological link between chronic effects of TBI and PD symptoms, as evidenced by significant overexpression and abnormal accumulation of α-synuclein in inflammation-infiltrated SN of rats subjected to chronic TBI. These results are in accordance with those reported in animal and clinical research in which TBI was found to induce overexpression of α-synuclein and PD-like symptoms in humans and animal models of TBI.[47–49] The link between TBI and PD was further investigated by quantifying the risk of PD after TBI compared to non-TBI trauma to eliminate the possibility of reverse-causation, where a patient may fall and sustain the TBI due to early motor symptoms of PD. The study reported that, among patients aged 55 years or older presenting to inpatient/emergency department settings with trauma, TBI is associated with a 44% increased risk of developing PD over 5–7 years that is unlikely to be due to confounding or reverse causation.[45] Furthermore, the risk of PD is equivalent after TBI due to falls versus non-falls but significantly higher with more severe or more frequent TBI. This strengthened the causal association and further reduced the possibility of reverse-causation. Although another study[50] could not replicate those findings, several limitations existed, namely, incomplete information on PD patient diagnosis and, in some cases, diagnostic misclassification. Although this study did not include milder single and repeated head injuries, Gardner et al.[45] reported that patients with mTBI were 24% more likely to develop PD than those with non-TBI trauma. This is in contrast to the findings of Marras et al.[51] where a causal association between mTBI and PD was not evident.

Previous epidemiological studies suggested that even a single TBI can raise a person's risk of developing AD or PD later in life,[49,52,53] and the more severe and frequent the TBI, the greater the disease risk. However, a recent study has reported that pooled clinical and neuropathologic data from three prospective cohort studies indicated that TBI with loss of consciousness for greater than 1 hour is associated with risk for Lewy body accumulation, progression of parkinsonism, and PD, but not dementia, AD, neuritic plaques, or NFTs.[54] This study calls into question the view that TBI is a significant risk factor for AD.

TBI and Amyotrophic Lateral Sclerosis

ALS, also known as Lou Gehrig's disease, is a progressive neurodegenerative disease that is less prevalent than AD and PD with an annual incidence of 2 per 100,000 per year.[55] ALS is the most common of the motor neuron diseases and causes the death of neurons that control voluntary muscles. ALS is characterized by stiff muscles, muscle twitching, and gradually worsening weakness due to muscles decreasing in size. This results in difficulty speaking, swallowing, and eventually breathing.[56]

Most people with ALS die between 2 and 4 years after the diagnosis. Around half of people with ALS die within 30 months of their symptoms beginning, and about 20% of people with ALS live between 5 years and 10 years after symptoms begin.[55] Several studies suggest that head trauma can be a risk factor for the development of ALS. There is a higher incidence of ALS later in life in professional athletes who play contact sports, which includes football and soccer. Retired National Football League (NFL) players had an ALS mortality rate four times higher than the general population.[16] In another study, professional Italian soccer players were 6.5 times more likely to develop ALS with a dose–response relationship between length of career and likelihood of disease.[57] ALS also occurs more often among US military veterans, which may be due to head injury.[58]

The defining feature of ALS is the death of both upper and lower motor neurons in the motor cortex of the brain, the brainstem, and the spinal cord. Prior to their destruction, motor neurons develop protein-rich inclusions in their cell bodies and axons. This may be partly due to defects in protein degradation. These inclusions often contain ubiquitin and generally incorporate one of the ALS-associated proteins: Cu–Zn superoxide dismutase (SOD1), TAR DNA binding protein (TDP-43, or TARDBP), or FUS.[59]

ALS is both a familial disease (10%) and a sporadic disease (90%). It is estimated that 90–95% of ALS cases are sporadic, and gene mutations in SOD1, senataxin, and dynactin account for some familial forms of the disease.[60] A common characteristic of ALS and other neurodegenerative disorders is the occurrence of a neuroinflammatory reaction consisting of activated glial cells, mainly microglia and astrocytes, and T cells. In addition, it has been previously demonstrated that increased microglial activation can be present up to 17 years after TBI. This suggests that TBI triggers a chronic inflammatory response particularly in subcortical regions.[11] Persistently activated microglia can be cytotoxic, and their persistent activation might predispose susceptible individuals to the development of neurodegenerative conditions.[61]

The connection between head trauma and ALS was described previously.[62] They reported that 10 of 12 brains of deceased athletes who had CTE also showed widespread TDP-43 proteinopathy affecting multiple areas of the brain. Three of the former athletes with CTE also had TDP-43 and abnormal tau protein in their spinal cords and had developed a progressive motor neuron disease several years before death. Two of the athletes were former football players and had been clinically diagnosed with ALS, and the third, an ex-boxer and military veteran, had been diagnosed with atypical ALS with dementia.

TBI and Frontotemporal Dementia

FTD is one of the leading causes of neurodegenerative dementia in people under 60 years of age.[63] It is a progressive degenerative brain disease having clinical diagnoses with symptoms attributable to frontal and temporal lobe atrophy. Second only to AD in prevalence, FTD accounts for 20% of young-onset dementia cases. Signs and symptoms typically manifest in late adulthood, more commonly between the ages of 55 and 65, approximately equally affecting men and women.[64] At autopsy, clinical diagnoses of FTD most often correlate with frontotemporal lobar degeneration (FTLD) neuropathology, including abnormal deposition of mutated tau (FTLD-tau), TDP-43 (FTLD-TDP), or FUS (FTLD-FUS) proteins in intraneuronal inclusion bodies.[63] While up to 50% of FTD cases are familial, involving genetic mutations in chromosome 9 open reading frame 72, progranulin (PGRN), microtubule-associated protein tau, valosin-containing protein, or chromatin-modifying protein 2B,[65] several studies have reported that TBI increases the risk for subsequent FTD.[66–68] TBI with extended (≥5 min) loss of consciousness (LOC) was reported to be a significant risk factor for a clinical diagnosis of FTD. TBI associated with extended LOC may increase the subsequent risk for FTD by approximately 67% and differentially affects both the pattern and severity of cognitive, behavioral, and functional symptomatology across clinical FTD subtypes.[68]

TBI may promote the development of FTD through its effects on microglial activation, which can lead to PGRN deficiency.[69] PGRN appears to play a role in neuronal growth and repair, and acquired PGRN deficiency could precipitate neurodegeneration, similar to the PGRN deficiency that arises from PGRN mutations associated with FTD.[70] Since the frontal and temporal lobes are particularly susceptible to damage in TBI, these regions may also be particularly susceptible to TBI-related PGRN depletion. Furthermore, TDP-43 deposition may be initiated by TBI since it has been observed in cases of CTE.[62]

TBI and Chronic Traumatic Encephalopathy

CTE is a progressive degenerative disease found in people who have had a severe blow or repeated blows to the head. A subtype of this is called "punch-drunk," a term coined by Martland[71] in 1928 to describe the chronic motor and psychiatric consequences of blows to the head as it was initially found in those with a history of boxing, and later renamed *dementia pugilistica*.[72] Subsequently, Critchley[73] examined boxers and described patients with unusual mental and physical symptoms including mood swings, irritability, paranoid depression, and, occasionally, uninhibited violent behavior. Motor findings included pyramidal, extrapyramidal, and cerebellar signs, with tremor and dysarthria. Sensory problems included deafness, poor vision, headaches, and unsteady gait. He described this progressive neurological disease in boxers as a chronic progressive traumatic encephalopathy of boxers.

The term CTE has been coined to encompass progressive neurodegenerative effects observed after multiple concussions sustained in any context.[74] CTE is usually described as a changing pattern of cognitive, psychiatric, and motor symptoms.[75]

CTE is characterized by the widespread accumulation of the abnormally phosphorylated (hyperphosphorylated) tau protein (p-tau) in the brain. Repeated mild traumatic injury can have numerous pathophysiological effects. The head trauma can damage axons and cause changes in membrane permeability leading to ionic shifts and calcium influx.[76] This results in caspase and calpain activation causing tau phosphorylation and aggregation leading to microtubule instability. Head injury can also activate microglia that release toxic levels of cytokines, chemokines, immune mediators, and excitotoxins (such as glutamate and aspartate). Excitotoxins inhibit phosphatases, resulting in p-tau in neurons and astrocytes and NFT deposition in particular areas of the brain.[77] CTE is distinguished from other neurodegenerative disorders by a distinctive topographic and cellular pattern of tau neurofibrillary pathology. As described by McKee et al.,[75] neuropathologically, the p-tau abnormalities begin focally as perivascular NFTs and neurites at the depths of the cerebral sulci and then spread to involve superficial layers of adjacent cortex before becoming a widespread degeneration affecting medial temporal lobe structures, diencephalon, and brainstem. CTE has been categorized into four stages (I–IV) describing the disease progression. These stages describe and correlate advancing clinical symptoms with the progressive neuropathology and are based on the increased severity of protein deposition, cerebral atrophy, and behavioral sequel.[75,78] A definitive diagnosis of CTE can only be confirmed at autopsy. The major risk factor for CTE appears to be mild, repetitive brain trauma, including repetitive concussions. CTE has been observed most often in professional athletes who are involved in contact sports (e.g., boxing, football, rugby, hockey, soccer, wrestling, skiing) and who have been subjected to repetitive blows to the head. CTE has been confirmed at autopsy in soldiers with histories of repetitive brain trauma returning from Iraq and Afghanistan. CTE has also been diagnosed in nonathletes who have experienced repetitive brain trauma, including epileptics and developmentally disabled individuals with head banging and domestic abuse victims.[75] It is unclear to what extent of severity or recurrence of head injury is required to initiate CTE.[75] Although CTE is similar to other neurodegenerative diseases, including AD, it is a distinct progressive tauopathy with unique neuropathological features. Aβ deposition and APP processing, production, and accumulation are increased after injury in experimental animal models and human brain.[79–88] In acute TBI, Aβ deposition is widely distributed throughout the neocortex without apparent association with the injury sites.[89] NFTs similar to AD are seen but the levels of senile plaques is reduced compared to AD. Irregular, multifocal, and perivascular tau-immunoreactive NFTs are now considered a CTE-specific pathology distinguishing it from other neurodegenerative diseases.[90] Aβ deposits are only identified in about 40% of those found to have CTE, as compared to extensive Aβ deposits present in nearly all those pathologically confirmed to have AD.[75] The predominant form of Aβ in acute TBI is Aβ42, whereas the Aβ40 form predominates in serum and cerebrospinal fluid, a situation similar to that in AD.[91] However, there is nevertheless confusion and inconsistency in the neuropathological findings for CTE due to the existence of overlapping neurodegenerative diseases (AD, PD, ALS) discovered at the time of death in those cases reported to be CTE.[92,93]

CTE Classification and Symptoms

The clinical symptoms of CTE usually begin at mid-life (~40–50 years of age) with a slower rate of progression compared to AD and FTD. Unlike AD or FTD, the clinical course of CTE is slow, progressing at a rate of 11–14 years between pathological stages. Thus, the symptoms of CTE, which gradually progress from changes in thinking, mood, and behavior to eventual dementia in advanced cases of CTE, begin years or even decades following exposure to repetitive blows to the head.[75] In addition, it is likely that axonal dysfunction and loss contribute to the production of clinical symptoms, especially in the early stages of CTE when tau pathology is focal and unlikely to account for the headache, attention and concentration loss, and memory difficulties experienced by patients with stage I or II disease. The spectrum of p-tau pathology ranged in severity from focal perivascular NFTs in the frontal cortex to severe tauopathy affecting widespread brain regions, including the medial temporal lobe. The different stages of pathological changes in patients correlated with the distinct behavioral abnormalities.[78] Furthermore, it is likely that CTE may not progress through all the disease stages or may not progress at the same rate in all patients.

Stage I

This first stage is characterized by headaches and loss of attention and concentration. In some patients there is short-term memory problems, depression, aggressive tendencies, and executive function difficulties (inability to connect experiences and memories). The neuropathology consists of limited focal areas of perivascular p-tau NFTs and astrocytic tangles predominantly in the sulci depths and frontal neocortex. Infrequent TDP-43 immunopositive neurites are found in the cerebral subcortical white matter in stages I through III.

Stage II

Depression, mood swings, headache, and short-term memory loss are more pronounced. Some patients experience executive dysfunction, suicidal thoughts, and language difficulties. There are multiple centralized brain regions of p-tau NFTs in the cerebral sulci and spread to the superficial layers of the cortex.

Stage III

Clinical symptoms continue to progress and include memory loss, executive dysfunction, attention and concentration issues, depression, mood swings, apathy, visuospatial difficulties, and aggression. Neuropathology consists of mild cerebral atrophy with widespread p-tau pathology and NFTs in the frontal and temporal lobes at the depths of the sulci. NFTs are also found in the amygdala, hippocampus, and entorhinal cortex.

Stage IV

Severe cognitive problems and memory loss are apparent, with many patients having progressed to full-blown dementia. Symptoms in this stage include profound loss of attention and concentration, paranoia, depression, gait and visuospatial difficulties, executive dysfunction, language difficulties, and aggression. Parkinsonism also affects physical movement for some. In this stage there is widespread brain atrophy, neuronal loss and gliosis of the cerebral cortex and hippocampus, and extensive p-tau pathology throughout the gray and white matter. TDP-43 immunoreactivity is severe, with intraneuronal and intraglial inclusions. At this stage of disease, CTE is often mistaken for AD or FTD.[94,95]

CTE and Genetics

The underlying genetics of CTE are unknown. However, not everyone with a history of repetitive brain trauma develops CTE, suggesting that there may be a genetic suscep-tibility in individuals who go on to develop the disease. Studies are now investigating the possible role of a genetic predisposition based on carrying the ApoE gene, which is carried on chromosome 19. For example, the link between ApoE4 and AD, where having the double allele is a risk factor for AD, may also apply to CTE. Studies have re-ported that the presence of the ApoE4 allele is associated with worse cognitive deficits in patients following severe head injury.[96,97] However, although 40% of those with AD have this type of allele, the association with CTE is less clear since the levels of Aβ plaques in CTE brain is much reduced compare to AD brain. In addition, no significant group differences appear between ApoE4 carriers in the CTE population and the gen-eral population,[98] which suggests that ApoE may not be a significant risk factor for the development of CTE. The result of this analysis is similar to findings by McKee et al.[78] who also reported nonsignificant differences between the ApoE genotype of the general population and the 68 cases of CTE.[99]

Pathological Dissemination of Neurodegenerative Diseases

Data continue to accumulate strengthening the link between TBI and processes identified as initiating factors associated with one or more forms of each of the neu-rodegenerative diseases (AD, PD, ALS, FTD, CTE) (see Figure 16.1). Although each of these diseases has distinct clinical phenotypes, they each share the common character-istic of having the accumulation of insoluble aggregates comprised of specific proteins (see Figure 16.1). For AD and CTE, aggregates of p-tau are found in NFTs and neu-ropil threads in addition to Aβ deposits (especially in sporadic AD). Familial FTLD-tau is due to tau gene mutations (FTLD-Tau). Neuronal accumulations of α-synuclein in Lewy bodies and Lewy neurites are the pathological signatures of sporadic PD and PD with dementia. ALS is associated with a mutant form of superoxide dismutase 1 and, along with a further subgroup of FTD (FTLD-TDP), is characterized by aggregates of TAR DNA-binding protein 43 (TDP-43). It has been proposed that cell-to-cell spread of disease pathology to interconnected neurons and adjacent glial cells involves a self-perpetuating pathogenic propagation that follows a similar mechanism reported for the spread of the transmissible prion diseases.[100] For prion diseases, the initial protein con-version mechanism that begins the entire process is still unknown. The molecular mech-anism described for propagation of prion diseases requires that the abnormal β-sheet conformation of the pathogenic form of the prion protein (PrP^{Sc}) functions as a seed and template to recruit more PrP^{Sc} by binding to and causing the conformational con-version (α-helical to β-sheet) of the normal, cellular prion protein (PrP^{C}). Thus, PrP^{Sc} induces a chain reaction–like process of protein misfolding and progressive aggrega-tion. This paradigm of pathological protein propagation in has been discussed for other

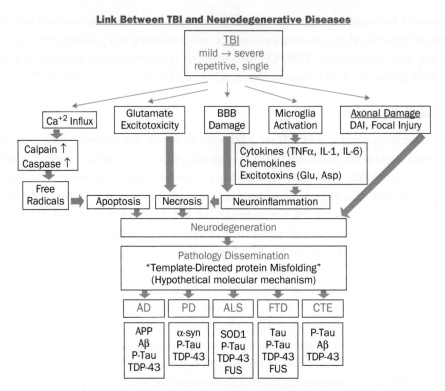

Figure 16.1 Diagram depicting various possible cascades of events associated with TBI-induced neuropathogenesis and their link to neurodegenerative diseases (NDs). A hypothetical mechanism for pathology dissemination leading to the NDs is also shown. Listed are major proteins currently associated with the respective NDs and which can serve as disease biomarkers.

abnormal protein-associated neurodegenerative diseases.[101] However, a major difference is that prion diseases, also known as transmissible spongiform encephalopathies, are infectious and can be transmitted from one host to another of similar PrP^C genotype. However, although there is no evidence of transmissibility from one host to another for the other neurodegenerative diseases, pathological propagation within a given host intraneuronally and interneuronally by a PrP-like mechanism has been reported in cell culture systems,[102–111] and in animal models.[112–116]

References

1. Sundman MH, Hall EE, Chen N-K. Examining the relationship between head trauma and neurodegenerative disease: a review of epidemiology, pathology and neuroimaging. *J Alzheimers Dis Parkinsonism*. 2014;4:137. doi:10.4172/2161-0460.1000137.

2. World Health Organization (WHO). *Traumatic Brain Injury: Neurological Disorders: Public Health Challenges*. Geneva, Switzerland: World Health Organization; 2006.

3. National Center for Injury Prevention and Control. *Report to Congress on Mild Traumatic Brain Injury in the United States: Steps to Prevent a Serious Public Health Problem*. Atlanta, GA: Centers for Disease Control and Prevention; 2003.

4. Coronado VG, McGuire LC, Faul M, Sugerman DE, Pearson WS. Traumatic brain injury epidemiology and public health issues. In: Zasler ND, Katz DI, Zafonte RD, eds. *Brain Injury Medicine: Principles and Practice*. New York: Demos Medical Publishing; 2012:84–100.

5. Langlois JA, Rutland-Brown W, Wald MM. The epidemiology and impact of traumatic brain injury: a brief overview. *J Head Trauma Rehabil.* 2006;21:375–378.

6. Sosin DM, Sniezek JE, Thurman DJ. Incidence of mild and moderate brain injury in the United States, 1991. *Brain Inj.* 1996;10:47–54.

7. Thurman DJ, Branche CM, Sniezek JE. The epidemiology of sports-related traumatic brain injuries in the United States: recent developments. *J Head Trauma Rehabil.* 1998;13:1–8.

8. Sayed TE, Mota A, Fraternali F, Ortiz M. Biomechanics of traumatic brain injury. *Comp Methods Applied Mech Eng.* 2008;197:4692–4701.

9. Smith DH, Uryu K, Saatman KE, Trojanowski JQ, McIntosh TK. Protein accumulation in traumatic brain injury. *Neuromolecular Med.* 2003;4:59–72.

10. Uryu K, Chen XH, Martinez D, et al. Multiple proteins implicated in neurodegenerative diseases accumulate in axons after brain trauma in humans. *Exp Neurol.* 2007;208:185–192.

11. Ramlackhansingh AF, Brooks DJ, Greenwood RJ, et al. Inflammation after trauma: microglial activation and traumatic brain injury. *Ann Neurol.* 2011;70:374–383.

12. Johnson VE, Stewart JE, Begbie FD, Trojanowski JQ, Smith DH, Stewart W. Inflammation and white matter degeneration persist for years after a single traumatic brain injury. *Brain.* 2013;136:28–42.

13. Gale SD, Johnson SC, Bigler ED, Blatter DD. Trauma-induced degenerative changes in brain injury: a morphometric analysis of three patients with preinjury and postinjury MR scans. *J Neurotrauma.* 1995;12:151–158. doi:10.1089/neu.1995.12.151.

14. Igarashi T, Potts MB, Noble-Haeusslein LJ. Injury severity determines Purkinje cell loss and microglial activation in the cerebellum after cortical contusion injury. *Exp Neurol.* 2007;203:258–268.

15. Chen H, Richard M, Sandler DP, Umbach DM, Kamel F. Head injury and amyotrophic lateral sclerosis. *Am J Epidemiol.* 2007;166:810–816.

16. Lehman EJ, Hein MJ, Baron SL, Gersic CM. Neurodegenerative causes of death among retired National Football League players. *Neurology.* 2012;79:1970–1974.

17. Shively S, Scher AI, Perl DP, Diaz-Arrastia R. Dementia resulting from traumatic brain injury: what is the pathology? *Arch Neurol.* 2012;69:1245–1251.

18. Jafari S, Etminan M, Aminzadeh F, Samii A. Head injury and risk of Parkinson disease: a systematic review and meta-analysis. *Mov Disord.* 2013;28:1222–1229.

19. Smith C, Gentleman SM, Leclercq PD, et al. The neuroinflammatory response in humans after traumatic brain injury. *Neuropathol Appl Neurobiol.* 2013;39:654–666. doi:10.1111/nan.12008.

20. Dardiotis E, Fountas KN, Dardioti M, et al. Genetic association studies in patients with traumatic brain injury. *Neurosurg Focus.* 2010;28:E9.

21. Fleminger S, Oliver DL, Lovestone S, Rabe-Hesketh S, Giora A. Head injury as a risk factor for Alzheimer's disease: the evidence 10 years on; a partial replication. *J Neurol Neurosurg Psychiatry.* 2003;74:857–862.

22. Sullivan P, Petitti D, Barbaccia J. Head trauma and age of onset of dementia of the Alzheimer type. *JAMA.* 1987;257:2289–2290.

23. Schofield PW, Tang M, Marder K, et al. Alzheimer's disease after remote head injury: an incidence study. *J Neurol Neurosurg Psychiatry.* 1997;62:119–124.

24. Mayeux R, Ottman R, Maestre G, et al. Synergistic effects of traumatic head injury and apolipoprotein-epsilon 4 in patients with Alzheimer's disease. *Neurology.* 1995;45:555–557.

25. Jiang X, Jia L-W, Li X-H, et al. Capsaicin ameliorates stress-induced Alzheimer's disease-like pathological and cognitive impairments in rats. *J Alzheimers Dis.* 2013;35:91–105.

26. Finder VH. Alzheimer's disease: a general introduction and pathomechanism. *J Alzheimers Dis.* 2010;22(suppl 3):5–19.

27. DeKosky ST, Abrahamson EE, Ciallella JR, et al. Association of increased cortical soluble abeta42 levels with diffuse plaques after severe brain injury in humans. *Arch Neurol.* 2007;64:541–544.

28. Yoshiyama Y, Uryu K, Higuchi M, et al. Enhanced neurofibrillary tangle formation, cerebral atrophy, and cognitive deficits induced by repetitive mild brain injury in a transgenic tauopathy mouse model. *J Neurotrauma.* 2005;22:1134–1141.

29. Finder VH, Glockshuber R. Amyloid-beta aggregation. *Neurodegener Dis.* 2007;4:13–27.

30. Chen XH, Johnson VE, Uryu K, Trojanowski JQ, Smith DH. A lack of amyloid beta plaques despite persistent accumulation of amyloid beta in axons of long-term survivors of traumatic brain injury. *Brain Pathol.* 2009;19:214–223.

31. Johnson VE, Stewart W, Smith DH. Widespread τ and amyloid-β pathology many years after a single traumatic brain injury in humans. *Brain Pathol.* 2012;22(2):142–149. doi:10.1111/j.1750-3639.2011.00513.x.

32. Johnson VE, Stewart W, Smith DH. Traumatic brain injury and amyloid-beta pathology: a link to Alzheimer's disease? *Nat Rev Neurosci.* 2010;11:361–370.

33. Breunig JJ, Guillot-Sestier MV, Town T. Brain injury, neuroinflammation and Alzheimer's disease. *Front Aging Neurosci.* 2013;5:26.

34. Scott G, Ramlackhansingh AF, Edison P, et al. Amyloid pathology and axonal injury after brain trauma. *Neurology.* 2016;86:821–828.

35. Thal DR, Rub U, Orantes M, Braak H. Phases of A beta-deposition in the human brain and its relevance for the development of AD. *Neurology.* 2002;58:1791–1800.

36. Chow VW, Mattson MP, Wong PC, Gleichmann M. An overview of APP processing enzymes and products. *Neuromolecular Med.* 2010;12:1–12.

37. Haass C, Kaether C, Thinakaran G, Sisodia S. Trafficking and proteolytic processing of APP. *Cold Spring Harb Perspect Med.* 2012;2:a006270.

38. Lin MT, Beal MF. Mitochondrial dysfunction and oxidative stress in neurodegenerative diseases. *Nature.* 2006;443:787–795.

39. Frugier T, Morganti-Kossmann MC, O'Reilly D, McLean CA. In situ detection of inflammatory mediators in post mortem human brain tissue after traumatic injury. *J Neurotrauma.* 2010;27:497–507.

40. Huang RQ, Cheng HL, Zhao XD, et al. Preliminary study on the effect of trauma-induced secondary cellular hypoxia in brain injury. *Neurosci Lett.* 2010;473:22–27.

41. Zhang X, Le W. Pathological role of hypoxia in Alzheimer's disease. *Exp Neurol.* 2010;223:299–303.

42. Sun X, He G, Qing H, et al. Hypoxia facilitates Alzheimer's disease pathogenesis by up-regulating BACE1 gene expression. *Proc Natl Acad Sci USA.* 2006;103:18727–18732.

43. Wen Y, Onyewuchi O, Yang S, Liu R, Simpkins JW. Increased beta-secretase activity and expression in rats following transient cerebral ischemia. *Brain Res.* 2004;1009:1–8.

44. Tesco G, Koh YH, Kang EL, et al. Depletion of GGA3 stabilizes BACE and enhances beta-secretase activity. *Neuron.* 2007;54:721–737.

45. Gardner RC, Burke JF, Nettiksimmons J, Goldman S, Tanner CM, Yaffe K. Traumatic brain injury in later life increases risk for Parkinson disease. *Ann Neurol.* 2015;77:987–995. doi:10.1002/ana.24396.

46. Acosta SA, Tajiri N, de la Pena I, et al. Alpha-synuclein as a pathological link between chronic traumatic brain injury and Parkinson's Disease. *J Cell Physiol*. 2015;230(5):1024–1032. doi:10.1002/jcp.24830.

47. Bower JH, Maraganore DM, Peterson BJ, McDonnell SK, Ahlskog JE, Rocca WA. 2003. Head trauma preceding PD: a case-control study. *Neurology*. 2003;60:1610–1615.

48. Goldman SM, Tanner CM, Oakes D, Bhudhikanok GS, Gupta A, Langston JW. Head injury and Parkinson's disease risk in twins. *Ann Neurol*. 2006;60:65–72.

49. Wong JC, Hazrati LN. Parkinson's disease, parkinsonism, and traumatic brain injury. *Crit Rev Clin Lab Sci*. 2013;50:103–106.

50. Rugbjerg K, Ritz B, Korbo L, Martinussen N, Olsen JH. Risk of Parkinson's disease after hospital contact for head injury: population based case-control study. *BMJ*. 2008;337:a2494. doi:10.1136/bmj.a2494.

51. Marras C, Hincapié CA, Kristman VL, et al. Systematic review of the risk of Parkinson's disease after mild traumatic brain injury: results of the International Collaboration on Mild Traumatic Brain Injury Prognosis. *Arch Phys Med Rehabil*. 2014;95(3 suppl):S238–244. doi:10.1016/j.apmr.2013.08.298.

52. Plassman BL, Havlik RJ, Steffens DC, et al. Documented head injury in early adulthood and risk of Alzheimer's disease and other dementias. *Neurology*. 2000;55(8):1158–1166.

53. Perry DC, Sturm VE, Peterson MJ, et al. Association of traumatic brain injury with subsequent neurological and psychiatric disease: a meta-analysis. *J Neurosurg*. 2016;124(2):511–526.

54. Crane PK, Gibbons LE, Dams-O'Connor K, et al. Association of traumatic brain injury with late-life neurodegenerative conditions and neuropathologic findings [published online ahead of print]. *JAMA Neurology*. 2016. doi:10.1001/jamaneurol.2016.1948.

55. Kiernan MC, Vucic S, Cheah BC, et al. Amyotrophic lateral sclerosis. *Lancet*. 2011;377(9769):942–955. doi:10.1016/s0140-6736(10)61156-7.

56. Zarei S, Carr K, Reiley L, et al. A comprehensive review of amyotrophic lateral sclerosis. *Surg Neurol Int*. 2015;6:171.

57. Chiò A, Benzi G, Dossena M, Mutani R, Mora G. Severely increased risk of amyotrophic lateral sclerosis among Italian professional football players. *Brain*. 2005;128:472–476.

58. Beard JD, Kamel F. Military service, deployments, and exposures in relation to amyotrophic lateral sclerosis etiology and survival. *Epidemiologic Rev*. 2015;37:55–70. doi:10.1093/epirev/mxu001.

59. Deng H-X, Zhai H, Bigio EH, et al. FUS-immunoreactive inclusions are a common feature in sporadic and non-SOD1 familial amyotrophic lateral sclerosis. *Annals Neurol*. 2010;67(6):739–748. doi:10.1002/ana.22051.

60. Shi P, Strom AL, Gal J, Zhu H. Effects of ALS-related SOD1 mutants on dynein- and KIF5-mediated retrograde and anterograde axonal transport. *Biochim Biophys Acta*. 2010;1802:707–716.

61. Gentleman SM, Leclercq PD, Moyes L, et al. Long-term intracerebral inflammatory response after traumatic brain injury. *Forensic Sci Int*. 2004;146(2-3):97–104.

62. McKee AC, Gavett BE, Stern RA, et al. TDP-43 proteinopathy and motor neuron disease in chronic traumatic encephalopathy. *J Neuropathol Exp Neurol*. 2010;69:918–929.

63. Perry DC, Miller BL. Frontotemporal dementia. *Semin Neurol*. 2013;33:336–341.

64. Snowden JS, Neary D, Mann DM. Frontotemporal dementia. *Br J Psychiatry*. 2002;180(2):140–143.

65. Onyike CU, Diehl-Schmid J. The epidemiology of frontotemporal dementia. *Int Rev Psychiatry.* 2013;25:130–137.

66. Rosso SM, Landweer EJ, Houterman M, Donker Kaat L, van Duijn CM, van Swieten JC. Medical and environmental risk factors for sporadic frontotemporal dementia: a retrospective case-control study. *J Neurol Neurosurg Psychiatry.* 2003;74:1574–1576.

67. Kalkonde YV, Jawaid A, Qureshi SU, et al. Medical and environmental risk factors associated with frontotemporal dementia: a case-control study in a veteran population. *Alzheimers Dement.* 2012;8:204–210.

68. Deutsch MB, Mendez MF, Teng E. Interactions between traumatic brain injury and frontotemporal degeneration. *Dement Geriatr Cogn Discord.* 2015;39:143–153.

69. Jawaid A, Rademakers R, Kass JS, Kalkonde Y, Schulz PE. Traumatic brain injury may increase the risk for frontotemporal dementia through reduced progranulin. *Neurodegener Dis.* 2009;6:219–220.

70. Finch N, Baker M, Crook R, et al. Plasma progranulin levels predict progranulin mutation status in frontotemporal dementia patients and asymptomatic family members. *Brain.* 2009;132:583–591.

71. Martland H. Punch drunk. *JAMA.* 1928;91:1103–1107. doi:10.1001/jama.1928.02700150029009.

72. Millspaugh J. Dementia pugilistica. *US Naval Med Bull.* 1937;35:297–303.

73. Critchley, M. Medical aspects of boxing, particularly from a neurological standpoint. *BMJ.* 1957;1:357–362. doi:10.1136/bmj.1.5015.357.

74. Miller H. Mental after-effects of head injury. *Proc Royal Soc Med.* 1966;59:257–261.

75. McKee AC, Cantu RC, Nowinski CJ, et al. Chronic traumatic encephalopathy in athletes: progressive tauopathy after repetitive head injury. *J Neuropathol Exp Neurol.* 2009;68:709–735. doi:10.1097/NEN.0b013e3181a9d503.

76. Giza, CC, Hovda DA. The neurometabolic cascade of concussion. *J Athl Train.* 2001;36:228–235.

77. Saulle M, Greenwald BD. Chronic traumatic encephalopathy: a review. *Rehabil Res Pract.* 2012;2012:816069. doi:10.1155/2012/816069.

78. McKee AC, Stern RA, Nowinski CJ, et al. The spectrum of disease in chronic traumatic encephalopathy. *Brain.* 2013;136:43–64. doi:10.1093/brain/aws307.

79. Roberts GW, Gentleman SM, Lynch A. βA4 amyloid protein deposition in brain after head trauma. *Lancet.* 1991;338:1422–1423.

80. Gentleman SM, Nash MJ, Sweeting CJ, Graham DI, Roberts GW. Beta-amyloid precursor protein (beta APP) as a marker for axonal injury after head injury. *Neurosci Lett.* 1993;160(2):139–144.

81. McKenzie JE, Gentleman SM, Roberts GW. Increased numbers of beta APP-immunoreactive neurones in the entorhinal cortex after head injury. *Neuroreport.* 1994;6:161–64.

82. Roberts GW, Gentleman SM, Lynch A. Beta amyloid protein deposition in the brain after severe head injury: implications for the pathogenesis of Alzheimer's disease. *J Neurol Neurosurg Psychiatry.* 1994;57:419–425.

83. Graham DI, Gentleman SM, Lynch A. Distribution of beta-amyloid protein in the brain following severe head injury. *Neuropathol Appl Neurobiol.* 1995;21:27–34.

84. Pierce JE, Trojanowski JQ, Graham DI. Immunohistochemical characterization of alterations in the distribution of amyloid precursor proteins and beta-amyloid peptide after experimental brain injury in the rat. *J Neurosci.* 1996;16:1083–1090.

85. Murakami N, Yamaki T, Iwamoto Y. Experimental brain injury induces expression of amyloid precursor protein, which may be related to neuronal loss in the hippocampus. *J Neurotrauma.* 1998;15:993–1003.

86. Smith DH, Chen XH, Nonaka M. Accumulation of amyloid beta and tau and the formation of neurofilament inclusions following diffuse brain injury in the pig. *J Neuropathol Exp Neurol.* 1999;58:982–992.

87. Masumura M, Hata R, Uramoto H. Altered expression of amyloid precursors proteins after traumatic brain injury in rats: in situ hybridization and immunohistochemical study. *J Neurotrauma.* 2000;17:123–134.

88. Uryu K, Laurer H, McIntosh T. Repetitive mild brain trauma accelerates Abeta deposition, lipid peroxidation, and cognitive impairment in a transgenic mouse model of Alzheimer amyloidosis. *J Neurosci.* 2002;22:446–454.

89. Graham DI, Gentleman SM, Nicoll JA. Altered beta-APP metabolism after head injury and its relationship to the aetiology of Alzheimer's disease. *Acta Neurochir Suppl.* 1996;66:96–102.

90. Omalu B, Bailes J, Hamilton RL, et al. Emerging histomorphologic phenotypes of chronic traumatic encephalopathy in American athletes. *Neurosurgery.* 2011;69:173–183. doi:10.1227/NEU.0b013e318212bc7b PMID: 21358359.

91. Gentleman SM, Greenberg BD, Savage MJ. Abeta 42 is the predominant form of amyloid beta-protein in the brains of short-term survivors of head injury. *Neuroreport.* 1997;8:1519–1522.

92. Gardner A, Iverson GL, McCrory P. Chronic traumatic encephalopathy in sport: a systematic review. *Br J Sports Med.* 2013;48:84–90. doi:10.1136/bjsports-2013-092646 PMID: 23803602.

93. Smith DH, Johnson VE, Stewart W. Chronic neuropathologies of single and repetitive TBI: substrates of dementia? *Nat Rev Neurol.* 2013;9:211–221. doi:10.1038/nrneurol.2013.29 PMID: 23458973.

94. Gavett BE, Stern RA, Cantu RC, Nowinski CJ, McKee AC. Mild traumatic brain injury: a risk factor for neurodegeneration. *Alzheimers Res Ther.* 2010;2:18.

95. Gavett BE, Stern RA, McKee AC. Chronic traumatic encephalopathy: a potential late effect of sport-related concussive and subconcussive head trauma. *Clin Sports Med.* 2011;30:179–188.

96. Jordan BD, Relkin NR, Ravdin LD, Jacobs AR, Bennett A, Gandy S. Apolipoprotein E ε4 associated with chronic traumatic brain injury in boxing. *JAMA.* 1997;278:136–140.

97. Kutner KC, Erlanger DM, Tsai J, Jordan B, Relkin NR. Lower cognitive performance of older football players possessing apoliopoprotein E eplison4. *Neurosurgery.* 2000;47:651–657.

98. Beydoun MA, Beydoun HA, Kaufman JS, et al. Apolipoprotein E e4 allele interacts with sex and cognitive status to influence all-cause and cause-specific mortality in US older adults. *J Am Geriatr Soc.* 2013;61:525–534. doi:10.1111/jgs.12156 PMID: 23581910.

99. McKee AC, Stein TD, Nowinski CJ, et al. The spectrum of disease in chronic traumatic encephalopathy. *Brain.* 2013;136:43–64. doi:10.1093/brain/aws307 PMID: 23208308.

100. Aguzzi A, Rajendran, L. The transcellular spread of cytosolic amyloids, prions, and prionoids. *Neuron.* 2009;64:783–790.

101. Brettschneider J, Del Tredici K, Lee, VM-Y, Trojanowski, JQ. Spreading of pathology in neurodegenerative diseases: a focus on human studies. *Nature Neurosci.* 2015;16:109–120.

102. Desplats P, Lee HJ, Bae EJ, et al. Inclusion formation and neuronal cell death through neuron-to-neuron transmission of α-synuclein. *Proc Natl Acad Sci USA.* 2009;106:13010–13015.

103. Frost B, Jacks RL, Diamond MI. Propagation of tau misfolding from the outside to the inside of a cell. *J Biol Chem*. 2009;284:12845–12852.

104. Nonaka T, Watanabe ST, Iwatsubo T, Hasegawa M. Seeded aggregation and toxicity of α-synuclein and tau: cellular models of neurodegenerative diseases. *J Biol Chem*. 2010;285:34885–34898.

105. Volpicelli-Daley LA, Luk KC, Patel TP, et al. Exogenous α-synuclein fibrils induce Lewy body pathology leading to synaptic dysfunction and neuron death. *Neuron*. 2011;72:57–71.

106. Munch C, O'Brien J, Bertolotti A. Prion-like propagation of mutant superoxide dismutase-1 misfolding in neuronal cells. *Proc Natl Acad Sci USA*. 2011;108:3548–3553.

107. Furukawa Y, Kaneko K, Watanabe S, Yamanaka K, Nukina N. A seeding reaction recapitulates intracellular formation of Sarkosyl-insoluble transactivation response element (TAR) DNA-binding protein-43 inclusions. *J Biol Chem*. 2011;286:18664–18672.

108. Freundt EC, Maynard N, Clancy EK, et al. Neuron-to-neuron transmission of α-synuclein fibrils through axonal transport. *Ann. Neurol*. 2012;72:517–524.

109. Nath S, Agholme L, Kurudenkandy FR, Granseth B, Marcusson J, Hallbeck M. Spreading of neurodegenerative pathology via neuron-to-neuron transmission of β-amyloid. *J Neurosci*. 2012;32:8767–8777.

110. Kfoury N, Holmes BB, Jiang H, Holtzman DM, Diamond MI. Trans-cellular propagation of Tau aggregation by fibrillar species. *J Biol Chem*. 2012;287:19440–19451.

111. Nonaka T, Masuda-Suzukake M, Arai T, et al. Prion-like properties of pathological TDP-43 aggregates from diseased brains. *Cell Rep*. 2013;4:124–134.

112. Clavaguera F, Bolmont T, Crowther RA, et al. Transmission and spreading of tauopathy in transgenic mouse brain. *Nature Cell Biol*. 2009;11:909–913.

113. Mougenot AL, Nicot S, Bencsik A, et al. Prion-like acceleration of a synucleinopathy in a transgenic mouse model. *Neurobiol Aging*. 2012;33:2225–2228.

114. Luk KC, Kehm VM, Zhang B, O'Brien P, Trojanowski JQ, Lee VM. Intracerebral inoculation of pathological α-synuclein initiates a rapidly progressive neurodegenerative α-synucleinopathy in mice. *J Exp Med*. 2012;209:975–986.

115. de Calignon A, Polydoro M, Suárez-Calvet M, et al. Propagation of tau pathology in a model of early Alzheimer's disease. *Neuron*. 2012;73:685–697.

116. Masuda-Suzukake M, Nonaka T, et al. Prion-like spreading of pathological α-synuclein in brain. *Brain*. 2013;136:1128–1138.

Section III

Neuroimaging and Biomarker Assessments in TBI

Neuroimaging and Its Application in the Diagnosis and Early Prognostication of TBI

Lijun Bai, Shan Wang, and Chuanzhu Sun

17

Traumatic brain injury (TBI) is a serious public health epidemic, and it is estimated that approximately 1.4 million people are affected by this disease in America every year.[1] According to information statistics, about 75–85% of TBI patients fall in the range of mild TBI (mTBI).[2] Due to the heterogeneous nature of the injury, which ranges widely from mild neurometabolic changes (that can recover quickly) to permanent continuous damage to either brain structure or function, the development of diagnostic tools for TBI faces challenges, as do the predictors of recovery.[3] It is too difficult for us to investigate directly the effects of brain damage after TBI by depending only on a patient's clinical manifestation; therefore, the development of neuroimaging techniques provides a clear view of TBI. Currently, nearly one-tenth of published reports about TBI use neuroimaging methods.[3] Since computed tomography (CT) and standard magnetic resonance imaging (MRI) cannot estimate the real extent of brain damage after TBI, until recently, abnormalities in TBI patients were generally detected through advanced neuroimaging techniques, such as diffusion tensor imaging (DTI) and blood oxygen level-dependent (BOLD)–based functional MRI (fMRI).[4,5]

fMRI is a widely used diagnostic imaging method to determine task-related dysfunction as well as cognitive assessment after TBI or any other brain injury occurring over a long, chronic phase. It can measure the fluctuations that exist in human brains during either active task states or in a resting state.[6,7] DTI, a relatively new MRI technique, allows the white matter tracts in the central network system (CNS) to be visualized. The advantage of DTI is its application in visualizing axonal injury and the major pathology of TBI. The degree and directionality of water diffusion in tissue can be measured by this technique so that color maps reveal the location and directionality of white matter tracts, thus making it possible to characterize brain abnormalities after TBI.[2,6]

Graph Theory Methods for the Analysis of Resting-State Functional Connectivity

In regarding the brain as a complex network, graph theory plays an increasingly popular role in neuroimaging research. For the purpose of investigating abnormalities of brain regions in patients with TBI, researchers usually employ resting-state fMRI data and graph theoretic analysis to detect the difference between TBI patients and healthy controls. Nodes of the intrinsic connectivity networks in normal brain are interrelated and interact, just as in a graph that consists of edges and every edge has its own weight. In graph theoretic analysis, by computing the Pearson's correlation coefficients between the time series from any pair of nodes in brain, we can calculate the individual's whole-brain functional connectivity matrix.[4,8,9] This method provides a particularly detailed framework for researchers working to understand brain network structure.

It is worth mentioning that the human brain typically shows a "small-world" characteristic in that simultaneous global and local parallel message processing is allowed, and the brain networks are optimized for information processing.[4,10] Random networks usually have a low clustering coefficient (C_{net}) and also a typically short path length. By comparison, brain small-world networks have similar path lengths but higher clustering coefficients (C_{net}). As reported in a previous study, the functional connectivity networks of healthy individuals have a small-world architecture, but TBI shifts these network functions and structures away from this organization. In TBI, diffuse axonal injury (DAI) to long white matter tracts is considered to be the leading cause of disruption in the brain's original small-world architecture.[11,12] Compared with healthy controls, functional connectivity was decreased after TBI, with longer path length between connected nodes; thus, the network efficiency of these patients is reduced.[4]

Analysis of graphs reveals the presence of *modules* (also called *systems*, reflecting different function modules in brain network) as well as *hub regions,* which have high connectivity within networks. The definition of hub regions is still controversial. One early definition is based on three nodal topological characteristics: nodal degree (S_i), efficiency (E_i), and betweenness centrality (B_i). The S_i provides an approach to quantify the extent that node i is relevant to the network. Nodes that have a high S_i must be information collection centers. The nodal efficiency E_i is a function of the minimum path length among regions. The betweenness centrality of a node i is defined as the number of shortest paths which passed through the node i between any two nodes. Based on these three topological characteristics, network hub regions are considered to be those nodes which have high weighted degree, high efficiency, and high betweenness centrality. It has been proved that hub regions change after TBI, and these changes may result in severe damage to a person's abilities.[13] Another definition was reported by Warren in 2014. He argued that nodal degree could not reflect its importance to network function because of its adjustability depending on network size. Warren and colleagues came up with two new measures for hub regions: system density and participation coefficient. System density is a measure reflecting the physical proximity of brain systems, and the participation coefficient value of a node judges the number of disparate systems that the node correlates strongly with. Hub regions are those locations with simultaneous high system density and a high participation coefficient. In their research, Warren et al. selected six target hubs (high system density and high participation coefficient) and two control hubs (high degree). They observed that damage to target hubs would produce severe cognitive deficits widely throughout brain networks such as memory, verbal function, and adaptive functions, whereas damage to control hubs only produced circumscribed cognitive injury, such as local perception loss.[14]

A general trend of fMRI studies reports decreased activity in the frontal regions following TBI, such as in the right precentral gyrus. Many previous studies have proved that the frontal regions are more vulnerable and that these regions always relate to cognitive function and executive control.[15] Some studies also report bilateral decreased activation in the dorsolateral prefrontal cortex (DLPFC). It is essential to note that there exists an unclear relationship between the DLPFC and working memory.[3] The cerebellum has been identified as implicated in executive control, such as behavior and working memory. Horak and Diener stated that cerebellar lesions could result in postural deficits,[16] which can be a prominent problem in TBI, especially for mTBI patients.[17]

The Theory and Application of Diffusion Tensor Imaging

Recently, several approaches have become widely used for DTI data processing. Region of interest (ROI)-based analysis can extract data from regions marked directly on the image and can be applied in seeking individual difference. The other methods are voxel-based morphometry (VBM), tract-based spatial statistics (TBSS), and tractography. Both VBM and TBSS rely on group normalized data that estimate tissue composition. Tractography is utilized to estimate white matter fibers' spatial location.[18,19] Compared with conventional MRI, DTI is more sensitive to microstructural abnormalities, especially in white matter.[20] Measurements from DTI help develop inferences about white matter by calculating the diffusion properties of water within tissue. The movement of water in an isotropic medium such as cerebrospinal fluid is not restricted, so that the water can diffuse similarly in all directions. In white matter, however, which is restricted by axonal membranes, myelin, and microtubules that are regarded as anisotropic media, the diffusion of water is no longer equal in all directions. Thus, a mathematical ellipsoidal diffusion model can be used to represent the diffusion of water in a voxel, if the voxel is the basic element in the MRI image.[21,22]

In the diffusion ellipsoid, *axial diffusivity* (AD) is defined as diffusion along the major axis. The average diffusion along the other two minor axes is *radial diffusivity* (RD).[23] Two common indices, fractional anisotropy (FA) and mean diffusivity (MD), are frequently used to characterize the properties of the diffusion ellipsoid. FA is a value ranging from 0 to 1, and tissue tends to be more anisotropic when the value of FA is higher. The mean of the three axes in the diffusion ellipsoid is the MD. Therefore, the value of MD reflects the rate of diffusion of water within tissue. The four parameters reflect different aspects of white matter integrity; different types of white matter injury will lead to different effects on these four parameters.[22] Findings of changes in the FA accompanied by various MD, RD, and AD values may add complexity to the characteristics of brain injury. For example, increased FA and decreased MD may indicate that swelling in axons occurred early after TBI and always correlates with poor clinical manifestation.[24] Eierud et al. have also suggested that poor neuropsychological performance is related to high FA values in the acute period after injury.[3] Another study suggests that simultaneously decreased FA and increased MD is an indicator of vasogenic edema, which may be resolved over time, and that simultaneously elevated FA and reduced MD is a feature of cytotoxic edema, with more conspicuous anisotropy and axonal swelling.[25] Some clinical research has detected those domains where the anisotropy of white matter tracts is abnormal. A method called *enhanced z-score microstructural assessment of pathology* (EZ-MAP) provides an approach to detect regional FA (or AD, RD, MD) abnormalities in TBI patients. The EZ-MAP compares a patient's FA values (or values for any of the other three metrics) to those of a normal, healthy group (reference group) at every voxel. The assessment of abnormality depends on the mean and standard deviation of the FA value from the chosen reference group. Thus, a bootstrap procedure must be employed to avoid sample-to-sample difference in z-scores. EZ-MAP provides a robust approach for detecting regional abnormal anisotropy in individuals with TBI.[26,27]

It is important to detect which type of injury TBI patients may have by analyzing changes in these parameters, especially because anisotropy (FA) changes have a strong correlation with time post-injury.[3,28] Based on the experiment carried out by Eierud, elevated FA values are more frequently detected during the acute phase (<2 weeks after mTBI), while decreased FA changes are more often reported after the acute phase (>2 weeks after mTBI).[3] One study of TBI selected patients within 5–14 days after injury who showed no abnormal findings based on clinical CT. Patients with mTBI showed decreased FA in the genu of the corpus callosum, but patients with moderate TBI show no such characteristic, although increased RD of the genu of the corpus callosum is found both in mTBI and in moderate TBI.[29] Similarly, some researchers reported that, compared with healthy controls, mTBI patients show decreased FA values in the splenium of the corpus callosum. By contrast, other domains of the corpus callosum in moderate TBI are also found to have reduced FA.[30] In addition, Kraus et al. investigated 13 brain regions from patients with various severities of TBI: mild, moderate, and severe. They found that FA decreases in all 13 brain regions in moderate and severe TBI patients, with accompanying increased AD and RD in several white matter tracts. For mTBI, only a few regions, such as the corticospinal tract and superior longitudinal fasciculus, show reduced FA and only with increased AD, indicating myelin damage occurring after moderate and severe TBI but not mTBI.[31] These results not only suggest that moderate and severe TBI shows more abnormalities, but they also provide a standard for the prognosis and assessment of TBI.

Despite the fact that DTI studies of TBI show a great deal of difference either in the time period after injury or in other controlled factors such as analysis methods and examined brain regions, many investigators conclude that DTI measures can be a significant early indicator for TBI, providing value prognosis for later injury.[2]

Developing Directions of Neuroimaging Research

Advanced imaging tools, either fMRI or DTI, are important for researchers to investigate the pathology of TBI, since traditional MRI and CT cannot provide effective evidence of cerebral injuries. These advances mean that the diagnosis of TBI can be based on neuroimaging biomarkers rather than on a single clinical manifestation. Although neuroimaging research on TBI has undergone great development during the past several decades, these methods still lack sensitivity at the level of individual patient study, as a kind of heterogeneous injury, mTBI makes it difficult to diagnose and predict one's injury. Hence, a personalized approach is needed. In addition, long-term studies are also needed to understand the later influence of brain injuries for the purpose of determining whether the function and structure of brain networks could change over time.[2] As for the pattern of imaging, Duhaime and Haacke have noted that it is essential to create more standardized protocols both in research and clinical examinations, including the application of multimodal imaging to detect brain lesions after TBI.[32,33]

Acknowledgments

This research was supported by the National Natural Science Foundation of China under Grant Nos. 81571752, 81371630, and Shanxi Nova Program (2014KJXX-34).

References

1. Langlois JA, Rutland BW, Thomas KE. *Traumatic Brain Injury in the United States: Emergency Department Visits, Hospitalizations, and Deaths.* Atlanta, GA: Centers for Disease Control and Prevention, National Center for Injury Prevention and Control; 2004.

2. Shenton ME, Hamoda HM, Schneiderman JS, et al. A review of magnetic resonance imaging and diffusion tensor imaging findings in mild traumatic brain injury. *Brain Imaging Behav.* 2012;6(2):137–192.

3. Eierud C, Craddock RC, Fletcher S, et al. Neuroimaging after mild traumatic brain injury: review and meta-analysis. *NeuroImage Clin.* 2014;4:283–294.

4. Sharp DJ, Gregory S, Robert L. Network dysfunction after traumatic brain injury. *Nature Reviews Neurology.* 2014;10(3):156–166.

5. Kihwan H, Christine MD, Ann MJ, et al. Disrupted modular organization of resting-state cortical functional connectivity in US military personnel following concussive 'mild' blast-related traumatic brain injury. *Neuroimage.* 2014;84:76–96.

6. Zwany M, Lars AR, Jacques DK. Structural and functional neuroimaging in mild-to-moderate head injury. *Neurology.* 2007;6:699–709.

7. Chang C, Leopold DA, Scholvinck ML, et al. Tracking brain arousal fluctuations with fMRI. *Proc Natl Acad Sci USA.* 2016;113(16):4518–4523.

8. Zhangjia D, Chaogan Y, Kuncheng L, et al. Identifying and mapping connectivity patterns of brain network hubs in Alzheimer's disease. *Cereb Cortex.* 2014:1–20.

9. Rubinov M, Sporns O. Complex network measures of brain connectivity: uses and interpretations. *Neuroimage.* 2010;52:1059–1069.

10. Bassett DS, Bullmore E. Small-world brain networks. *Neuroscientist,* 2006;12:512–523.

11. Caeyenberghs K. Altered structural networks and executive deficits in traumatic brain injury patients. *Brain Struct.* 2014;219:193–209.

12. Pandit AS. Traumatic brain injury impairs small-world topology. *Neurology.* 2013;80:1826–1833.

13. Zhiqiang Z, Wei L, Huafu C, et al. Altered functional-structural coupling of large-scale brain networks in idiopathic generalized epilepsy. *Brain.* 2011;134:2912–2928.

14. Warren DE, Power JD, Bruss J, et al. Network measures predict neuropsychological outcome after brain injury. *Proc Natl Acad Sci USA.* 2014;111(39):11247–11252.

15. McCrea M, Guskiewica KM, Marshall SW, et al. Acute effects and recovery time following concussion in collegiate football players: the NCAA Concussion Study. *JAMA.* 2003;290:2556–2563.

16. Horak FB, Diener HC. Cerebellar control of postural scaling and central set in stance. *J. Neurophysiol.* 1994;72:479–493.

17. Krivitzky LS, Roebuck-Spencer TM, Roth RM, et al. Functional magnetic resonance imaging of working memory and response inhibition in children with mild traumatic brain injury. *J Int Neuropsychol Soc.* 2011;17:1143–1152.

18. Emsell L, Van Hecke W, Tournier J-D. *Introduction to Diffusion Tensor Imaging.* Amsterdam, Netherlands: Elsevier; 2007; 66(4):61A.

19. Smith SM, Jenkinson, M, Johansen-Berg H, et al. Tract-based spatial statistics: voxelwise analysis of multi-subject diffusion data. *Neuroimage*. 2006;31(4):1487–1505.

20. Basser PJ, Mattiello J, LeBihan D. MR diffusion tensor spectroscopy and imaging. *Biophys J*. 1994;66(1):259–267.

21. Basser PJ. Inferring microstructural features and the physiological state of tissues from diffusion-weighted images. *NMR Biomed*. 1995;8:333–344.

22. Madden DJ, Bennett IJ, Burzynska A, et al. Diffusion tensor imaging of cerebral white matter integrity in cognitive aging. *Biochimica Biophysica Acta*. 2012;1822:386–400.

23. Pierpaoli C, Basser PJ. Toward a quantitative assessment of diffusion anisotropy. *Magn Reson Med*. 1996;36:893–906.

24. Bazarian JJ, Zhong J. DTI detects clinically important axonal damage after mild TBI: a pilot study. *J Neurotrauma*. 2007;24(9):1447–1459.

25. Kou Z, Tong KA. The role of advanced MR imaging findings as biomarkers of TBI. *J Head Trauma Rehabil*. 2010;25(4):267–282.

26. Lipton ML, Kim N, Park YK, et al. Robust detection of traumatic axonal injury in individual mild traumatic brain injury patients: intersubject variation, change over time and bidirectional changes in anisotropy. *Brain Imaging and Behavior*. 2012;6:329–342.

27. Kim N, Branch CA, Kim M, Lipton ML. Whole brain approaches for identification of microstructural abnormalities in individual patients: comparison of techniques applied to mild traumatic brain injury. *Plos One*. 2013;8(3):1–14.

28. Niogi SN, Mukherjee P. Diffusion tensor imaging of mild traumatic brain injury[J]. *J Head Trauma Rehabil*. 2010;25(4):241.

29. Kumar R, Gupts RK. Comparative evaluation of corpus callosum DTI metrics in acute mild and moderate traumatic brain injury: its correlation with neuropsychometric tests. *Brain Inj*. 2009;23(7):675–685.

30. Matsushita M, Hosoda K. Utility of diffusion tensor imaging in the acute stage of mild to moderate traumatic brain injury for detecting white matter lesions and predicting long-term cognitive function in adults. *J Neurosurg*. 2011;115(1):130–139.

31. Kraus MF, Susmaras T. White matter integrity and cognition in chronic traumatic brain injury: a diffusion tensor imaging study. *Brain*. 2007;130(10):2508–2519.

32. Duhaime AC, Gean AD. Common data elements in radiologic imaging of traumatic brain injury. *Arch Phys Med Rehabil*. 2010;91(11):1661–1666.

33. Haacke EM, Mittal S. Susceptibility-weighted imaging: technical aspects and clinical applications, part 1. *AJNR Am J Neuroradiol*. 2009;30(1):19–30.

The Potential of Brain-Specific Blood Biomarkers for TBI Patient Management, Diagnosis, and Clinical Research

Olena Y. Glushakova, Alex B. Valadka, Ronald L. Hayes, and Alexander V. Glushakov

18

Introduction

Traumatic brain injury (TBI) is a major health and socioeconomic problem representing the leading cause of death and disability in the United States and worldwide; it has no effective treatment.[1-3] In the United States alone, around 1.7 million people sustain TBI annually, resulting in 52,000 deaths and more than 90,000 long-term disabilities in TBI survivors.[4-6] TBI is a heterogeneous disorder involving a complex cascade of several primary and secondary mechanisms associated with acute and chronic excitotoxic damage, oxidative stress, and neuroinflammation. Primary injury mechanisms associated with mechanical damage to the brain are generally irreversible, whereas secondary injury associated with delayed pathophysiological pathways involving different cell types in the brain are potentially treatable and are extensively studied for development of therapeutic strategies for TBI. However, these multifactorial disturbances in neuronal, glial, and microvascular cellular function are largely not addressed by current clinical TBI management.[7]

Current Diagnostics and Management of TBI in Intensive Care: Accomplishments and Limitations

Over the several past decades, improvements have been made in the diagnosis and management of TBI. This has resulted in advances in the care of TBI patients, decreases in mortality, and improvements in overall patient outcome. Current TBI diagnosis is commonly based on a neurological examination using the Glasgow Coma Scale (GSC), pupillary reactivity,[8-14] and neuroimaging.[14,15] However, several reports indicate that correlation of GSC score with injury severity is age-dependent,[16] which may limit its prognostic power,[17] and even that GCS assessments are not sensitive enough to predict its correlation with either functional outcome[10,18,19] or anatomical damage.[20-22]

Computed tomography (CT) is currently the most commonly used objective measurements of injury.[23] However, due to substantial patient exposure to potentially harmful ionizing radiation during CT scan,[24,25] and taking into account its limited sensitivity and predictive value,[26] the health risks of performing of CT examination can outweigh benefits, especially in mild to moderate TBI cases.[27-30] There is ongoing research to include modalities of magnetic resonance imaging (MRI) for TBI assessment, including diffusion tensor imaging (DTI), susceptibility weighted imaging (SWI), and functional MRI (fMRI), as well as positron-emission tomography (PET) and high-definition fiber tracking (HDFT).[14,15] However, neuroimaging is not readily available everywhere, and even advanced MRI modalities are only specific for certain types of brain injury (e.g., diffuse axonal injury [DAI], hemorrhage, neuronal lesions) and often might not completely reflect the injury phenotype of a particular TBI patient.

Current management of TBI patients in the ICU is mainly focused on management of the primary injuries to the brain and skull that are directly associated with acute mechanical damage including surgical interventions, stabilizing the patient's status, and monitoring and managing intracranial pressure (ICP), pyrexia, cerebral perfusion, and brain oxygenation.[31–33]

Overall, effective treatment and management of TBI is hampered by lack of evidence-based TBI diagnostic categories to determine anatomical brain injury severity and phenotype as well as prognosis.

Surrogate Endpoints and Selection of Brain-Specific Protein Biomarkers for TBI Diagnosis and Management

As discussed, current TBI diagnostic methods are primarily based on neurological assessments using GCS scores, pupillary reactivity, and CT imaging studies, which are useful predictors of the extent of brain damage especially in severe TBI cases. However, these indices have limited sensitivity in mild TBI and have poor predictive value for secondary injuries or adverse events. Current clinical and experimental research suggests that repetitive assessments of certain biomarkers associated with secondary injury mechanisms in an individual patient could provide valuable information regarding a patient's status and potential response to treatment focusing on preventing or minimizing secondary injuries.[34]

The Promise of Brain-Specific Biomarkers in Management of TBI Patients and Clinical Trials

Numerous brain-specific proteins synthesized in astrocytes, such as glial fibrillary acidic protein (GFAP) and calcium binding protein B (S100β), and in neurons or neuronal processes such as ubiquitin C-terminal hydrolase L1 (UCH-L1), microtubule-associated protein 2 (MAP-2), myelin basic protein (MBP), neuron-specific enolase (NSE), and tau are released into the cerebrospinal fluid (CSF) and blood following cellular damage by different brain injuries including TBI. These proteins have been studied as diagnostic and prognostic biomarkers associated with neuropathology and functional outcome following these injuries. Several cell-specific protein biomarkers released in CSF and blood following neurological injury are produced by proteolytic activity of calpain and caspase proteases, including α-II spectrin breakdown products (SBDPs), caspase-cleaved tau, and of caspase-cleaved cytokeratin-18.[35] In addition, many other protein biomarkers (e.g., cytokines) that represent systemic inflammation are thought to originate in the brain following injury. Studies have implicated all of these proteins as prospective biomarkers of TBI. Numerous clinical studies provided evidence of strong correlations of concentrations of these biomarkers in blood and CSF with several clinically important TBI outcome measures such as GCS, ICP, injury phenotype (i.e., focal vs. diffuse), and short- and long-term patient outcome.[36] Recent studies also suggest the clinical utility of biomarker applications to pediatric TBI.[37,38] In addition to CSF and blood, some of the biomarkers associated with brain injury are present in other biofluids including urine,[39–46] saliva,[47,48] and exhaled breath condensate[49] in patients with neurological injury, thus suggesting their potential applications for noninvasive diagnostics in TBI. Moreover, recent studies provide evidence for the use of several protein biomarkers as prognostic markers for secondary neuronal and systemic injuries, thereby advancing a personalized approach for the management of TBI patients and stratification of patients for clinical trials.[14,36,50,51]

Brain-Specific Biomarkers Potentially Useful in TBI Management and Clinical Trials

It is widely recognized that increased levels of that several CNS-specific neuronal and glial protein biomarkers in CSF and serum including GFAP, S100β, UCH-L1, SBDPs (i.e., SBDP150, SBDP145 and SBDP120), MAP-2, and tau are associated with neurological and neurodegenerative conditions such as mild and severe TBI, sport-related head injury, stroke, epilepsy, neurotoxicity, Parkinson disease (PD), and Alzheimer disease (AD).[52–73] However, the concentration and temporal changes of these biomarkers depend on the neurological injury phenotype, suggesting that serial sampling of different biomarkers in serum results in distinguishably different temporal trajectories in TBI patients presenting different injury phenotypes.[34] For example, a recent study by Meier and colleagues reported significant increases in serum levels of UCH–L1 and S100β following sport-related concussion, whereas GFAP levels were not different.[72] In contrast, GFAP can be significantly elevated in mild TBI patients presenting to emergency rooms but not reporting a sport concussion.[72,74]

One of the most important aspects of TBI diagnosis is the potential ability to identify injury phenotypes. Biomarkers including S100β, NSE, and GFAP have been reported to be promising candidates for assessments of cerebral hypoxia, a common condition following TBI associated with increased morbidity.[75] Moreover, recent clinical studies have provided strong evidence that blood-based biomarker profiles can discriminate between focal and diffuse brain injury detected by CT in severe TBI patients,[76] as well as discriminate between patients with positive and negative CT findings.[55,63,74,77–79] Clinical studies demonstrated that the levels of some of these biomarkers including GFAP, S100β, UCH-L1, and tau are correlated with patient outcome after TBI.[53,76,77,80–92] Although a recent report by Posti et al. questioned the clinical utility of UCH-L1 and GFAP for acute diagnosis of TBI,[93] Papa and Wang reviewed significant deficiencies in the design and interpretation of the Posti study.[94]

Glial Biomarkers Associated with TBI

Because astrogliosis is one of the important hallmarks of brain injuries, specific proteins expressed in astrocytes which are also often upregulated in different neurological conditions have long been studied as biomarkers of TBI. GFAP and S100β are among most promising glial biomarkers of TBI.

S100β, a member of the S100 protein family expressed in the central nervous system (CNS), is one of the most studied astrocytic markers associated with neurological disorders.[95–97] Increases in cerebrospinal fluid (CSF) and serum S100β concentrations have been reported at acute stages of severe TBI[98–107] and closed head injury in children.[108,184] Serum levels of S100β were associated with different types of traumatic intracranial lesions[109] and blood–brain barrier (BBB) damage[88,89] and were correlated with brain injury severity,[99] ICP,[100–103] CT findings,[98,100,101,104,105] and neurological deficits.[106] A correlation between both serum and CSF levels of S100β and ICP was observed at both early and late phases of TBI, whereas the NSE levels, another biomarker used in the study, were only weakly associated with increased ICP in only the late phase, suggesting the utility of S100β as a more accurate predictor of increased ICP.[102,107] However, studies have reported that serum levels of S100β in combination with the levels of NSE and GFAP might have improved predictive values for overall TBI outcome.[56,86,87,110,111] Numerous studies have reported correlations of the S100β levels with clinical outcome (e.g., Glasgow Outcome Scale [GOS] or Glasgow Outcome Scale-Extended [GOS-E]) and discussing S100β as a potential prognostic serum biomarker in severe TBI.[39,99,112–115]

GFAP is another CNS-specific astrocytic marker primarily expressed in mature astrocytes[116] that has been extensively studied as a biomarker in brain injury studies[34,96] and clinical trials.[117] GFAP is also considered a brain-specific marker for malignant gliomas.[118] Elevated concentrations of GFAP and its breakdown products (GFAP-BDP) mainly resulted from calpain proteolysis[58] in CSF and serum and were reported in adult mild, moderate, and severe TBI patients; these elevated concentrations were correlated with TBI magnitude and outcome in adults[55,56,63,77,79,84,87,99,119,120] and children.[80,121,122] A prospective study also showed that serum concentration of GFAP was significantly higher in patients with increased ICP.[101,123] Studies in severe TBI patients provided evidence that serum levels of GFAP, along with its ratio to a neuronal biomarker UCH-L1, could distinguish focal from diffuse injury.[76,82,123] Importantly, a recent preclinical study demonstrated a significant correlation of serum and CSF levels of GFAP to the value of the GFAP-to-UCH-L1 ratio following experimental TBI; no significant correlations were observed for UCH-L1 alone, thus suggesting the validity of serum GFAP analyses to assess changes of this biomarker in the brain.[124] These findings are consistent with results of a study by Papa and colleagues that focused on the diagnostic accuracy of GFAP and UCH-L1; this study demonstrated that GFAP performed most consistently in detecting mild to moderate TBI and in predicting CT lesions and neurosurgical intervention.[74] Although serum GFAP is a widely recognized marker of severe TBI that increases during the first days following injury,[84,101,123,125–127] a recent study by Bogoslovsky and colleagues[128] demonstrated increased plasma GFAP levels for up to 90 days after TBI, suggesting that GFAP might be useful as a biomarker in both acute and subacute TBI phases. Moreover, recent data suggest that GFAP outperforms S100β in detecting traumatic intracranial lesions on CT scans in patients with mild TBI.[87]

Biomarkers Associated with Axonal and Neuronal Injury

Several proteins present in neurons and axonal processes have been studied as biomarkers of TBI, including neuron-specific enzymes (i.e., UCH-L1, NSE); structural proteins and products of their degradation, including members of the MAP family (e.g., tau and its isoforms and *MAP-2*), SBDP, neurofilaments (NF); and proteins associated with myelin (e.g., MBP).

UCH-L1 is a highly abundant neuron-specific protein[129] and has been documented as a therapeutic and diagnostic target for CNS injuries and neurodegeneration.[96,117,130] Clinical studies have shown that CSF and serum levels of UCH-L1 are elevated after TBI, and these levels are significantly associated with measures of injury severity and outcome in adults[52–54,64,131,132] and in children.[53] These findings are consistent with preclinical studies demonstrating increases of UCH-L1 concentrations in CSF and serum in animals following acute experimental TBI.[124,133] Several clinical studies have demonstrated a strong correlation of UCH-L1 in CSF and serum with TBI severity at acute TBI phase and clinical outcome.[74,76,78,99,131] Interestingly, a recent TBI study suggests that serum UCH-L1 concentrations might be able to discriminate TBI patients with abnormal and normal CT findings.[77] In addition, assessment of UCH-L1 along with GFAP has been suggested to differentiate between diffuse and focal injuries and CT positive and negative findings.[64,76]

Tau is a CNS protein that belongs to MAP family and is predominantly expressed in neurons that play a critical role in normal physiological function; its abnormal processing is implicated in the pathophysiology of many neurodegenerative disorders such AD.[134–136] Different tau isoforms in the CSF have long been considered as promising markers to discriminate neurodegenerative disorders from healthy aging.[137,138] CSF levels of tau protein were also increased following acute brain injuries such as stroke[139–141] and TBI.[142,143] Similarly, increased serum and plasma levels of tau protein have been demonstrated in patients following stroke and mild and severe TBI.[92,144–146] Interestingly, these studies have also shown that CSF and serum concentrations of tau protein in TBI patients measured acutely after injury are correlated with short- and long-term outcome.[143,146] Total tau levels in acute and chronic TBI were correlated with clinical and radiological variables of TBI severity.[92,128] In addition to total tau protein levels, its phosphorylated form and products of its enzymatic proteolysis have been suggested as biomarkers of both acute brain injuries and degenerative disease.[35] Limited studies suggest that elevated levels of proteolytically cleaved fragments after TBI were associated with an increased risk of CT lesions[147] and increased ICP.[148] In sports-related concussion patients, serum levels of specific tau fragments generated by a disintegrin and metalloproteinase domain-containing protein 10 (ADAM10) and caspase-3 were significantly higher in postconcussion samples compared with pre-season samples, and the levels of ADAM10-cleved tau were correlated with the duration of postconcussive symptoms.[149] A preclinical study documented that caspase-3-cleaved tau in the brain is detectable as early as 24 hours following TBI and forms perivascular aggregates at chronic time points, thus suggesting its possible role in chronic neurodegeneration following TBI.[150] Plasma levels of hyperphosphorylated tau and its ratio to total tau were elevated in patients with chronic TBI compared to controls, suggesting that these indices can serve as diagnostic and prognostic biomarkers for both acute and chronic TBI.[92] Recent studies by Wang and colleagues revealed that preclinical AD subjects with self-reported mild TBI had a smaller cortical thickness that was correlated with CSF total tau levels.[151]

MAP-2, a brain-specific member of the MAP family, is considered a dendritic marker[152] and a prospective marker of brain injuries. An increase in MAP-2 concentration was observed in the serum of severe TBI patients, and this increase was associated with TBI severity and correlated with long-term cognitive outcome.[60] In TBI patients, early elevated CSF levels of MAP-2 were associated with severity of diffuse brain injury and predicted 2-week mortality.[71,153]

α-II spectrin is a major structural component in the cytoskeletons of neurons, and it is especially abundant in axons. It is a major substrate for proteolysis by calpain and caspase-3 proteases resulting in the accumulation of its several signature cleavage products, notably calpain-specific 150 kDa and 145 kDa SBDPs (SBDP150 and SBDP145, respectively) and caspase-3-specific 120 kDa SBDP (SBDP120).[154] Numerous studies have demonstrated that temporal levels of SBDPs correlated with acute diagnosis of severe TBI patients,[131] and their increased levels in CSF and/or serum in severe TBI patients were correlated with the severity of brain injury[81,155–157] and clinical outcome.[53,81,84,157–159] A study by Pineda and colleagues documented that CSF levels of SBDP150, SBDP145, and SBDP120 were higher in a diffuse brain injury group compared to a focal TBI group, although significant changes were observed only for SBDP150.[157] A positive correlation between SBDP levels in CSF and ICP has been found in a cohort of TBI patients with prolonged elevations of ICP.[155]

MBP is a structural hydrophilic protein that plays a critical role in myelin organization in the CNS, and it has long been considered a marker of demyelination.[160] Significant increases in serum MBP levels were observed in severe TBI patients at the time of admission and up to 2 weeks after injury, and the highest MBP levels were associated with poor outcome.[161] Further studies suggested a prospective prognostic value of serum MBP levels in both adult and pediatric TBI.[162–164]

NSE is a neuron-specific isoform of the glycolytic enzyme enolase. Several studies documented elevated NSE concentrations in CSF and blood samples following different brain disorders, including TBI and stroke, and found correlation of NSE levels with clinical outcome in adults and children[162,165–168] (see also a systematic review by Mercier and colleagues[166]). Increased NSE levels have been also demonstrated in the preclinical models of brain injuries.[169–173]

NF isoforms are major cytoskeletal components of axons including light (68 kDa), medium (150 kDa), and heavy (190–210 kDa) NF chains (NF-L, NF-M, and NF-H, respectively)[174,175] Elevated levels of NF-L in CSF have been reported in different chronic neurodegenerative disorders such as AD and following acute brain injuries, including ischemic stroke, subarachnoid hemorrhage (SAH) and TBI; NF-L levels remained elevate for months after brain injury, suggesting ongoing axonal degeneration in these patients.[176–178] Acute increases in the CSF levels of phosphorylated NFL-H have been reported in amateur boxers following a bout.[179] Acute serum levels of NF-H in adult and pediatric patients with TBI were correlated with CT findings, and these levels were significantly higher in patients with DAI.[180–182]

Clinical Studies of TBI Using Brain Specific Protein Biomarkers

Several clinical studies listed in the ClinicalTrials.gov registry and World Health Organization (WHO) International Clinical Trials Registry Platform (ICTRP) are seeking to determine the utility of different protein biomarkers associated with brain injuries (Table 18.1). These studies are examining relationships between biomarker levels and injury severity in the prediction of clinical outcome and the assessment of the efficacy of therapeutic interventions. The conduct of such studies reflects the emerging

Table 18.1:

Reported results from clinical trials of serum brain-specific protein biomarkers in traumatic brain injury (TBI)

Trial Number and References	Study Type and Design	Patient/Control Groups (Size) in Published Studies	Time Points	Biomarker Outcomes	Clinical Outcomes Tested
NCT00545662 (COBRIT)[128]	Interventional, randomized, double-blind, placebo-controlled phase 3	Mild TBI (34)/control (19)	Within 24 hours, 30 and 90 days	GFAP, tau, Amyloid-β	GOS-E
NCT01295346 (ATO-04b)[77]	Observational prospective multicenter	Mild, moderate TBI (273)	6 hours	GFAP, S100β, UCH-L1	CT
NCT01363583[183]	Interventional, randomized, prospective, double-blind, phase 1	Severe TBI (48)	Serial 1–5 days	NSE, S100β	CPP, CT, ICP, Morris-Marshall score
NCT01565551 (TRACK-TBI)[63,64,79,92]	Observational, prospective, multicenter, cohort study	Mild, moderate and severe TBI (215),[63,79] TBI (206)/control (175),[64] and TBI (217)[92]	24 hours and 44.5 days	GFAP GFAP-BDP, UCH-L1, Tau	CDE, CT, GOS-E
CT2014042017356N1[185,186]	Interventional, single-center, randomized, blinded controlled, phase 2	DAI (with and without o progesterone treatment)	24 hours	NSE, S100β	GCS
IRCT2013022610178N4[187]	Interventional prospective, randomized, not blinded	TBI (68) (with and without o memantine treatment)	7 days	NSE	GCS
NCT02021877	Observational prospective	TBI (389)/orthopedic control (81)	7 days	GFAP, UCHL-1	GCS, CT

CDE, common data elements; CT, computed tomography; DAI, diffuse axonal injury; GCS, Glasgow Coma Scale; GFAP, glial fibrillary acidic protein; GOS-E, Glasgow Outcome Scale-Extended; NSE, neuron-specific enolase; S100β, calcium binding protein B; UCHL-1, ubiquitin C-terminal hydrolase L1.

interest of using biomarkers as ancillary or even surrogate outcome measures. The most used brain-specific protein biomarkers in clinical trials include S100β, NSE, SBDPs, GFAP, and UCH-L1. Several of these trials have been focusing on the association of biomarker levels with conventional outcome measures such as GOS or GOS-E, ICP, cerebral perfusion pressure (CPP), and CT imaging. To date, only a limited number of studies have published results. Notably, the results of clinical trial TBI NCT01565551 (TRACK-TBI) have been reported in several publications describing in greater details different aspects of the diagnostic utility of several biomarkers used in this trial (e.g., GFAP, GFAP-BDP, UCH-L1, tau), which allows a side-by-side comparison of their diagnostic significance in the same patient population.[63,64,79,92] Current trends in biomarker research in clinical trials are summarized in Figure 18.1.

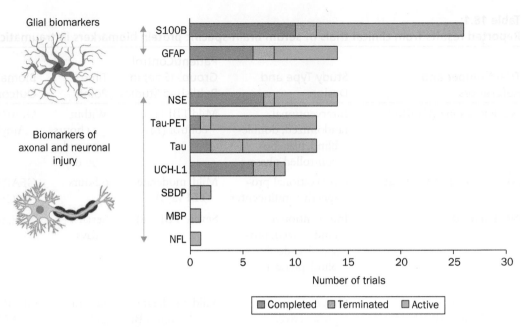

Figure 18.1 Current trends of biomarker research in clinical trials.

Association of Biomarkers with TBI Severity and Outcome in Clinical Trials

Several trials demonstrated an association of GFAP and UCH-L1 levels with TBI severity and outcome (NCT01565551 [TRACK-TBI][64] and NCT02021877).[78,85] Nevertheless, neither of these biomarkers (i.e., GFAP and UCH-L1) has adequate sensitivity and specificity for their association with outcome assessed at 3 months after injury using a GOS-E threshold.[64] In severe TBI patients, NSE levels had the highest prediction power of mortality (NCT01363583).[183,184] Elevated levels of plasma GFAP-BDP in mild, moderate, and severe TBI demonstrated very good predictive value for discrimination of injury severity.[79]

Several current ongoing clinical trials are focusing on evaluating the diagnostic utility of blood levels of S100β in patients with different types of TBI in adult (NCT01619293, NCT02650765) and pediatric (NCT02855034, NCT02819778) populations. In a prospective multicenter observational study, blood concentrations of S100β along with UCH-L1 and GFAP have been tested to determine their relationships with clinical measures of injury severity, occurrence of complications, and outcome (NCT01295346 [ATO-04b]) Interestingly, an ongoing clinical trial is evaluating the utility of salivary levels of brain-specific biomarkers (i.e., GFAP, S100β, and NSE) as a diagnostic tool for acute pediatric TBI to detect injuries that may not be detectable by conventional neuroimaging studies (NCT02609568). Other current clinical trials are investigating the role of concentrations of S100β and NSE in serum in mild and moderate TBI (NCT02988102, NTR5409, NCT01122212). Three clinical trials aimed to investigate the prognostic potential of prehospital and repeated in-hospital measurements of S100β, NSE, and GFAP as predictors of neurological outcome in patients suffering severe TBI (NCT03062566) and the potential of prehospital S100β and GFAP measurements to predict the need for neurosurgical interventions in moderate TBI and to rule-in high-risk patients (NCT02867137 [PreTBI I], NCT03028376 [PreTBI II]).

In addition, blood biomarkers of chronic TBI outcome can be used in the assessment of risk of developing neurodegenerative diseases such as chronic traumatic encephalopathy (CTE) following TBI. These trial have been mainly focused on different tau isoforms due to their well-established roles in pathophysiology of neurodegeneration as well as their prospective diagnostic and prognostic values in both chronic and acute phases of TBI. These trials include assessments of changes in concentrations of tau protein and its phosphorylated isoform in CSF, blood, brain microdialysate, and postmortem tissue and their correlation with neuroimaging and chronic TBI outcome, as well as the correlation of tau with risk of CTE, AD, and posttraumatic stress disorder (PTSD) (NCT01687153, NCT02191267, NCT02997371, NCT01952288, NCT01687153, NCT02191267). In addition, several trials are examining relationships between tau aggregate deposition in TBI and CTE patients using tau positron emission tomography (PET) imaging. Some of these studies seek to establish correlations between tau assessed by PET and tau concentrations in CSF (NCT01687153, NCT01952288, NCT02003183, NCT02079766, NCT02103894, NCT02191267, NCT02266563, NCT02278367, NCT02512029, NCT02798185, NCT02997371, NCT03218332, ChiCTR-OPC-16008982, CTRI/2017/04/008412, IRCT2013022610178N4, IRCT201410312582N9, IRCT201410312582N9, JPRN-UMIN000014785, JPRN-UMIN000013517).

Association of Biomarkers with ICP, CPP, and CT Findings in Clinical Studies

S100β levels in severe TBI patients were associated with ICP and CPP and reflected different aspects of brain injury as evaluated by CT scan (NCT01363583).[183] The results of a trial reported by Welch and colleagues documented that levels of GFAP and UCH-L1 demonstrated a potential to predict acute intracranial lesions detected by CT with high sensitivity and sufficient specificity to afford objective decision-making power for reduction in CT use (NCT01295346 [ATO-04b]).[77]

Several other ongoing trials have been directed toward establishing a relationship between biomarker levels in biofluid with neuroimaging, with the aim of reducing CT use. These trials are focusing on evaluating the levels of different blood biomarkers including UCH-L1 and GFAP in adult TBI subjects (NCT02541123 [VIGILANT]) and S100β in both adults (NCT00717301, NCT00822445) and children (NCT02819778) as well as S100β and tau (NCT03280485) with acute intracranial lesions detectable with CT scan. Several trials suggested potential roles of plasma or serum concentrations of UCH-L1 and GFAP (NCT02021877)[78,85] and GFAP-BDP[63] as prognostic indicators to distinguish mass lesions from diffuse injuries evident on CT scans. A recent clinical study indicated that plasma levels of total and phosphorylated tau, as well as their ratio, allow significant discrimination between patients with positive and negative CT findings (NCT01565551 [TRACK-TBI]).[92] A completed trial employed S100β and tau versus CT findings (NCT03280485). A currently active trial is aimed to correlate several blood biomarkers including GFAP, SBDP, and MBP with myelin damage as assessed by DTI (ACTRN12615000543583).

Potential Role of Biomarkers for Assessment of Cell-Specific Injuries Following TBI in Clinical Studies

The association of cell-specific biomarkers UCHL-1 and GFAP with neuronal glial injury is widely recognized. Two recently completed trials performed clinical testing of a specific biomarker assay (i.e., the Banyan UCH-L1/GFAP Detection assay) to detect specific glial and neuronal brain-specific proteins UCHL-1 and GFAP in the blood from patients following TBI (NCT01426919 [ALERT-TBI] and NCT02439736 [ALERT-TBIx]). Another ongoing clinical trial aims to evaluate serum levels of several brain-specific proteins including tau, GFAP, S100β, and NFL as novel biomarkers of traumatic microvascular injury and BBB dysfunction (NCT03139682). A current clinical trial tests several brain-specific proteins in serum including tau, GFAP, S100β, and NFL as novel biomarkers for the assessment of microvascular injury and BBB dysfunction in TBI (NCT03139682).

Use of Biomarkers for Assessing Treatment Efficacy in Clinical Trials

Different blood-based brain-specific biomarkers have been used in several completed and ongoing clinical trials to assess treatment efficacy in TBI. Plasma levels of GFAP, tau, and amyloid-β after TBI were used to evaluate the treatment efficacy of citicoline (NCT00545662 [COBRIT]),[128] serum levels of NSE and S100β were used to evaluate the treatment efficacy of progesterone (CT2014042017356N1),[185,186] and serum levels of NSE were used to evaluate the treatment efficacy of memantine (IRCT2013022610178N4).[187]

In addition, there are several trials with no published results. A previous trial, which has been terminated due to lack of clinical benefit of treatment, employed serum levels of glial and neuronal biomarkers (i.e., S100β, GFAP, UCH-L1, and SBDP150) to evaluate patient response to progesterone treatment (NCT01730443 [BIO-ProTECT]). An ongoing randomized, double-blind, placebo-controlled clinical trial used levels of protein biomarkers including SBDP150, S100, GFAP, and UCH-L1 as secondary outcomes to determine the tolerability and safety of NNZ-2566 as treatment in mild TBI (NCT02100150). Currently, two erythropoietin trials in severe TBI are using blood and CSF levels of NSE and S100β as outcome measures (NCT00260052, NCT00375869). Serum S100β concentrations have been used in a completed trial aimed to test the efficacy of epigallocatechin-3-gallate supplementation (NCT02731495) and the comparative evaluation of hypertonic saline formulations (IRCT201011055107N1) in TBI patients. S100β and NSE levels have been used for assessment of remote ischemic conditioning as a TBI treatment (NCT03176823). NSE has also been used in a clinical trial aimed to study the neuroprotective effect of atorvastatin in patient with TBI (IRCT2013041910178N5).

Improving Clinical Study Designs Using Blood-Based Biomarkers in Combination with Other Outcomes Measures

Numerous studies in TBI suggest that brain-specific protein biomarkers might be useful in a wide range of clinical applications including development of evidence-based patient management, improvement of clinical trial design, drug development, and assessment of therapeutic strategies. The majority of TBI biomarker studies have been focused on correlating biomarker profiles with clinical outcomes and imaging results and suggest insufficient sensitivity or specificity of individual biomarker in terms of diagnosis. However, the addition of biomarker measures to clinical endpoints and imaging may provide valuable information on injury phenotype to help identify and target subpopulations for interventions based on underlying injury mechanisms, improve outcome prediction, and serve as surrogate markers of recovery. For example, using a combination of neuronal and glial biomarkers such as UCH-L1 and GFAP and their ratio allowed researchers to distinguish focal and diffuse injury based on CT findings and suggested their association with TBI outcome.[59,82] Studies also suggested that the levels of brain injury biomarkers in blood and CSF may improve the predictive power of the IMPACT outcome calculator.[84,153]

At the time of this book's publication, there are no biomarkers formally approved by the US Food and Drug Administration (FDA) either for diagnosis of TBI or for use in clinical trials. However, the FDA and its nonprofit sister institution, the Critical Path Institute (https://c-path.org/) have shown strong interest in pursuing this option. During the first half of 2016, both organizations held workshops focusing on accelerating the integration of CNS biomarkers into the development of therapies for TBI and assessments of neurotoxicity. Undoubtedly, potential future FDA approvals of biomarkers for diagnosis of TBI will further facilitate their use in clinical trials.

References

1. Leo P, McCrea M. Epidemiology. In: Laskowitz D, Grant G, eds. *Translational Research in Traumatic Brain Injury*. Boca Raton, FL: Taylor & Francis; 2016. https://www.ncbi.nlm.nih.gov/books/NBK326730/

2. Hyder AA, Wunderlich CA, Puvanachandra P, Gururaj G, Kobusingye OC. The impact of traumatic brain injuries: a global perspective. *Neuro Rehabilitation*. 2007;22(5):341–353.

3. Langlois JA, Rutland-Brown W, Wald MM. The epidemiology and impact of traumatic brain injury: a brief overview. *J Head Trauma Rehabil*. 2006;21(5):375–378.

4. Pearson WS, Sugerman DE, McGuire LC, Coronado VG. Emergency department visits for traumatic brain injury in older adults in the United States: 2006–08. *West J Emerg Med*. 2012;13(3):289–293.

5. Adams JH, Jennett B, Murray LS, Teasdale GM, Gennarelli TA, Graham DI. Neuropathological findings in disabled survivors of a head injury. *J Neurotrauma*. 2011;28(5):701–709.

6. Laskowitz D, Grant G (eds.). *Translational Research in Traumatic Brain Injury*. Boca Raton, FL: Taylor & Francis; 2016.

7. Galgano M, Toshkezi G, Qiu X, Russell T, Chin L, Zhao LR. Traumatic brain injury: current treatment strategies and future endeavors. *Cell Transplant*. 2017;26(7):1118–1130.

8. Sternbach GL. The Glasgow coma scale. *J Emerg Med*. 2000;19(1):67–71.

9. Teasdale G, Jennett B. Assessment of coma and impaired consciousness. A practical scale. *Lancet*. 1974;2(7872):81–84.

10. Chamoun RB, Robertson CS, Gopinath SP. Outcome in patients with blunt head trauma and a Glasgow Coma Scale score of 3 at presentation. *J Neurosurg*. 2009;111(4):683–687.

11. Jennett B, Bond M. Assessment of outcome after severe brain damage. *Lancet*. 1975;1(7905):480–484.

12. Woischneck D, Firsching R, Ruckert N, et al. Clinical predictors of the psychosocial long-term outcome after brain injury. *Neurol Res*. 1997;19(3):305–310.

13. Majdan M, Steyerberg EW, Nieboer D, Mauritz W, Rusnak M, Lingsma HF. Glasgow coma scale motor score and pupillary reaction to predict six-month mortality in patients with traumatic brain injury: comparison of field and admission assessment. *J Neurotrauma*. 2015;32(2):101–108.

14. Reis C, Wang Y, Akyol O, et al. What's new in traumatic brain injury: update on tracking, monitoring and treatment. *Int J Mol Sci*. 2015;16(6):11903–11965.

15. Currie S, Saleem N, Straiton JA, Macmullen-Price J, Warren DJ, Craven IJ. Imaging assessment of traumatic brain injury. *Postgrad Med J*. 2016;92(1083):41–50.

16. Salottolo K, Levy AS, Slone DS, Mains CW, Bar-Or D. The effect of age on Glasgow Coma Scale score in patients with traumatic brain injury. *JAMA Surg*. 2014;149(7):727–734.

17. Woischneck D, Firsching R, Schmitz B, Kapapa T. The prognostic reliability of the Glasgow coma score in traumatic brain injuries: evaluation of MRI data. *Eur J Trauma Emerg Surg*. 2013;39(1):79–86.

18. Chaudhuri K, Malham GM, Rosenfeld JV. Survival of trauma patients with coma and bilateral fixed dilated pupils. *Injury*. 2009;40(1):28–32.

19. Udekwu P, Kromhout-Schiro S, Vaslef S, Baker C, Oller D. Glasgow Coma Scale score, mortality, and functional outcome in head-injured patients. *J Trauma*. 2004;56(5):1084–1089.

20. Firsching R, Woischneck D, Klein S, Ludwig K, Dohring W. Brain stem lesions after head injury. *Neurol Res*. 2002;24(2):145–146.

21. Weiss N, Galanaud D, Carpentier A, Naccache L, Puybasset L. Clinical review: prognostic value of magnetic resonance imaging in acute brain injury and coma. *Crit Care (London, England)*. 2007;11(5):230.

22. Weiss N, Galanaud D, Carpentier A, et al. A combined clinical and MRI approach for outcome assessment of traumatic head injured comatose patients. *J Neurol*. 2008;255(2):217–223.

23. Korley FK, Kelen GD, Jones CM, Diaz-Arrastia R. Emergency department evaluation of traumatic brain injury in the United States, 2009–2010. *J Head Trauma Rehabil*. 2016;31(6):379–387.

24. Smith-Bindman R, Lipson J, Marcus R, et al. Radiation dose associated with common computed tomography examinations and the associated lifetime attributable risk of cancer. *Arch Intern Med*. 2009;169(22):2078–2086.

25. Brenner DJ, Hall EJ. Computed tomography—an increasing source of radiation exposure. *N Engl J Med*. 2007;357(22):2277–2284.

26. Sherer M, Stouter J, Hart T, et al. Computed tomography findings and early cognitive outcome after traumatic brain injury. *Brain Inj*. 2006;20(10):997–1005.

27. Stiell IG, Wells GA, Vandemheen K, et al. The Canadian CT Head Rule for patients with minor head injury. *Lancet*. 2001;357(9266):1391–1396.

28. Haydel MJ, Preston CA, Mills TJ, Luber S, Blaudeau E, DeBlieux PM. Indications for computed tomography in patients with minor head injury. *N Engl J Med*. 2000;343(2):100–105.

29. Melnick ER, Szlezak CM, Bentley SK, Dziura JD, Kotlyar S, Post LA. CT overuse for mild traumatic brain injury. *Jt Comm J Qual Patient Saf*. 2012;38(11):483–489.

30. Korley FK, Morton MJ, Hill PM, et al. Agreement between routine emergency department care and clinical decision support recommended care in patients evaluated for mild traumatic brain injury. *Acad Emerg Med*. 2013;20(5):463–469.

31. Chakraborty S, Skolnick B, Narayan RK. Neuroprotection trials in traumatic brain injury. *Curr Neurol Neurosci Rep.* 2016;16(4):29.

32. Haddad SH, Arabi YM. Critical care management of severe traumatic brain injury in adults. *Scand J Trauma Resusc Emerg Med.* 2012;20(1):1–15.

33. Whitaker-Lea WA, Valadka AB. Acute management of moderate-severe traumatic brain injury. *Phys Med Rehabil Clin N Am.* 2017;28(2):227–243.

34. Thelin EP, Zeiler FA, Ercole A, et al. Serial sampling of serum protein biomarkers for monitoring human traumatic brain injury dynamics: a systematic review. *Front Neurol.* 2017;8:300.

35. Glushakova O, Glushakov A, Wijesinghe D, Valadka A, Hayes R, Glushakov A. Prospective clinical biomarkers of caspase-mediated apoptosis associated with neuronal and neurovascular damage following stroke and other severe brain injuries: Implications for chronic neurodegeneration. *Brain Circ.* 2017;3(2):87–108.

36. Yokobori S, Hosein K, Burks S, Sharma I, Gajavelli S, Bullock R. Biomarkers for the clinical differential diagnosis in traumatic brain injury: a systematic review. *CNS Neurosci Ther.* 2013;19(8):556–565.

37. Papa L, Mittal MK, Ramirez J, et al. Neuronal biomarker ubiquitin C-terminal hydrolase detects traumatic intracranial lesions on computed tomography in children and youth with mild traumatic brain injury. *J Neurotrauma.* 2017;34(13):2132–2140.

38. Hayes R, Glushakova O, Glushakov A. Finding effective biomarkers for pediatric traumatic brain injury. *Brain Circ.* 2016;2(3):129–132.

39. Rodriguez-Rodriguez A, Egea-Guerrero JJ, Leon-Justel A, et al. Role of S100B protein in urine and serum as an early predictor of mortality after severe traumatic brain injury in adults. *Clin Chim Acta.* 2012;414:228–233.

40. Risso FM, Serpero LD, Zimmermann LJ, et al. Urine S100 BB and A1B dimers are valuable predictors of adverse outcome in full-term asphyxiated infants. *Acta Paediatr.* 2013;102(10):e467–472.

41. Gazzolo D, Frigiola A, Bashir M, et al. Diagnostic accuracy of S100B urinary testing at birth in full-term asphyxiated newborns to predict neonatal death. *PloS One.* 2009;4(2):e4298.

42. Liu L, Zheng CX, Peng SF, et al. Evaluation of urinary S100B protein level and lactate/creatinine ratio for early diagnosis and prognostic prediction of neonatal hypoxic-ischemic encephalopathy. *Neonatology.* 2010;97(1):41–44.

43. Florio P, Luisi S, Moataza B, et al. High urinary concentrations of activin A in asphyxiated full-term newborns with moderate or severe hypoxic ischemic encephalopathy. *Clin Chem.* 2007;53(3):520–522.

44. Gazzolo D, Marinoni E, Di Iorio R, et al. Measurement of urinary S100B protein concentrations for the early identification of brain damage in asphyxiated full-term infants. *Arch Pediatr Adolesc Med.* 2003;157(12):1163–1168.

45. Bashir M, Frigiola A, Iskander I, et al. Urinary S100A1B and S100BB to predict hypoxic ischemic encephalopathy at term. *Front Biosci (Elite ed).* 2009;1:560–567.

46. Gazzolo D, Marinoni E, Di Iorio R, et al. Urinary S100B protein measurements: a tool for the early identification of hypoxic-ischemic encephalopathy in asphyxiated full-term infants. *Crit Care Med.* 2004;32(1):131–136.

47. Hicks SD, Johnson J, Carney MC, et al. Overlapping microRNA expression in saliva and cerebrospinal fluid accurately identifies pediatric traumatic brain injury. *J Neurotrauma.* 2018 Jan 1;35(1):64–72.

48. Gazzolo D, Pluchinotta F, Bashir M, et al. Neurological abnormalities in full-term asphyxiated newborns and salivary S100B testing: the "Cooperative Multitask against Brain Injury of Neonates" (CoMBINe) international study. *PloS One.* 2015;10(1):e0115194.

49. Korovesi I, Papadomichelakis E, Orfanos SE, et al. Exhaled breath condensate in mechanically ventilated brain-injured patients with no lung injury or sepsis. *Anesthesiology.* 2011;114(5):1118–1129.

50. Gao J, Zheng Z. Development of prognostic models for patients with traumatic brain injury: a systematic review. *Int J Clin Exp Med.* 2015;8(11):19881–19885.

51. Bogoslovsky T, Gill J, Jeromin A, Davis C, Diaz-Arrastia R. Fluid biomarkers of traumatic brain injury and intended context of use. *Diagnostics (Basel, Switzerland).* 2016;6(4):37.

52. Papa L, Lewis LM, Silvestri S, et al. Serum levels of ubiquitin C-terminal hydrolase distinguish mild traumatic brain injury from trauma controls and are elevated in mild and moderate traumatic brain injury patients with intracranial lesions and neurosurgical intervention. *J Trauma Acute Care Surg.* 2012;72(5):1335–1344.

53. Berger RP, Hayes RL, Richichi R, Beers SR, Wang KK. Serum concentrations of ubiquitin C-terminal hydrolase-L1 and alphaII-spectrin breakdown product 145 kDa correlate with outcome after pediatric TBI. *J Neurotrauma.* 2012;29(1):162–167.

54. Papa L, Akinyi L, Liu MC, et al. Ubiquitin C-terminal hydrolase is a novel biomarker in humans for severe traumatic brain injury. *Crit Care Med.* 2010;38(1):138–144.

55. Papa L, Lewis LM, Falk JL, et al. Elevated levels of serum glial fibrillary acidic protein breakdown products in mild and moderate traumatic brain injury are associated with intracranial lesions and neurosurgical intervention. *Ann Emerg Med.* 2012;59(6):471–483.

56. Vos PE, Jacobs B, Andriessen TM, et al. GFAP and S100B are biomarkers of traumatic brain injury: an observational cohort study. *Neurology.* 2010;75(20):1786–1793.

57. Ren C, Zoltewicz S, Guingab-Cagmat J, et al. Different expression of ubiquitin C-terminal hydrolase-L1 and alphaII-spectrin in ischemic and hemorrhagic stroke: Potential biomarkers in diagnosis. *Brain Res.* 2013;1540:84–91.

58. Zoltewicz JS, Scharf D, Yang B, Chawla A, Newsom KJ, Fang L. Characterization of antibodies that detect human GFAP after traumatic brain injury. *Biomark Insights.* 2012;7:71–79.

59. Mondello S, Linnet A, Buki A, et al. Clinical utility of serum levels of ubiquitin C-terminal hydrolase as a biomarker for severe traumatic brain injury. *Neurosurgery.* 2012;70(3):666–675.

60. Mondello S, Gabrielli A, Catani S, et al. Increased levels of serum MAP-2 at 6-months correlate with improved outcome in survivors of severe traumatic brain injury. *Brain Inj.* 2012;26(13-14):1629–1635.

61. Mondello S, Constantinescu R, Zetterberg H, Andreasson U, Holmberg B, Jeromin A. CSF alpha-synuclein and UCH-L1 levels in Parkinson's disease and atypical parkinsonian disorders. *Parkinsonism Relat Disord.* 2014;20(4):382–387.

62. Mondello S, Palmio J, Streeter J, Hayes RL, Peltola J, Jeromin A. Ubiquitin carboxy-terminal hydrolase L1 (UCH-L1) is increased in cerebrospinal fluid and plasma of patients after epileptic seizure. *BMC Neurol.* 2012;12(1):85.

63. Okonkwo DO, Yue JK, Puccio AM, et al. GFAP-BDP as an acute diagnostic marker in traumatic brain injury: results from the Prospective Transforming Research and Clinical Knowledge in Traumatic Brain Injury Study. *J Neurotrauma.* 2013;30(17):1490–1497.

64. Diaz-Arrastia R, Wang KK, Papa L, et al. Acute biomarkers of traumatic brain injury: relationship between plasma levels of ubiquitin C-terminal hydrolase-L1 and glial fibrillary acidic protein. *J Neurotrauma.* 2014;31(1):19–25.

65. Glushakova OY, Jeromin A, Martinez J, et al. Cerebrospinal fluid protein biomarker panel for assessment of neurotoxicity induced by kainic acid in rats. *Toxicol Sci.* 2012;130(1):158–167.

66. Fink EL, Berger RP, Clark RS, et al. Exploratory study of serum ubiquitin carboxyl-terminal esterase L1 and glial fibrillary acidic protein for outcome prognostication after pediatric cardiac arrest. *Resuscitation.* 2016;101:65–70.

67. Fink EL, Berger RP, Clark RS, et al. Serum biomarkers of brain injury to classify outcome after pediatric cardiac arrest. *Crit Care Med.* 2014;42(3):664–674.

68. Yan XX, Jeromin A, Jeromin A. Spectrin Breakdown Products (SBDPs) as potential biomarkers for neurodegenerative diseases. *Current translational geriatrics and experimental gerontology reports.* 2012;1(2):85–93.

69. Cai Y, Zhu HX, Li JM, et al. Age-related intraneuronal elevation of alphaII-spectrin breakdown product SBDP120 in rodent forebrain accelerates in 3xTg-AD mice. *PloS One.* 2012;7(6):e37599.

70. Pritt ML, Hall DG, Jordan WH, et al. Initial biological qualification of SBDP-145 as a biomarker of compound-induced neurodegeneration in the rat. *Toxicol Sci.* 2014;141(2):398–408.

71. Papa L, Robicsek SA, Brophy GM, et al. Temporal profile of Microtubule Associated Protein (MAP-2)—a novel indicator of diffuse brain injury severity and early mortality after brain trauma. *J Neurotrauma.* 2018;35(1):32–40.

72. Meier TB, Nelson LD, Huber DL, Bazarian JJ, Hayes RL, McCrea MA. Prospective Assessment of Acute Blood Markers of Brain Injury in Sport-Related Concussion. *J Neurotrauma.* 2017;34(22):3134–3142.

73. Lewis LM, Schloemann D, Papa L, et al. Utility of serum biomarkers in the diagnosis and stratification of mild traumatic brain injury. *Acad Emerg Med.* 2017;24(6):710–720.

74. Papa L, Brophy GM, Welch RD, et al. Time course and diagnostic accuracy of glial and neuronal blood biomarkers GFAP and UCH-L1 in a large cohort of trauma patients with and without mild traumatic brain injury. *JAMA Neurol.* 2016;73(5):551–560.

75. Stein DM, Lindell AL, Murdock KR, et al. Use of serum biomarkers to predict cerebral hypoxia after severe traumatic brain injury. *J Neurotrauma.* 2012;29(6):1140–1149.

76. Mondello S, Papa L, Buki A, et al. Neuronal and glial markers are differently associated with computed tomography findings and outcome in patients with severe traumatic brain injury: a case control study. *Crit Care (London, England).* 2011;15(3):R156.

77. Welch RD, Ayaz SI, Lewis LM, et al. Ability of serum glial fibrillary acidic protein, ubiquitin C-terminal hydrolase-L1, and S100B to differentiate normal and abnormal head computed tomography findings in patients with suspected mild or moderate traumatic brain injury. *J Neurotrauma.* 2016;33(2):203–214.

78. Posti JP, Takala RS, Runtti H, et al. The levels of glial fibrillary acidic protein and ubiquitin C-terminal hydrolase-L1 during the first week after a traumatic brain injury: correlations with clinical and imaging findings. *Neurosurgery.* 2016 Sep;79(3):456–64.

79. McMahon PJ, Panczykowski DM, Yue JK, et al. Measurement of the glial fibrillary acidic protein and its breakdown products GFAP-BDP biomarker for the detection of traumatic brain injury compared to computed tomography and magnetic resonance imaging. *J Neurotrauma.* 2015;32(8):527–533.

80. Mannix R, Eisenberg M, Berry M, Meehan WP 3rd, Hayes RL. Serum biomarkers predict acute symptom burden in children after concussion: a preliminary study. *J Neurotrauma.* 2014;31(11):1072–1075.

81. Mondello S, Robicsek SA, Gabrielli A, et al. AlphaII-spectrin breakdown products (SBDPs): diagnosis and outcome in severe traumatic brain injury patients. *J Neurotrauma.* 2010;27(7):1203–1213.

82. Mondello S, Jeromin A, Buki A, et al. Glial neuronal ratio: a novel index for differentiating injury type in patients with severe traumatic brain injury. *J Neurotrauma.* 2012;29(6):1096–1104.

83. Kou Z, Gattu R, Kobeissy F, et al. Combining biochemical and imaging markers to improve diagnosis and characterization of mild traumatic brain injury in the acute setting: results from a pilot study. *PloS One.* 2013;8(11):e80296.

84. Czeiter E, Mondello S, Kovacs N, et al. Brain injury biomarkers may improve the predictive power of the IMPACT outcome calculator. *J Neurotrauma.* 2012;29(9):1770–1778.

85. Takala RS, Posti JP, Runtti H, et al. GFAP and UCH-L1 as outcome predictors in traumatic brain injury. *World neurosurgery.* 2016;87:8–20.

86. Goyal A, Failla MD, Niyonkuru C, et al. S100b as a prognostic biomarker in outcome prediction for patients with severe traumatic brain injury. *J Neurotrauma.* 2013;30(11):946–957.

87. Papa L, Silvestri S, Brophy GM, et al. GFAP out-performs S100beta in detecting traumatic intracranial lesions on computed tomography in trauma patients with mild traumatic brain injury and those with extracranial lesions. *J Neurotrauma.* 2014;31(22):1815–1822.

88. Koh SX, Lee JK. S100B as a marker for brain damage and blood-brain barrier disruption following exercise. *Sports Med.* 2014;44(3):369–385.

89. Li X, Wilder-Smith CH, Kan ME, Lu J, Cao Y, Wong RK. Combat-training stress in soldiers increases S100B, a marker of increased blood-brain-barrier permeability, and induces immune activation. *Neuro Endocrinol Lett.* 2014;35(1):58–63.

90. Sanchez-Pena P, Pereira AR, Sourour NA, et al. S100B as an additional prognostic marker in subarachnoid aneurysmal hemorrhage. *Crit Care Med.* 2008;36(8):2267–2273.

91. Marchi N, Bazarian JJ, Puvenna V, et al. Consequences of repeated blood-brain barrier disruption in football players. *PloS One.* 2013;8(3):e56805.

92. Rubenstein R, Chang B, Yue JK, et al. Comparing plasma phospho tau, total tau, and phospho tau-total tau ratio as acute and chronic traumatic brain injury biomarkers. *JAMA Neurol.* 2017;74(9):1063–1072.

93. Posti JP, Hossain I, Takala RS, et al. Glial fibrillary acidic protein and ubiquitin C-terminal hydrolase-L1 are not specific biomarkers for mild CT-negative traumatic brain injury. *J Neurotrauma.* 2017 Jan 27. doi:10.1089/neu.2016.4442. [Epub ahead of print].

94. Papa L, Wang KKW. Raising the bar for traumatic brain injury biomarker research: methods make a difference. *J Neurotrauma.* 2017;34(13):2187–2189.

95. Yardan T, Erenler AK, Baydin A, Aydin K, Cokluk C. Usefulness of S100B protein in neurological disorders. *JPMA J Paki Med Assoc.* 2011;61(3):276–281.

96. Glushakova O, Glushakov A, Miller E, Valadka A, Hayes R. Biomarkers for acute diagnosis and management of stroke in neurointensive care units. *Brain Circ.* 2016;2(1):28–47.

97. Rezaei O, Pakdaman H, Gharehgozli K, et al. S100 B: a new concept in neurocritical care. *Iranian J Neurol.* 2017;16(2):83–89.

98. Raabe A, Kopetsch O, Woszczyk A, et al. Serum S-100B protein as a molecular marker in severe traumatic brain injury. *Restor Neurol Neurosci.* 2003;21(3-4):159–169.

99. Lee JY, Lee CY, Kim HR, Lee CH, Kim HW, Kim JH. A role of serum-based neuronal and glial markers as potential predictors for distinguishing severity and related outcomes in traumatic brain injury. *J Korean Neurosurg Soc.* 2015;58(2):93–100.

100. Raabe A, Grolms C, Sorge O, Zimmermann M, Seifert V. Serum S-100B protein in severe head injury. *Neurosurgery*. 1999;45(3):477–483.

101. Pelinka LE, Kroepfl A, Leixnering M, Buchinger W, Raabe A, Redl H. GFAP versus S100B in serum after traumatic brain injury: relationship to brain damage and outcome. *J Neurotrauma*. 2004;21(11):1553–1561.

102. Kirchhoff C, Buhmann S, Braunstein V, et al. Cerebrospinal s100-B: a potential marker for progressive intracranial hemorrhage in patients with severe traumatic brain injury. *Eur J Med Res*. 2008;13(11):511–516.

103. Hayakata T, Shiozaki T, Tasaki O, et al. Changes in CSF S100B and cytokine concentrations in early-phase severe traumatic brain injury. *Shock (Augusta, Ga)*. 2004;22(2):102–107.

104. Raabe A, Grolms C, Keller M, Dohnert J, Sorge O, Seifert V. Correlation of computed tomography findings and serum brain damage markers following severe head injury. *Acta Neurochir*. 1998;140(8):787–791; discussion 791–792.

105. Nylen K, Ost M, Csajbok LZ, et al. Serum levels of S100B, S100A1B and S100BB are all related to outcome after severe traumatic brain injury. *Acta Neurochir*. 2008;150(3):221–227; discussion 227.

106. Elting JW, de Jager AE, Teelken AW, et al. Comparison of serum S-100 protein levels following stroke and traumatic brain injury. *J Neurol Sci*. 2000;181(1-2):104–110.

107. Stein DM, Kufera JA, Lindell A, et al. Association of CSF biomarkers and secondary insults following severe traumatic brain injury. *Neurocrit Care*. 2011;14(2):200–207.

108. Berger RP, Pierce MC, Wisniewski SR, Adelson PD, Kochanek PM. Serum S100B concentrations are increased after closed head injury in children: a preliminary study. *J Neurotrauma*. 2002;19(11):1405–1409.

109. Wolf H, Frantal S, Pajenda G, Leitgeb J, Sarahrudi K, Hajdu S. Analysis of S100 calcium binding protein B serum levels in different types of traumatic intracranial lesions. *J Neurotrauma*. 2015;32(1):23–27.

110. Bohmer AE, Oses JP, Schmidt AP, et al. Neuron-specific enolase, S100B, and glial fibrillary acidic protein levels as outcome predictors in patients with severe traumatic brain injury. *Neurosurgery*. 2011;68(6):1624–1630; discussion 1630–1631.

111. Papa L, Robinson G, Oli M, et al. Use of biomarkers for diagnosis and management of traumatic brain injury patients. *Expert Opin Med Diagn*. 2008;2(8):937–945.

112. Townend WJ, Guy MJ, Pani MA, Martin B, Yates DW. Head injury outcome prediction in the emergency department: a role for protein S-100B? *J Neurol Neurosurg Psychiatry*. 2002;73(5):542–546.

113. Woertgen C, Rothoerl RD, Brawanski A. Early S-100B serum level correlates to quality of life in patients after severe head injury. *Brain Inj*. 2002;16(9):807–816.

114. Rainey T, Lesko M, Sacho R, Lecky F, Childs C. Predicting outcome after severe traumatic brain injury using the serum S100B biomarker: results using a single (24h) time-point. *Resuscitation*. 2009;80(3):341–345.

115. Thelin EP, Johannesson L, Nelson D, Bellander BM. S100B is an important outcome predictor in traumatic brain injury. *J Neurotrauma*. 2013;30(7):519–528.

116. Eng LF. Glial fibrillary acidic protein (GFAP): the major protein of glial intermediate filaments in differentiated astrocytes. *J Neuroimmunol*. 1985;8(4-6):203–214.

117. Glushakova OY, Glushakov AV, Mannix R, Miller E, Valadka AB, Hayes RL. The use of blood-based biomarkers to improve the design of clinical trials of traumatic brain injury. In: Skolnick B, Alves W, eds. *Handbook of Neuroemergency Clinical Trials*. 2nd ed. 2018:139–166.

118. Foerch C, Pfeilschifter W, Zeiner P, Brunkhorst R. [Glial fibrillary acidic protein in patients with symptoms of acute stroke: diagnostic marker of cerebral hemorrhage]. *Der Nervenarzt.* 2014;85(8):982–989.

119. Honda M, Tsuruta R, Kaneko T, et al. Serum glial fibrillary acidic protein is a highly specific biomarker for traumatic brain injury in humans compared with S-100B and neuron-specific enolase. *J Trauma.* 2010;69(1):104–109.

120. Halford J, Shen S, Itamura K, et al. New astroglial injury-defined biomarkers for neurotrauma assessment. *J Cereb Blood Flow Metabol.* 2017;37(10):3278–3299.

121. Fraser DD, Close TE, Rose KL, et al. Severe traumatic brain injury in children elevates glial fibrillary acidic protein in cerebrospinal fluid and serum. *Pediatr Crit Care Med.* 2011;12(3):319–324.

122. Hayes RL, Mondello S, Wang K. Glial fibrillary acidic protein: a promising biomarker in pediatric brain injury. *Pediatr Crit Care Med.* 2011;12(5):603–604.

123. Pelinka LE, Kroepfl A, Schmidhammer R, et al. Glial fibrillary acidic protein in serum after traumatic brain injury and multiple trauma. *J Trauma.* 2004;57(5):1006–1012.

124. Huang XJ, Glushakova O, Mondello S, Van K, Hayes RL, Lyeth BG. Acute temporal profiles of serum levels of UCH-L1 and GFAP and relationships to neuronal and astroglial pathology following traumatic brain injury in rats. *J Neurotrauma.* 2015;32(16):1179–1189.

125. Nylen K, Ost M, Csajbok LZ, et al. Increased serum-GFAP in patients with severe traumatic brain injury is related to outcome. *J Neurol Sci.* 2006;240(1-2):85–91.

126. Vos PE, Lamers KJ, Hendriks JC, et al. Glial and neuronal proteins in serum predict outcome after severe traumatic brain injury. *Neurology.* 2004;62(8):1303–1310.

127. Zurek J, Fedora M. The usefulness of S100B, NSE, GFAP, NF-H, secretagogin and Hsp70 as a predictive biomarker of outcome in children with traumatic brain injury. *Acta Neurochir.* 2012;154(1):93–103; discussion 103.

128. Bogoslovsky T, Wilson D, Chen Y, et al. Increases of plasma levels of glial fibrillary acidic protein, tau, and amyloid beta up to 90 days after traumatic brain injury. *J Neurotrauma.* 2017;34(1):66–73.

129. Day IN, Thompson RJ. UCHL1 (PGP 9.5): neuronal biomarker and ubiquitin system protein. *Prog Neurobiol.* 2010;90(3):327–362.

130. Wang KK, Yang Z, Sarkis G, Torres I, Raghavan V. Ubiquitin C-terminal hydrolase-L1 (UCH-L1) as a therapeutic and diagnostic target in neurodegeneration, neurotrauma and neuro-injuries. *Exp Opin Thera Targets.* 2017;21(6):627–638.

131. Brophy GM, Mondello S, Papa L, et al. Biokinetic analysis of ubiquitin C-terminal hydrolase-L1 (UCH-L1) in severe traumatic brain injury patient biofluids. *J Neurotrauma.* 2011;28(6):861–870.

132. Puvenna V, Brennan C, Shaw G, et al. Significance of ubiquitin carboxy-terminal hydrolase l1 elevations in athletes after sub-concussive head hits. *PloS One.* 2014;9(5):e96296.

133. Liu MC, Akinyi L, Scharf D, et al. Ubiquitin C-terminal hydrolase-L1 as a biomarker for ischemic and traumatic brain injury in rats. *Eur J Neurosci.* 2010;31(4):722–732.

134. Avila J, Lucas JJ, Perez M, Hernandez F. Role of tau protein in both physiological and pathological conditions. *Physiol Rev.* 2004;84(2):361–384.

135. Grundke-Iqbal I, Iqbal K, Tung YC, Quinlan M, Wisniewski HM, Binder LI. Abnormal phosphorylation of the microtubule-associated protein tau (tau) in Alzheimer cytoskeletal pathology. *Proc Nat Acad Sci USA.* 1986;83(13):4913–4917.

136. Grundke-Iqbal I, Iqbal K, Quinlan M, Tung YC, Zaidi MS, Wisniewski HM. Microtubule-associated protein tau. A component of Alzheimer paired helical filaments. *J Biol Chem.* 1986;261(13):6084–6089.

137. Andreasen N, Minthon L, Clarberg A, et al. Sensitivity, specificity, and stability of CSF-tau in AD in a community-based patient sample. *Neurology.* 1999;53(7):1488–1494.

138. Hampel H, Blennow K, Shaw LM, Hoessler YC, Zetterberg H, Trojanowski JQ. Total and phosphorylated tau protein as biological markers of Alzheimer's disease. *Exp Gerentol.* 2010;45(1):30–40.

139. Hesse C, Rosengren L, Vanmechelen E, et al. Cerebrospinal fluid markers for Alzheimer's disease evaluated after acute ischemic stroke. *J Alzheimer's Dis: JAD.* 2000;2(3-4):199–206.

140. Hesse C, Rosengren L, Andreasen N, et al. Transient increase in total tau but not phospho-tau in human cerebrospinal fluid after acute stroke. *Neurosci Lett.* 2001;297(3):187–190.

141. Bielewicz J, Kurzepa J, Czekajska-Chehab E, Stelmasiak Z, Bartosik-Psujek H. Does serum Tau protein predict the outcome of patients with ischemic stroke? *J Mol Neurosci: MN.* 2011;43(3):241–245.

142. Franz G, Beer R, Kampfl A, et al. Amyloid beta 1-42 and tau in cerebrospinal fluid after severe traumatic brain injury. *Neurology.* 2003;60(9):1457–1461.

143. Ost M, Nylen K, Csajbok L, et al. Initial CSF total tau correlates with 1-year outcome in patients with traumatic brain injury. *Neurology.* 2006;67(9):1600–1604.

144. Bulut M, Koksal O, Dogan S, et al. Tau protein as a serum marker of brain damage in mild traumatic brain injury: preliminary results. *Adv Ther.* 2006;23(1):12–22.

145. Kavalci C, Pekdemir M, Durukan P, et al. The value of serum tau protein for the diagnosis of intracranial injury in minor head trauma. *Am J Emerg Med.* 2007;25(4):391–395.

146. Liliang PC, Liang CL, Weng HC, et al. Tau proteins in serum predict outcome after severe traumatic brain injury. *Surg Res.* 2010;160(2):302–307.

147. Shaw GJ, Jauch EC, Zemlan FP. Serum cleaved tau protein levels and clinical outcome in adult patients with closed head injury. *Ann Emerg Med.* 2002;39(3):254–257.

148. Zemlan FP, Jauch EC, Mulchahey JJ, et al. C-tau biomarker of neuronal damage in severe brain injured patients: association with elevated intracranial pressure and clinical outcome. *Brain Res.* 2002;947(1):131–139.

149. Shahim P, Linemann T, Inekci D, et al. Serum tau fragments predict return to play in concussed professional ice hockey players. *J Neurotrauma.* 2016;33(22):1995–1999.

150. Glushakova OY, Glushakov AO, Borlongan CV, Valadka AB, Hayes RL, Glushakov AV. Role of caspase-3-mediated apoptosis in chronic caspase-3-cleaved tau accumulation and blood-brain barrier damage in the corpus callosum after traumatic brain injury in rats. *J Neurotrauma.* 2018 Jan 1;35(1):157–173.

151. Wang ML, Wei XE, Yu MM, Li PY, Li WB. Self-reported traumatic brain injury and in vivo measure of AD-vulnerable cortical thickness and AD-related biomarkers in the ADNI cohort. *Neurosci Lett.* 2017;655:115–120.

152. Olmsted JB. Microtubule-associated proteins. *Ann Rev Cell Biol.* 1986;2:421–457.

153. Papa L, Robertson CS, Wang KK, et al. Biomarkers improve clinical outcome predictors of mortality following non-penetrating severe traumatic brain injury. *Neurocrit Care.* 2015;22(1):52–64.

154. Zhang Z, Larner SF, Liu MC, Zheng W, Hayes RL, Wang KK. Multiple alphaII-spectrin breakdown products distinguish calpain and caspase dominated necrotic and apoptotic cell death pathways. *Apoptosis.* 2009;14(11):1289–1298.

155. Brophy GM, Pineda JA, Papa L, et al. AlphaII-Spectrin breakdown product cerebrospinal fluid exposure metrics suggest differences in cellular injury mechanisms after severe traumatic brain injury. *J Neurotrauma.* 2009;26(4):471–479.

156. Lewis SB, Velat GJ, Miralia L, et al. Alpha-II spectrin breakdown products in aneurysmal subarachnoid hemorrhage: a novel biomarker of proteolytic injury. *J Neurosurg.* 2007;107(4):792–796.

157. Pineda JA, Lewis SB, Valadka AB, et al. Clinical significance of alphaII-spectrin breakdown products in cerebrospinal fluid after severe traumatic brain injury. *J Neurotrauma.* 2007;24(2):354–366.

158. Cardali S, Maugeri R. Detection of alphaII-spectrin and breakdown products in humans after severe traumatic brain injury. *J Neurosurg Sci.* 2006;50(2):25–31.

159. Chen S, Shi Q, Zheng S, et al. Role of alpha-II-spectrin breakdown products in the prediction of the severity and clinical outcome of acute traumatic brain injury. *Exp Ther Med.* 2016;11(5):2049–2053.

160. Cohen SR, Herndon RM, McKhann GM. Myelin basic protein in cerebrospinal fluid as an indicator of active demyelination. *Trans Am Neurol Assoc.* 1976;101:45–47.

161. Thomas DG, Palfreyman JW, Ratcliffe JG. Serum-myelin-basic-protein assay in diagnosis and prognosis of patients with head injury. *Lancet.* 1978;1(8056):113–115.

162. Berger RP, Beers SR, Richichi R, Wiesman D, Adelson PD. Serum biomarker concentrations and outcome after pediatric traumatic brain injury. *J Neurotrauma.* 2007;24(12):1793–1801.

163. Beers SR, Berger RP, Adelson PD. Neurocognitive outcome and serum biomarkers in inflicted versus non-inflicted traumatic brain injury in young children. *J Neurotrauma.* 2007;24(1):97–105.

164. Su E, Bell MJ, Kochanek PM, et al. Increased CSF concentrations of myelin basic protein after TBI in infants and children: absence of significant effect of therapeutic hypothermia. *Neurocrit Care.* 2012;17(3):401–407.

165. Cunningham RT, Young IS, Winder J, et al. Serum neurone specific enolase (NSE) levels as an indicator of neuronal damage in patients with cerebral infarction. *Eur J Clin Invest.* 1991;21(5):497–500.

166. Mercier E, Boutin A, Shemilt M, et al. Predictive value of neuron-specific enolase for prognosis in patients with moderate or severe traumatic brain injury: a systematic review and meta-analysis. *CMAJ Open.* 2016;4(3):E371–E382.

167. Wilkinson AA, Dennis M, Simic N, et al. Brain biomarkers and pre-injury cognition are associated with long-term cognitive outcome in children with traumatic brain injury. *BMC Pediatr.* 2017;17(1):173.

168. Nakhjavan-Shahraki B, Yousefifard M, Oraii A, Sarveazad A, Hosseini M. Meta-analysis of neuron specific enolase in predicting pediatric brain injury outcomes. *EXCLI J.* 2017;16:995–1008.

169. Steinberg R, Gueniau C, Scarna H, Keller A, Worcel M, Pujol JF. Experimental brain ischemia: neuron-specific enolase level in cerebrospinal fluid as an index of neuronal damage. *J Neurochem.* 1984;43(1):19–24.

170. Hardemark HG, Persson L, Bolander HG, Hillered L, Olsson Y, Pahlman S. Neuron-specific enolase is a marker of cerebral ischemia and infarct size in rat cerebrospinal fluid. *Stroke.* 1988;19(9):1140–1144.

171. Hardemark HG, Ericsson N, Kotwica Z, et al. S-100 protein and neuron-specific enolase in CSF after experimental traumatic or focal ischemic brain damage. *J Neurosurg*. 1989;71(5 Pt 1):727–731.

172. Hatfield RH, McKernan RM. CSF neuron-specific enolase as a quantitative marker of neuronal damage in a rat stroke model. *Brain Res*. 1992;577(2):249–252.

173. Barone FC, Clark RK, Price WJ, et al. Neuron-specific enolase increases in cerebral and systemic circulation following focal ischemia. *Brain Res*. 1993;623(1):77–82.

174. Petzold A. Neurofilament phosphoforms: surrogate markers for axonal injury, degeneration and loss. *J Neurol Sci*. 2005;233(1-2):183–198.

175. Frappier T, Stetzkowski-Marden F, Pradel LA. Interaction domains of neurofilament light chain and brain spectrin. *Biochem J*. 1991;275(Pt 2):521–527.

176. Van Geel WJ, Rosengren LE, Verbeek MM. An enzyme immunoassay to quantify neurofilament light chain in cerebrospinal fluid. *J Immunol Meth*. 2005;296(1-2):179–185.

177. Rosengren LE, Karlsson JE, Karlsson JO, Persson LI, Wikkelso C. Patients with amyotrophic lateral sclerosis and other neurodegenerative diseases have increased levels of neurofilament protein in CSF. *J Neurochem*. 1996;67(5):2013–2018.

178. Bagnato S, Grimaldi LME, Di Raimondo G, et al. Prolonged cerebrospinal fluid neurofilament light chain increase in patients with post-traumatic disorders of consciousness. *J Neurotrauma*. 2017;34(16):2475–2479.

179. Neselius S, Zetterberg H, Blennow K, Marcusson J, Brisby H. Increased CSF levels of phosphorylated neurofilament heavy protein following bout in amateur boxers. *PloS One*. 2013;8(11):e81249.

180. Gatson JW, Barillas J, Hynan LS, Diaz-Arrastia R, Wolf SE, Minei JP. Detection of neurofilament-H in serum as a diagnostic tool to predict injury severity in patients who have suffered mild traumatic brain injury. *J Neurosurg*. 2014;121(5):1232–1238.

181. Zurek J, Bartlova L, Fedora M. Hyperphosphorylated neurofilament NF-H as a predictor of mortality after brain injury in children. *Brain Inj*. 2011;25(2):221–226.

182. Vajtr D, Benada O, Linzer P, et al. Immunohistochemistry and serum values of S-100B, glial fibrillary acidic protein, and hyperphosphorylated neurofilaments in brain injuries. *Soudni lekarstvi/casopis Sekce soudniho lekarstvi Cs lekarske spolecnosti J Ev Purkyne*. 2012;57(1):7–12.

183. Olivecrona Z, Bobinski L, Koskinen LO. Association of ICP, CPP, CT findings and S-100B and NSE in severe traumatic head injury. Prognostic value of the biomarkers. *Brain Inj*. 2015;29(4):446–454.

184. Bouvier D, Fournier M, Dauphin JB, et al. Serum S100B determination in the management of pediatric mild traumatic brain injury. *Clin Chem*. 2012;58(7):1116–1122.

185. Shahrokhi N, Soltani Z, Khaksari M, Karamouzian S, Mofid B, Asadikaram G. The serum changes of neuron-specific enolase and intercellular adhesion molecule-1 in patients with diffuse axonal injury following progesterone administration: a randomized clinical trial. *Arch Trauma Res*. 2016;5(3):e37005.

186. Mofid B, Soltani Z, Khaksari M, et al. What are the progesterone-induced changes of the outcome and the serum markers of injury, oxidant activity and inflammation in diffuse axonal injury patients? *Int Immunopharmacol*. 2016;32:103–110.

187. Mokhtari M, Nayeb-Aghaei H, Kouchek M, et al. Effect of memantine on serum levels of neuron-specific enolase and on the Glasgow Coma Scale in patients with moderate traumatic brain injury. *J Clin Pharmacol*. 2018;58(1):42–47.

The Role of Inflammation in Traumatic Brain Injury

Sarah C. Hellewell, Bridgette D. Semple, Jenna M. Ziebell, Nicole Bye, and Cristina Morganti-Kossmann

19

Introduction

Decades ago, the brain was thought to be refractory to immune activation due to its isolation from the bloodstream. Despite being modest compared to the immune activation occurring in peripheral organs or in infectious diseases of the nervous system (e.g., meningitis), the brain is capable of eliciting a significant immune response acutely following trauma. This complex process involves soluble immune mediators including cytokines and *chemo*tactic cyto*kines* (chemokines), as well as the activation of immune-competent cells originating from the central nervous system (CNS) and the peripheral immune system. The migration of resident glial cells to regions of cerebral damage leads to the secretion of a multitude of cytokines, which have been detected as early as a few minutes following traumatic brain injury (TBI) in both animal and human brain.[1]

Within the first 48 hours after TBI, peripheral leukocytes, mostly neutrophils and macrophages, cross the blood–brain barrier (BBB) to invade the damaged brain, ultimately propagating and sustaining the inflammatory response. Although this acute phase subsides rapidly, studies from our group and others demonstrated a protracted cytokine production in cerebrospinal fluid (CSF), albeit declining over the course of 3 weeks post-TBI.[2] These findings support substantial differences in timing of neuroinflammation when comparing human data with animal data; in rodents, the time frame from initiation to resolution of inflammatory processes is rather rapid (days to weeks), a fact that should be taken into consideration when establishing the timing of antiinflammatory intervention.

In recent years, chronic neuroinflammation has been acknowledged in postmortem brains of individuals who died months to decades after TBI.[3–6] The cell type mostly activated is microglia—not only in the vicinity of injury but also globally. Chronic microglial activation has been associated with long-term neuropsychiatric symptoms such as depression, epilepsy, dementia, and chronic traumatic encephalopathy (CTE), a condition that has received much attention recently in sport-related repetitive concussion.[7] The opportunity to visualize microglia with positron emission tomography (PET) via labeling the receptor translocator protein (TSPO) permits assessment of the degree of inflammation in live individuals, providing novel insight into this multifaceted process.[8] Based on the dual role of microglia, further investigations are required to fully dissect different stages of activation, the cellular differentiation phenotypes with their relative molecular patterns, and the contribution of these phenotypes to posttraumatic neuropathology.[9]

Although diffuse and focal brain injury coexist in varying degrees in each case, experimental studies have helped to clarify that inflammatory processes differ significantly in these types of TBI. Focal brain injury is characterized by a compact accumulation of neutrophils, macrophages, and astrocytes around the lesion with a sudden, marked increase in localized cytokine production.[10,11] Conversely, diffuse axonal damage presents a subtle inflammatory response with lower cytokine concentrations and absence of neutrophils, but with discrete accumulation of macrophages in white matter regions where axonal injury is predominant, such as the corpus callosum and brainstem.[12,13]

The varying intensity of immune responses reported in individuals affected by brain trauma has spurred several investigations that support a predisposition to higher and prolonged cytokine production in female patients.[14] In addition, the characterization of single nucleotide polymorphisms (SNPs) proved that the genetic make-up of individuals carrying two tumor necrosis factor (TNF) or interleukin (IL)-1 alleles exacerbates cytokine synthesis and predisposes to a poorer outcome after TBI.[15,16]

Cytokines and Neuroinflammation

The immune response to TBI is orchestrated by an array of pro- and antiinflammatory cytokines, preformed peptides that are rapidly released and newly synthesized following injury[17,18] (Table 19.1). Cytokines bind to high-affinity receptors on their target cells, inducing upregulation of cell adhesion molecules and facilitating the transmigration of immune cells to the injured tissue.[19] Cytokines signal further cytokine production in a positive feedback loop, propagating the immune response.[20] This initial activity is largely favorable by clearance of cellular debris to promote repair. However, without adequate control, this response may become ungovernable and support a cytotoxic environment, augmenting cell death and prolonging mechanisms of secondary brain injury.[21] As such, the temporal profile of cytokine production should be considered in parallel to the concentration when assessing the inflammatory response to TBI (Figure 19.1).

Tumor Necrosis Factor

A true pleiotropic cytokine, TNF is upregulated within hours of experimental injury by resident glial cells and infiltrating leukocytes.[22–24] Early pharmacological studies found TNF to be detrimental in the acute phase after moderate to severe TBI [25,26]; however, subsequent experiments suggest that TNF is required for long-term recovery.[27,28] Elucidation of TNF's role has been complicated by a seemingly model- and severity-dependent response, with reports of low or no upregulation in some experimental paradigms, particularly in mild injuries. Clinically, TNF mRNA has been detected in postmortem brain of individuals who died within minutes of injury,[29] with elevated CSF and serum concentrations increased by 24 hours.[2,30–32] Compared to other cytokines (e.g., IL-6), the concentrations of TNF in human CSF have been found to be considerably lower.[33]

Table 19.1:
Key observations on the role of proinflammatory cytokines and chemokines in traumatic brain injury (TBI)

Tumor necrosis factor (TNF)

Rapidly upregulated by glia[22–24]

mRNA in human brain within minutes of injury[29]

Evident in human CSF and serum by 24 hours[2,30–32]

Detrimental acutely after experimental injury[25,26]

Potential role in tissue recovery[27,28]

Interleukin (IL-1β)

mRNA within minutes, protein within 2 hours[13,24,34–37]

Peak levels at 6–12 hours[11,38–40]

IL-1ra studies highlight deleterious role of IL-1β[45–47]

Therapeutic potential of IL-1ra administration[48–50]

Interleukin (IL-6)

Prominent role in leukocyte extravasation[53]

Observable increase in brain tissue between 3–8 hours of injury[23,36,54,55]

Maximal levels at 3 days in human CSF[41,42,63,64]

May be evident in CSF for up to 3 weeks[63]

Beneficial and deleterious roles[58–62]

Chemokines

Regulate leukocyte activation and transmigration into the injured brain[83–85]

Peak levels within 4–8 hours in experimental TBI[40,90–94]

Rapidly released in human CSF (Il-8, CCL2/MCP-1)[40,86–89]

CCL2/CXCR2-KO mice have improved outcomes[40,96–99]

Interleukin-1

IL-1 is present in both membrane-bound (IL-1α) and secreted (IL-1β) forms, with IL-1β being one of the most studied cytokines in TBI. IL-1β plays a central role by stimulating target cells to produce proinflammatory cytokines.[18] IL-1β mRNA is upregulated within minutes of experimental injury, followed by increased protein levels within the first 2 hours.[13,24,34–37] IL-1β protein is short-lived, typically peaking around 6–12 hours post-TBI with resolution by 72 hours.[11,38–40] In postmortem brains of TBI patients, IL-1β mRNA increased within minutes of injury,[29] while blood and CSF elevations have been detected within hours of clinical TBI[30,31,41] in brain extracellular space.[42–44]

The role of IL-1β in TBI-induced inflammation has been found to be largely deleterious. Administration of its natural antagonist, the IL-1 receptor antagonist (IL-1ra), reduced neuronal damage, minimized tissue loss,[45–47] and reduced cognitive, but not behavioral, deficits.[48,49] Consistently, mice with transgenic overexpression of IL-1ra demonstrated improved neurological function.[50] Treatment with IL-1β neutralizing antibody also dampened the neuroinflammatory response, reduced lesion volumes, and improved cognitive function.[51,52] Thus far, IL-1β is the only cytokine to show a coherent

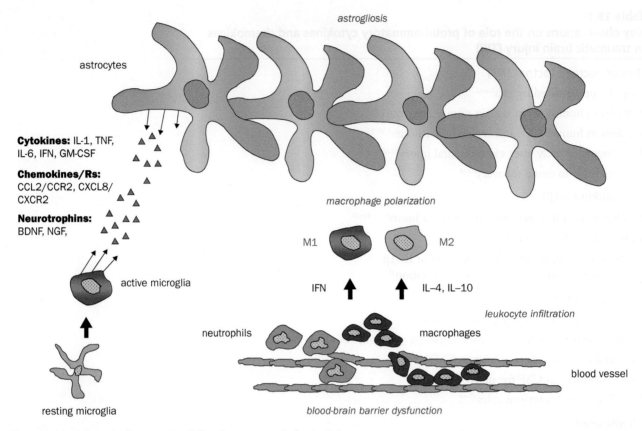

Figure 19.1 Neuroinflammation following traumatic brain injury.

impact on the pathophysiology of TBI when investigated under different experimental approaches.

Interleukin-6

IL-6 is a potent immune modulator, controlling production of chemokines and enhancing leukocyte extravasation via upregulation of cell adhesion molecules.[53] Brain elevation of IL-6 occurs between 3 and 8 hours post-TBI[24] in various injury paradigms.[23,36,54,55] The dual action of IL-6 is supported in IL-6 overexpressing mice showing decreased apoptosis and oxidative stress alongside increased wound healing,[56] while deleterious long-term consequences have been demonstrated in IL-6 overexpression.[57] In contrast, mice deficient for IL-6 have impaired inflammatory responses and increased neurodegeneration.[58,59] However, the ability of IL-6 to inhibit TNF synthesis[60] and dampen N-methyl-D-aspartate (NMDA)-mediated toxicity[61] suggest IL-6 to be largely protective. Also, IL-6 induces the synthesis of the neurotrophic growth factor (NGF) in astrocytes, thus implying a direct role in promoting neuronal survival.[62] Clinically, IL-6 is the cytokine secreted at highest concentrations in CSF, with maximal levels detected 2 days after TBI,[41,42,63,64] while its secretion is prolonged in serum and CSF for up to 3 weeks post-TBI.[63]

The Impact of Hypoxia on TBI-Induced Neuroinflammation

While the role of inflammation in TBI has been widely investigated, less is known about the impact of posttraumatic insults on the magnitude and progression of this response. Hypoxia is a frequent secondary insult aggravating secondary brain damage and is unequivocally associated with adverse outcome.[65,66] Hypoxia displays an intrinsic capability to elicit an inflammatory response.[67] Experimentally, posttraumatic hypoxia heightened and prolonged IL-1β production,[13,37] as well as increased tissue and plasma IL-6, a finding associated with aggravated motor/cognitive deficits and axonal pathology after traumatic axonal injury.[13,68,69] Hypoxia also exacerbated the production of IL-6 and TNF after TBI, compared to normoxic TBI animals.[13] Increased proinflammatory response coincided with amplified leukocyte infiltration to the injured tissue,[12] suggesting a proportional mechanism to injury severity, possibly aimed to combat heightened tissue damage. Few studies have examined the production of proinflammatory cytokines in TBI patients with posttraumatic hypoxia. A recent profiling of eight cytokines in CSF from TBI-hypoxic patients found that only GM-CSF was significantly higher, whereas GM-CSF, interferon-γ (IFNγ), and, to a lower extent, TNF had a prolonged profile when compared to normoxic TBI patients.[70]

Interaction of Chemokines, Leukocyte Recruitment, and Blood–Brain Barrier Dysfunction

The invasion of immune cells from the peripheral circulation is characteristic of the inflammatory response, particularly after focal TBI.[71,72] Neutrophils accumulate in cerebral vasculature and subarachnoid spaces within hours of injury, then enter the brain parenchyma in peak numbers within 24–48 hours.[73] Blood-borne monocytes are delayed responders, reaching a high abundance around 1 week after injury.[12,74] These cells persist in the brain parenchyma for weeks to months after TBI.[75,76] Small numbers of T-lymphocytes infiltrate the injured brain, although their contribution to neuropathology remains unclear.[77]

Under physiological conditions, the passage of cells and molecules into the CNS is limited by the BBB, comprised of astrocytes, pericytes, and microvascular endothelial cells. This barrier is activated acutely after TBI involving a plethora of peripheral and centrally derived mediators to create an inflammatory microenvironment.[78,79] Transmigration of leukocytes across the BBB is a sequential, tightly regulated process[80,81] requiring signaling by chemokines to G-protein-coupled receptors on circulating leukocytes; the upregulation and binding of complementary cell adhesion receptor-ligand pairs; and reversible interactions between leukocytes, endothelial cells and neighboring astrocytes.[71,82]

By initiating and mediating this process, chemokines are key mediators in cerebral inflammation after injury (Table 19.1).[83–85] A wide range of chemokines and their receptors are rapidly upregulated after TBI in both patients[40,86–89] and experimental models,[40,90–94] including CCL2, CCL3, CCL4, CCL5, CXCL8, and CX3CL1. Most chemokines exhibit considerable promiscuity, targeting more than one receptor in vivo.[95] However, gene-deficient and transgenic mouse models have identified the nonredundant role of CCL2 (also known as monocyte chemoattractant protein-1) and its cognate receptor CCR2 in monocyte recruitment and macrophage differentiation after CNS injury.[40,96–99]

Similarly, neutrophil transmigration depends on signaling of CXCL8 (or IL-8) via the CXCR2 receptor[11,94,100–103]

Macrophage Polarization

Abundant evidence from experimental TBI suggests that the extent of leukocyte infiltration is dependent upon injury severity and that its reduction is associated with improved outcomes and amelioration of neurodegenerative processes.[104] Infiltrated macrophages and neutrophils contribute to secondary tissue damage by releasing factors promoting neuronal death, oxidative stress, and neuroinflammatory cascades.[72,105] However, leukocytes also contribute to reparative processes, supporting axonal and vascular regrowth by inducing antiinflammatory cytokines and the removal of cellular debris.[106,107]

This dual functionality reflects the heterogeneous populations of macrophages infiltrating the injured brain and their polarization to distinct activation states. In vitro, different subsets have been identified with discrete functional phenotypes (Table 19.2). Classically activated or "M1" macrophages are induced by toll-like receptors, lipopolysaccharide (LPS), and IFNγ and are defined as proinflammatory cells releasing neurotoxic cytokines and reactive oxidative metabolites. Alternatively activated or "M2" macrophages, a phenotype induced by the antiinflammatory cytokines IL-4 and IL-10, seem to promote axonal regrowth and suppression of the inflammatory response.[108,109] A large panel of cell markers have now been identified to distinguish and characterize discrete functions of these subsets.[110]

In vivo, however, the injured brain is a considerably more complex signaling environment, yielding a dynamic mix of phenotypes that cannot be readily simplified into binary categorization.[111–113] Overall, activated microglia and infiltrated macrophages express both M1- and M2-like activation markers early after injury, with the M2 phenotype being transient and dwarfed by a predominant M1 phenotype persisting to at

Table 19.2:
Key features of M1 and M2 phenotype macrophages

Phenotype	Activation via	Release	Role	Reference
M1	LPS, IFNγ	IL-1β, IL-6, IL-18, IFNγ	Proinflammatory: Release neurotoxic cytokines and oxidative metabolites; inhibit NSPC proliferation, differentiation and survival	108,109,166,170–173,192
M2	IL-4, IL-10	CXCL12, CCL2, BDNF, EGF	Antiinflammatory; Support axonal regeneration; promote NSPC proliferation, neuronal differentiation and survival	108,109,174,175,192

BDNF, brain-derived neurotrophic factor; CCL, C-C motif ligand; CXCL, C-X-C motif ligand; EGF, epidermal growth factor; IFN, interferon; IL, interleukin; LPS, lipopolysaccharide; NSPC, neural stem/progenitor cell.

least 7 days post-injury.[114–116] Recent findings have identified phenotypes intermediate between the M1 and M2 classifications,[112] cells that express both M1 and M2 markers simultaneously,[113] and the ability of macrophages to reversibly change their phenotype in response to the evolving microenvironment.[117] Ongoing research in this arena continues to provide new insight into the dynamics of leukocyte activation and function after TBI.

Glial Responses to TBI

Resident glia play a major role in inflammatory processes after TBI. Astrocytes and microglia are considered to be key initiators of the inflammatory response following injury. Indeed, these cells are capable of secreting a plethora of cytokines, chemokines, and growth factors, as well as undergoing morphological changes.[118–123] Ultimately, these changes can influence the local microenvironment and determine the extent of damage and repair.

Astrocytes

Astrogliosis, or the increase of astrocyte activity, is a common response to focal and diffuse TBI. It involves changes to cell morphology, increased expression of the intermediate filament proteins (GFAP and vimentin), and increased proliferation, as well as the secretion of inflammatory mediators and growth factors.[124] In focal injury, glial scar formation consists mainly of astrocytes along with microglia, endothelial cells, and fibroblasts.[125] Although the exact purpose of the scar is unclear, it is hypothesized to act as a physical barrier to encapsulate damaged tissue in order to prevent toxic molecules and danger-associated molecular patterns (DAMPs) from leaking into healthy tissue, as well as preventing access to invading immune cells.

The response of astrocytes to TBI is controversial. Astrocytes sequester and metabolize excess glutamate, help reduce edema, and uphold the BBB; however, reactive astrocytes can influence the responses of other cell types within the brain and the periphery. Following stab wound injury, ablation of astrocytes resulted in increased leukocyte infiltration leading to neurodegeneration.[126] However, recent research with transgenic mice demonstrated essential protective roles of astrocytes in focal TBI.[127] Astrocytes work in concert with microglia. In fact, microglia can heighten their activity as a compensatory mechanism for depleted astrocytic numbers, and excessive activation of astrocytes can dampen microglial responses.[128,129]

Microglia

Microglia form the immune cells of the CNS, having an established role in inflammatory processes including systemic infections and localized injury.[120] However, with studies on real-time cellular interactions, more diverse roles and relationships for microglia have been proposed.[130,131] Microglia are rapidly activated in response to changes in the microenvironment, with emerging data suggesting a function as effectors of plasticity by acting on synapses.[119,130,131]

For decades, research focused on the changes in microglial morphology reflecting function. However, recent data suggest that the immune phenotype, or inflammatory marker profile (either pro- or anti-) may dictate microglial function more than morphology alone. Supporting recent experimental and clinical evidence reports long-lasting changes in the profile of microglia after TBI. Even after resolution of acute inflammation, microglial markers including OX-6, MHCII, CD68, and CD11b remain up-regulated for weeks to months.[3,132] For example, rats subjected to diffuse TBI displayed microglial activation with immunophenotype changes for at least 1 month following injury.[121,133] These are also detected years after clinical TBI.[134] In focal brain injury, mice had higher expression MHCII, CD68, and NOX2 markers in the cortex and thalamus for 12 months.[135] Overall, the increase of these inflammatory genes represents a distinct change in microglia profile.

Role of Inflammation in Posttraumatic Neurogenesis

Recent research supports a role for neuroinflammation in promoting CNS repair and regeneration by stimulating the production of new neurons (neurogenesis) from neural stem/progenitor cells (NSPCs). Constitutive neurogenesis persists in discrete regions of the normal adult brain from NSPCs residing in the subventricular zone (SVZ) lining the lateral ventricles and the subgranular zone (SGZ) of the hippocampal dentate gyrus.[136–139] In rodent brain, SVZ NSPCs give rise to immature neurons (neuroblasts) that migrate along the rostral migratory stream (RMS) to the olfactory bulb where they mature into the appropriate neuronal subtype and integrate within existing neural networks.[137,140,141] NSPCs are also present in human brain in a region comparable to the rodent SVZ,[142,143] and new neuroblasts have been detected migrating to the olfactory bulb,[144,145] although the existence of a human RMS remains controversial.[146] Intriguingly, in humans and higher primates, but not in rodents, SVZ NSPCs may also contribute to neurogenesis in the striatum—a brain region involved in movement coordination, cognition, and emotion.[147] Within the hippocampus of rodents and humans, SGZ NSPCs generate functional, mature neurons within the dentate gyrus granule cell layer,[140,148,149] with an annual turnover rate of 1.75%, which equates to approximately 700 new hippocampal neurons per day in humans.[149]

Compelling evidence has shown that neurogenesis from NSPCs in the SVZ and SGZ is enhanced in response to acute TBI, ischemia, and chronic neurodegenerative diseases,[150–153] as well as following stroke in humans.[154,155] New cells generated in the SVZ migrate to the injured brain region, differentiate into the neuronal phenotype specific to the area,[156–158] and establish long-distance connections.[158] However, the ability of proliferating NSPCs to replace lost neurons is limited since only a few precursors differentiate into neurons, and most new neurons die shortly after generation,[156,159] presumably due to the pathological environment in which they were formed. Likewise, in the hippocampus—which is particularly vulnerable to brain insults[160]—neurogenesis is stimulated following injury, but the majority of new neurons do not survive.[161,162]

This abortive attempt at brain repair seems to depend on the inflammatory response to injury, with inflammation playing a dual role. While many factors released by activated glia appear largely responsible for stimulating the early stages of neurogenesis, including NSPC proliferation, neuroblast migration, and neuronal differentiation, other inflammatory factors generate the pathological environment responsible for inhibiting new-neuron survival.[9,163–165]

Early work investigating the contribution of activated microglia to injury-induced neurogenesis found a primarily deleterious role for these cells, whereby inhibiting microglia with minocycline and indomethacin resulted in enhanced hippocampal neurogenesis in models of cranial irradiation, epilepsy, and stroke,[166–169] which was associated with improved functional outcome.[168] However, more recent studies have revealed that neurogenesis may depend on microglial activation, with M1 phenotype being inhibitory and M2 microglia being supportive, and these diverse characteristics may be linked to the soluble factors that are selectively released[9,164] (Table 19.2). For example, following LPS or IL-6 stimulation or during status epilepticus, the cytokines expressed by acutely activated M1 microglia, including IL-1β, IL-6, IL-18, IFNγ, and TNF, specifically inhibit NSPC proliferation, neuronal differentiation, or survival of new neurons.[166,170–173] Conversely, microglia with an M2 phenotype activated via an adaptive immunity response to low levels of IFNγ can instruct neuronal differentiation and survival.[174] The chemokines, including CXCL12 and CCL2, and growth factors, such as brain-derived neurotrophic factor (BDNF) and epidermal growth factor (EGF)[175] produced by microglia in turn promote multiple neurogenic stages, including NSPC proliferation and neuronal differentiation and survival, as well as the redirected migration of neuroblasts to the damaged brain region.[163,176–179] While the concept of brain regeneration following TBI is quite new, it is clear that by elucidating the interaction between inflammation and neurogenesis, new potential therapies could be developed to further support brain repair.

Therapies Modulating Immune Activation

Although neuroinflammation is a pathogenic reaction to TBI through its proportional associations to brain lesions, neuronal loss, axonal damage, and motor/cognitive dysfunction, its abolishment via high-dose antiinflammatory therapies (corticosteroids, ibuprofen, minocycline) or genetic deletion of critical inflammatory mediators (TNF) limits neurological recovery.[1] The failure of such aggressive therapies underlies the intrinsic beneficial properties of neuroinflammation. Cytokines play a crucial role in regulating the neurotrophic factors necessary to promote neuronal survival. Animal studies also demonstrated that administration of antiinflammatory cytokine IL-10 or IL-1ra and G-CSF stimulates neurogenesis through the induction of neurotrophins. Also, the activation of microglia in the proximity of injured axons in a mild TBI micro-pig model seems necessary to repair injured axons via induction of BDNF, as shown after spinal cord injury.[34]

A number of antiinflammatory strategies have been tested experimentally, leading to mixed results. Such therapies are distinguished between those with a broad spectrum of effects as opposed to those that directly target single immune mediators with established "neurotoxic" properties. Among the broad-spectrum immunosuppressants reported to show benefit to the injured brain are corticosteroids, minocycline, melatonin, ibuprofen, and erythropoietin (EPO).[1,162,180,181] However, clinical trials have failed to substantiate neuroprotection following corticosteroid administration[182,183] or, more recently, erythropoietin (EPO) therapy.[184,185] In regards to hypothermia, preclinical studies showed that a mild reduction in temperature reduced brain damage and neurological deficit.[186,187] Among the secondary injury pathways affected by hypothermia is neuroinflammation. A number of hypothermia clinical trials have been concluded with promising findings to date, and larger trials are expected in the near future.[188] It seems that specifically those patients with focal TBI and evacuated mass lesions may benefit from hypothermia as a promising therapy.

Over the past decades, many preclinical studies have successfully inhibited TNF with the administration of TNF-binding protein, indomethacin, and the nonpsychotic cannabinoid HU-211.[50] However, these optimistic pharmacological reports were contradicted by experimental TBI data on TNF-knockout mice, whose full recovery was impaired with the deletion of TNF as compared to wild-type counterparts.[27,189] Recently, TNF action has been neutralized with a newer drug, etanercept, a decoy fusion receptor formed by a human α-receptor dimer bound to IgG1, that prevents binding of TNF to its receptor. Etanercept has been trialed in stroke and TBI patients with promising results in improving neurological dysfunction.[190] Currently, when addressing specific cytokine inhibition, much potential lies in the role of IL-1ra, which has been tested in preclinical studies.[191]

Conclusion

The duality of neuroinflammation relative to the pathophysiology of TBI is a widely accepted concept. Over the past decades, plentiful studies have reported unequivocal as well as conflicting results that need to be reconciled with robust experimental research alongside clinical evidence. The heterogeneity of the pathology in itself makes it difficult to compare studies and draw definite conclusions. We face investigations reporting significant correlations of inflammatory mediators and clinical parameters and others that fail to detect any associations. The comparison of such reports is impaired by the variability of data in chronically insufficient population sizes in both observational studies and clinical trials, as well as the intercenter variations in which TBI patients are cared for. However, thus far, the accumulation of data clearly support the existence of detrimental effects exhibited by inflammatory processes that need to be neutralized, as well as beneficial properties that may be supported and boosted. Ongoing research will be able to identify therapeutic modalities that will prove beneficial for the treatment of this devastating disease.

References

1. Hellewell S, Semple BD, Morganti-Kossmann MC. Therapies negating neuroinflammation after brain trauma. *Brain Res.* 2016;1640:36–56.

2. Csuka E, Morganti-Kossmann MC, Lenzlinger PM, Joller H, Trentz O, Kossmann T. IL-10 levels in cerebrospinal fluid and serum of patients with severe traumatic brain injury. relationship to IL-6, TNF-alpha, TGF-beta 1 and blood-brain barrier function. *J Neuroimmunol.* 1999;101(2):211–221.

3. Johnson VE, Stewart JE, Begbie FD, Trojanowski JQ, Smith DH, Stewart W. Inflammation and white matter degeneration persist for years after a single traumatic brain injury. *Brain.* 2013;136(Pt 1):28–42.

4. Faden AI, Loane DJ. Chronic neurodegeneration after traumatic brain injury. Alzheimer disease, chronic traumatic encephalopathy, or persistent neuroinflammation? *Neurotherapeutics.* 2015;12(1):143–150.

5. Smith C, Gentleman SM, Leclercq PD, et al. The neuroinflammatory response in humans after traumatic brain injury. *Neuropathol Appl Neurobiol.* 2013;39(6):654–666.

6. Faden AI, Wu J, Stoica BA, Loane DJ. Progressive inflammation-mediated neurodegeneration after traumatic brain or spinal cord injury. *Br J Pharmacol.* 2016;173(4):681–691.

7. Ojo JO, Mouzon B, Greenberg MB, Bachmeier C, Mullan M, Crawford F. Repetitive mild traumatic brain injury augments tau pathology and glial activation in aged hTau mice. *J Neuropathol Exp Neurol.* 2013;72(2):137–151.

8. Papadopoulos V, Lecanu L. Translocator protein (18 kDa) TSPO. an emerging therapeutic target in neurotrauma. *Exp Neurol.* 2009;219(1):53–57.

9. Loane DJ, Kumar A. Microglia in the TBI brain: the good, the bad, and the dysregulated. *Exp Neurol.* 2016;275(3):316–327.

10. Bye N, Habgood MD, Callaway JK, et al. Transient neuroprotection by minocycline following traumatic brain injury is associated with attenuated microglial activation by no changes in cell apoptosis or neutrophil infiltration. *Exp Neurol.* 2007;204:220–233.

11. Semple BD, Bye N, Ziebell JM, Morganti-Kossmann MC. Deficiency of the chemokine receptor CXCR2 attenuates neutrophil infiltration and cortical damage following closed head injury. *Neurobiol Dis.* 2010;40:394–403.

12. Hellewell SC, Yan EB, Agyapomaa DA, Bye N, Morganti-Kossmann MC. Post-traumatic hypoxia exacerbates brain tissue damage. analysis of axonal injury and glial responses. *J Neurotrauma.* 2010;27(11):1997–2010.

13. Yan EB, Hellewell SC, Bellander BM, Agyapomaa DA, Morganti-Kossmann MC. Post-traumatic hypoxia exacerbates neurological deficit, neuroinflammation and cerebral metabolism in rats with diffuse traumatic brain injury. *J Neuroinflamm.* 2011;8:147.

14. Mellergård P, Åneman O, Sjögren F, Säberg C, Hillman J. Differences in cerebral extracellular response of interleukin-1β, interleukin-6, and interleukin-10 after subarachnoid hemorrhage or severe head trauma in humans. *Neurosurgery.* 2011;68(1):12–19.

15. Waters RJ, Murray GD, Teasdale GM, et al. Cytokine gene polymorphisms and outcome after traumatic brain injury. *J Neurotrauma.* 2013;30(20):1710–1760.

16. Hadjigeorgiou GM, Paterakis K, Dardiotis E, et al. IL-1RN and IL-1B gene polymorphisms and cerebral hemorrhagic events after traumatic brain injury. *Neurology.* 2005;65(7):1077–1082.

17. Lucas S-M, Rothwell NJ, Gibson R. The role of inflammation in CNS injury and disease. *Br J Pharmacol.* 2006;147:S232–S240.

18. Rothwell NJ. Cytokines—killers in the brain? *J Physiol.* 1999;514:3–17.

19. Cederberg D, Siesjö P. What has inflammation to do with traumatic brain injury? *Childs Nerv Syst.* 2010;26:221–226.

20. Turrin NP, Plata-Salamán CR. Cytokine-cytokine interactions and the brain. *Brain Res Bull.* 2000;51(1):3–9.

21. Lenzlinger PM, Morganti-Kossmann MC, Laurer HL, McIntosh T. The duality of the inflammatory response to traumatic brain injury. *Mol Neurobiol.* 2001;24(1-3):169–181.

22. Knoblach SM, Fan L, Faden AI. Early neuronal expression of tumor necrosis factor-α after experimental brain injury contributes to neurological impairment. *J Neuroimmunol.* 1999;95:115–125.

23. Shohami E, Novikov M, Bass R, Yamin A, Gallily R. Closed head injury triggers early production of TNF-α and IL-6 by brain tissue. *J Cereb Blood Flow Metab.* 1994;14:615–619.

24. Taupin V, Toulmond S, Serrano A, Benavides J, Zavala F. Increase in Il-6, Il-1 and Tnf levels in rat-brain following traumatic lesion—influence of pre-traumatic and posttraumatic

treatment with Ro5 4864;a Peripheral-Type (P-Site) Benzodiazepine Ligand. *J Neuroimmunol.* 1993;42(2):177–185.

25. Kim KS, Wass CA, Cross AS, Opal SM. Modulation of blood-brain barrier permeability by tumor necrosis factor and antibody to tumor necrosis factor in the rat. *Lymphokine Cytokine Res.* 1992;11(6):293–298.

26. Shohami E, Bass R, Wallach D, Yamin A, Gallily R. Inhibition of tumor necrosis factor alpha (TNFα) activity in rat brain is associated with cerebroprotection after closed head injury. *J Cereb Blood Flow Metab.* 1996;16:378–384.

27. Scherbel U, Raghupathi R, Nakamura M, et al. Differential acute and chronic responses of tumor necrosis factor-deficient mice to experimental brain injury. *PNAS.* 1999;96(15):8721–8726.

28. Sullivan PG, Bruce-Keller AJ, Rabchevsky AG, et al. Exacerbation of damage and altered NF-κB activation in mice lacking tumor necrosis factor receptors after traumatic brain injury. *J Neurosci.* 1999;19(5):6248–6256.

29. Frugier T, Morganti-Kossmann MC, O'Reilly D, McLean CA. In situ detection of inflammatory mediators in post mortem human brain tissue after traumatic injury. *J Neurotrauma.* 2010;27(3):497–507.

30. Hayakata T, Shiozaki T, Tasaki O, et al. Changes in CSF S100B and cytokine concentrations in early-phase severe traumatic brain injury. *Shock.* 2004;22(2):102–107.

31. Shiozaki T, Hayakata T, Tasaki O, et al. Cerebrospinal fluid concentrations of anti-inflammatory mediators in early-phase severe traumatic brain injury. *Shock.* 2005;23(5):406–410.

32. Morganti-Kossmann MC, Lenzlinger PM, Hans VH, et al. Production of cytokines following brain injury: Beneficial and deleterious for the damaged tissue. *Mol Psychiatry.* 1997;2(2):133–136.

33. Csuka E, Morganti-Kossmann MC, Lenzlinger PM, Joller H, Trentz O, Kossmann T. IL-10 levels in cerebrospinal fluid and serum patients with severe traumatic brain injury: relationship to IL-6, TNF-α, TGF-β and blood-brain barrier function. *J Neuroimmunol.* 1999;101(2):211–221.

34. Fassbender K, Schneider S, Bertsch T, et al. Temporal profile of release of interleukin-1 beta in neurotrauma. *Neurosci Lett.* 2000;284(3):135–138.

35. Kamm K, VanderKolk W, Lawrence C, Jonker M, Davis AT. The effect of traumatic brain injury upon the concentration and expression of interleukin-1β and interleukin-10 in the rat. *J Trauma.* 2006;60:152–157.

36. Woodroofe MN, Sarna GS, Wadhwa M, et al. Detection of Interleukin-1 and Interleukin-6 in adult-rat brain, following mechanical injury, by invivo microdialysis—evidence of a role for microglia in cytokine production. *J Neuroimmunol.* 1991;33(3):227–236.

37. Hellewell SC, Yan EB, Alwis DS, Bye N, Morganti-Kossmann MC. Erythropoietin improves motor and cognitive deficit, axonal pathology, and neuroinflammation in a combined model of diffuse traumatic brain injury and hypoxia, in association with upregulation of the erythropoietin receptor. *J Neuroinflammation.* 2013;10(156).

38. Knoblach SM, Faden AI. Administration of either anti-intercellular adhesion molecule-1 or a nonspecific control antibody improves recovery after traumatic brain injury in the rat. *J Neurotrauma.* 2002;19(9):1039–1050.

39. Ciallella JR, Ikonomovic MD, Paljug WR, et al. Changes in expression of amyloid precursor protein and interleukin-1 beta after experimental traumatic brain injury in rats. *J Neurotrauma.* 2002;19(12):1555–1567.

40. Semple BD, Bye N, Rancan M, Ziebell JM, Morganti-Kossmann MC. Role of CCL2 (MCP-1) in traumatic brain injury (TBI): evidence from severe TBI patients and CCL2-/- mice. *J Cereb Blood Flow Metab.* 2010;30(4):769–782.

41. Singhal A, Baker AJ, Hare GMT, Reinders FX, Schlichter LC, Moulton RJ. Association between cerebrospinal fluid interleukin-6 concentrations and outcome after severe human traumatic brain injury. *J Neurotrauma.* 2002;19(8):929–937.

42. Helmy A, Carpenter KL, Menon DK, Pickard JD, Hutchinson PJ. The cytokine response to human traumatic brain injury: temporal profiles and evidence for cerebral parenchymal production. *J Cereb Blood Flow Metab.* 2011;31:658–670.

43. Mellergård P, Åneman O, Sjögren F, Pettersson P, Hillman J. Changes in extracellular concentrations of some cytokines, chemokines, and neurotrophic factors after insertion of intracerebral microdialysis catheters in neurosurgical patients. *Neurosurgery.* 2008;62:151–158.

44. Hutchinson PJ, O'Connell MT, Rothwell NJ, et al. Inflammation in human brain injury: intracerebral concentrations of IL-1 alpha, IL-1 beta, and their endogenous inhibitor IL-1r. *J Neurotrauma.* 2007;24(10):1545–1557.

45. Toulmond S, Rothwell NJ. Interleukin-1 receptor antagonist inhibits neuronal damage caused by fluid percussion injury in the rat. *Brain Res.* 1995;671(2):261–266.

46. Jones NC, Prior MJW, Burden-Teh E, Marsden CA, Morris PG, Murphy S. Antagonism of the interleukin-1 receptor following traumatic brain injury in the mouse reduces the number of nitric oxide synthase-2-positive cells and improves anatomical and functional outcomes. *Eur J Neurosci.* 2005;22(1):72–78.

47. Lu KT, Wang YW, Wo YY, Yang YL. Extracellular signal-regulated kinase-mediated IL-1-induced cortical neuron damage during traumatic brain injury. *Neurosci Lett.* 2005;386:40–45.

48. Knoblach SM, Susan MKC. Cortical interleukin-1 beta elevation after traumatic brain injury in the rat: no effect of two selective antagonists on motor recovery. *Neurosci Lett.* 2000;289:5–8.

49. Sanderson KL, Raghupathi R, Saatman KE, Martin D, Miller G, McIntosh TK. Interleukin-1 receptor antagonist attenuates regional neuronal cell death and cognitive dysfunction after experimental brain injury. *J Cereb Blood Flow Metab.* 1999;19(10):1118–1125.

50. Tehranian R, Andell-Jonsson S, Beni SM, et al. Improved recovery and delayed cytokine induction after closed head injury in mice with central overexpression of the secreted isoform of the interleukin-1 receptor antagonist. *J Neurotrauma.* 2002;19(8):939–951.

51. Clausen F, Hånell A, Israelsson C, et al. Neutralization of interleukin-1β reduces cerebral edema and tissue loss and improves late cognitive outcome following traumatic brain injury in mice. *Eur J Neurosci.* 2011;34(1):110–123.

52. Clausen F, Hanell A, Bjork M, et al. Neutralization of interleukin-1 beta modifies the inflammatory response and improves histological and cognitive outcome following traumatic brain injury in mice. *Eur J Neurosci.* 2009;30(3):385–396.

53. Romano M, Sironi M, Toniatti C, et al. Role of IL-6 and its soluble receptor in induction of chemokines and leukocyte recruitment. *Immunity.* 1997;6(3):315–325.

54. Ziebell JM, Bye N, Semple BD, Kossmann T, Morganti-Kossmann MC. Attenuated neurological deficit, cell death and lesion volume in Fas-mutant mice is associated with altered neuroinflammation following traumatic brain injury. *Brain Res.* 2011;1414:94–105.

55. Williams AJ, Wei HH, Dave JR, Tortella FC. Acute and delayed neuroinflammatory response following experimental penetrating ballistic brain injury in the rat. *J Neuroinflamm.* 2007;4:17–29.

56. Penkowa M, Giralt M, Lago N, et al. Astrocyte-targeted expression of IL-6 protects the CNS against a focal brain injury. *Exp Neurol.* 2003;181(2):130–148.

57. Campbell IL, Abraham CR, Masliah E, et al. Neurologic disease induced in transgenic mice by cerebral overexpression of interleukin-6. *Proc Nat Acad Sci USA.* 1993;90(21):10061–10065.

58. Penkowa M, Giralt M, Carrasco J, Hadberg H, Hidalgo J. Impaired inflammatory response and increased oxidative stress and neurodegeneration after brain injury in interleukin-6-deficient mice. *Glia.* 2000;32(3):271–285.

59. Raivich G, Jones LL, Werner A, Bluthmann H, Doetschmann T, Kreutzberg GW. Molecular signals for glial activation: Pro- and anti-inflammatory cytokines in the injured brain. In: A Baethmann, N Plesnila, F Ringel, J Eriskat (Eds.), *Current Progress in the Understanding of Secondary Brain Damage from Trauma and Ischemia.* Vol.73. Vienna, Austria: Springer-Verlag; 1999:21–30.

60. Aderka D, Le JM, Vilcek J. Il-6 inhibits lipopolysaccharide-induced tumor necrosis factor production in cultured human-monocytes, U937 cells, and in mice. *J Immunol.* 1989;143(11):3517–3523.

61. Wang XQ, Peng YP, Lu JH, Cao BB, Qiu YH. Neuroprotection of interleukin-6 against NMDA attack and its signal transduction by JAK and MAPK. *Neurosci Lett.* 2009;450(2):122–126.

62. Kossmann T, Hans VH, Imhof HG, Trentz O, Morganti-Kossmann MC. Interleukin-6 released in human cerebrospinal fluid following traumatic brain injury may trigger nerve growth factor production in astrocytes. *Brain Res.* 1996;713(1-2):143–152.

63. Kossmann T, Hans VH, Imhof HG, et al. Intrathecal and serum interleukin-6 and the acute-phase response in patients with severe traumatic brain injuries. *Shock.* 1995;4(5):311–317.

64. Buttram SDW, Wisniewski SR, Jackson EK, et al. Multiplex assessment of cytokine and chemokine levels in cerebrospinal fluid following severe pediatric traumatic brain injury. Effects of moderate hypothermia. *J Neurotrauma.* 2007;24(11):1707–1717.

65. McHugh GS, Engel DC, Butcher I, et al. Prognostic value of secondary insults in traumatic brain injury: results from the IMPACT study. *J Neurotrauma.* 2007;24(2):287–293.

66. Chi JH, Knudson MM, Vassar MJ, et al. Prehospital hypoxia affects outcome in patients with traumatic brain injury: a prospective multicenter study. *J Trauma.* 2006;61(5):1134–1141.

67. Jellema RK, Lima Passos V, Zwanenburg A, et al. Cerebral inflammation and mobilization of the peripheral immune system following global hypoxia-ischemia in preterm sheep. *J Neuroinflammation.* 2013;10:13.

68. Goodman MD, Makley AT, Huber NL, et al. Hypobaric hypoxia exacerbates the neuroinflammatory response to traumatic brain injury. *J Surg Res.* 2011;165(1):30–37.

69. Chatzipanteli K, Vitarbo E, Alonso OF, Bramlett HM, Dietrich WD. Temporal profile of cerebrospinal fluid, plasma, and brain interleukin-6 after normothermic fluid-percussion brain injury: effect of secondary hypoxia. *Ther Hypothermia Temp Manag.* 2012;2(4):167–175.

70. Yan EB, Satgunaseelan L, Paul E, et al. Post-traumatic hypoxia is associated with prolonged cerebral cytokine production, higher serum biomarker levels, and poor outcome in patients with severe traumatic brain injury. *J Neurotrauma.* 2014;31(7):618–629.

71. Man S, Ubogu EE, Ransohoff RM. Inflammatory cell migration into the central nervous system: a few new twists on an old tale. *Brain Pathol.* 2007;17(2):243–250.

72. Morganti-Kossmann MC, Satgunaseelan L, Bye N, Kossmann T. Modulation of immune response by head injury. *Injury.* 2007;38(12):1392–1400.

73. Carlos TM, Clark RS, Franicola-Higgins D, Schiding JK, Kochanek PM. Expression of endothelial adhesion molecules and recruitment of neutrophils after traumatic brain injury in rats. *J Leukoc Biol.* 1997;61(3):279–285.

74. Fujita T, Yoshimine T, Maruno M, Hayakawa T. Cellular dynamics of macrophages and microglial cells in reaction to stab wounds in rat cerebral cortex. *Acta Neurochir.* 1998;140(3):275–279.

75. Rodriguez-Paez AC, Brunschwig JP, Bramlett HM. Light and electron microscopic assessment of progressive atrophy following moderate traumatic brain injury in the rat. *Acta Neuropathol.* 2005;109:603–616.

76. Gentleman SM, Leclercq PD, Moyes L, et al. Long-term intracerebral inflammatory response after traumatic brain injury. *Forensic Sci Int.* 2004;146:97–104.

77. Tobin RP, Mukherjee S, Kain JM, et al. Traumatic brain injury causes selective, CD74-dependent peripheral lymphocyte activation that exacerbates neurodegeneration. *Acta Neuropathol Comm.* 2014;2:143.

78. Habgood MD, Bye N, Dziegielewska KM, et al. Changes in blood-brain barrier permeability to large and small molecules following traumatic brain injury in mice. *Eur J Neurosci.* 2007;25(1):231–238.

79. Lu J, Moochhala S, Kaur C, Ling E. Cellular inflammatory response associated with breakdown of the blood-brain barrier after closed head injury in rats. *J Neurotrauma.* 2001;18(4):399–408.

80. Bernardes-Silva M, Anthony DC, Issekutz AC, Perry VH. Recruitment of neutrophils across the blood-brain barrier: the role of E- and P-selectins. *J Cereb Blood Flow Metab.* 2001;21:1115–1124.

81. Szmydynger-Chodobska J, Strazielle N, et al. Posttraumatic invasion of monocytes across the blood-cerebrospinal fluid barrier. *J Cereb Blood Flow Metab.* 2012;32(1):93–104.

82. Engelhardt B. Immune cell entry into the central nervous system: involvement of adhesion molecules and chemokines. *J Neurol Sci.* 2008;274:23–26.

83. Eugenin EA, Berman JW. Chemokine-dependent mechanisms of leukocyte trafficking across a model of the blood-brain barrier. *Methods.* 2003;29(4):351–361.

84. Ransohoff RM. Chemokines in neurological disease models: correlation between chemokine expression patterns and inflammatory pathology. *J Leukoc Biol.* 1997;62:645–652.

85. Ransohoff RM, Tani M. Do chemokines mediate leukocyte recruitment in post-traumatic CNS inflammation? *Trends Neurosci.* 1998;21(4):154–159.

86. Buttram SD, Wisniewski SR, Jackson EK, et al. Multiplex assessment of cytokine and chemokine levels in cerebrospinal fluid following severe pediatric traumatic brain injury: effects of moderate hypothermia. *J Neurotrauma.* 2007;24(11):1707–1717.

87. Rancan M, Bye N, Otto VI, et al. The chemokine fractalkine in patients with severe traumatic brain injury and a mouse model of closed head injury. *J Cereb Blood Flow Metab.* 2004;24(10):1110–1118.

88. Kossmann T, Stahel PF, Lenzlinger PM, et al. Interleukin-8 released into the cerebrospinal fluid after brain injury is associated with blood-brain barrier dysfunction and nerve growth factor production. *J Cereb Blood Flow Metab.* 1997;17(3):280–289.

89. Whalen MJ, Carlos TM, Kockanek PM, et al. Interleukin-8 is increased in cerebrospinal fluid of children with severe head injury. *Crit Care Med.* 2000;28:929–934.

90. Muessel MJ, Berman NEJ, Klein RM. Early and specific expression of monocyte chemoattractant protein-1 in the thalamus induced by cortical injury. *Brain Res.* 2000;870:211–221.

91. Ma M, Wei T, Boring L, Charo IF, Ransohoff RM, Jakeman LB. Monocyte recruitment and myelin removal are delayed following spinal cord injury in mice with CCR2 chemokine receptor deletion. *J Neurosci Res.* 2002;68:691–702.

92. Rancan M, Otto VI, Hans VHJ, et al. Upregulation of ICAM-1 and MCP-1 but not of MIP-2 and sensorimotor deficit in response to traumatic axonal injury in rats. *J Neurosci Res.* 2001;63:438–446.

93. Glabinski AR, Balasingam V, Tani M, et al. Chemokine monocyte chemoattractant protein-1 is expressed by astrocytes after mechanical injury to the brain. *J Immunol.* 1996;156:4363–4368.

94. Rhodes JKJ, Sharkey J, Andrews PJD. The temporal expression, cellular localisation, and inhibition of the chemokines MIP-2 and MCP-1 after traumatic brain injury in the rat. *J Neurotrauma.* 2009;26:1–19.

95. Zlotnik A, Yoshie O. Chemokines. A new classification system and their role in immunity. *Immunity.* 2000;12:121–127.

96. Muessel MJ, Klein RM, Wilson AM, Berman NEJ. Ablation of the chemokine monocyte chemoattractant protein-1 delays retrograde neuronal degeneration, attenuates microglial activation, and alters expression of cell death molecules. *Mol Brain Res.* 2002;103:12-27.

97. Hsieh CL, Niemi EC, Wang SH, et al. CCR2 deficiency impairs macrophage infiltration and improves cognitive function after traumatic brain injury. *J Neurotrauma.* 2014;31(20):1677–1688.

98. Gyoneva S, Kim D, Katsumoto A, Kokiko-Cochran ON, Lamb BT, Ransohoff RM. Ccr2 deletion dissociates cavity size and tau pathology after mild traumatic brain injury. *J Neuroinflammation.* 2015;12:228.

99. Morganti JM, Jopson TD, Liu S, et al. CCR2 antagonism alters brain macrophage polarization and ameliorates cognitive dysfunction induced by traumatic brain injury. *J Neurosci.* 2015;35(2):748–760.

100. Otto VI, Stahel PF, Rancan M, et al. Regulation of chemokines and chemokine receptors after experimental closed head injury. *Neuro Report.* 2001;12(9):2059–2064.

101. Valles A, Grijpink-Ongering L, de Bree FM, Tuinstra T, Ronken E. Differential regulation of the CXCR2 chemokine network in rat brain trauma: Implications for neuroimmune interactions and neuronal survival. *Neurobiol Dis.* 2006;22:312–322.

102. Wu F, Zhao Y, Jiao T, et al. CXCR2 is essential for cerebral endothelial activation and leukocyte recruitment during neuroinflammation. *J Neuroinflammation.* 2015;12:98.

103. Connell BJ, Gordon JR, Saleh TM. ELR-CXC chemokine antagonism is neuroprotective in a rat model of ischemic stroke. *Neurosci Lett.* 2015;606:117–122.

104. Hellewell S, Semple BD, Morganti-Kossmann MC. Therapies negating neuroinflammation after brain trauma. *Brain Res.* 2016; 1640(Pt A):36–56.

105. Nguyen HX, O'Barr TJ, Anderson AJ. Polymorphonuclear leukocytes promote neurotoxicity through release of matrix metalloproteinases, reactive oxygen species and TNF-alpha. *J Neurochem.* 2007;102:900–912.

106. Giulian D, Chen J, Ingeman JE, George JK, Noponen M. The role of mononuclear phagocytes in wound healing after traumatic injury to adult mammalian brain. *J Neurosci.* 1989;9(12):4416–4429.

107. Lenzlinger PM, Morganti-Kossmann MC, Laurer HL, McIntosh TK. The duality of the inflammatory response to traumatic brain injury. *Mol Neurobiol.* 2001;24(1-3):169–181.

108. Auffray C, Sieweke MH, Geissmann F. Blood monocytes: development, heterogeneity, and relationship with dendritic cells. *Ann Rev Immunol.* 2009;27:669–692.

109. Geissmann F, Jung S, Littman DR. Blood monocytes consist of two principal subsets with distinct migratory properties. *Immunity.* 2003;19(1):71–82.

110. Jablonski KA, Amici SA, Webb LM, et al. Novel markers to delineate murine M1 and M2 macrophages. *PloS One.* 2015;10(12):e0145342.

111. Martinez FO, Gordon S. The M1 and M2 paradigm of macrophage activation: time for reassessment. *F1000Prime Rep.* 2014;6:13.

112. Hsieh CL, Kim CC, Ryba BE, et al. Traumatic brain injury induces macrophage subsets in the brain. *Eur J Immunol.* 2013;43(8):2010–2022.

113. Morganti JM, Riparip LK, Rosi S. Call off the dog(ma): M1/M2 polarization is concurrent following traumatic brain injury. *PloS One.* 2016;11(1):e0148001.

114. Kumar A, Alvarez-Croda DM, Stoica BA, Faden AI, Loane DJ. Microglial/macrophage polarization dynamics following traumatic brain injury. *J Neurotrauma.* 2016; 33(19):1732–1750.

115. Kigerl KA, Gensel JC, Ankeny DP, Alexander MP, Donnelly DJ. Identification of two distinct macrophage subsets with divergent effects causing either neurotoxicity or regeneration in the injured mouse spinal cord. *J Neurosci.* 2009;29(43):13435–13444.

116. Wang G, Zhang J, Hu X, et al. Microglia/macrophage polarization dynamics in white matter after traumatic brain injury. *J Cereb Blood Flow Metab.* 2013;33(12):1864–1874.

117. Stout RD, Jiang C, Matta B, Tietzel I, Watkins SK, Suttles J. Macrophages sequentially change their functional phenotype in response to changes in microenvironmental influences. *J Immunol.* 2005;175:342–349.

118. Ziebell JM, Rowe RK, Muccigrosso MM, et al. Aging with a traumatic brain injury: could behavioral morbidities and endocrine symptoms be influenced by microglial priming? *Brain Behav Immun.* 2017; 59:1–7.

119. Evilsizor MN, Ray-Jones HF, Ellis TW Jr, Lifshitz J, Ziebell JM. Microglia in experimental brain injury: implications on neuronal injury and circuit remodeling. In: Kobeissy FH, ed. *Brain Neurotrauma: Molecular, Neuropsychological, and Rehabilitation Aspects.* Boca Raton, FL; CRC Press/Taylor & Francis 2015. Chapter 8.

120. Ziebell JM, Adelson PD, Lifshitz J. Microglia: dismantling and rebuilding circuits after acute neurological injury. *Metab Brain Dis.* 2015;30(2):393–400.

121. Cao T, Thomas TC, Ziebell JM, Pauly JR, Lifshitz J. Morphological and genetic activation of microglia after diffuse traumatic brain injury in the rat. *Neuroscience.* 2012;225:65–75.

122. Ziebell JM, Bye N, Semple BD, Kossmann T, Morganti-Kossmann MC. Attenuated neurological deficit, cell death and lesion volume in Fas-mutant mice is associated with altered neuroinflammation following traumatic brain injury. *Brain Res.* 2011;1414:94–105.

123. Ziebell JM, Morganti-Kossmann MC. Involvement of pro- and anti-inflammatory cytokines and chemokines in the pathophysiology of traumatic brain injury. *Neurotherapeutics.* 2010;7(1):22–30.

124. Karve IP, Taylor JM, Crack PJ. The contribution of astrocytes and microglia to traumatic brain injury. *Br J Pharmacol.* 2016;173(4):692–702.

125. Silver J, Miller JH. Regeneration beyond the glial scar. *Nat Rev Neurosci.* 2004;5(2):146–156.

126. Bush TG, Puvanachandra N, Horner CH, et al. Leukocyte infiltration, neuronal degeneration, and neurite outgrowth after ablation of scar-forming, reactive astrocytes in adult transgenic mice. *Neuron.* 1999;23(2):297–308.

127. Myer DJ, Gurkoff GG, Lee SM, Hovda DA, Sofroniew MV. Essential protective roles of reactive astrocytes in traumatic brain injury. *Brain.* 2006;129(Pt 10):2761–2772.

128. Kim JH, Min KJ, Seol W, Jou I, Joe EH. Astrocytes in injury states rapidly produce anti-inflammatory factors and attenuate microglial inflammatory responses. *J Neurochem.* 2010;115(5):1161–1171.

129. Robel S, Bardehle S, Lepier A, Brakebusch C, Gotz M. Genetic deletion of cdc42 reveals a crucial role for astrocyte recruitment to the injury site in vitro and in vivo. *J Neurosci.* 2011;31(35):12471–12482.

130. Tremblay ME, Lowery RL, Majewska AK. Microglial interactions with synapses are modulated by visual experience. *PLoS Biol.* 2010;8(11):e1000527.

131. Wake H, Moorhouse AJ, Jinno S, Kohsaka S, Nabekura J. Resting microglia directly monitor the functional state of synapses in vivo and determine the fate of ischemic terminals. *J Neurosci.* 2009;29(13):3974–3980.

132. VanGuilder HD, Bixler GV, Brucklacher RM, et al. Concurrent hippocampal induction of MHC II pathway components and glial activation with advanced aging is not correlated with cognitive impairment. *J Neuroinflammation.* 2011;8:138.

133. Ziebell JM, Taylor SE, Cao T, Harrison JL, Lifshitz J. Rod microglia. elongation, alignment, and coupling to form trains across the somatosensory cortex after experimental diffuse brain injury. *J Neuroinflammation.* 2012;9:247.

134. Gentleman SM, Leclercq PD, Moyes L, et al. Long-term intracerebral inflammatory response after traumatic brain injury. *Forensic Sci Int.* 2004;146(2-3):97–104.

135. Loane DJ, Kumar A, Stoica BA, Cabatbat R, Faden AI. Progressive neurodegeneration after experimental brain trauma: association with chronic microglial activation. *J Neuropathol Exp Neurol.* 2014;73(1):14–29.

136. Eriksson PS, Perfilieva E, Bjork-Eriksson T, et al. Neurogenesis in the adult human hippocampus. *Nat Med.* 1998;4(11):1313–1317.

137. Lois C, Alvarez-Buylla A. Proliferating subventricular zone cells in the adult mammalian forebrain can differentiate into neurons and glia. *Proc Nat Acad Sci USA.* 1993;90(5):2074–2077.

138. Reynolds BA, Weiss S. Generation of neurons and astrocytes from isolated cells of the adult mammalian central nervous system. *Science.* 1992;255(5052):1707–1710.

139. Richards LJ, Kilpatrick TJ, Bartlett PF. De novo generation of neuronal cells from the adult mouse brain. *PNAS.* 1992;89(18):8591–8595.

140. Abrous DN, Koehl M, Le Moal M. Adult neurogenesis. from precursors to network and physiology. *Physiol Rev.* 2005;85(2):523–569.

141. Doetsch F, Alvarez-Buylla A. Network of tangential pathways for neuronal migration in adult mammalian brain. *Proc Nat Acad Sci USA.* 1996;93(25):14895–14900.

142. Quinones-Hinojosa A, Sanai N, Gonzalez-Perez O, Garcia-Verdugo JM. The human brain subventricular zone: stem cells in this niche and its organization. *Neurosurg Clin N Am.* 2007;18(1):15–20, vii.

143. Sanai N, Nguyen T, Ihrie RA, et al. Corridors of migrating neurons in the human brain and their decline during infancy. *Nature.* 2011;478(7369):382–386.

144. Curtis MA, Kam M, Nannmark U, et al. Human neuroblasts migrate to the olfactory bulb via a lateral ventricular extension. *Science.* 2007;315(5816):1243–1249.

145. Wang C, Liu F, Liu YY, et al. Identification and characterization of neuroblasts in the subventricular zone and rostral migratory stream of the adult human brain. *Cell Res.* 2011;21(11):1534–1550.

146. Sanai N, Tramontin AD, Quinones-Hinojosa A, et al. Unique astrocyte ribbon in adult human brain contains neural stem cells but lacks chain migration. *Nature.* 2004;427(6976):740–744.

147. Ernst A, Alkass K, Bernard S, et al. Neurogenesis in the striatum of the adult human brain. *Cell.* 2014;156(5):1072–1083.

148. Hastings NB, Gould E. Rapid extension of axons into the CA3 region by adult-generated granule cells.[erratum appears in *J Comp Neurol.* 1999 Dec 6;415(1):144]. *J Comp Neurol.* 1999;413(1):146–154.

149. Spalding KL, Bergmann O, Alkass K, et al. Dynamics of hippocampal neurogenesis in adult humans. *Cell.* 2013;153(6):1219–1227.

150. Kernie SG, Parent JM. Forebrain neurogenesis after focal ischemic and traumatic brain injury. *Neurobiol Dis.* 2010;37(2):267–274.

151. Richardson RM, Sun D, Bullock MR. Neurogenesis after traumatic brain injury. *Neurosurg Clin N Am.* 2007;18(1):169–+.

152. Winner B, Kohl Z, Gage FH. Neurodegenerative disease and adult neurogenesis. *Eur J Neurosci.* 2011;33(6):1139–1151.

153. Yu TS, Washington PM, Kernie SG. Injury-induced neurogenesis: mechanisms and relevance. *Neuroscientist.* 2016;22(1):61–71.

154. Macas J, Nern C, Plate KH, Momma S. Increased generation of neuronal progenitors after ischemic injury in the aged adult human forebrain. *J Neurosci.* 2006;26(50):13114–13119.

155. Marti-Fabregas J, Romaguera-Ros M, Gomez-Pinedo U, et al. Proliferation in the human ipsilateral subventricular zone after ischemic stroke. *Neurology.* 2010;74(5):357–365.

156. Arvidsson A, Collin T, Kirik D, Kokaia Z, Lindvall O. Neuronal replacement from endogenous precursors in the adult brain after stroke. *Nat Med.* 2002;8(9):963–970.

157. Jiang W, Gu W, Brannstrom T, Rosqvist R, Wester P. Cortical neurogenesis in adult rats after transient middle cerebral artery occlusion. *Stroke.* 2001;32(5):1201–1207.

158. Magavi SS, Leavitt BR, Macklis JD. Induction of neurogenesis in the neocortex of adult mice [see comment]. *Nature.* 2000;405(6789):951–955.

159. Parent JM, Vexler ZS, Gong C, Derugin N, Ferriero DM. Rat forebrain neurogenesis and striatal neuron replacement after focal stroke. *Ann Neurol.* 2002;52(6):802–813.

160. Nikonenko AG, Radenovic L, Andjus PR, Skibo GG. Structural features of ischemic damage in the hippocampus. *Anat Rec (Hoboken).* 2009;292(12):1914–1921.

161. Bye N, Carron S, Han X, et al. Neurogenesis and glial proliferation are stimulated following diffuse traumatic brain injury in adult rats. *J Neurosci Res.* 2011;89(7):986–1000.

162. Ng SY, Semple BD, Morganti-Kossmann MC, Bye N. Attenuation of microglial activation with minocycline is not associated with changes in neurogenesis after focal traumatic brain injury in adult mice. *J Neurotrauma.* 2012;29(7):1410–1425.

163. Bye N, Turnley AM, Morganti-Kossmann MC. Inflammatory regulators of redirected neural migration in the injured brain. *NeuroSignals.* 2012;20(3):132–146.

164. Ekdahl CT, Kokaia Z, Lindvall O. Brain inflammation and adult neurogenesis: the dual role of microglia. *Neuroscience.* 2009;158(3):1021–1029.

165. Whitney NP, Eidem TM, Peng H, Huang Y, Zheng JC. Inflammation mediates varying effects in neurogenesis: relevance to the pathogenesis of brain injury and neurodegenerative disorders. *J Neurochem.* 2009;108(6):1343–1359.

166. Ekdahl CT, Claasen J-H, Bonde S, Kokaia Z, Lindvall O. Inflammation is detrimental for neurogenesis in adult brain. *Proc Nat Acad Sci USA.* 2003;100(23):13632–13637.

167. Hoehn BD, Palmer TD, Steinberg GK. Neurogenesis in rats after focal cerebral ischemia is enhanced by indomethacin. *Stroke.* 2005;36(12):2718–2724.

168. Liu Z, Fan Y, Won SJ, Neumann M, Hu D, Zhou L, Weinstein PR, Liu J. Chronic treatment with minocycline preserves adult new neurons and reduces functional impairment after focal cerebral ischemia. *Stroke*. 2007;38(1):146–152.

169. Monje ML, Mizumatsu S, Fike JR, Palmer TD. Irradiation induces neural precursor-cell dysfunction. *Nat Med*. 2002;8(9):955–962.

170. Iosif RE, Ekdahl CT, Ahlenius H, et al. Tumor necrosis factor receptor 1 is a negative regulator of progenitor proliferation in adult hippocampal neurogenesis. *J Neurosci*. 2006;26(38):9703–9712.

171. Liu Y-P, Lin H-I, Tzeng S-F. Tumor necrosis factor-alpha and interleukin-18 modulate neuronal cell fate in embryonic neural progenitor culture. *Brain Res*. 2005;1054(2):152–158.

172. Monje ML, Toda H, Palmer TD. Inflammatory blockade restores adult hippocampal neurogenesis. *Science*. 2003;302(5651):1760–1765.

173. Vallieres L, Campbell IL, Gage FH, Sawchenko PE. Reduced hippocampal neurogenesis in adult transgenic mice with chronic astrocytic production of interleukin-6. *J Neurosci*. 2002;22(2):486–492.

174. Butovsky O, Ziv Y, Schwartz A, et al. Microglia activated by IL-4 or IFN-gamma differentially induce neurogenesis and oligodendrogenesis from adult stem/progenitor cells. *Mol Cell Neurosci*. 2006;31(1):149–160.

175. Rock RB, Gekker G, Hu S, et al. Role of microglia in central nervous system infections. *Clin Microbiol Rev*. 2004;17(4):942–964.

176. Craig CG, Tropepe V, Morshead CM, Reynolds BA, Weiss S, van der Kooy D. In vivo growth factor expansion of endogenous subependymal neural precursor cell populations in the adult mouse brain. *J Neurosci*. 1996;16(8):2649–2658.

177. Imitola J, Raddassi K, Park KI, et al. Directed migration of neural stem cells to sites of CNS injury by the stromal cell-derived factor 1alpha/CXC chemokine receptor 4 pathway. *Proc Natl Acad Sci USA*. 2004;101(52):18117–18122.

178. Pencea V, Bingaman KD, Wiegand SJ, Luskin MB. Infusion of brain-derived neurotrophic factor into the lateral ventricle of the adult rat leads to new neurons in the parenchyma of the striatum, septum, thalamus, and hypothalamus. *J Neurosci*. 2001;21(17):6706–6717.

179. Yan Y-P, Sailor KA, Lang BT, Park S-W, Vemuganti R, Dempsey RJ. Monocyte chemoattractant protein-1 plays a critical role in neuroblast migration after focal cerebral ischemia. *J Cereb Blood Flow Metab*. 2007;27(6):1213–1224.

180. Hellewell SC, Morganti-Kossmann MC. Guilty molecules, guilty minds? The conflicting roles of the innate immune response to traumatic brain injury. *Mediators Inflamm*. 2012;2012:18.

181. Lin C, Chao H, Li Z, et al. Melatonin attenuates traumatic brain injury-induced inflammation: A possible role for mitophagy. *J Pineal Res*. 2016;61(2):177–186.

182. Bergold PJ. Treatment of traumatic brain injury with anti-inflammatory drugs. *Exp Neurol*. 2015;275(3):367–380.

183. Muzha I, Filipi N, Lede R. Effect of intravenous corticosteroids on death within 14 days in 10008 adults with clinically significant head injury (MRC CRASH trial): randomised placebo-controlled trial. *Lancet*. 2004;364(9442):1321–1328.

184. Nichol A, French C, Little L, et al. Erythropoietin in traumatic brain injury (EPO-TBI): a double-blind randomised controlled trial. *Lancet*. 2015;386(10012):2499–2506.

185. Robertson CS, Hannay HJ, Yamal JM, Gopinath S, Goodman JC, Tilley BC. Effect of erythropoietin and transfusion threshold on neurological recovery after traumatic brain injury: a randomized clinical trial. *JAMA*. 2014;312(1):36–47.

186. Yokobori S, Yokota H. Targeted temperature management in traumatic brain injury. *J Intensive Care*. 2016;4:28.

187. Dietrich WD, Bramlett HM. Therapeutic hypothermia and targeted temperature management in traumatic brain injury: Clinical challenges for successful translation. *Brain Res*. 2016;1(1640):94–103.

188. Yokobori S, Yokota H. Targeted temperature management in traumatic brain injury. *J Intensive Care*. 2016;4(28).

189. Shohami E, Ginis I, Hallenbeck JM. Dual role of tumor necrosis factor alpha in brain injury. *Cytokine Growth Factor Rev*. 1999;10(2):119–130.

190. Ignatowski TA, Spengler RN, Dhandapani KM, Folkersma H, Butterworth RF, Tobinick E. Perispinal etanercept for post-stroke neurological and cognitive dysfunction: scientific rationale and current evidence. *CNS Drugs*. 2014;28(8):679–697.

191. Helmy A, Guilfoyle MR, Carpenter KL, Pickard JD, Menon DK, Hutchinson PJ. Recombinant human interleukin-1 receptor antagonist in severe traumatic brain injury: a phase II randomized control trial. *J Cereb Blood Flow Metab*. 2014;34(5):845–851.

192. Karve IP, Taylor JM, Crack PJ. The contribution of astrocytes and microglia to traumatic brain injury. *Br J Pharmacol*. 2016;173:692–702.

Glutamate Receptor Peptides in Acute Neurotrauma

S. A. Dambinova, J. D. Mullins, and Thomas Gennarelli

20

Introduction

External mechanical forces can cause acute neurotrauma (mild, moderate, or severe) to the brain (traumatic brain injury, or TBI) and the spinal cord (spinal cord injury, or SCI). The impact causes alterations in neuronal cells, leading to primary focal and/or diffuse axonal damage, followed by secondary injuries to cerebrovascular autoregulation.[1] The latter is associated with transitory or persistent edema formation and rapid deterioration in clinical symptoms, thus increasing mortality.[2,3] The majority of research is currently focusing on biomarkers for neuronal injury, while the search for biomarkers that can identify the risk of regional and global cerebral blood flow (CBF) dysfunctions remains challenging. Identifying brain biomarkers sensitive to neuronal damage as well as edema formation after an acute brain impact to prevent delayed, or secondary, cerebral ischemia remains an unmet medical need.

Cerebral edema is a dramatic alteration in intra- and extracellular ion and water balance, causing increased brain tissue volume and intracranial pressure (ICP) as the major immediate consequences of neurotrauma.[3] Vasogenic (develops within 48 hours after TBI) and cytotoxic (beyond 48 hours after neurotrauma) edemas are two broad categories of varying stages of edema, from transitory to permanent change of regional vascular permeability, depending on time course, localization, and severity of injury. Global edema resulting from severe neurotrauma is accompanied primarily by subarachnoid hemorrhage or delayed cerebral ischemia and stroke.[4,5]

The difficulty of diagnosing and predicting outcome after acute TBI is associated with limitations of clinical assessment and neuroimaging. Neuroimaging techniques can provide additional clinical information, but the diagnostic capabilities of these techniques are limited by their sensitivities and high capital costs and service requirements. Furthermore, magnetic resonance imaging (MRI) and computed tomography (CT) often do not provide information that can predict the consequences and outcome of neurotrauma, particularly in mild TBI.[4,6]

Brain biomarkers detected by a rapid blood test would have important diagnostic/prognostic capabilities in mild TBI and SCI, which affect an estimated 80% of the 2.5–6.5 million individuals who suffer from life-long impairment as a result of neurotrauma.[7] The most important challenge is having the ability to predict delayed cerebral ischemic events after an injury. This can be accomplished using a blood test based on a panel of specific brain-borne biomarkers of neurotoxicity in the hospital and emergency settings.

233

Emergent management of neurotrauma in the field, prior to neuroimaging, is essential to ensure that patients receive timely personalized treatment, especially if the CT scan is normal or MRI is contraindicated or not available. The ability to speed up ruling-in DAI and reversible or persistent edema formation using a blood test (i.e., tissue-based evidence)—for example, in the ambulance—would also be extremely important in this critical assessment interval.

Patients who experience multiple neurotrauma may face an increased risk of developing a stroke,[5,8] brain-related seizures,[3] or both in severe cases. A blood test panel detecting brain-relevant biomarkers to classify patients as having low-, moderate-, or high-risk of CBF dysfunction could single out a target group for appropriate intervention by specialists, to whom patients with the highest risk of delayed ischemia should immediately be directed. Thus, there is need for a panel of biochemical markers to recognize early neuronal and cerebral vascular injuries that would provide accurate assessment and prediction of outcome after neurotrauma.

This review focuses on neurotoxicity (excitotoxicity) biomarkers for the α-amino-3-hydroxy-5-methyl-4-isoxazolepropionic acid (AMPA) receptor (AMPAR), the N-methyl-D-aspartate (NMDA) receptor (NMDAR), and the kainate receptor (KAR) peptides as detected in the biological fluids of subjects who suffered repetitive mild neurotrauma, from subtle to more serious. The main objective is to reveal a connection between various anatomical locations of glutamate receptors (GluR) and neuronal injury/CBF dysfunction through correlation with clinical scores and injury localization defined by advanced neuroimaging. The potential role of AMPAR, NMDAR, and KAR peptides in the regulation of acute and semi-acute neuronal injuries accompanied by arteriovenous impairment is also explored.

Glutamate Receptor Peptides as Key Neurotoxicity Biomarkers

A mechanical impact alters electrical signal transduction and cerebral blood circulation in restricted brain areas, launching an excitotoxicity (neurotoxicity) cascade.[9] The latter is involved in the mechanism of progressive transitory and/or persistent edema formation that can worsen a patient's condition, requiring emergent actions.

Excitotoxicity is a pathological process caused by the excitatory neurotransmitter glutamate—an abundant substance that regulates up to 90% of signal transductions in the brain—overactivating AMPAR, NMDAR, and KAR.[10] Ionotropic GluR represent more than 25 membrane proteins that mediate 80% of pre- and postsynaptic neurotransmission in cortical, subcortical, and brainstem areas. These proteins regulate long- and short-term synaptic plasticity through adaptation of corresponding gene expression.[11] In addition, vessel vasoconstriction/vasodilatation and CBF velocity primarily depend on GluR, which causes peptide fragments to be released into nervous tissue and peripheral fluids.[11–14] Abnormal trafficking of these peptides into extracellular fluids may cause a build-up of osmotic pressure gradient, leading to formation of secondary vasogenic and cytotoxic edema. Worsening cerebral conditions after neurotrauma can cause loss of consciousness, a vegetative state, or even coma.[1]

These assumptions are supported by a recent study of neuronal excitotoxicity, which showed differing amounts of glutamate circulating in arterial and venous blood,[15] perhaps explaining the different subtypes of ionotropic GluR engaged in neurotrauma.

Therefore, GluR biomarkers values, combined with imaging data and clinical evaluation, could assist in estimating the severity of the consequences of neuronal and CBF dysfunction.

Increased ICP and glutamate overload may activate a neurotoxicity cascade, causing alterations in the NR2 NMDAR subtypes that regulate cerebral arterial microvessel functions,[16] the kainate receptors (GluR5/6, GluR6/7) that potentially affect venous circulation, and the ionotropic AMPAR subtypes, reflecting dendrite-axonal injury in white matter.[17] Based on structural tractography[18] and GluR localizations,[19] it is known that NMDAR subtypes are mostly located in the cortical area of ascending fiber tracts, while KAR are substantially distributed in the descending commissural fibers of brainstem,[20] and AMPARs belong to longitudinal nerve fibers in subcortical structures such as the hippocampus.[19]

As soon as excitotoxicity affects GluR, a number of receptor fragments are cleaved by numerous enzymes, and it is these substructures that are involved in the neurodegradomic cascade that implicates the blood–brain barrier (BBB), brain microvessels, and microglia. To understand how, when, and which subtype of GluR peptide maybe released into peripheral fluids in response to neurotrauma, a neurodegradomic approach may be used.[11]

Glutamate neuroreceptor biomarkers generally represent N-terminal peptide fragments of AMPAR, NMDAR, or KAR, with certain immune-active epitopes that are severed from synaptic membrane surfaces by serine proteases.[11] When the BBB is compromised due to brain injury or disorders, peptides and proteins are released into biological fluids and accumulate in the blood in detectable amounts. These neurodegradomic products, which are released into the bloodstream or CSF, are measured using specific antibodies attached to magnetic particles.

GluR peptide feasibility studies have been conducted to measure peptide fragments using direct or peptide capture assays. The direct assay uses specific antibodies against synthetic peptide (capture antibody) and enzyme-labeled antibodies (detection antibodies) to the peptide for the quantitative measurements of unknown peptide concentrations in human plasma. Blood tests for a panel of GluR peptides have been manufactured and donated for research by GRACE Laboratories, LLC (Atlanta, GA).

AMPAR Peptides in DAI of Subcortical Areas After Mild TBI

It is known that AMPAR subtypes (GluR1, GluR2/3, and GluR4) are primarily distributed in the forebrain and subcortical pathways, including the hippocampus, amygdala, thalamus, hypothalamus, and brainstem.[12,20] This architecture supports the noncortical nature of subtle brain injury (Table 20.1). These regions of the brain are predictable sources of biomarkers, given the functional spatial-temporal coherence, developmental pathways, and cerebral plasticity subjected to mild brain injury.[21] It was demonstrated that the GluR1 subtype of AMPAR was mainly located in dendrites and axons of brain white matter, while GluR2/3 and GluR4 belong to spinal cord white matter.[17]

During the acute phase of mild TBI or following axonal injury, a massive release of glutamate, which up-regulates excitotoxic AMPARs, has been detected.[22,23] The GluR1-subunit of N-terminal AMPAR fragments is rapidly cleaved by extracellular proteases and released into the bloodstream, where this degradation product

Table 20.1:
Ionotropic glutamate receptor family

Ionotropic Glutamate Receptor Type	Subtype	Functions	Localization
NMDAR	NR1, NR2A, NR2B, NR3, NR4	Postsynaptic depolarization, STP microvessel regulation	*Cortical*: Forebrain, visual, motor, verbal areas, microvessel surfaces
AMPAR	GluR1, GluR2, GluR3, GluR4	Fast postsynaptic EPSP, LTP, spiking activity	*Subcortical*: Hippocampus, cerebellum, brainstem
Kainate receptors	GluR5, GluR6, KA1/KA2	Pre-/postsynaptic miniature IPSP GABA transmission modulation	*Brainstem*: Basal ganglia nucleus, dorsal root ganglions, cervical area of spinal cord

EPSP, excitatory postsynaptic potential; GABA, γ-aminobutyric acid; IPSP, inhibitory postsynaptic potential; LTP, long-term potentiation.

can be detected directly (peptide fragment of 5–7 kD). In addition, astrocytes and oligodendrocytes, as well as myelin, could be involved in glutamate-induced activation of GluR breakdown products. However, mechanisms of acute damage to CNS white matter are poorly understood and should be studied in details for immediate TBI treatment optimization.[17]

AMPAR peptide detection in active duty personnel ($n = 173$) as a part of postdeployment mild TBI screening yielded an optimal cutoff value of 1.0 ng/mL (92% sensitivity, 81% specificity), at which a positive predictive value of 93% was achieved.[24] In the civilian setting, a clinical study ($n = 155$) in a trauma unit (violence-related events, motor vehicle crashes, and incidental falls) showed an AMPAR peptide sensitivity of 84% and specificity of 93%, corresponding to a cutoff of 0.4 ng/mL with a significant positive likelihood ratio of 11.6 to diagnose mild TBI versus three distinct control groups comprising healthy volunteers, persons with spinal cord ischemia and strokelike symptoms, in addition to severe TBI and polytrauma.

The AMPAR peptide plasma concentrations for concussion and contusion[25] (the mild TBI group) are shown in Figure 20.1. Subjects with mild concussions ($n = 21$) had AMPAR peptide concentrations within 0.54–1.37 ng/mL. Increased AMPAR peptide levels, with a median concentration of 2.37 ng/mL (range, 1.98–3.26 ng/mL), identified 28 patients with moderate concussions. More severe cases of mild TBI/contusion ($n = 15$) showed a median value of 4.93 ng/mL (range, 3.52–12.46 ng/mL) and areas of subcortical injuries on MRI (Figure 20.2A).[26] Group comparison of median values of the AMPAR peptide concentration demonstrated significant differences ($P < 0.001$, independent samples t-test, Welch-test, 95% CI) for the entire mild TBI group compared with controls. A sensitivity of 85% and a specificity of 80%, with a positive predictive value of 81% for the AMPAR peptide assay to diagnose chronic contusion, were achieved at an optimal cutoff value of 1.4 ng/mL.[26]

Traumatic cerebral vascular injury (TCVI) is common feature of the immediate consequences of neurotrauma that is accountable for CBF disturbances and cerebral microvessel damage, with the latter being a part of the neurovascular unit that couples local cerebral flow with neuronal metabolism and leads to development of secondary ischemic events.[27]

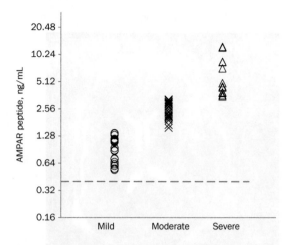

Figure 20.1 Distribution of α-amino-3-hydroxy-5-methyl-4-isoxazolepropionic acid receptor (AMPAR) peptide depending on severity of mild traumatic brain injury. Red dotted line shows cut off 0.4 ng/mL.

NMDAR Peptides in Delayed Cerebral Ischemia After Neurotrauma

NMDAR contain NR1 and NR2 subunits that determine the biophysical and pharmacological properties of the receptor (Table 20.1). The NR2 subunits NR2A, NR2B, NR2C, and NR2D are responsible for the Ca^{2+} permeability regulation underlying several nervous disorders.[28,29] NR2 subunits of the NMDA receptor can be modified by edema/cerebral ischemia, regulating cell damage or survival under these pathological conditions.[11]

Of 84 athletes enrolled in a study, 22 (26%) had increased NR2 peptide amounts compared to levels for the age- and gender-matched groups representing low distributions of NR2 peptide. Conversely, significant differences were observed for the concussion group. Highly elevated NMDAR biomarker values indicated the possibility of vasogenic edema due to secondary injury in the acute phase post-injury (Figure 20.2B). This finding was supported by diffusion tensor imaging (DTI) findings of cytotoxic edema in a semi-acute phase of mild TBI.[30] In a study of semi-acute to chronic phases of concussions in club sport athletes, biomarker assays and IMPACT testing was useful for assigning subjects in the neuroimaging study. Out of 84 athletes, 7 were recommended for MRI. In general, it seems plausible to consider a "three circles" approach to assessment of short- and long-term consequences after concussions and mild TBI in otherwise healthy persons. The "three circles" approach comprises detection of neurotoxicity biomarkers in conjunction with advanced neuroimaging (3 T or 9 T MRI, DTI, and functional MRI) and neuropsychological testing.[14] Results showed the opportunity for gradual return to play and/or direct assignment of selected athletes to treatment optimized to prevent encephalopathy development and to avoid risk of further neurological complications.

KAR Peptides in CBF Autoregulation Following TBI and Incomplete SCI

KARs (GluR5/6, GluR6/7) are located mostly in the hippocampus, subcortical areas, spinal cord tract, and brainstem,[31] with effects on cerebral venous circulation (Table 20.1).

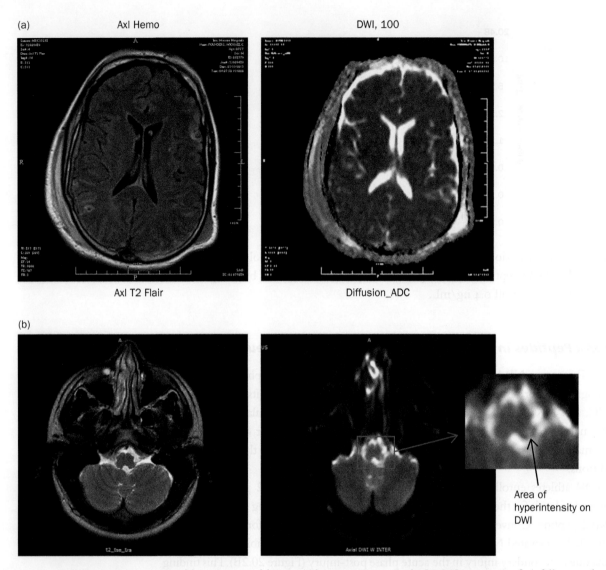

Figure 20.2 (A) Contusion acquired by 53-year-old man (Glasgow Coma Scale [GCS] score, 8) after fall caused multiple hematomas registered by magnetic resonance imaging (MRI) within 48 hours after contusion. The subcortical areas of multiple bleeding are seen on axial Hemo and T2-weighed scans and cortical edema on diffusion ADC image. α-amino-3-hydroxy-5-methyl-4-isoxazolepropionic acid receptor (AMPAR) peptide, 12.5 ng/mL (cutoff of 0.4 ng/mL), NR2 peptide, 12.0 ng/mL (cutoff of 0.5 ng/mL). (B) Concussion with temporary loss of consciousness acquired by 22-year-old male football player (GCS scores, 14) with normal T2-weighted MRI scans and areas of hyperintensity in brainstem area registered by diffusion weighted image (DWI) within 2 weeks after the impact. N-methyl-D-aspartate receptor (NMDAR) peptide, 2.7 ng/mL (cutoff of 0.5 ng/mL), KAR peptide, 7.9 ng/mL (Norm <1.5 ng/mL).

It has been shown that KARs are involved in the development of intractable epilepsy[32] as well a number of neuromediator systems in the medulla[33] that regulate involuntary life-sustaining functions (breathing, swallowing, and heart rate), with functional execution through neuronal glutamatergic networking, mainly KAR.[14]

KAR peptide detection in active-duty personnel (*n* = 53) as a part of post-deployment mild TBI screening yielded in optimal cutoff value of 1.0 ng/mL (90% sensitivity, 83%

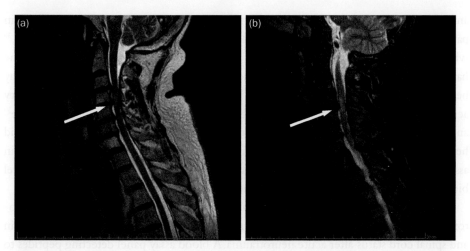

Figure 20.3 Spinal cord ischemia on C4–C5 level acquired by 67-year-old man after incomplete spinal cord injury registered by Sag T2 (A) and Sag STIR within 24 hours of the onset. Kainite peptide, 6.8 ng/mL (preliminary cutoff of 1.5 ng/mL), α-amino-3-hydroxy-5-methyl-4-isoxazolepropionic acid receptor (AMPAR) peptide, 4.4 ng/mL (cutoff of 0.5 ng/mL).

specificity), at which a positive predictive value of 93% was achieved. The study in the civilian trauma unit ($n = 45$) showed abnormal KAR concentrations (range, 1.5–7.7 ng/mL) accompanied by values of AMPAR and NR2 peptides that were increased above the cutoff, reflecting the combination of DAI with global edema involving cortical, subcortical, and brainstem areas. Preliminary calculations of KAR peptide assay performance characteristics to assess mild TBI estimated a sensitivity of 83% and specificity of 92%, at a cutoff of 0.5 ng/mL.

Preliminary assessment of KAR peptide in patients with SCI ($n = 10$) demonstrated the highest peptide levels (range, 1.9–6.8 ng/mL) within 1–6 months following the injury, with ischemia presented on MRI (Figure 20.3). Lower KAR peptide concentrations (<1.5 ng/mL) were detected in healthy volunteers/radiculopathy ($p < 0.02$) and ischemic stroke ($p = 0.003$). KARs were higher after spinal cord injury (3.0–6.8 ng/mL) than spinal cord infarction (1.8–2.5 ng/mL). This pilot investigation indicated a trend for higher KAR peptide amounts in SCI localized to cervical area of the spinal cord. That could serve as an additional support to the critical role of kainate-induced structural damage to myelin sheath slowing or shutting down the signal transduction after SCI.[17]

Discussion

The traumatized brain has increased sensitivity to secondary ischemic events triggered by a neurotransmitter storm evoked by the initial injury.[3,27] Recently, mild TBI has been suggested as an independent major predictor for stroke.[5] Despite this, the involvement of vascular components in mild TBI pathology remains underestimated, especially for the severe state of reinjuries. Biomarkers capable of recognizing poor arterial and/or venous circulations connected to vasogenic/cytotoxic edema are needed.

Blood-borne cellular proteins, secreted proteins, peptides, and proteolytic fragments may be considered first-generation neuronal and glial biomarkers for TBI.[34] Higher amounts of cleaved tau and α-II spectrin degradation products have been detected in patients with an unfavorable outcome[35] and secondary deterioration in clinical status,[36] while examination of neuron-specific enolase (NSE) in relation to clinical outcome has resulted in conflicting results.[37] In addition, calcium binding protein B (S100β) may be a valuable indicator of brain damage in polytrauma,[38] while serum glial fibrillary acidic protein (GFAP) can detect intracerebral hemorrhage in the acute phase of stroke[39] and provide information about brain injury severity and outcome after subarachnoid hemorrhage.[40] The lack of sufficient sensitivity and specificity of these biomarkers in assessment of mild to severe neurotrauma, however, has stimulated a search for novel biomarkers with better performance characteristics.[41]

This review highlights the potential use of metabolic brain biomarkers of neurotoxicity/excitotoxicity that could be integrated into current clinical evaluation of brain and spinal cord status after acute neurotrauma. A blood assay panel detecting peptides to GluR subunits AMPAR, NMDAR, and KAR might increase actionable information by anticipating edema formation as a secondary or delayed injury in cortical, subcortical, and brainstem areas.

The consequences of cerebral edema can be lethal and include cerebral ischemia from compromised regional or global CBF and intracranial compartmental shifts due to ICP gradients that result in compression of vital brain structures. Cerebrovascular dysfunction can deteriorate a patient's condition rapidly, and emergent medical assistance is required to maintain regional and global CBF to meet CNS metabolic requirements and prevent secondary neuronal injury from cerebral ischemia.

Possible brain biomarker candidates could include NR2 NMDAR subtypes, which regulate cerebral arterial circulation, and KARs, which affect venous functions. It seems that an NR2-to-KAR ratio might be able to indicate the type of edema: an increase in KAR peptide values would indicate development of cytotoxic edema and point to a more severe brain state.

These biomarkers represent a second generation of brain "tracers" that could be used to decipher the microstructural abnormalities observed on CT/MRI. Abnormal values of several GluR peptides may assist in staging edema formation and assist in decision-making for further medical assistance. Subjects with abnormal concentrations of multiple metabolic biomarkers should be directed to neuroimaging to assess the type of edema and a subsequent personalized treatment plan. Moreover, the use of neurotoxicity biomarkers may assist radiologists with additional information concerning the area of interest, such as where microstructural changes might be located (cortical, subcortical, or brainstem injuries).

Accurate assessment of neurotrauma for personalized management of brain and spinal cord injuries to prevent premature return to work, play, or duty is vital to protecting the long-term wellness of athletes and others at risk of reinjury. Structural and metabolic biomarkers can be used to complement the neuropsychological testing currently used to assess mild neurotrauma to facilitate decision-making in return to play, work, or duty.

Data from the feasibility research described in this review should be expanded and confirmed by further clinical investigations on wider population groups with neurotrauma, including SCI. The primary limitations of preliminary research are insufficient statistical power in groups, especially in SCI; various time intervals between an impact and blood draws for assays; and worsening conditions affecting secondary ischemic events, as described earlier for NR2 peptide biomarkers.[11] Additionally, different assays representing biomarkers for neuronal injury and for cerebral arterial and venous circulations should be compared in the same study to be able to select the specific panel of biomarkers with the best performance characteristics in relation to clinical evaluation and neuroimaging, particularly with advanced 3 T DTI/DWI modalities.

References

1. Gennarelli TA. Mechanisms of brain injury. *J Emerg Med*. 1993;11(suppl 1):5–11.

2. Sobrino J, Shafi S. Timing and causes of death after injuries. *Proc (Bayl Univ Med Cent)*. 2013;26(2):120–123.

3. Iffland PH II, Grant GA, Janigro D. Mechanisms of cerebral edema leading to early seizures after traumatic brain injury. In: Lo EH, Lok J, Ning M, Whalen M, eds. *Vascular Mechanisms in CNS Trauma*. New York: Springer Science; 2014:29–45.

4. Beaumont A, Gennarelli T. CT prediction of contusion evolution after closed head injury: the role of pericontusional edema. *Acta Neurochir Suppl*. 2006;96:30–32.

5. Burke JF, Stulc JL, Skolarus LE, et al. Traumatic brain injury may be an independent risk factor for stroke *Neurology*. 2013;81(1):33–39.

6. Mechtler LL, Dhadtri KK, Crutchfield KE. Advanced neuroimaging of mild traumatic brain injury. *Neurol Clin*. 2014; 32:31–58.

7. Center for Disease Control. *Report to Congress on Traumatic Brain Injury in the United States: Epidemiology and Rehabilitation*. National Center for Injury Prevention and Control; Division of Unintentional Injury Prevention. Atlanta, GA; 2015.

8. Chen YH, Kang JH, Lin HC. Patients with traumatic brain injury: population-based study suggests increased risk of stroke. *Stroke*. 2011;42:2733–2739.

9. Blaylock RL, Maroon JC. Imminoexcitotoxicity as a central mechanism in chronic traumatic encephalopathy—a unifying hypothesis. In: Dambinova SA, Hayes RL, Wang KKW, eds. *Biomarkers for TBI*. London, UK: RSC Publishing, RSC Drug Discovery Series; 2012:45–65.

10. Olney JW, Sharpe LG. Brain lesions in an infant rhesus monkey treated with monsodium glutamate. *Science*. 1969;166(3903):386–388.

11. Dambinova SA. Neurodegradomics: the source of biomarkers for mild TBI. In: Dambinova SA, Hayes RL, Wang KKW, eds. *Biomarkers for TBI*. London, UK: RSC Publishing, RSC Drug Discovery Series, 2012:66–86.

12. Hammond JC, McCullumsmith RE, Funk AJ, et al. Evidence for abnormal forward trafficking of AMPA receptors in frontal cortex of elderly patients with schizophrenia. *Neuropsychopharmacol*. 2010;35:2110–2119.

13. Dambinova SA, Bettermann K, Glynn T, et al. Diagnostic potential of the NMDA receptor peptide assay for acute ischemic stroke. *PLoS One*. 2012;7:e42362.

14. Dambinova SA, Sowell RL, Maroon J. Gradual return to play: potential role of neurotoxicity biomarkers in assessment of concussions severity. *J Mol Biomar Diagn*. 2013;S3:003.

15. Nombela F, Blanco M, Pérez de la Ossa N, et al. Neuronal excitotoxicity after carotid angioplasty and stent placement procedures. *Radiology*. 2013;268(2):515–520.

16. Sharp CD, Fowler M, Jackson TH, et al. Human neuroepithelial cells express NMDA receptors. *BMC Neurosci*. 2003;4:28–32.

17. Li S, Stys PK. Mechanisms of ionotropic glutamate receptor-mediated excitotoxicity in isolated spinal cord white matter. *J Neurosci*. 2000;20(3):1190–1198.

18. Wedeen VJ, Rosene DL, Wang R, et al. The geometric structure of the brain fiber pathways. *Science*. 2012;335(6076):1628–1634.

19. Monyer H, Jonas P, Rossier J. Molecular determinants controlling functional properties of AMPARs and NMDARs in the mammalian CNS. In P Jonas, H Monyer (Eds.), *Ionotropic glutamate receptors in the CNS*. New York, USA: Springer-Verlag, Handbook of experimental Pharmacology, 1999;141:309–330.

20. Lai M, Hughes EG, Peng X, et al. AMPA receptor antibodies in limbic encephalitis alter synaptic receptor location. *AnnNeurol*. 2009;65:424–434.

21. Shrey DW, Griesbach GS, Giza CC. The pathophysiology of concussions in youth. *Phys Med Rehabil Clin N Am*. 2011;22:577–602.

22. Dambinova SA. Diagnostic challenges in traumatic brain injury. *IVD Technology* 2007;3:3–7.

23. Dimou S, Lagopoulos J. Toward objective markers of concussion in sport: a review of white matter and neurometabolic changes in the brain after sports-related concussion. *J Neurotrauma*. 2014;31(5):413–424.

24. Shikuev AV, Skoromets TA, Skulyabin DI, et al. Feasibility studies of neurotoxicity biomarkers for assessment of traumatic brain injury. In SA Dambinova, RL Hayes, KKW Wang (Eds.), *Biomarkers for TBI*. London, UK: RSC Publishing, RSC Drug Discovery Series, 2012:148–163.

25. Mullins JD, Shikuev AV, Danilenko UI, Dambinova SA. AMPAR Peptide values in sport-related concussions. In: *2012 Military Health System Research Symposium; 2012 Aug 13-16;* Ft. Lauderdale (2012). p. 134.

26. Mullins JD. Biomarkers of TBI: implications for diagnosis and management of contusions. In: *AMSUS 118ᵗʰ Annual Continuing Education Meeting;*2013 Nov 3-8; Seattle, WA (2013). p. 147. http://amsusce.org/wp-content/uploads/2015/05/Abstract-Summaries-10.22.13.2.pdf

27. Kenney K, Amyot F, Haber M, et al. Cerebral vascular injury in traumatic brain injury. *J Exp Neurol*. 2016;275(Pt 3):353–366.

28. Gagliardi RJ. Neuroprotection, excitotoxicity and NMDA antagonists. *Arq Neuropsiquiatr*. 2000;58:583–588.

29. Meldrum BS. The role of glutamate in epilepsy and other CNS disorders. *Neurology*. 1994;44(11 Suppl 8):S14–23.

30. Mayer AR, Ling J, Mannell MV, et al. A prospective diffusion tensor imaging study in mild traumatic brain injury. *Neurology*. 2010;74(8):643–650.

31. Jin XT, Smith Y. Localization and functions of kainate receptors in the basal ganglia. In A Rodriguez-Moreno, TS Sihra (Eds.), *Kainate Receptors*. New York, USA: Springer, 2011: 27.

32. Vincent A, Bien CG, Irani SR, Waters P. Autoantibodies associated with diseases of the CNS: new developments and future challenges. *Lancet Neurol*. 2011;10:759–772.

33. Alexandrova EV, Zaitsev OS, Potapov AA. Neurotransmitter basis of consciousness and unconsciousness states. *Zh Vopr Neirokhir Im NN Burdenko*. 2014;78:26–32.

34. Zhang J, Puvenna V, Janigro D. Biomarkers of Traumatic Brain Injury and their relationship to pathology. In D Laskowitz, G Grant (Eds.), *Translational Research in Traumatic Brain Injury*. Boca Raton, FL: CRC Press/Taylor and Francis Group, 2016, Chapter 12.

35. Chen S, Shi Q, Zheng S, et al. Role of α-II-spectrin breakdown products in the prediction of the severity and clinical outcome of acute traumatic brain injury. *Exp Ther Med*. 2016;11(5):2049–2053.

36. Siman R, Giovannone N, Hanten G, et al. Evidence that the blood biomarker SNTF predicts brain imaging changes and persistent cognitive dysfunction in mild TBI patients. *Front Neurol.* 2013;4:190.

37. Cheng F, Yuan Q, Yang J, et al. The prognostic value of serum neuron-specific enolase in traumatic brain injury: systematic review and meta-analysis. *PLoS One.* 2014;9(9):e106680.

38. Woodcock T, Morganti-Kossmann MC. The role of markers of inflammation in traumatic brain injury. *Front Neurol.* 2013;4:18.

39. Mayer CA, Brunkhorst R, Niessner M, et al. Blood levels of glial fibrillary acidic protein (GFAP) in patients with neurological diseases. *PLoS One.* 2013;8(4):e62101.

40. Schiff L, Hadker N, Weiser S, Rausch C. A literature review of the feasibility of glial fibrillary acidic protein as a biomarker for stroke and traumatic brain injury. *Mol Diagn Ther.* 2012;16(2):79–92.

41. Buonora JE, Yarnell AM, Lazarus RC, Mousseau M, Latour LL, Rizoli SB, Baker AJ, Rhind SG, Diaz-Arrastia R, Mueller GP. Multivariate analysis of traumatic brain injury: development of an assessment score. *Front Neurol.* 2015;6:68.

Serum Markers of Subclinical Brain Damage in Low-Grade Chronic Concussion and Asymptomatic Cerebral Small Vessel Disease

Sergio González-García, Alina González-Quevedo,
Zenaida Hernández-Díaz, Melany Betancourt-Loza,
and Anay Cordero-Eiriz

21

Introduction

The identification of subclinical brain damage (SBD) remains challenging, and its frequency is widely underestimated. In the absence of clinical symptoms, the diagnosis and clinical assessment of asymptomatic low-grade chronic concussion and asymptomatic cerebral small vessel disease (ACSVD) in subjects with vascular preexisting conditions are rarely performed.

However, the identification of subjects who sustain multiple asymptomatic concussions and subjects with ACSVD is an urgent task in order to evaluate the cumulative effects of both on the brain—the first induced by low-grade chronic brain trauma and the second by sustained vascular load over the course of decades. These patients with SBD are at a greater risk of developing neurodegenerative and vascular diseases; therefore, the identification of both entities in their subclinical state and their follow-up is crucial, and serum markers could aid in this direction.

To date, no serum marker has achieved an effective clinical application to detect SBD due to asymptomatic concussion or asymptomatic small vessel disease (SVD) in spite of their cost-effectiveness, minimally invasive nature, and possible advantages, not only as diagnostic tools, but also as predictors of eventual neurodegenerative and vascular diseases during follow-up.

A comparison between low-grade concussion and asymptomatic SVD as subclinical brain damage is described in Table 21.1.

Brief Pathophysiological Cascade

Low-Grade Chronic Concussion

Concussion is defined as a complex pathophysiological process affecting the brain, induced by biomechanical forces with associated traumatically induced alteration in mental status with or without loss of consciousness.[1-2] Low-grade chronic concussion is a slight and continuous damage of the brain tissue without clinical symptoms.

Its prevalence is increasing over recent years and it is underestimated because many people with concussion may not seek medical attention. It is likely that the true global

Table 21.1:
Brief comparison between low-grade chronic concussion and asymptomatic small vessel disease

Comparisons	Low-Grade Chronic Concussion	Asymptomatic Small Vessel Disease
Main cause	Slight brain trauma	Vascular load
Frequency/diagnostic	Rising/underestimated	Rising/underestimated
Main chronic effects	Neurodegenerative diseases	Vascular diseases
Imaging studies as diagnostic tools	Advanced MRI techniques (DTI, SWI, SPECT, and fMRI)	MRI-specific sequences (T_1, T_2, FLAIR, $T_2\star$)
Brain-derived protein or autoantibodies as serum markers of subclinical brain damage		
Main advantage	Neurochemical expression of the subtle damage	
Clinical application	Decision-making for return to duty or play in chronically concussed subjects	Cost-effective mass population screening
Approved serum marker	None	None
Main biases which could affect the results	Presence of the blood–brain barrier, reactive response of the brain to injury, extracerebral sources of brain-derived protein, different experimental timing, and technical procedures.	
Other advantages for their implementation	Cost effectiveness, noninvasive sample collection, reference for neuroimaging referrals, and optimal patient follow-up.	
Future approach	Point-of-care tests/devices	

population incidence of mild traumatic brain injury (mTBI) exceeds 600 per 100,000 people annually (or roughly 42 million people worldwide every year).[3]

In concussion, the brain is exposed to rapid acceleration, deceleration, or rotational forces, and tissue is elongated and deformed, stretching individual neurons, glial cells, and blood vessels with altered membrane permeability.[4] In addition, there is a rapid release of neurotransmitters, an influx of calcium, an efflux of potassium, and acceleration of the cellular sodium–potassium (Na^+–K^+) pump to maintain membrane homeostasis, requiring large increases in glucose metabolism. These changes are referred to as the "neurometabolic cascade of concussion,"[5] and this hypermetabolism, in conjunction with a decreased cerebral blood flow, produces a disparity between glucose supply and demand and, consequently, a cellular energy crisis.[5] Axons in the white matter are especially susceptible to this acceleration–deceleration injury causing diffuse axonal injury (DAI), mainly due to their viscoelastic nature, anisotropic arrangement in tracts, and linear arrangement of microtubules and neurofilaments.[6]

The glial, neuronal soma, and axonal injuries due to mechanical deformation and stretching causes the release of cytoplasmic and bound-membrane proteins which could be used to monitor neurochemical expression of the slight damage occurring during concussion.

Asymptomatic Small Vessel Disease

Cerebral SVD refers to a syndrome that comprises clinical and imaging findings that are thought to result from pathologies in perforating cerebral arterioles, capillaries, and venules,[7] which could be described as "silent" lesions or ACSVD in patients without clinical symptoms. Because small vessel damage cannot be readily visualized in vivo, the effect of SVD on the brain parenchyma is usually inferred from findings on magnetic resonance imaging (MRI), and these changes are considered the hallmarks of the disease.[8] Changes in white matter and subcortical gray matter include small subcortical infarcts, lacunes, white matter hyperintensities (WMHs), prominent perivascular spaces (PVS), cerebral microbleeds (CMBs), and atrophy (9). The prevalence of silent brain infarcts (SBI) varies from 8% to 28%,[10] but microscopic brain infarcts have been found in up to 68% of community studies,[11] whereas the prevalence of WMHs is 80% or greater in those 60 years or older.[12]

The underlying pathology of ACSVD remains imprecise. Pathologically, it is characterized by partial loss of myelin, axons, and oligodendroglial cells; mild reactive astrocytic gliosis; and sparsely distributed macrophages, as well as stenosis resulting from hyaline fibrosis of arterioles and smaller vessels.[13,14] In this process, the disruption of the blood–brain barrier (BBB) results in leakage of fluid, plasma components, and cells and eventually leads to perivascular inflammation, demyelination, and gliosis.[15]

Chronic Effects

Low-Grade Chronic Concussion

The neurometabolic cascade of concussion promotes the accumulation, misfolding, and aggregation of multiple abnormal proteins associated with neurodegeneration, including tau, β-amyloid, α-synuclein, and TAR DNA binding 43 proteins.[16] All these promote the development of postconcussive syndrome (PCS), a potentially debilitating syndrome that consists of physical symptoms (headache, dizziness, fatigue), cognitive disturbances (impaired concentration and memory), or emotional problems including depression and anxiety[17,18] and can lead to an increased risk for suicide or development of psychiatric illness.[19] In fact, repetitive concussions increase by threefold memory impairment, by fivefold mild cognitive impairment (MCI),[20] and by threefold diagnosed depression.[21] In addition, repetitive concussions are risk factors for progressive tauopathy and chronic traumatic encephalopathy (CTE), with its clinical symptoms such as behavioral disturbances including lack of insight and judgment, disinhibition, euphoria, hypomania, irritability, and aggressiveness.[22] In addition to CTE, repetitive mTBI increases the risk of Alzheimer' disease, frontotemporal lobar degeneration. and other neurodegenerative processes, such as Parkinson disease.[23–25]

Asymptomatic Small Vessel Disease

There is increasing evidence showing that ACSVD is more dynamic than originally thought, with lesions progressing over time and the outcome and impact on brain damage varying.[15] Symptoms of ACSVD develop insidiously with cognitive impairment, dementia, and depression; the presence of WMHs almost triples the risk of stroke, doubles the risk of dementia, and increases the risk of death.[26]

Consequences of SVD in the brain parenchyma include a wide range of lesions whose prevalence varies across study populations, imaging techniques, and the age of the studied subjects; but most of the reports agree that ACSVD as a clinical-pathological condition is responsible for up to 45% of dementia cases and accounts for about 20% of all stroke worldwide.[26–28] Silent brain infarcts have been extensively associated with the occurrence of future clinical stroke,[29,30] cognitive decline, and dementia.[27,28] In the past several years, there has been a growing interest in the clinical significance of deep brain infarcts and WMLs as causes of vascular cognitive impairment (VCI). Particularly, small, deep brain infarcts are known to cause so-called strategic infarct dementia, and the lesion burden has also been associated with dementia risk,[31] cognitive decline, dementia, gait disturbance, urinary incontinence, and disability.[32–34]

Diagnostic Imaging Tools

Low-Grade Chronic Concussion

Concussion is generally regarded as functional, rather than structural damage, therefore brain findings with conventional neuroimaging tools are normal,[35] in particular in regard to the recognition of DAI.[36] However, advanced magnetic resonance imaging (MRI) methods have demonstrated the ability to detect and localize pathophysiological consequences of concussion.

DAI and microhemorrhages caused by concussion are best detected with diffusion tensor imaging (DTI), which provides information related to the integrity of fiber tracts and white matter microstructure.[35,37] Other techniques that support the clinical diagnoses of concussions are susceptibility-weighted imaging (SWI), magnetic resonance spectroscopy,[38] single-proton emission computed tomography (SPECT) imaging,[39] and functional MRI (fMRI).[40]

Despite increased sensitivity, current clinical guidelines make no recommendations regarding MRI in the diagnosis of concussions.[41]

Asymptomatic Small Vessel Disease

MRI methods are capable of detecting slight changes in white matter and subcortical gray matter as a result of pathologies in perforating cerebral arterioles, capillaries, and venules. In particular, deep brain infarcts appear hypointense on T1 sequences and fluid-attenuated inversion recovery (FLAIR) sequences,[42] and WMH appear as hypointensities on T1-weighted imaging and as hyperintensities on T2-weighted imaging, proton density, and FLAIR MRI.[43,44] The T2$\star$ gradient echo sequence and the newer susceptibility-weighted imaging (SWI) provide sensitive methods for detecting microbleeds.[45,46] These lesions correspond to small collections of hemosiderin-laden macrophages around small perforating vessels.[43,44]

MRI-based DTI provides a measure of water diffusion in white matter tracts, allowing researchers to examine the integrity of the white matter outside WMH lesions,[47] thus suggesting that visible lesions are indicative of wider injury. Additional promising MRI-based techniques for the study of WMLs in SVD include magnetization transfer (MTI) and high-field-MRI[48,49] as the severity of tissue changes associated with incidental WMLs in these patients cannot be sufficiently determined by conventional MRI.

Serum Brain-Derived Markers

Clinical application of blood biomarkers for concussion and ACSVD is not only cost-effective and minimally invasive, but may also help in identifying patients who require referrals for neuroradiological assessment or follow-up examination. Unfortunately, highly sensitive and specific serum markers for subclinical brain damage do not exist.

First, it is important to mention how brain-derived proteins reach the bloodstream. Two main paths are present: first, following damage to the neurovascular unit (NVU), particularly at the capillary level, and, second, through the glymphatic system.[50]

The slight and continuous injury resulting from low-grade concussion and/or ACSVD damages the entire NVU (neurons, glial cells, and endothelium) through mechanical deformation of the BBB through shear stress forces that alter the tight junctions of the barrier.[51,52] A second mechanism may also increase the permeability of the BBB based on fluctuations in cerebral blood flow, brain edema, elevated intracranial pressure, and immune activation.[50] When cells in the NVU are damaged as a result of these injuries, cytosolic and membrane-bound proteins are released into the cerebrospinal fluid (CSF) and interstitial fluid (ISF); from there they could pass across the damaged tight junctions of the BBB or could be driven into the paravenous space by astrocytic water systems and cerebral arterial pulse pressure,[53–56] and finally be transported into the peripheral bloodstream through arachnoid villi of the dural sinuses and deep cervical lymph nodes.[50,57]

Low-Grade Chronic Concussion

There is a mounting body of research supporting the use of biomarkers to detect concussion,[58–63] however no serum marker has been approved yet. It is a challenge to identify serum markers for the diagnosis of slight and diffuse brain damage as a consequence of concussion because the cell stretching and cell disruption may seem transient. Unlike other organ-based diseases where rapid diagnosis employing biomarkers from blood tests are clinically essential to guide clinical diagnosis and treatment, there are no rapid, definitive diagnostic blood tests for concussion.

More than 11 different biomarkers have been measured in several studies,[64] with calcium binding protein B (S100β) most frequently assessed, followed by glial fibrillary acidic protein (GFAP), neuron-specific enolase (NSE), tau, neurofilament light protein (NFL), and amyloid protein.[65] As indicators of astroglial injury, S100β and GFAP are two of the most extensively studied biomarkers. Raised levels of S100β have been associated with increased incidence of PCS and problems with cognition,[66,67] with altered MRI, and with neuropsychological examination disturbances after concussion.[66–68] Other studies have shown an increase in serum S100β levels after concussion and even after subconcussive head impacts.[69,70] Although these reports have produced consistent data, some datasets have failed to differentiate athletes with concussion from extraneous exercise groups.[71–74] This may be a result of significant increases in S100β levels after exhaustive sports training due to the presence of extracerebral sources of S100β, such as adipocytes, chondrocytes, and melanocytes.[75,76]

GFAP is a promising brain-specific glial-derived biomarker for concussion.[64,65,77–79] Compared with S100β, serum GFAP levels distinguish concussed patients from trauma patients without concussion, and GFAP is released into serum following a concussion during the first hour of injury and remains elevated for several days after injury.[64,65,78]

In the expression of neuronal injury, several markers have been explored, and NSE and ubiquitin C-terminal hydrolase are the most reviewed. Several reports on serum NSE levels in mTBI have already been published.[80–83] In the setting of DAI, levels of NSE at 72 hours after injury have shown an association with unfavorable outcome.[84] Elevated serum levels of NSE were found in amateur boxers even after an extended resting period[85]; nevertheless, Shahim et al. reported that in 35 concussed ice hockey players, there was no difference in serum NSE from pre-season baseline levels to post-concussion values,[86] thus limiting its clinical utility in mTBI. An important limitation of NSE in mTBI is the occurrence of false-positive results in the setting of hemolysis.[87,88]

A promising biomarker for concussions currently under investigation is ubiquitin C-terminal hydrolase L1 (UCH-L1).[59,64,89,90] Increases in serum UCH-L1 have also been found in children with mild and moderate TBI[83] and with severe TBI.[91] However, recent studies have identified significant elevations in serum UCH-L1 levels in individuals with non–sport-related concussion (e.g., motor vehicle accidents, falls) compared to healthy controls.[92,93]

As axonal injury markers, α-II spectrin breakdown products (SBDP), tau-protein, and neurofilaments have been studied. α-II spectrin (280 kDa) is the major structural component of the cortical membrane cytoskeleton and is particularly abundant in axons and presynaptic terminals.[94] It is also a major substrate for both calpain and caspase-3 cysteine proteases, and their breakdown products (i.e., SBDP) have been associated with TBI.[95,96] Levels of SBDPs and SBDP150 (marker of necrosis) have been examined in patients with mTBI and have shown a significant association with acute measures of injury severity, such as Glasgow Coma Scale score, intracranial injuries on CT, and neurosurgical intervention.[97] In this study, serum SBDP150 levels were much higher in patients with mTBI/concussion than in trauma patients who did not have a head injury.[97] However, serum SBDP145 has also been measured in children with TBI. Levels were significantly greater in subjects with moderate and severe TBI than in controls, but were not elevated in mild TBI.[91]

After a concussion, axons appear to be most susceptible to damage, and because tau is a protein that is highly enriched in axons, abnormalities in tau are the most consistent feature found in CTE[98] related to axonal disruption.[99,100] A recent report demonstrated that tau measured in blood could provide the opportunity to assess neurologic injury shortly after concussion, as well as facilitate monitoring of recovery over time.[101] Looking only at those athletes who sustained a concussion, those with a longer return to play had higher tau concentrations overall, as well as an acute increase in plasma tau levels.[101] There are, however, inconsistencies in the performance of tau in the form of cleaved-tau (c-tau), total-tau (t-tau), and phosphorylated-tau (p-tau) in trauma,[64] although Shahim reported higher serum levels of these tau species in professional hockey players after concussion and the association of these levels with the duration of postconcussion symptoms.[70,86]

Neurofilaments are heteropolymeric components of the neuron cytoskeleton that consist of a 68-kDa light neurofilament subunit (NF-L) backbone with either 160-kDa medium (NF-M) or 200-kDa heavy subunit (NF-H) side arms.[102]

NF-H was significantly higher in those children with DAI on initial CT scan.[103] For more than 10 days after admission, patients with DAI/ have higher serum NF-H in comparison with subjects with focal injuries.[104] NFL-L has also been shown to be elevated in boxers with mTBI after a bout.[62,105] The levels were associated with the number of hits to the head received, as well as subjective and objective estimates of the intensity of the fight.[62]

Asymptomatic Small Vessel Disease

The detection of early brain deterioration requires imaging techniques too scarce and costly for routine use in general practice; however, the brain is one of the main affected organs as a consequence of vascular risk factors.[106,107] Techniques to measure brain-derived proteins in serum in order to detect asymptomatic SVD are cost-effective for mass population screening due to their potential for providing a more accessible, rapid, and less expensive solution requiring minimal expertise to interpret.[108]

Blood biomarkers for systemic inflammation,[109–113] endothelial dysfunction,[110–113] and oxidative stress[112,113] have been explored in relation to subclinical brain damage during the past years in the general population and also in hypertensive patients and in those with diabetes mellitus.[108] Serum markers for cardiovascular disorders have been studied as well, specifically in the Atherosclerosis Risk in Communities (ARIC) study. Brain natriuretic peptide (BNP) and N-terminal pro-B natriuretic peptide (NT-proBNP) were associated with WMH and SBI.[114] Similar results from an MRI study (ISSYS) revealed that NT-proBNP is independently associated with silent cerebrovascular lesions and could be a surrogate marker of vascular brain damage in hypertension.[115]

Two different subsamples from the community-based Northern Manhattan Study (NOMAS) studied blood-based biomarkers with SBD. The first, posits an association between the hormone fibroblast growth factor 23 (FGF23) and subclinical cerebrovascular damage.[116] The second found an independent association between procalcitonin, a marker of bacterial infection, and midregional proatrial natriuretic peptide (MRproANP), a marker for cardiac dysfunction with SBIs and WMHs.[117]

However, more specific serum markers to brain damage tissue have been less thoroughly investigated, and there is little information regarding the association between brain-derived serum markers and asymptomatic SVD. The idea of employing brain-derived proteins as markers of SBD is plausible because, as a result of the slight and maintained injury to brain tissue caused by hypertension and other vascular comorbidities, brain cells are damaged and the BBB is compromised, thus making it easier for cytosolic contents released from injured brain tissue to reach the bloodstream.[108] These proteins, peptides, and their autoantibodies could be a more accurate neurochemical expression of brain damage. A pilot study conducted in Havana demonstrated an association between higher NSE serum levels with more severe WML.[118] The follow-up of a larger cohort supported these results, indicating that serum NSE levels could be useful in identifying hypertensive patients with putative subclinical brain damage for subsequent brain MRI scanning. The longitudinal study of this cohort provided additional information suggesting that increased NSE could be a useful prognostic marker for central nervous system vascular events in asymptomatic hypertensive patients.[119] In addition to this biomarker, serum autoantibodies against the subunit NR2 of the N-methyl-D-aspartate (NMDA) receptor (NR2Ab) were explored as indicators of SBD in HT subjects with vascular preexisting conditions. Higher serum NR2Ab levels were related with more severe brain MRI lesions, particularly WMH, denoting cerebral asymptomatic SVD.[120]

The idea of employing blood-based biomarkers of brain damage for predicting subclinical brain damage in neurologically asymptomatic subjects is supported by the previously mentioned findings and should be investigated in more depth.

Future Approaches

Although research in the field of concussion serum markers has increased exponentially over the past 20 years,[121–123] there are still inconsistencies and lack of reproducibility in some results. On the other hand, initial reports relating serum brain-derived markers as predictors of subclinical brain damage in ASCVD[119,120] need further confirmation in larger cohorts of patients. There are many biases that can affect the results when investigating circulating biomarkers in subclinical brain damage as a consequence of concussion or ASCVD, and great care must be taken when designing a blood-based biomarker assay and in the interpretation of these results. Among the main issues to consider are (1) the imaging/neurological assessment procedures used, (2) the presence of the BBB and the reactive response of the brain to injury, (3) extracerebral sources of the brain-derived marker, (4) experimental timing, and (5) the technical procedures used to produce biomarker measurements.

Brain-derived proteins as markers for subclinical brain damage are attractive for several reasons[50]: they are cost effective, they require minimally invasive sample collection, they can provide a reference for neuroimaging referrals, they may be used to identify various types of brain injury, and fluctuations in blood levels may help to classify injury severity and indicate the resolution of brain damage.

Brain-derived proteins—or the autoantibodies directed against these—when used as markers for subclinical brain damage, should be available as point-of-care (POC) tests in order to detect a concussion in the field and make rapid decisions relating to the trauma. Also, as a prehospital screening tool to identify ASCVD, these tests should allow rapid vascular-risk assessment and filtering of patients for neuroimaging studies and preventive/therapeutic interventions.[108, 120]

Conclusion

ACSVD and low-grade chronic concussion can affect brain tissue through different mechanisms, but the final neurochemical expression can be the same in terms of the release into the bloodstream of brain-specific proteins or autoantibodies directed against these. Routine imaging assessment in these cases is generally not informative, and other more advanced techniques are not readily available and very expensive. Blood-based biomarkers could be very useful for the early detection of asymptomatic brain damage in these situations due to their cost-effectiveness, minimally invasive nature, and possible advantages, not only as diagnostic tools, but also as predictors of eventual neurodegenerative and vascular diseases during follow-up.

References

1. McCrory P, Meeuwisse WH, Aubry M, et al. Consensus statement on concussion in sport: the 4th International Conference on Concussion in Sport, Zurich, November 2012. *J Athl Train.* 2013;48(4):554–575.

2. Kulbe J, Geddes JW. Current status of fluid biomarkers in mild traumatic brain injury. *Exp Neurol.* 2016;275(03):334–352.

3. Gardner RC, Yaffe K. Epidemiology of mild traumatic brain injury and neurodegenerative disease. *Mol Cell Neurosci.* 2015;66(Pt B):75–80. doi:10.1016/j.mcn.2015.03.001.

4. McKee AC, Daneshvar DH, Alvarez VE, Stein TD. The neuropathology of sport. *Acta Neuropathol.* 2014;127(1):29–51. doi:10.1007/s00401-013-1230-6.

5. Giza CC, Hovda DA. The new neurometabolic cascade of concussion. *Neurosurgery.* 2014;75(suppl 4):S24–S33. doi:10.1227/NEU.0000000000000505.

6. Johnson VE, Stewart JE, Begbie FD, Trojanowski JQ, Smith DH, Stewart W. Inflammation and white matter degeneration persist for years after a single traumatic brain injury. *Brain.* 2013;136(Pt 1):28–42. doi:10.1093/brain/aws322.

7. Moody DM, Brown WR, Challa VR, Anderson RL. Periventricular venous collagenosis: association with leukoaraiosis. *Radiology.* 1995;194(2):469–476.

8. Rincon F, Wright CB. Current pathophysiological concepts in cerebral small vessel disease. *Front Aging Neurosci.* 2014;6:24. doi:10.3389/fnagi.2014.00024.

9. Wardlaw JM, Smith EE, Biessels GJ, et al. Neuroimaging standards for research into small vessel disease and its contribution to ageing and neurodegeneration. *Lancet Neurol.* 2013;12:822–838.

10. Vermeer SE, Longstreth WT Jr, Koudstaal PJ. Silent brain infarcts: a systematic review. *Lancet Neurol.* 2007;6(7):611–619.

11. Launer LJ, Hughes TM, White LR. Microinfarcts, brain atrophy, and cognitive function: the Honolulu Asia Aging Study Autopsy Study. *Ann Neurol.* 2011;70(5):774–780. doi:10.1002/ana.22520.

12. de Leeuw FE, de Groot JC, Achten E, et al. Prevalence of cerebral white matter lesions in elderly people: a population based magnetic resonance imaging study. The Rotterdam Scan Study. *J Neurol Neurosurg Psychiatry.* 2001;70(1):9–14.

13. Madden DJ, Bennett IJ, Burzynska A, Potter GG, Chen NK, Song AW. Diffusion tensor imaging of cerebral white matter integrity in cognitive aging. *Biochim Biophys Acta.* 2012 Mar;1822(3):386–400.

14. Black S, Gao F, Bilbao J. Understanding white matter disease: imaging-pathological correlations in vascular cognitive impairment. *Stroke.* 2009;40:S48–52.

15. Shi Y, Wardlaw JM. Update on cerebral small vessel disease: a dynamic whole-brain disease. *Stroke and Vascular Neurology.* 2016;1:e000035. doi:10.1136/svn-2016-00003.

16. Iverson GL, Gardner AJ, McCrory P, Zafonte R, Castellani RJ. A critical review of chronic traumatic encephalopathy. *Neurosci Biobehav Rev.* 2015;56:276–293.

17. Arciniegas DB, Anderson CA, Topkoff J, McAllister TW. Mild traumatic brain injury: a neuropsychiatric approach to diagnosis, evaluation, and treatment. *Neuropsychiatr Dis Treat.* 2005;1:311–27.

18. Ryan LM, Warden DL. Post concussion syndrome. *Int Rev Psychiatry.* 2003;15:310–16.

19. Carroll LJ, Cassidy JD, Cancelliere C, et al. Systematic review of the prognosis after mild traumatic brain injury in adults: cognitive, psychiatric, and mortality outcomes: results of

the International Collaboration on Mild Traumatic Brain Injury Prognosis. *Arch Phys Med Rehabil.* 2014;95:S152–S173.

20. Guskiewicz KM, Marshall SW, Bailes J, McCrea M, Cantu RC, Randolph C, Jordan BD. Association between recurrent concussion and late-life cognitive impairment in retired professional football players. *Neurosurgery.* 2005;57(4):719–726

21. Guskiewicz KM, Marshall SW, Bailes J, et al. Recurrent concussion and risk of depression in retired professional football players. *Med Sci Sports Exerc.* 2007;39(6):903–909.

22. Mckee AC, Daneshvar DH. The neuropathology of traumatic brain injury. *Handb Clin Neurol.* 2015;127:45–66. doi:10.1016/B978-0-444-52892-6.00004-0.

23. Blennow K, Zetterberg H, Fagan AM. Fluid biomarkers in Alzheimer disease. *Cold Spring Harb Perspect Med.* 2012;2(9):a006221. doi:10.1101/cshperspect.a006221.

24. Young JS, Hobbs JG, Bailes JE. the impact of traumatic brain injury on the aging brain. *Curr Psychiatry Rep.* 2016;18(9):81. doi:10.1007/s11920-016-0719-9.

25. Hobbs JG, Young JS, Bailes JE. Sports-related concussions: diagnosis, complications, and current management strategies. *Neurosurg Focus.* 2016;40(4):E5.

26. Pantoni L. Cerebral small vessel disease: from pathogenesis and clinical characteristics to therapeutic challenges. *Lancet Neurol.* 2010;9:689–701.

27. Debette S, Markus HS. The clinical importance of white matter hyperintensities on brain magnetic resonance imaging: systematic review and meta-analysis. *BMJ.* 2010;341: c3666. doi:10.1136/bmj.c3666.

28. Debette S, Beiser A, DeCarli C, et al. Association of MRI markers of vascular brain injury with incident stroke, mild cognitive impairment, dementia, and mortality: the Framingham Offspring Study. *Stroke.* 2010;41(4):600–606.

29. Gupta S. Burden of multiple chronic conditions in Delaware, 2011-2014. *Prev Chronic Dis.* 2016;13:E160. doi:10.5888/pcd13.160264.

30. Gupta A, Giambrone AE, Gialdini G, Finn C, Delgado D, Gutierrez J, et al. Silent brain infarction and risk of future stroke: a systematic review and meta-analysis. *Stroke.* 2016;47(3):719–725. doi:10.1161/STROKEAHA.115.011889.

31. Koga H, Takashima Y, Murakawa R, Uchino A, Yuzuriha T, Yao H. Cognitive consequences of multiple lacunes and leukoaraiosis as vascular cognitive impairment in community-dwelling elderly individuals. *J Stroke Cerebrovasc Dis.* 2009;18(1):32–37. doi:10.1016/j.jstrokecerebrovasdis.2008.07.010.

32. Vermeer SE, Prins ND, den Heijer T, Hofman A, Koudstaal PJ, Breteler MM. Silent brain infarcts and the risk of dementia and cognitive decline. *N Engl J Med.* 2003;348(13):1215–1222

33. Vermeer SE, Longstreth WT Jr, Koudstaal PJ. Silent brain infarcts: a systematic review. *Lancet Neurol.* 2007;6(7):611–619.

34. Baezner H, Blahak C, Poggesi A, et al; LADIS Study Group. Association of gait and balance disorders with age-related white matter changes: the LADIS study. *Neurology.* 2008;70(12):935–942.

35. Meaney DF, Smith DH. Biomechanics of concussion. *Clin Sports Med.* 2011;30(1):19–31, vii. doi:10.1016/j.csm.2010.08.009.

36. Metting Z, Wilczak N, Rodiger LA, Schaaf JM, van der Naalt J. GFAP and S100B in the acute phase of mild traumatic brain injury. *Neurology.* 2012;78:1428–1433.

37. Oni MB, Wilde EA, Bigler ED, et al. Diffusion tensor imaging analysis of frontal lobes in pediatric traumatic brain injury. *J Child Neurol.* 2010;25(8):976–984. doi:10.1177/0883073809356034.

38. Vagnozzi R, Signoretti S, Cristofori L, et al. Assessment of metabolic brain damage and recovery following mild traumatic brain injury: a multicentre, proton magnetic resonance spectroscopic study in concussed patients. *Brain*. 2010;133(11):3232–3242. doi:10.1093/brain/awq200

39. Harch PG, Andrews SR, Fogarty EF, Amen D, Pezzullo JC, Lucarini J, et al. A phase I study of low-pressure hyperbaric oxygen therapy for blast-induced post-concussion syndrome and post-traumatic stress disorder. *J Neurotrauma*. 2012;29(1):168–185.

40. Gosselin N, Bottari C, Chen JK, et al. Electrophysiology and functional MRI in post-acute mild traumatic brain injury. *J Neurotrauma*. 2011;28(3):329–341. doi:10.1089/neu.2010.1493.

41. Jagoda AS, Bazarian JJ, Bruns JJ Jr, et al. Clinical policy: neuroimaging and decision making in adult mild traumatic brain injury in the acute setting. *J Emerg Nurs*. 2009;35:e5–e40.

42. Patel B, Markus HS. Magnetic resonance imaging in cerebral small vessel disease and its use as a surrogate disease marker. *Int J Stroke*. 2011;6:47–59.

43. Valdés Hernández MC, Piper RJ, Bastin ME, et al. Morphologic, distributional, volumetric, and intensity characterization of periventricular hyperintensities. *AJNR Am J Neuroradiol*. 2014;35(1):55–62. doi:10.3174/ajnr.A3612.

44. Wardlaw JM, Smith EE, Biessels GJ, et al; Standards for Reporting Vascular changes on neuroimaging (STRIVE v1). Neuroimaging standards for research into small vessel disease and its contribution to ageing and neurodegeneration. *Lancet Neurol*. 2013;12(8):822–838. doi:10.1016/S1474-4422(13)70124-8.

45. Yamashiro K, Tanaka R, Okuma Y, et al. Cerebral microbleeds are associated with worse cognitive function in the nondemented elderly with small vessel disease. *Cerebrovasc Dis Extra*. 2014;4(3):212–220. doi:10.1159/000369294.

46. Miwa K, Tanaka M, Okazaki S, Yagita Y, Sakaguchi M, Mochizuki H, Kitagawa K. Multiple or mixed cerebral microbleeds and dementia in patients with vascular risk factors. *Neurology*. 2014;83(7):646–653. doi:10.1212/WNL.0000000000000692.

47. Lockhart SN, Mayda AB, Roach AE, et al. Episodic memory function is associated with multiple measures of white matter integrity in cognitive aging. *Front Hum Neurosci*. 2012;6:56. doi:10.3389/fnhum.2012.00056. eCollection 2012.

48. Fazekas F, Ropele S, Enzinger C, et al. MTI of white matter hyperintensities. *Brain*. 2005;128(Pt 12):2926–2932.

49. Bastin ME, Clayden JD, Pattie A, Gerrish IF, Wardlaw JM, Deary IJ. Diffusion tensor and magnetization transfer MRI measurements of periventricular white matter hyperintensities in old age. *Neurobiol Aging*. 2009;30(1):125–136.

50. Kawata K, Liu CY, Merkel SF, Ramirez SH, Tierney RT, Langford D. Blood biomarkers for brain injury: what are we measuring? *Neurosci Biobehav Rev*. 2016;68:460–473. doi:10.1016/j.neubiorev.2016.05.009.

51. Rodriguez-Baeza A, Reina-de la Torre F, Poca A, Marti M, Garnacho A. Morphological features in human cortical brain microvessels after head injury: a three-dimensional and immunocytochemical study. *Anat Rec A Discov Mol Cell Evol Biol*. 2003;273:583–93.

52. Vajtr D, Benada O, Kukacka J, Prusa R, Houstava L, Toupalik P, Kizek R. Correlation of ultrastructural changes of endothelial cells and astrocytes occurring during blood brain barrier damage after traumatic brain injury with biochemical markers of BBB leakage and inflammatory response. *Physiol Res*. 2009;58:263–268.

53. Iliff JJ, Wang M, Liao Y, et al. A paravascular pathway facilitates CSF flow through the brain parenchyma and the clearance of interstitial solutes, including amyloid beta. *Sci Transl Med.* 2012;4:147ra111.

54. Iliff JJ, Lee H, Yu M, et al. Brain-wide pathway for waste clearance captured by contrast-enhanced MRI. *J Clin Invest.* 2013a;123:1299–1309. [PubMed: 23434588]

55. Iliff JJ, Wang M, Zeppenfeld DM, et al. Cerebral arterial pulsation drives paravascular CSF-interstitial fluid exchange in the murine brain. *J Neurosci.* 2013b;33:18190–18199. [PubMed: 24227727]

56. Iliff JJ, Chen MJ, Plog BA, et al. Impairment of glymphatic pathway function promotes tau pathology after traumatic brain injury. *J Neurosci.* 2014;34:16180–16193.

57. Aspelund A, Antila S, Proulx ST, et al. A dural lymphatic vascular system that drains brain interstitial fluid and macromolecules. *J Exp Med.* 2015;212:991–999.

58. Lewis LM, Schloemann D, Papa L, et al. Utility of serum biomarkers in the diagnosis and stratification of mild traumatic brain injury [published online ahead of print February 7, 2017]. *Acad Emerg Med.* doi:10.1111/acem.13174.

59. Papa L, Edwards D, Ramia M. exploring serum biomarkers for mild traumatic brain injury. In: Kobeissy FH, ed. Boca Raton, FL: CRC Press/Taylor & Francis; 2015:299–307.

60. Papa L, Ramia MM, Edwards D, Johnson BD, Slobounov SM. Systematic review of clinical studies examining biomarkers of brain injury in athletes after sports-related concussion. *J Neurotrauma.* 2015;32(10):661–673. doi:10.1089/neu.2014.3655.

61. Zetterberg H, Tanriverdi F, Unluhizarci K, Selcuklu A, Kelestimur F, Blennow K. Sustained release of neuron-specific enolase to serum in amateur boxers. *Brain Inj.* 2009;23(9):723–726. doi:10.1080/02699050903120399.

62. Zetterberg H, Hietala MA, Jonsson M, et al. Neurochemical aftermath of amateur boxing. *Arch Neurol.* 2006;63(9):1277–1280.

63. Graham MR, Myers T, Evans P, et al. Direct hits to the head during amateur boxing is associated with a rise in serum biomarkers for brain injury. *Int J Immunopathol Pharmacol.* 2011;24(1):119–125.

64. Papa L. Potential blood-based biomarkers for concussion. *Sports Med Arthrosc.* 2016;24(3):108–115. doi:10.1097/JSA.0000000000000117.

65. Papa L, Brophy GM, Welch RD, et al. Time course and diagnostic accuracy of glial and neuronal blood biomarkers GFAP and UCH-L1 in a large cohort of trauma patients with and without mild traumatic brain injury. *JAMA Neurol.* 2016;73(5):551–560. doi:10.1001/jamaneurol.2016.0039.

66. Ingebrigtsen T, Romner B. Management of minor head injuries in hospitals in Norway. *Acta Neurol Scand.* 1997;95(1):51–55.

67. Waterloo K, Ingebrigtsen T, Romner B. Neuropsychological function in patients with increased serum levels of protein S-100 after minor head injury. *Acta Neurochir (Wien).* 1997;139(1):26–31

68. Ingebrigtsen T, Waterloo K, Jacobsen EA, Langbakk B, Romner B. Traumatic brain damage in minor head injury: relation of serum S-100 protein measurements to magnetic resonance imaging and neurobehavioral outcome. *Neurosurgery.* 1999;45(3):468–475.

69. Kiechle K, Bazarian JJ, Merchant-Borna K, et al. Subject-specific increases in serum S-100B distinguish sports-related concussion from sports-related exertion. *PLoS One.* 2014;9: e84977.

70. Shahim P, Tegner Y, Wilson DH, et al. Blood biomarkers for brain injury in concussed professional ice hockey players. *JAMA Neurol.* 2014;71:684–692.

71. Otto M, Holthusen S, Bahn E, Sohnchen N, Wiltfang J, et al. Boxing and running lead to a rise in serum levels of S-100B protein. *Int J Sports Med*.2000;21: 551–555.

72. Hasselblatt M, Mooren FC, Von Ahsen N, et al. Serum S100beta increases in marathon runners reflect extracranial release rather than glial damage. *Neurology*. 2004;62:1634–1636.

73. Stalnacke BM, Tegner Y, Sojka P. Playing ice hockey and basketball increases serum levels of S-100B in elite players: a pilot study. *Clin J Sport Med*. 2003;13:292–302.

74. Stalnacke BM, Tegner Y, Sojka P. Playing soccer increases serum concentration of the biochemical markers of brain damage S-100B and neuron- specific enolase in elite players: a pilot study. *Brain Injury*. 2004;18:899–909.

75. Anderson RE, Hansson LO, Nilsson O, Liska J, Settergren G, Vaage J. Increase in serum S100A1-B and S100BB during cardiac surgery arises from extracerebral sources. *Ann Thorac Surg*. 2001;71(5):1512–1517.

76. Wolf H, Krall C, Pajenda G, et al. Preliminary findings on biomarker levels from extracerebral sources in patients undergoing trauma surgery: Potential implications for TBI outcome studies. *Brain Inj*. 2016;30(10):1220–1225. doi:10.3109/02699052.2016.1170883.

77. Wang KK, Yang Z, Yue JK, et al. Plasma anti-glial fibrillary acidic protein autoantibody levels during the acute and chronic phases of traumatic brain injury: a transforming research and clinical knowledge in traumatic brain injury pilot study. *J Neurotrauma*. 2016;33(13):1270–1277.

78. Papa L, Silvestri S, Brophy GM, et al. GFAP out-performs S100β in detecting traumatic intracranial lesions on computed tomography in trauma patients with mild traumatic brain injury and those with extracranial lesions. *J Neurotrauma*. 2014;31(22):1815–1822. doi:10.1089/neu.2013.3245.

79. Bogoslovsky T, Wilson D, Chen Y, et al. Increases of plasma levels of glial fibrillary acidic protein, tau, and amyloid β up to 90 days after traumatic brain injury. *J Neurotrauma*. 2017;34(1):66–73. doi:10.1089/neu.2015.4333.

80. de Kruijk JR, Leffers P, Menheere PP, Meerhoff S, Twijnstra A. S-100B and neuron-specific enolase in serum of mild traumatic brain injury patients. A comparison with health controls. *Acta Neurol Scand*. 2001;103(3):175–179.

81. Shahim P, Blennow K, Zetterberg H. Tau, s-100 calcium-binding protein B, and neuron-specific enolase as biomarkers of concussion-reply. *JAMA Neurol*. 2014;71(7):926–927. doi:10.1001/jamaneurol.2014.1160.

82. Stålnacke BM, Björnstig U, Karlsson K, Sojka P. One-year follow-up of mild traumatic brain injury: post-concussion symptoms, disabilities and life satisfaction in relation to serum levels of S-100B and neurone-specific enolase in acute phase. *J Rehabil Med*. 2005;37(5):300–305.

83. Papa L, Mittal MK, Ramirez J, et al. Neuronal biomarker ubiquitin C-terminal hydrolase (uch-l1) detects traumatic intracranial lesions on CT in children and youth with mild traumatic brain injury. *J Neurotrauma*. 2017. doi:10.1089/neu.2016.4806.

84. Chabok SY, Moghadam AD, Saneei Z, Amlashi FG, Leili EK, Amiri ZM. Neuron-specific enolase and S100BB as outcome predictors in severe diffuse axonal injury. *J Trauma Acute Care Surg*. 2012;72(6):1654–1657. doi:10.1097/TA.0b013e318246887e.

85. Zetterberg H, Tanriverdi F, Unluhizarci K, Selcuklu A, Kelestimur F, Blennow K. Sustained release of neuron-specific enolase to serum in amateur boxers. *Brain Inj*. 2009;23(9):723–726. doi:10.1080/02699050903120399.

86. Shahim P, Linemann T, Inekci D, et al. Serum tau fragments predict return to play in concussed professional ice hockey players. *J Neurotrauma*. 2015;33:1–5.

87. Johnsson P, Blomquist S, Lührs C, et al. Neuron-specific enolase increases in plasma during and immediately after extracorporeal circulation. *Ann Thorac Surg.* 2000;69(3):750–754.

88. Ramont L, Thoannes H, Volondat A, Chastang F, Millet MC, Maquart FX. Effects of hemolysis and storage condition on neuron-specific enolase (NSE) in cerebrospinal fluid and serum: implications in clinical practice. *Clin Chem Lab Med.* 2005;43(11):1215–1217.

89. Diaz-Arrastia R, Wang KK, Papa L, et al.; TRACK-TBI Investigators. Acute biomarkers of traumatic brain injury: relationship between plasma levels of ubiquitin C-terminal hydrolase-L1 and glial fibrillary acidic protein. *J Neurotrauma.* 2014;31(1):19–25. doi:10.1089/neu.2013.3040.

90. Puvenna V, Brennan C, Shaw G, et al. Significance of ubiquitin carboxy-terminal hydrolase L1 elevations in athletes after sub-concussive head hits. *PLoS One.* 2014;9(5):e96296.

91. Berger RP, Hayes RL, Richichi R, Beers SR, Wang KK. Serum concentrations of ubiquitin C-terminal hydrolase-L1 and αII-spectrin breakdown product 145 kDa correlate with outcome after pediatric TBI. *J Neurotrauma.* 2012;29(1):162–167.

92. Rhine T, Babcock L, Zhang N, Leach J, Wade SL. Are UCH-L1 and GFAP promising biomarkers for children with mild traumatic brain injury? Brain Inj. 2016;30(10):1231–1238. doi:10.1080/02699052.2016.1178396.

93. Kou Z, Gattu R, Kobeissy F, et al. Combining biochemical and imaging markers to improve diagnosis and characterization of mild traumatic brain injury in the acute setting: results from a pilot study. *PLoS One.* 2013;8(11):e80296. doi:10.1371/journal.pone.0080296.

94. Chen S, Shi Q, Zheng S, et al. Role of α-II-spectrin breakdown products in the prediction of the severity and clinical outcome of acute traumatic brain injury. *Exp Ther Med.* 2016;11(5):2049–2053.

95. Cardali S, Maugeri R. Detection of alphaII-spectrin and breakdown products in humans after severe traumatic brain injury. *J Neurosurg Sci.* 2006;50(2):25–31.

96. Pineda JA, Lewis SB, Valadka AB, et al. Clinical significance of alphaII-spectrin breakdown products in cerebrospinal fluid after severe traumatic brain injury. *J Neurotrauma.* 2007;24(2):354–366.

97. Mondello S, Papa L, Buki A, et al. Neuronal and glial markers are differently associated with computed tomography findings and outcome in patients with severe traumatic brain injury: a case control study. *Crit Care.* 2011;15:R156.

98. Neselius S, Zetterberg H, Blennow K, et al. Olympic boxing is associated with elevated levels of the neuronal protein tau in plasma. *Brain Inj.* 2013;27:425–433.

99. Kosik KS, Finch EA. MAP2 and tau segregate into dendritic and axonal domains after the elaboration of morphologically distinct neurites: an immunocytochemical study of cultured rat cerebrum. *J Neurosci.* 1987;7(10):3142–3153.

100. Holleran L, Kim JH, Gangolli M, et al. Axonal disruption in white matter underlying cortical sulcus tau pathology in chronic traumatic encephalopathy. *Acta Neuropathol.* 2017;133(3):367–380. doi:10.1007/s00401-017-1686-x.

101. Gill J, Merchant-Borna K, Jeromin A, Livingston W, Bazarian J. Acute plasma tau relates to prolonged return to play after concussion. *Neurology.* 2017;88(6):595–602. doi:10.1212/WNL.0000000000003587.

102. Julien JP, Mushynski WE. Neurofilaments in health and disease. *Prog Nucleic Acid Res Mol Biol.* 1998;61:1–23.

103. Žurek J, Fedora M. The usefulness of S100B, NSE, GFAP, NF-H, secretagogin and Hsp70 as a predictive biomarker of outcome in children with traumatic brain injury. *Acta Neurochir (Wien)*. 2012;154(1):93–103; discussion 103. doi:10.1007/s00701-011-1175-2.

104. Vajtr D, Benada O, Linzer P, et al. Immunohistochemistry and serum values of S-100B, glial fibrillary acidic protein, and hyperphosphorylated neurofilaments in brain injuries. *Soud Lek*. 2012;57(1):7–12.

105. Neselius S, Brisby H, Theodorsson A, Blennow K, Zetterberg H, Marcusson J. CSF-biomarkers in Olympic boxing: diagnosis and effects of repetitive head trauma. *PLoS One*. 2012;7(4):e33606. doi:10.1371/journal.pone.0033606.

106. Mancia G, Fagard R, Narkiewicz K, et al. ESH/ESC practice guidelines for the management of arterial hypertension. Task force for the management of arterial hypertension of the European society of hypertension and the European society of cardiology. *Blood Press*. 2014;23(1):3–16.

107. Henskens LH, van Oostenbrugge RJ, Kroon AA, Hofman PA, Lodder J, de Leeuw PW. Detection of silent cerebrovascular disease refines risk stratification of hypertensive patients. *J Hypertens*. 2009;27(4):846–853. doi:10.1097/HJH.0b013e3283232c96.

108. González-Quevedo A, González-García S, Peña-Sánchez M, Menéndez-Saínz C, Fernández-Carriera R, Cordero-Einz A. Blood-based biomarkers could help identify subclinical brain damage caused by arterial hypertension. *MEDICC Review*. 2016;18(1–2):46–53.

109. Mitaki S, Nagai A, Oguro H, Yamaguchi S. C-reactive protein levels are associated with cerebral small vessel-related lesions. *Acta Neurol Scand*. 2016;133(1):68–74. doi:10.1111/ane.12440.

110. Shoamanesh A, Preis SR, Beiser AS, et al. Inflammatory biomarkers, cerebral microbleeds, and small vessel disease: Framingham Heart Study. *Neurology*. 2015;84(8):825–832. doi:10.1212/WNL.0000000000001279.

111. Wiseman SJ, Doubal FN, Chappell FM, et al. Plasma biomarkers of inflammation, endothelial function and hemostasis in cerebral small vessel disease. *Cerebrovasc Dis*.2015;40(3–4):157–164. doi:10.1159/000438494.

112. Maschirow L, Khalaf K, Al-Aubaidy HA, Jelinek HF. Inflammation, coagulation, endothelial dysfunction and oxidative stress in prediabetes: biomarkers as a possible tool for early disease detection for rural screening. *Clin Biochem*. 2015;48(9):581–585.

113. Wiseman S, Marlborough F, Doubal F, Webb DJ, Wardlaw J. Blood markers of coagulation, fibrinolysis, endothelial dysfunction and inflammation in lacunar stroke versus non-lacunar stroke and non-stroke: systematic review and meta-analysis. *Cerebrovasc Dis*. 2014;37(1):64–75. doi:10.1159/000356789.

114. Dadu RT, Fornage M, Virani SS, et al. Cardiovascular biomarkers and subclinical brain disease in the atherosclerosis risk in communities study. *Stroke*. 2013;44(7):1803–1808. doi:10.1161/STROKEAHA.113.001128.

115. Vilar-Bergua A, Riba-Llena I, Penalba A, et al. N-terminal pro-brain natriuretic peptide and subclinical brain small vessel disease. *Neurology*. 2016;87(24):2533–2539.

116. Wright CB, Shah NH, Mendez AJ, et al. fibroblast growth factor 23 is associated with subclinical cerebrovascular damage: the Northern Manhattan Study. *Stroke*. 2016;47(4):923–928. doi:10.1161/STROKEAHA.115.012379.

117. Katan M, Moon Y, von Eckardstein A, et al. Procalcitonin and midregional proatrial natriuretic peptide as biomarkers of subclinical cerebrovascular damage: the Northern Manhattan Study. *Stroke*. 2017;48(3):604–610. doi:10.1161/STROKEAHA.116.014945.

118. Gonzalez-Quevedo A, González García S, Fernández Concepción O, et al. Increased serum S-100B and neuron specific enolase—potential markers of early nervous system involvement in essential hypertension. *Clinical Biochemistry* (2011) 44(2–3) 154–159.

119. González-Quevedo A, Gonzalez-Garcia S, Hernández-Díaz Z, et al. Serum neuron specific enolase could predict subclinical brain damage and the subsequent occurrence of brain related vascular events during follow up in essential hypertension. *J Neurol Sci.* 2016;363:158–163.

120. González-García S, González-Quevedo A, Cordero Eiriz A, et al. Circulating autoantibodies against the NR2 peptide of the NMDA receptor are associated with subclinical brain damage in hypertensive patients with other pre-existing conditions for vascular risk. *J Neurol Sci.* 2017;375:324–330. doi:10.1016/j.jns.2017.02.028.

121. Kochanek PM, Berger RP, Bayir H, Wagner AK, Jenkins LW, Clark RS. Biomarkers of primary and evolving damage in traumatic and ischemic brain injury: diagnosis, prognosis, probing mechanisms, and therapeutic decision making. *Curr Opin Crit Care.* 2008;14(2):135–141. doi:10.1097/MCC.0b013e3282f57564.

122. Papa L, Ramia MM, Kelly JM, Burks SS, Pawlowicz A, Berger RP. Systematic review of clinical research on biomarkers for pediatric traumatic brain injury. *J Neurotrauma.* 2013;30(5):324–338. doi:10.1089/neu.2012.2545.

123. Papa L, Mendes ME, Braga CF. mild traumatic brain injury among the geriatric population. *Curr Transl Geriatr Exp Gerontol Rep.* 2012;1(3):135–142.

MicroRNA Biomarkers in Traumatic Brain Injury

*Manish Bhomia, Nagaraja S. Balakathiresan, Kevin K. W. Wang,
and Barbara Knollmann-Ritschel*

22

Introduction

Traumatic brain injury (TBI) is defined as an injury to the brain by external forces that
leads to a disruption in the normal function of the brain. Worldwide, TBI is currently
considered one of the major of causes of disability and death, as well as a leading cause
of injury-related deaths in the United States (US). Nearly 1.7 million civilians are affected by brain injury every year, and 5.3 million live with TBI-related disabilities. The
incidence of TBI in military service members has seen a significant increase in the past
decade with operations in Iraq and Afghanistan. More than 330,000 service members
have been diagnosed with some form of TBI since 2000. Among these injuries, more
than 75% of TBI is classified as mild (mTBI). In terms of the economic burden, it is
estimated that, in the US alone, the annual cost associated with the management of TBI
is approximately $10 billion.[1] The high incidence of TBI-related deaths and prolonged
disability is primarily due to an incomplete understanding of the mechanisms of TBI pathology because the cellular and molecular changes are dynamic and complex, and there
is a tremendous heterogeneity in clinical TBI causes and symptoms. In the past decade,
significant progress has been made at the molecular, cellular, and behavioral levels due
to the introduction of novel techniques and the development of new animal models for
studying brain injury.

Molecular changes after TBI have been studied in both in vitro and in vivo models.
Gene expression studies at the posttranscriptional and posttranslational levels have
identified several key molecules that have been shown to play a critical role in TBI pathology. In particular, microRNAs (miRNA) have been extensively studied for their
role in TBI pathology and as a biomarker for TBI.[2] MiRNAs are small endogenous
RNA segments that regulate transcription in eukaryotic cells at the posttranscriptional
level. Mature miRNAs are approximately 22 nucleotides in length and are evolutionary
well conserved across different species. MiRNAs are expressed from both the protein
coding and noncoding regions of the DNA. Evidence from recent studies suggests that
almost all cellular functions, such as development, proliferation, and differentiation,
are regulated by miRNAs. More than 1,000 unique miRNAs have been identified in
humans, and this number is expected to increase with the availability of new genomic
sequencing technologies, such as next-generation sequencing. Several miRNAs are
expressed abundantly in both the developing and mature central nervous system (CNS),
where they play an important role in regulating protein expression. Many brain-specific
or enriched miRNAs are shown to express a specific temporal and spatial pattern during

different developmental stages of the CNS. MiRNAs have been shown to be present both within the neuron and in different types of supporting cells, such as astrocytes and microglial cells. Enriched miRNAs in certain brain regions play specific roles in physiological function. These observations indicate that miRNAs are key regulators of complex brain functions such as memory and learning through their action in modulating dendrite spine formations, synaptic plasticity, learning, and memory-associated genes. In addition, accumulating evidence strongly suggests that altered expression of miRNAs is associated with several brain diseases, brain disorders, and brain injury.[3]

In this chapter, we focus on recent developments in the field of neurotrauma with an emphasis on the role of miRNAs. The development of different animal models to study the potential use of miRNAs as diagnostic biomarkers, to differentiate the severity of the injury, and to understand the role of miRNAs in TBI pathophysiology is discussed.

MiRNAs in TBI Pathology and Treatment

TBI is an acquired brain injury caused by instantaneous mechanical forces like a jolt, bump, or blow to the head or a penetrating head injury that disrupts the normal function of the brain. TBI is classified as mild, moderate, or severe based on scoring using the Glasgow Coma Scale (GCS). The GCS is a standard measure of ascertaining initial severity and prognosis by examining the eye movements and verbal and motor responses of the patient.[4] Primary mechanical force is responsible for the onset of histopathological TBI hallmarks seen across multiple brain regions and resulting from damaged cellular membranes, axons, and vasculature. Subsequent secondary molecular, biochemical, and cellular events create further neuronal, glial, and vascular injuries. Cellular and molecular events, including changes in membrane permeability and reactive oxygen generation, occur during the acute stage, whereas apoptotic cell death and neurogenesis develop over a prolonged period of time.[5] To understand the pathophysiology of heterogeneous mTBI, several animal models have been developed: the weight-drop model, the controlled cortical impact (CCI) injury, and the blast overpressure (BOP) injury model. In the BOP models, the primary blast waves induce tissue deformity due to compression and stretching, axonal injury, microglial activation, and numerous behavioral deficits. In the closed head injury model, the weight-drop yields widespread axonal injury, minimal focal neuronal damage, brain edema, microglial activation, and motor, cognitive, emotional, and visual deficits. CCI injury mainly produces severe TBI (sTBI) with significant neuron loss at the site of impact and commonly associated subdural hemorrhage, vascular damage, microglial activation, and axonal injury.[6]

Recent studies have shown that miRNAs are important in regulating both CNS homeostasis and TBI pathology. MiRNA expression profiling studies in brain tissue in rodent models of TBI have suggested the involvement of miRNAs in inflammation and apoptosis, as well as in regulation of pro-survival pathways. The in vitro scratch injury model examining rat primary cortical neurons identified a key role of miR-22 in regulating apoptosis. Scratch injury in these cells resulted in reduced expression of miR-22. Exogenously added miR-22 in the form of agomirs protected these cells by targeting Bax and Pten and promoted phosphorylation of Akt-1, thus suggesting that miR-22 has a neuroprotective role in TBI.[7] Glial cells are the immune cells of the CNS. MiRNAs have been shown to regulate the inflammatory cascade in glial cells following their activation. Oxygen glucose deprivation (OGD) in vitro resulted in damage to astrocytes, which was reversed by treatment with miR-7. It was shown that miR-7 targeted endoplasmic reticulum stress proteins and prevented oxidative damage to the astrocytes following OGD.[8] In contrast to the neuroprotective role of miRNAs, miR-711 has been implicated in contributing to neuronal cell death. In the rodent model of CCI, it was shown that miR-711 expression increased rapidly after CCI injury along with a decrease in Akt levels. Therefore, by targeting Akt, miR-711 up-regulates the pro-apoptotic bcl-2 protein, which results in cellular apoptosis.[9] In the same model, expression of miR-27a and miR-27b decreased rapidly, which was associated with increased expression of the bcl-2 family of proteins leading to apoptosis in the neuronal cells.[10]

To identify the role of these miRNAs in cellular function, bioinformatic analysis has revealed that these miRNAs may regulate the expression levels of proteins involved in a variety of cellular processes including intracellular signaling, cellular architecture, inflammation, metabolism, cell death, and survival.[11,12] Analysis of miRNA expression in rat cerebral cortex after TBI has shown that miR-21 could also be involved in the intricate process of TBI.[13] In vitro studies on miR-21 indicate that it can reduce neuronal apoptosis through activating the PTEN-Akt signaling pathway. In vivo administration of exogenous miR-21 in animals improved their outcome after TBI. Similarly, miR-21 administration in rats alleviated secondary blood–brain barrier damage after TBI by activating the Ang-1/Tie-2 axis in brain microvascular endothelial cells.[14–16] In the mouse CCI model, differentially expressed miRNAs were identified in the brain at the site of injury at 24 hours and 7 days post-injury. Pathway analysis using computational tools identified canonical pathways like calcium signaling, synaptic pathways, and axon guidance to be the major targets of modulated miRNAs.[17] The altered miRNAs in TBI provide a high-level network perspective on global patterns of cellular and molecular changes that occur after injury. The analysis of altered miRNAs and their targets indicates that these will be useful in identifying the major pathophysiological processes in TBI, such as apoptosis, inflammation, and cell proliferation, and may lead to miRNA-based therapeutic interventions.

TBI Biomarkers

Moderate to severe TBI can be easily diagnosed by the presence of clinical symptoms and through imaging methods such as computed tomography (CT) and magnetic resonance imaging (MRI). CT and MRI are both useful tools to detect intracranial lesions in moderate to severe TBI. mTBI, on the other hand, may not have immediate clinical symptoms, which can lead to missed diagnosis, and patients often do not seek immediate medical attention, instead presenting to a primary care clinician weeks later. TBI is currently assessed using the patient's GCS score and loss or alterations of consciousness to determine the severity of the brain injury. However, due to the complex nature of the injury, which may include polytrauma, alcohol abuse, use of sedatives, and psychological stress, the usefulness of the GCS score may become very limited.[18]

In response, blood-based biomarkers have been extensively studied for TBI diagnostics due to their ease of use and the low cost of measurements.[19] Biomarkers have several advantages as diagnostic tools because they can be measured from biofluids such as blood, urine, cerebrospinal fluid (CSF), and saliva and can easily be quantitated using standard biochemical and molecular methods. Several studies over the past decade have identified promising protein-based biomarkers for detecting mTBI such as calcium binding protein β (S100β), glial fibrillary acidic protein (GFAP), and ubiquitin c-terminal hydrolase-L1 (UCH-L1). Despite several clinical studies, however, most of these protein-based biomarkers lacks sensitivity and specificity to detect mTBI, and currently there are no approved diagnostic tests for detecting mTBI.

By contrast, blood-based miRNA biomarkers are very stable at variable pH conditions and resistant to repeated freeze–thaw and enzymatic degradation, which makes them a suitable biomarker candidate for TBI, including mTBI. MiRNAs can be detected in the serum and can be an indicator of disease pathology in the cell of origin, including neuronal cells. This property of reflecting a disease condition at a distant site has increased the possibility of using miRNAs as biomarkers of central nervous system (CNS) pathology.

We have studied the possible use of miRNAs for mTBI in both the rodent model of TBI and in clinical cases in the human. Our lab reported that expression of miRNA let-7i was up-regulated in both serum and CSF after exposure to mild to moderate BOP wave injury in a rodent model.[20] The serum expression of miRNAs in response to a concussive mild injury in a closed head injury model was similarly reported. A signature of 13 miRNAs was found to be modulated in the serum immediately after injury.[21] In addition, MiRNA modulation was analyzed in a rodent model of traumatic stress. A signature of nine miRNAs was identified that are up-regulated in the serum and amygdala of the animals 2 weeks after exposure to traumatic stress. Interestingly, the 9 miRNAs from the traumatic stress study and the 13 miRNAs from the TBI study were unique, suggesting that miRNA expression in serum may be a specific indicator of the altered physical state of the brain.[22] Redell and colleagues also studied miRNA expression in human serum samples of TBI. Their results identified miR-16, miR-92a, and miR-765 as potential biomarkers of sTBI with good diagnostic accuracy; however, the diagnostic accuracy of these markers for mTBI was limited.[23] In a follow-up study from our group, we identified a panel of 10 serum miRNAs as biomarkers of mild to severe TBI. This panel was validated in the CSF samples from sTBI patients.[18]

Comparison of the results from the clinical study with the earlier rodent studies showed a good correlation between these studies. Serum miRNA from blast-induced mTBI in rats showed several common miRNAs such as miR-20a, miR-362-3p, miR-195, miR-451, and miR-92a. MiR-362-3p identified in the human study was likewise found to be modulated in a rodent model of closed head injury. MiR-16 and miR-92a identified by Redell et al. were significantly up-regulated in both mTBI and sTBI. However, miR-16 was also found to be significantly up-regulated in an orthopedic injury group, suggesting that miR-16 may not be specific for TBI. In summary, some miRNAs identified in the human study correlate with the previously identified miRNAs in the rodent model; however, many miRNAs were unique to the human study and were not previously reported as potential TBI biomarkers. Differences in the expression of serum miRNAs in rodent and human studies may be due to the heterogeneity of TBI in humans in comparison to a controlled TBI, such as blast injury, in animal studies. In another study, miR-91, miR-191, and miR-499 were found to be elevated in the serum of sTBI patients, and their increased expression in patients correlates with poor clinical outcome.[24] Most studies so far have screened and identified miRNA candidate biomarkers for TBI (Table 22.1), but further studies are required to validate these candidates for clinical use.

Table 22.1:
MicroRNA biomarker for traumatic brain injury (TBI) in animal and human studies

Tissue	Organism and Injury Type	Altered miRNAs	References
Serum, CSF	Human, mTBI	hsa-miR-151-5P, hsa-miR-195, hsa-miR-20a, hsa-miR-30d, hsa-miR-328, hsa-miR-362-3p, hsa-miR-486, hsa-miR-505★, hsa-miR-92a	Bhomia et al. 2016[18]
Brain	Mouse, closed head injury model	mmu-miR-369-3p, rno-miR-224, mmu-miR-18a, mmu-miR-668, mmu-miR-423-5p, mmu-miR-494, mmu-miR-466j, mmu-miR-465a-5p	Chandran et al. 2016[17]
Serum	Mouse, closed head injury model	mmu-miR-376a, hsa-miR-214, mmu-miR-214, mmu-miR-337-5p, mmu-miR-574-3p, mmu-miR-434-3p, mmu-miR-671-3p, mmu-miR-218, mmu-miR-199a-3p, hsa-miR-106b★, mmu-miR-106b, mmu-miR-31, rno-miR-196c	Sharma et al. 2014[21]
CSF	Human, severe TBI	hsa-miR-9, hsa-miR-451	Patz et al. 2013[25]
Serum, CSF	Rat, repetitive blast overpressure exposures	mmu-let-7i, mmu-miR-122, mmu-miR-200b★, mmu-miR-340-5p, mmu-miR-874	Balakathiresan et al. 2012[20]
PBMCs	Human (OEF/OIF Veterans), mTBI	hsa-miR-671-5p	Pasinetti et al. 2012[26]
Plasma	Human, mTBI and sTBI	hsa-miR-16, hsa-miR-92a	Redell et al. 2010[23]
Brain (Hippocampus)	Rat, controlled cortical impact injury	mmu-miR-144, mmu-miR-136, mmu-miR-148b-5p, mmu-miR-342-5p, mmu-miR-23a★	Hu et al. 2012[27]
Brain (Hippocampus)	Rat, controlled cortical impact injury	mmu-miR-107, mmu-miR-130a, mmu-miR-223, mmu-miR-292-5p, mmu-miR-433-3p, mmu-miR-451, mmu-miR-541, mmu-miR-711	Redell et al. 2009[11]

CSF, cerebrospinal fluid; OEF, Operation Enduring Freedom; OIF, Operation Iraqi Freedom.

Conclusion

The role of noncoding RNA regions, especially miRNAs, has been studied in many neurodegenerative disorders such as Alzheimer disease, Parkinson disease, and stroke. Several reports in the literature suggest the use of miRNAs for the clinical diagnosis of TBI and the elucidation of its pathology, and their possible use as therapeutic interventions. However, most of these studies are conducted in rodent models, and their role in human TBI pathology is yet to be firmly established. MiRNAs are a promising tool for the diagnosis of mTBI because multiple possible candidate miRNAs have been identified. Further studies in a large clinical trial including both civilian and military TBI are needed to substantiate the clinical usefulness of these miRNAs as biomarkers of TBI.

Disclaimer

The opinions expressed herein are those of the authors and are not necessarily representative of those of the Uniformed Services University of the Health Sciences, Department of Defense or the United States Army, Navy, or Air Force and DMRDP.

References

1. Rubiano AM, Carney N, Chesnut R, Puyana JC. Global neurotrauma research challenges and opportunities. *Nature.* 2015;527;S193–197. doi:10.1038/nature16035.
2. Yu B, Zhou S, Yi S, Gu X. The regulatory roles of non-coding RNAs in nerve injury and regeneration. *Prog Neurobiol.* 2015;134:122–139. doi:10.1016/j.pneurobio.2015.09.006).
3. Su W, Aloi MS, Garden GA. MicroRNAs mediating CNS inflammation: small regulators with powerful potential. *Brain Behav Immun.* 2016;52:1–8. doi:10.1016/j.bbi.2015.07.003.
4. McGinn MJ, Povlishock JT. Pathophysiology of traumatic brain injury. *Nuerosurg Clin N Am.* 2016;27:397–407. doi:10.1016/j.nec.2016.06.002.
5. Quillinan N, Herson PS, Traystman RJ. Neuropathophysiology of brain injury. *Anesthesiol Clin.* 2016;34:453–464. doi:10.1016/j.anclin.2016.04.011.
6. Shultz SR, McDonald SJ, Vonder Haar C, et al. The potential for animal models to provide insight into mild traumatic brain injury: translational challenges and strategies [published online ahead of print September 19, 2016]. *Neurosci Biobehav Rev.* doi:10.1016/j.neubiorev.2016.09.014.
7. Ma, J. Shaofeng S, Xinwei H, et al. MicroRNA-22 attenuates neuronal cell apoptosis in a cell model of traumatic brain injury. *Am J Translat Res.* 2016;8:1895–1902.
8. Dong YF, Chen ZZ, Zhao Z, et al. Potential role of microRNA-7 in the anti-neuroinflammation effects of nicorandil in astrocytes induced by oxygen-glucose deprivation. *J Neuroinflammation.* 2016;13:60. doi:10.1186/s12974-016-0527-5.
9. Sabirzhanov B, Stoica BA, Zhao Z, et al. miR-711 upregulation induces neuronal cell death after traumatic brain injury. *Cell Death Differ.* 2016;23:654–668. doi:10.1038/cdd.2015.132.
10. Sabirzhanov B, Zhao Z, Stoica BA, et al. Downregulation of miR-23a and miR-27a following experimental traumatic brain injury induces neuronal cell death through activation of proapoptotic Bcl-2 proteins. *J Neurosci.* 2014;34:10055–10071. doi:10.1523/jneurosci.1260-14.2014.
11. Redell JB, Liu Y, Dash PK. Traumatic brain injury alters expression of hippocampal microRNAs: potential regulators of multiple pathophysiological processes. *J Neurosci Res.* 2009;87:1435–1448. doi:10.1002/jnr.21945.
12. Redell JB, Zhao J, Dash PK. Altered expression of miRNA-21 and its targets in the hippocampus after traumatic brain injury. *J Neurosci Res.* 2011;89:212–221. doi:10.1002/jnr.22539.
13. Lei P, Li Y, Chen X, et al. Microarray based analysis of microRNA expression in rat cerebral cortex after traumatic brain injury. *Brain Res.* 2009;1284:191–201. doi:10.1016/j.brainres.2009.05.074.
14. Han Z, Chen F, Ge X, et al. miR-21 alleviated apoptosis of cortical neurons through promoting PTEN-Akt signaling pathway in vitro after experimental traumatic brain injury. *Brain Res.* 2014;1582:12–20. doi:10.1016/j.brainres.2014.07.045.
15. Ge XT, Lei P, Wang HC, et al. miR-21 improves the neurological outcome after traumatic brain injury in rats. *Sci Rep.* 2014;4:6718. doi:10.1038/srep06718.
16. Ge X, Han Z, Chen F, et al. MiR-21 alleviates secondary blood-brain barrier damage after traumatic brain injury in rats. *Brain Res.* 2015;1603:150–157. doi:10.1016/j.brainres.2015.01.009.

17. Chandran R, Sharma A, Bhomia M, et al. Differential expression of microRNAs in the brains of mice subjected to increasing grade of mild traumatic brain injury. *Brain Inj.* 2016;1–14. doi:10.1080/02699052.2016.1213420.

18. Bhomia M, Balakathiresan NS, Wang KK, et al. A panel of serum MiRNA biomarkers for the diagnosis of severe to mild traumatic brain injury in humans. *Sci Rep.* 2016;6:28148. doi:10.1038/srep28148.

19. Kawata K, Liu CY, Merkel SF, et al. Blood biomarkers for brain injury: what are we measuring? *Neurosci Biobehav Rev.* 2016;68:460–473. doi:10.1016/j.neubiorev.2016.05.009.

20. Balakathiresan N, Bhomia M, Chandran R, et al. MicroRNA let-7i is a promising serum biomarker for blast-induced traumatic brain injury. *J Neurotrauma.* 2012;29:1379–1387. doi:10.1089/neu.2011.2146.

21. Sharma A, Chandran R, Barry ES, et al. Identification of serum microRNA signatures for diagnosis of mild traumatic brain injury in a closed head injury model. *PLoS One.* 2014;9: e112019. doi:10.1371/journal.pone.0112019.

22. Balakathiresan NS, Chandran R, Bhomia M, et al. Serum and amygdala microRNA signatures of posttraumatic stress: fear correlation and biomarker potential. *J Psychiatr Res.* 2014;57:65–73. doi:10.1016/j.jpsychires.2014.05.020.

23. Redell JB, Moore AN, Ward NH 3rd, et al. Human traumatic brain injury alters plasma microRNA levels. *J Neurotrauma.* 2010;27:2147–2156. doi:10.1089/neu.2010.1481.

24. Yang T, Song J, Bu X, et al. Elevated serum miR-93, miR-191, and miR-499 are noninvasive biomarkers for the presence and progression of traumatic brain injury. *J Neurochem.* 2016;137:122–129. doi:10.1111/jnc.13534.

25. Patz S, Trattnig C, Grünbacher G, et al. More than cell dust: microparticles isolated from cerebrospinal fluid of brain injured patients are messengers carrying mRNAs, miRNAs, and proteins. *J Neurotrauma.* 2013;30:1232–1242. doi:10.1089/neu.2012.2596.

26. Pasinetti GM, Ho L, Dooley C, et al. Select non-coding RNA in blood components provide novel clinically accessible biological surrogates for improved identification of traumatic brain injury in OEF/OIF veterans. *Am J Nondegen Dis.* 2012;1:88–98.

27. Hu Z, Yu D, Almeida-Suhett C, et al. Expression of miRNAs and their cooperative regulation of the pathophysiology in traumatic brain injury. *PLoS One.* 2012;7:e39357. doi:10.1371/journal.pone.0039357.

Section IV

Translational Animal Studies of TBI

Translational Mild Traumatic Brain Injury Research: Bridging the Gap Between Models and Clinical Uncertainty

Eugene Park and Andrew J. Baker

23

Clinical TBI Versus Translational Research

A critical hurdle in translational studies of mild traumatic brain injury (mTBI) stems from ambiguity around a precise clinical definition of mTBI. Extending interpretation of this imprecise definition into clinically relevant animal models becomes a chicken-or-egg exercise in validating translational model results with clinical uncertainty. Studies in animal models are further constrained by obvious anatomical, metabolic, and genetic differences between human and rodents (Table 23.1).[1] These differences have important implications regarding pathophysiology and outcome. For example, diffuse axonal injury to white matter is a common pathological finding in both clinical and animal mTBI. However, white matter to gray matter ratios weigh predominantly toward white matter in humans (60:40) while in rodents the ratio of white to gray matter favors the opposite (10:90). By the same token, rodent brains are lissencephalic whereas human brains are gyrencephalic. These constitutional differences have an impact on the biomechanics of injury transduction and extrapolation of pathophysiological processes between species. This reinforces disconnects between our understanding of human mTBI, which relies on clinical diagnosis and identifies neuroanatomical abnormalities on a macroscopic scale, and animal models, which have identified microscopic and molecular-level changes in structure and function. Nonetheless, animal models have proved to be useful in identifying numerous underlying pathophysiologies not readily detectable or accessible in the living patient.

What Constitutes mTBI? Bedside to Bench

The clinical definition of mTBI continues to evolve with our understanding of the pathophysiological processes involved. The earliest commonly adopted system of severity classification in clinical use is the 15-point Glasgow Coma Scale (GCS).[2] Much of the underlying pathophysiology is wholly lumped into a single category termed "mild" based on the patient's level of consciousness. More recently, with mainstream focus on the long-term effect of concussions in athletes and military personnel, there has been adoption of a subclinical category of mTBI. "Subconcussion" has been used to describe traumatic impacts that have no immediate clinical symptoms[3] but can result in neurodegenerative pathology.[4] There is strong clinical evidence that a significant proportion of mTBI patients who have otherwise no detectable abnormalities on imaging have

Table 23.1:
Species differences and implications in mild traumatic brain injury (mTBI) research

Gray vs. white matter ratios	The human brain has a gray-to-white matter ratio of approximately 60:40. The rodent gray-to-white matter ratio is approximately 90:10. How do these differences relate to overall injury progression and pathophysiology?
Skull thickness	Pigs and human share closer brain mass and body weight ratio in comparison to rodents. However, the pig skull is thicker than the human skull and may affect energy transfer in primary blast injuries.
Brain mass	Differences in brain mass have implications for the translation of mechanical forces into shear and stretch injuries. Exponentially higher rotational forces are required to induce comparable levels of shear stress with decreasing brain mass.
Brain anatomy	The human brain has considerable increase in overall surface area due to numerous sulci and gyri (gyrencephaly), whereas rodent brains lack the gyri (lissencephaly) with the exception of the cerebellum.
Aging and metabolism	Rodents have much shorter average life spans (2–3 years) compared to humans. How this protracted timeline correlates to progression of injury between species is not entirely known. This has implications for interpretation of windows of vulnerability from repeat injuries as well as treatment strategies.

reduced quality of life and persistent neurological symptoms.[5] Criteria for mTBI established by the American Congress of Rehabilitation Medicine, the Centers for Disease Control and Prevention, the Department of Defense/Department of Veterans Affairs, and the World Health Organization share similar inclusion criteria. Most common elements include some form of loss of consciousness (LOC) and posttraumatic amnesia coupled with no obvious anatomical abnormalities on medical imaging.[6] Despite increased resolution and sensitivity of evolving magnetic resonance imaging (MRI) technologies, computed tomography (CT), a less sensitive, more accessible, and less expensive imaging modality, is the conventional imaging approach in diagnosis of mTBI.[7] From a translational perspective, animal models have been used to study micropathology and pathophysiology at cellular and molecular levels. Numerous models have included adaptations of well-established systems including the fluid percussion injury device,[8–10] controlled cortical impact,[11–15] various weight-drop techniques,[16–18] and, more recently, blast injuries. Outcome measures using these models have employed titrated levels of injury severity such that outcomes share histopathological continuity with clinical imaging (i.e., no obvious cerebral contusions or hemorrhage), but also quantifiable surrogate behavioral endpoints (e.g., impaired righting reflex, tests of anxiety) that bear resemblance to clinical neurological symptoms in mTBI patients. The criteria for LOC is difficult to recreate in a lab environment given that most if not all mTBI procedures require anesthesia for reasons of restraint, reproducibility, and ethics. In this regard, the development of surrogate measures such as time to recovery from anesthesia or multipoint evaluations scales such as the neurological severity score (NSS) represent the research correlate of the GCS.

Development of Objective Diagnostics for mTBI

A fundamental shortcoming of mTBI diagnosis is the lack of a truly objective readout that reflects underlying pathophysiological processes and correlates with injury severity.[19] Toward this end, there has been work on the development of serum and cerebrospinal fluid (CSF) biomarkers to diagnose and potentially prognosticate outcome after TBI.[20] While the majority of this work has focused on moderate and severe TBI, limited studies have addressed biomarkers in mTBI.[21,22] Protein candidates investigated in human mTBI and animal models include calcium binding protein B (S100β), glial fibrillary acidic protein (GFAP), neuron-specific enolase (NSE), spectrin breakdown products (SBPD), and phosphorylated neurofilament expression. The investigation of these serum and CSF biomarkers is based on a clinical hypothesis-driven approach using the assumption that these candidate biomarkers are likely to be abundantly expressed, brain-relevant, and vulnerable following mTBI. There are only a handful of studies performed in translational mTBI research to validate the many clinical trials reporting the sometimes conflicting or nonsignificant contributions of these biomarkers as diagnostics or prognosticators of injury. An alternate and comprehensive approach involves microRNA array[23–26] and proteomic[27–29] technologies to screen large groups of biomarkers with no predetermined links to mTBI pathophysiology. This approach utilizes laboratory-based tools that have begun to translate toward bedside application. This is an area of research in its infancy. Due to the complexity and heterogeneity of mTBI, it is likely that a biomarker profile consisting of numerous relevant biomarkers will be needed to accurately diagnose injuries.

Models of mTBI

There are numerous modifications and variations of existing devices to induce various forms of mTBI in animal models. The lack of a standardized model in mTBI research is perhaps unavoidable given the heterogeneity of mild brain injuries owing to pre-injury factors, genetics, and mechanisms of injury.[30] This in turn provokes discussion about the role of animal models and whether they represent a recapitulation of injury mechanics or pathophysiological processes. The key goal of translational research is to provide information on the pathophysiological mechanisms and potential treatments for mTBI in well-controlled settings that could not otherwise be performed in human patients. In this regard, histopathology, molecular analysis, and electrophysiological approaches in animal models have been useful in elucidating underlying pathophysiological mechanisms linking the clinical observations of altered white matter integrity and impaired function (Table 23.2).[31,32]

The methodological approaches of studying mTBI can be categorized into two philosophies: (1) a model can be designed to mimic the injury on a biomechanical level, or (2) a model can be designed with the intention to reproduce pathophysiological processes with relevance to the overall injury process. For example, rotational/acceleration models of mTBI[33,34] may be considered more relevant to the mechanical

Table 23.2:
Injury models and considerations in translational mild traumatic brain injury (mTBI) research

Injury Model	Considerations in Translational mTBI Research
Fluid percussion injury (FPI)	Surgical preparation involving craniotomy. Combination of contusion and diffuse loading on the brain.
Controlled cortical impact (CCI)	Surgical preparation involving craniotomy. No standardized injury parameters.
Weight-drop	Variability in method used to induce injury (e.g., head stabilization with foam cushion vs. free fall)
Rotational/acceleration	Limited to larger animals (swine and rabbits) with the exception of the CHIMERA model.
Primary blast	Scaling parameters are highly variable between studies. What constitutes mTBI due to blast? Potential confounding effects from blast wind, excessive durations, or overpressures. Scaling issues and uncertainties around the mechanism of brain injury due to primary blast waves.

reproduction of injury seen in motor vehicle or sports-related concussions. However, anatomical and size differences between species leave this approach open to criticism in regards to the biomechanical scaling of injury from small mammal to primate. By contrast, the fluid percussion injury model, despite being mechanically isolated from real-world scenarios, has been invaluable in our understanding of white matter and neuronal susceptibility and inflammation following mTBI.[9,10,35,36] Furthermore, comparisons between different mechanical models of mTBI demonstrate variability in outcome within the same set of outcome measures.[18,37] Thus, the biological question being addressed must be matched with an appropriate model in order to be properly investigated (Figure 23.1).

mTBIs arising from blast have come to the research forefront with the recognition that 10–20% of returning military personnel have sustained a TBI event most commonly attributable to blast exposure.[38–41] Extensive research has gone into modeling and understanding the biomechanical transfer of energy from a primary blast wave (shock wave) to human tissues using human cadavers, animal models, and computer simulations. The field of blast research represents a prime example of the intersection between translational research and implications for clinical application of the research findings.

There is ample evidence, but conflicting theories, on how primary blast waves result in brain injury. Competing theories include increases in intracranial pressure (ICP) due to thoracic transfer for of pressure,[42] shear stresses from wave propagation within the brain,[43] inertial injury due to head movement,[44] CSF cavitation,[45] and skull flexure.[46] However, the precise causal mechanism is difficult to isolate in real-world scenarios due to a multitude of factors including body and head displacement from blast wind (also

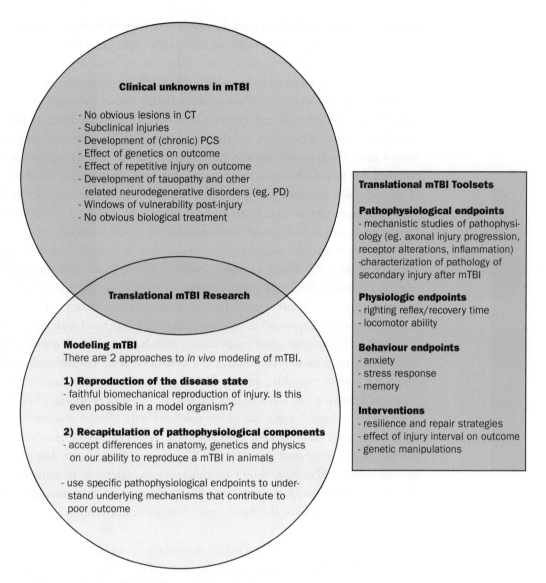

Clinical unknowns in mTBI

- No obvious lesions in CT
- Subclinical injuries
- Development of (chronic) PCS
- Effect of genetics on outcome
- Effect of repetitive injury on outcome
- Development of tauopathy and other
  related neurodegenerative disorders (eg. PD)
- Windows of vulnerability post-injury
- No obvious biological treatment

Translational mTBI Research

Modeling mTBI
There are 2 approaches to *in vivo* modeling of mTBI.

1) Reproduction of the disease state
- faithful biomechanical reproduction of injury. Is this
  even possible in a model organism?

2) Recapitulation of pathophysiological components
- accept differences in anatomy, genetics and physics
  on our ability to reproduce a mTBI in animals

- use specific pathophysiological endpoints to understand underlying mechanisms that contribute to
  poor outcome

Translational mTBI Toolsets

Pathophysiological endpoints
- mechanistic studies of pathophysiology (eg. axonal injury progression,
receptor alterations, inflammation)
-characterization of pathology of
secondary injury after mTBI

Physiologic endpoints
- righting reflex/recovery time
- locomotor ability

Behaviour endpoints
- anxiety
- stress response
- memory

Interventions
- resilience and repair strategies
- effect of injury interval on outcome
- genetic manipulations

Figure 23.1 Schematic of translational approach to mild traumatic brain injury (mTBI).

known as tertiary injuries) and secondary concussions arising from impact against hard surfaces. Dynamic and highly volatile combat environments lead to loss of critical information, such as standoff distance from explosion and type or quantity of ordnance. Given that so many factors cannot be determined with certainty, and because imaging of suspected mTBI blast patients do not present with abnormal CT findings, mTBI remains a clinical diagnosis.[47] How does one correlate the pathophysiological processes derived from an animal model of injury when the underlying mechanisms of injury in human scenarios are still not fully understood?

The majority of primary blast studies to date have been performed in rats and mice, which opens discussion about scaling of injury severity.[48] There is no common consensus on what level of overpressure exposure constitutes mTBI, particularly for a small rodent. To date, models have tended to be built around pathophysiological response rather than the physics contributing to injury, which brings into question the overall relevance of some of the blast models, which may have excessively high pressure levels or durations more comparable to atomic blasts rather than blasts from explosives.[48] There are clear differences in survivability from blast that are mass dependent; animals with smaller masses (e.g., rodents) have lower survivability at comparable blast levels than do larger mammalian species.[48–50] Whether these fatality curves also apply to the extent of brain injury is not yet fully understood. Other factors, including direction of placement, also affects severity of outcome, and the means by which blast waves are generated (compressed gases vs. explosives) are also variably reported and may have different effects on outcome due to differences in shock wave parameters. Parsing out whether the effects of primary blast exposure are specifically related to energy transfer across the brain, ICP changes, or inertial injury due to head movement may be a function of the blast parameters as well as how models are being applied to test subjects.

Studies have reported neurocognitive impairment, ICP swells, and delayed cytoskeletal proteolysis at subclinical exposure levels.[51,52] Other "mild" overpressure exposures result in increased GFAP expression, evidence of apoptotic cell death, behavioral deficits, and axonal injury.[53,54] These research findings have some consistency with observed white matter abnormalities reported in veterans with mTBI associated with blast exposure,[47,55] but a lack of histopathological confirmation with human tissues leaves the findings in blast models open to interpretation. On a behavioral level, translational mTBI animal studies are able to reproduce anxiety-like or posttraumatic stress disorder (PTSD)-like behaviors following low levels of blast exposure,[35,56–58] thus providing a behavioral endpoint for neurological status that shares similarity with clinical observation suggesting that blast-injured patients who have sustained an mTBI have higher rates of PTSD, depression, and stress than non-blast mTBI patients.[59–62] However, data are conflicting because other studies have found no difference in outcomes in symptom reporting or rates of PTSD in blast versus non-blast patients who have sustained mTBIs.[63,64] Cognitive outcomes have also been reported to be uniform regardless of blast or non-blast injury.[61,65]

Complicating the diagnosis of mTBI, particularly in military settings, is the association of comorbidities with overlapping symptoms of mTBI with other neurological disorders including PTSD and postconcussive syndrome (PCS). This makes accurate diagnosis of the underlying cause of neurological dysfunction difficult to determine. PCS is a loosely defined condition in which patients exhibit deficits in attention, speed of information processing, sleep disturbance, fatigue, irritability, and memory impairment[66–69] at least 3 months after initial trauma.[70] Some studies suggest that health status or comorbidities have equal if not greater roles to play in the persistence of PCS reporting in chronic mTBI cases.[71–73] This brings into question whether persistent mTBI symptoms being reported are a result of actual physiological damage or change within the brain, or whether the illness falls under the domain of a psychiatric disorder. Given the requirements of psychological assessment, PCS in translational research remains unexplored in animal models.

Development of mTBI models with sufficient severity to produce quantifiable outcomes is a delicate balance between clinical relevance and translational feasibility. The majority of mTBIs resolve over time, with only a subset of patients having persistent neurological deficits. An ideal model should have predictive validity and reproducibility in outcome.[74] However, developing a model to reproduce the pathophysiology of this select injury subgroup that demonstrates persistent neurological impairment brings into question whether these models truly represent the clinical definition of "mild" TBI. For example, a model that reproduces persistent neurological impairment may fail to address underlying factors, such as genetics, that may be influencing outcome.

Investigation of Genetic Contribution to Outcome and Resilience

There are known genetic contributors to outcome in TBI. Apolipoprotein (ApoE) is the best known example of a genetic contribution to outcome. ApoE is involved in numerous homeostatic processes, including cell membrane and repair, dendrite and synapse formation, cytoskeletal maintenance, intracellular calcium homeostasis, immunomodulation, enzymatic regulation, neural synaptic transmission, regulation of oxidative stress, and coagulation.[75] Given these diverse roles, the genetic contribution of ApoE to outcome after TBI is a plausible avenue for investigation. The ε4 (ApoEε4) isoform, in particular, is associated with worse outcome following TBI in several clinical studies.[76,77] However, the data seem to support a greater risk for poor outcome in severe TBI and limited if any prognostic value in mTBI.[75]

Animal studies in ApoE-deficient mice suggest a neuroprotective role for ApoEε4 in single concussive[78] or repetitive mTBI paradigms.[79] It is not clear whether these contradictory findings are due to the use of ApoE knock-out KO mice, which may have unintended consequences on other homeostatic pathways affecting outcome. There are transgenic strains of mice with differential cellular- and isoform-specific expression levels of ApoE4, but these have yet to be applied in mTBI translational studies.[80] These further highlight discrepancies between translational research and clinical findings that must be interpreted with caution.

Repetitive mTBI

Postmortem findings demonstrating evidence of tauopathies in deceased professional sports athletes[81] and risks associated with development of dementia-related disorders are a relatively novel area of investigation in translational mTBI research.[82] Two clinical unknowns that have potential to be addressed with animal models relate to the temporal windows of vulnerability between mTBI events and the long-term implications of repetitive head traumas on the development of other neurodegenerative diseases. On the clinical front, return-to-play guidelines are variable and depend on neurological diagnosis[83] but may not take into account the pathophysiological processes underlying the injury. Cortical impact models demonstrate increased susceptibility within a vulnerable window that leads to worse outcome.[84] However, it is unclear how the injury interval used in animal studies translates to human physiology. Furthermore, studies in animals involve far fewer concussive events than those typically sustained by athletes. For example,[85] football athletes can receive up to 1,000 subconcussive hits within a season,[86] while animal models are generally limited to only several repeated events. There are histopathological differences between models as well as differences in outcome to consider. For example, a weight-drop model of repetitive mTBI produced no evidence of gross histopathological damage, but animals still demonstrated persistent neurological deficits that were also dependent on the post-injury interval.[87] Reports of higher frequencies of modeled impact in animals correspond to worse outcome[88] and is consistent with reports in human studies indicating that more incidences of concussion result in persistent or greater neurological deficits.[89,90] Collectively, the translational studies support the concept that inter-injury period plays a role in overall outcome.

The role of repetitive mTBI on development of neurological degenerative diseases is in its infancy. There is recognition of a potential increased risk in the development of neurodegenerative diseases such as Parkinson disease.[91] Other reports cite mixed results in terms of the development of dementia or chronic cognitive impairment, suggesting that further work is needed to clarify the contribution of mTBI in these areas.[92]

One area of particular interest is the development of *chronic traumatic encephalopathy* (CTE). The first clinical description of CTE (colloquially referred to as "punch drunk") was in 1928, through postmortem analysis of a boxer's brain.[93] Numerous studies have since described similar pathologies in soldiers and in athletes involved in contact sports.[94] The pathology is distinguishable from other tauopathies, such as Alzheimer disease (AD), by the differential distribution of phosphorylated-tau (p-tau) protein deposits found in neurofibrillary and astrocytic tangles in the superficial layers of the cortex.[95] Translational animal models used to study CTE employ various methods to induce brain trauma.[94] However, the examination of repetitive mTBI in these models has produced varied results, with a subset of studies demonstrating the evolution of p-tau deposition[96–99] while others fail to find such evidence.[87,100–102] Single blast exposure in mice has been shown to result in hyperphosphorylated tau deposition, akin to findings in blast-exposed war veterans.[44] However, the veteran cases had previous histories of concussions, which raises concerns about the accuracy of modeling CTE-linked pathologies with a single concussive blow. Furthermore, clinical data indicate that CTE is a progressive phenomenon that develops over years, whereas animal models, though generally accepted to have protracted timelines given their shorter life spans, tend to develop tau depositions within much shorter time frames.

Although clinical diagnosis of CTE can only be confirmed through postmortem pathology, there are associated behavioral impairments believed to accompany CTE including irritability, impulsivity, aggression, heightened suicide behaviors, depression, and short-term memory loss.[81] Interestingly, some studies in animal models that demonstrate increases in p-tau fail to demonstrate impaired behavior[96] or vice versa.[100] Similarly in clinical cases, some individuals who display CTE-associated behavioral disorders fail to demonstrate neuropathologic evidence of CTE neuropathology.[103] There is also potential selection bias in reported human studies of CTE, raising concerns as to whether p-tau is a universal causal mechanism in the development of CTE.

Translational research has been a necessary component of understanding the pathophysiological processes associated with mTBI. It is clear, however, that interpretation of results and extrapolation of these findings warrants caution. Furthermore, a thorough evaluation of animal models and their relevance to the clinical condition must be appropriately evaluated to avoid erroneous conclusions about the injury process.

References

1. Ventura-Antunes L, Mota B, Herculano-Houzel S. Different scaling of white matter volume, cortical connectivity, and gyrification across rodent and primate brains. *Front Neuroanat.* 2013;7:3.

2. Teasdale G, Jennett B. Assessment of coma and impaired consciousness. A practical scale. *Lancet.* 1974;2(7872):81–84.

3. Spiotta AM, Shin JH, Bartsch AJ, Benzel EC. Subconcussive impact in sports: a new era of awareness. *World Neurosurg.*75(2):175–178.

4. Bailes JE, Petraglia AL, Omalu BI, Nauman E, Talavage T. Role of subconcussion in repetitive mild traumatic brain injury. *J Neurosurg.* 2013;119(5):1235–1245.

5. McMahon P, Hricik A, Yue JK, et al. Symptomatology and functional outcome in mild traumatic brain injury: results from the prospective TRACK-TBI study. *J Neurotrauma.* 2014;31(1):26–33.

6. Elder GA, Stone JR, Ahlers ST. Effects of low-level blast exposure on the nervous system: is there really a controversy? *Front Neurol.* 2014;5:269.

7. Jagoda AS, Bazarian JJ, Bruns JJ Jr, et al. Clinical policy: neuroimaging and decision making in adult mild traumatic brain injury in the acute setting. *J Emerg Nurs.* 2009;35(2):e5–40.

8. Sullivan HG, Martinez J, Becker DP, Miller JD, Griffith R, Wist AO. Fluid-percussion model of mechanical brain injury in the cat. *J Neurosurg.* 1976;45(5):521–534.

9. Shultz SR, MacFabe DF, Foley KA, Taylor R, Cain DP. A single mild fluid percussion injury induces short-term behavioral and neuropathological changes in the Long-Evans rat: support for an animal model of concussion. *Behav Brain Res.* 2011;224(2):326–335.

10. Park E, McKnight S, Ai J, Baker AJ. Purkinje cell vulnerability to mild and severe forebrain head trauma. *J Neuropathol Exp Neurol.* 2006;65(3):226–234.

11. Dixon CE, Clifton GL, Lighthall JW, Yaghmai AA, Hayes RL. A controlled cortical impact model of traumatic brain injury in the rat. *J Neurosci Methods.* 1991;39(3):253–262.

12. Lighthall JW. Controlled cortical impact: a new experimental brain injury model. *J Neurotrauma.* 1988;5(1):1–15.

13. Mao H, Zhang L, Yang KH, King AI. Application of a finite element model of the brain to study traumatic brain injury mechanisms in the rat. *Stapp Car Crash J.* 2006;50:583–600.

14. Milman A, Rosenberg A, Weizman R, Pick CG. Mild traumatic brain injury induces persistent cognitive deficits and behavioral disturbances in mice. *J Neurotrauma.* 2005;22(9):1003–1010.

15. Ucar T, Tanriover G, Gurer I, Onal MZ, Kazan S. Modified experimental mild traumatic brain injury model. *J Trauma.* 2006;60(3):558–565.

16. Foda MA, Marmarou A. A new model of diffuse brain injury in rats. Part II: morphological characterization. *J Neurosurg.* 1994;80(2):301–313.

17. Marmarou A, Foda MA, van den Brink W, Campbell J, Kita H, Demetriadou K. A new model of diffuse brain injury in rats. Part I: pathophysiology and biomechanics. *J Neurosurg.* 1994;80(2):291–300.

18. Viano DC, Hamberger A, Bolouri H, Saljo A. Evaluation of three animal models for concussion and serious brain injury. *Ann Biomed Eng.* 2012;40(1):213–226.

19. Bakay RA, Ward AA Jr. Enzymatic changes in serum and cerebrospinal fluid in neurological injury. *J Neurosurg.* 1983;58(1):27–37.

20. Jeter CB, Hergenroeder GW, Hylin MJ, Redell JB, Moore AN, Dash PK. Biomarkers for the diagnosis and prognosis of mild traumatic brain injury/concussion. *J Neurotrauma.* 2013;30(8):657–670.

21. Kulbe JR, Geddes JW. Current status of fluid biomarkers in mild traumatic brain injury. *Exp Neurol.* 2015;275(Pt 3):334–352.

22. Zetterberg H, Smith DH, Blennow K. Biomarkers of mild traumatic brain injury in cerebrospinal fluid and blood. *Nat Rev Neurol.* 2013;9(4):201–210.

23. Balakathiresan N, Bhomia M, Chandran R, Chavko M, McCarron RM, Maheshwari RK. MicroRNA let-7i is a promising serum biomarker for blast-induced traumatic brain injury. *J Neurotrauma.* 2012;29(7):1379–1387.

24. Redell JB, Moore AN, Ward NH 3rd, Hergenroeder GW, Dash PK. Human traumatic brain injury alters plasma microRNA levels. *J Neurotrauma.* 2010;27(12):2147–2156.

25. Pasinetti GM, Ho L, Dooley C, Abbi B, Lange G. Select non-coding RNA in blood components provide novel clinically accessible biological surrogates for improved identification of traumatic brain injury in OEF/OIF Veterans. *Am J Neurodegener Dis.* 2012;1(1):88–98.

26. Redell JB, Moore AN, Grill RJ, et al. Analysis of functional pathways altered after mild traumatic brain injury. *J Neurotrauma.* 2013;30(9):752–764.

27. Crawford F, Crynen G, Reed J, et al. Identification of plasma biomarkers of TBI outcome using proteomic approaches in an APOE mouse model. *J Neurotrauma.* 2012;29(2):246–260.

28. Siman R, McIntosh TK, Soltesz KM, Chen Z, Neumar RW, Roberts VL. Proteins released from degenerating neurons are surrogate markers for acute brain damage. *Neurobiol Dis.* 2004;16(2):311–320.

29. Gao W, Lu C, Kochanek PM, Berger RP. Serum amyloid A is increased in children with abusive head trauma: a gel-based proteomic analysis. *Pediatr Res.* 2014;76(3):280–286.

30. Rosenbaum SB, Lipton ML. Embracing chaos: the scope and importance of clinical and pathological heterogeneity in mTBI. *Brain Imaging Behav.* 2012;6(2):255–282.

31. Bigler ED. Neuroimaging biomarkers in mild traumatic brain injury (mTBI). *Neuropsychol Rev.* 2013;23(3):169–209.

32. Shin SS, Pathak S, Presson N, et al. Detection of white matter injury in concussion using high-definition fiber tractography. *Prog Neurol Surg.* 2014;28:86–93.

33. Browne KD, Chen XH, Meaney DF, Smith DH. Mild traumatic brain injury and diffuse axonal injury in swine. *J Neurotrauma.* 2011;28(9):1747–1755.

34. Namjoshi DR, Cheng WH, McInnes KA, et al. Merging pathology with biomechanics using CHIMERA (Closed-Head Impact Model of Engineered Rotational Acceleration): a novel, surgery-free model of traumatic brain injury. *Mol Neurodegener.* 2014;9:55.

35. Park E, Eisen R, Kinio A, Baker AJ. Electrophysiological white matter dysfunction and association with neurobehavioral deficits following low-level primary blast trauma. *Neurobiol Dis.* 2013;52:150–159.

36. Shultz SR, MacFabe DF, Foley KA, Taylor R, Cain DP. Sub-concussive brain injury in the Long-Evans rat induces acute neuroinflammation in the absence of behavioral impairments. *Behav Brain Res.* 2011;229(1):145–152.

37. Mychasiuk R, Hehar H, Candy S, Ma I, Esser MJ. The direction of the acceleration and rotational forces associated with mild traumatic brain injury in rodents effect behavioural and molecular outcomes. *J Neurosci Methods.* 2016;257:168–178.

38. Hoge CW, McGurk D, Thomas JL, Cox AL, Engel CC, Castro CA. Mild traumatic brain injury in US soldiers returning from Iraq. *N Engl J Med.* 2008;358(5):453–463.

39. Terrio H, Brenner LA, Ivins BJ, et al. Traumatic brain injury screening: preliminary findings in a US Army Brigade Combat Team. *J Head Trauma Rehabil.* 2009;24(1):14–23.

40. Eskridge SL, Macera CA, Galarneau MR, et al. Injuries from combat explosions in Iraq: injury type, location, and severity. *Injury*. 2012;43(10):1678–1682.

41. Okie S. Traumatic brain injury in the war zone. *N Engl J Med*. 2005;352(20):2043–2047.

42. Courtney AC, Courtney MW. A thoracic mechanism of mild traumatic brain injury due to blast pressure waves. *Med Hypotheses*. 2009;72(1):76–83.

43. Chen Y, Huang W. Non-impact, blast-induced mild TBI and PTSD: concepts and caveats. *Brain Inj*. 2011;25(7-8):641–650.

44. Goldstein LE, Fisher AM, Tagge CA, et al. Chronic traumatic encephalopathy in blast-exposed military veterans and a blast neurotrauma mouse model. *Sci Transl Med*. 2012;4(134):134ra160.

45. Taylor PA, Ludwigsen JS, Ford CC. Investigation of blast-induced traumatic brain injury. *Brain Inj*. 2014;28(7):879–895.

46. Moss WC, King MJ, Blackman EG. Skull flexure from blast waves: a mechanism for brain injury with implications for helmet design. *Phys Rev Lett*. 2009;103(10):108702.

47. Mac Donald CL, Johnson AM, Cooper D, et al. Detection of blast-related traumatic brain injury in US military personnel. *N Engl J Med*. 2011;364(22):2091–2100.

48. Bass CR, Panzer MB, Rafaels KA, Wood G, Shridharani J, Capehart B. Brain injuries from blast. *Ann Biomed Eng*. 2012;40(1):185–202.

49. Bowen IG, Fletcher ER, Richmond DR, Hirsch FG, White CS. Biophysical mechanisms and scaling procedures applicable in assessing responses of the thorax energized by air-blast overpressures or by nonpenetrating missiles. *Ann NY Acad Sci*. 1968;152(1):122–146.

50. Richmond DR, Damon EG, Fletcher ER, Bowen IG, White CS. The relationship between selected blast-wave parameters and the response of mammals exposed to air blast. *Ann NY Acad Sci*. 1968;152(1):103–121.

51. Park E, Gottlieb JJ, Cheung B, Shek PN, Baker AJ. A model of low-level primary blast brain trauma results in cytoskeletal proteolysis and chronic functional impairment in the absence of lung barotrauma. *J Neurotrauma*. 2011;28(3):343–357.

52. Saljo A, Svensson B, Mayorga M, Hamberger A, Bolouri H. Low-level blasts raise intracranial pressure and impair cognitive function in rats. *J Neurotrauma*. 2009;26(8):1345–1352.

53. Kamnaksh A, Kovesdi E, Kwon SK, et al. Factors affecting blast traumatic brain injury. *J Neurotrauma*. 2011;28(10):2145–2153.

54. Long JB, Bentley TL, Wessner KA, Cerone C, Sweeney S, Bauman RA. Blast overpressure in rats: recreating a battlefield injury in the laboratory. *J Neurotrauma*. 2009;26(6):827–840.

55. Jorge RE, Acion L, White T, et al. White matter abnormalities in veterans with mild traumatic brain injury. *Am J Psychiatry*. 2012;169(12):1284–1291.

56. Elder GA, Dorr NP, De Gasperi R, et al. Blast exposure induces post-traumatic stress disorder-related traits in a rat model of mild traumatic brain injury. *J Neurotrauma*. 2012;29(16):2564–2575.

57. Cernak I, Merkle AC, Koliatsos VE, et al. The pathobiology of blast injuries and blast-induced neurotrauma as identified using a new experimental model of injury in mice. *Neurobiol Dis*. 2011;41(2):538–551.

58. Zuckerman A, Ram O, Ifergane G, et al. Controlled low-pressure blast-wave exposure causes distinct behavioral and morphological responses modelling mild traumatic brain injury, post-traumatic stress disorder, and comorbid mild traumatic brain injury-post-traumatic stress disorder. *J Neurotrauma*. 2017;34 (1):145–164.

59. Sayer NA, Chiros CE, Sigford B, et al. Characteristics and rehabilitation outcomes among patients with blast and other injuries sustained during the global War on Terror. *Arch Phys Med Rehabil*. 2008;89(1):163–170.

60. Lippa SM, Pastorek NJ, Benge JF, Thornton GM. Postconcussive symptoms after blast and nonblast-related mild traumatic brain injuries in Afghanistan and Iraq war veterans. *J Int Neuropsychol Soc.* 2010;16(5):856–866.

61. Lange RT, Pancholi S, Brickell TA, et al. Neuropsychological outcome from blast versus non-blast: mild traumatic brain injury in US military service members. *J Int Neuropsychol Soc.* 2012;18(3):595–605.

62. Mendez MF, Owens EM, Reza Berenji G, Peppers DC, Liang LJ, Licht EA. Mild traumatic brain injury from primary blast vs. blunt forces: post-concussion consequences and functional neuroimaging. *NeuroRehabilitation.* 2013;32(2):397–407.

63. Belanger HG, Proctor-Weber Z, Kretzmer T, Kim M, French LM, Vanderploeg RD. Symptom complaints following reports of blast versus non-blast mild TBI: does mechanism of injury matter? *Clin Neuropsychol.* 2011;25(5):702–715.

64. Mac Donald CL, Johnson AM, Wierzechowski L, et al. Prospectively assessed clinical outcomes in concussive blast vs nonblast traumatic brain injury among evacuated US military personnel. *JAMA Neurol.* 2014;71(8):994–1002.

65. Belanger HG, Kretzmer T, Yoash-Gantz R, Pickett T, Tupler LA. Cognitive sequelae of blast-related versus other mechanisms of brain trauma. *J Int Neuropsychol Soc.* 2009;15(1):1–8.

66. Kraus J, Schaffer K, Ayers K, Stenehjem J, Shen H, Afifi AA. Physical complaints, medical service use, and social and employment changes following mild traumatic brain injury: a 6-month longitudinal study. *J Head Trauma Rehabil.* 2005;20(3):239–256.

67. Lundin A, de Boussard C, Edman G, Borg J. Symptoms and disability until 3 months after mild TBI. *Brain Inj.* 2006;20(8):799–806.

68. Vanderploeg RD, Curtiss G, Belanger HG. Long-term neuropsychological outcomes following mild traumatic brain injury. *J Int Neuropsychol Soc.* 2005;11(3):228–236.

69. Yang CC, Tu YK, Hua MS, Huang SJ. The association between the postconcussion symptoms and clinical outcomes for patients with mild traumatic brain injury. *J Trauma.* 2007;62(3):657–663.

70. Carroll LJ, Cassidy JD, Peloso PM, et al. Prognosis for mild traumatic brain injury: results of the WHO Collaborating Centre Task Force on Mild Traumatic Brain Injury. *J Rehabil Med.* 2004(43 suppl):84–105.

71. McLean SA, Kirsch NL, Tan-Schriner CU, et al. Health status, not head injury, predicts concussion symptoms after minor injury. *Am J Emerg Med.* 2009;27(2):182–190.

72. Meares S, Shores EA, Batchelor J, et al. The relationship of psychological and cognitive factors and opioids in the development of the postconcussion syndrome in general trauma patients with mild traumatic brain injury. *J Int Neuropsychol Soc.* 2006;12(6):792–801.

73. Meares S, Shores EA, Taylor AJ, et al. Mild traumatic brain injury does not predict acute postconcussion syndrome. *J Neurol Neurosurg Psychiatry.* 2008;79(3):300–306.

74. Levin HS, Robertson CS. Mild traumatic brain injury in translation. *J Neurotrauma.* 2012;30(8):610–617.

75. Lawrence DW, Comper P, Hutchison MG, Sharma B. The role of apolipoprotein E epsilon (epsilon)-4 allele on outcome following traumatic brain injury: A systematic review. *Brain Inj.* 2015;29(9):1018–1031.

76. Zhou W, Xu D, Peng X, Zhang Q, Jia J, Crutcher KA. Meta-analysis of APOE4 allele and outcome after traumatic brain injury. *J Neurotrauma.* 2008;25(4):279–290.

77. Zeng S, Jiang JX, Xu MH, et al. Prognostic value of apolipoprotein E epsilon4 allele in patients with traumatic brain injury: a meta-analysis and meta-regression. *Genet Test Mol Biomarkers*. 2014;18(3):202–210.

78. Han SH, Chung SY. Marked hippocampal neuronal damage without motor deficits after mild concussive-like brain injury in apolipoprotein E-deficient mice. *Ann N Y Acad Sci*. 2000;903:357–365.

79. Namjoshi DR, Martin G, Donkin J, et al. The liver X receptor agonist GW3965 improves recovery from mild repetitive traumatic brain injury in mice partly through apolipoprotein E. *PLoS One*. 2013;8(1):e53529.

80. Mannix R, Meehan WP III. Evaluating the effects of APOE4 after mild traumatic brain injury in experimental models. 2015. In FH Kobeissy (Ed.), *Brain Neurotrauma: Molecular, Neuropsychological, and Rehabilitation Aspects*. Boca Raton (FL): CRC Press/Taylor & Francis; 2015. Chapter 9. Frontiers in Neuroengineering.

81. McKee AC, Cantu RC, Nowinski CJ, et al. Chronic traumatic encephalopathy in athletes: progressive tauopathy after repetitive head injury. *J Neuropathol Exp Neurol*. 2009;68(7):709–735.

82. Gardner RC, Yaffe K. Epidemiology of mild traumatic brain injury and neurodegenerative disease. *Mol Cell Neurosci*. 2015;66(Pt B):75–80.

83. Putukian M. Repeat mild traumatic brain injury: how to adjust return to play guidelines. *Curr Sports Med Rep*. 2006;5(1):15–22.

84. Huang L, Coats JS, Mohd-Yusof A, et al. Tissue vulnerability is increased following repetitive mild traumatic brain injury in the rat. *Brain Res*. 2013;1499:109–120.

85. Laurer HL, Bareyre FM, Lee VM, et al. Mild head injury increasing the brain's vulnerability to a second concussive impact. *J Neurosurg*. 2001;95(5):859–870.

86. Gysland SM, Mihalik JP, Register-Mihalik JK, Trulock SC, Shields EW, Guskiewicz KM. The relationship between subconcussive impacts and concussion history on clinical measures of neurologic function in collegiate football players. *Ann Biomed Eng*. 2012;40(1):14–22.

87. Mannix R, Meehan WP, Mandeville J, et al. Clinical correlates in an experimental model of repetitive mild brain injury. *Ann Neurol*. 2013;74(1):65–75.

88. Longhi L, Saatman KE, Fujimoto S, et al. Temporal window of vulnerability to repetitive experimental concussive brain injury. *Neurosurgery*. 2005;56(2):364–374; discussion 364–374.

89. Vagnozzi R, Signoretti S, Tavazzi B, et al. Temporal window of metabolic brain vulnerability to concussion: a pilot 1H-magnetic resonance spectroscopic study in concussed athletes: part III. *Neurosurgery*. 2008;62(6):1286–1295; discussion 1295–1296.

90. Cancelliere C, Hincapie CA, Keightley M, et al. Systematic review of prognosis and return to play after sport concussion: results of the International Collaboration on Mild Traumatic Brain Injury Prognosis. *Arch Phys Med Rehabil*. 2014;95(3 suppl):S210–229.

91. Marras C, Hincapie CA, Kristman VL, et al. Systematic review of the risk of Parkinson's disease after mild traumatic brain injury: results of the International Collaboration on Mild Traumatic Brain Injury Prognosis. *Arch Phys Med Rehabil*. 2014;95(3 suppl):S238–244.

92. Godbolt AK, Cancelliere C, Hincapie CA, et al. Systematic review of the risk of dementia and chronic cognitive impairment after mild traumatic brain injury: results of the International Collaboration on Mild Traumatic Brain Injury Prognosis. *Arch Phys Med Rehabil*. 2014;95(3 suppl):S245–256.

93. Martland J. Punch drunk. *JAMA*. 1928;91:1103–1107.

94. Ojo JO, Mouzon BC, Crawford F. Repetitive head trauma, chronic traumatic encephalopathy and tau: challenges in translating from mice to men. *Exp Neurol.* 2016;275(Pt 3):389–404.

95. McKee AC, Stern RA, Nowinski CJ, et al. The spectrum of disease in chronic traumatic encephalopathy. *Brain.* 2013;136(Pt 1):43–64.

96. Kane MJ, Angoa-Perez M, Briggs DI, Viano DC, Kreipke CW, Kuhn DM. A mouse model of human repetitive mild traumatic brain injury. *J Neurosci Methods.* 2012;203(1):41–49.

97. Arun P, Abu-Taleb R, Oguntayo S, et al. Distinct patterns of expression of traumatic brain injury biomarkers after blast exposure: role of compromised cell membrane integrity. *Neurosci Lett.* 2013;552:87–91.

98. Zhang J, Teng Z, Song Y, Hu M, Chen C. Inhibition of monoacylglycerol lipase prevents chronic traumatic encephalopathy-like neuropathology in a mouse model of repetitive mild closed head injury. *J Cereb Blood Flow Metab.* 2015;35(3):443–453.

99. Luo J, Nguyen A, Villeda S, et al. Long-term cognitive impairments and pathological alterations in a mouse model of repetitive mild traumatic brain injury. *Front Neurol.* 2014;5:12.

100. Mouzon BC, Bachmeier C, Ferro A, et al. Chronic neuropathological and neurobehavioral changes in a repetitive mild traumatic brain injury model. *Ann Neurol.* 2014;75(2):241–254.

101. Bolton AN, Saatman KE. Regional neurodegeneration and gliosis are amplified by mild traumatic brain injury repeated at 24-hour intervals. *J Neuropathol Exp Neurol.* 2014;73(10):933–947.

102. Xu L, Nguyen JV, Lehar M, et al. Repetitive mild traumatic brain injury with impact acceleration in the mouse: multifocal axonopathy, neuroinflammation, and neurodegeneration in the visual system. *Exp Neurol.* 2014;275(Pt 3):436–449.

103. Gardner A, Iverson GL, McCrory P. Chronic traumatic encephalopathy in sport: a systematic review. *Br J Sports Med.* 2013;48(2):84–90.

Military-Relevant Rodent Models of Blast-Induced Traumatic Brain Injuries

Ibolja Cernak

24

Importance and Complexity of Blast-Induced Traumatic Brain Injuries

Need for Blast Injury Models

Traumatic brain injury (TBI) is a problem of significant concern for military populations, particularly in the United States. Recent reports estimate that approximately 348,000 US military personnel experienced a TBI during Operations Iraqi Freedom (OIF) and Enduring Freedom (OEF)[1] with that number equivalent to roughly 13% of the deployed forces.[2] More than 83% of all TBIs have been classified as mild, 9% as moderate, 1% severe, and 1.4% penetrating. The majority (more than 78%) of the head injuries had been inflicted by explosive weaponry, thus by blast.[3] Recent data demonstrated that the number of reports on postconcussion symptoms increased as a function of cumulative blast exposures among service members exposed to blast.[4] This information supports previous clinical[5–7] and experimental findings suggesting summative effects of repeated, low-intensity blast exposures.[8,9]

In both civilian and military environments, exposure to a blast may inflict injuries on a continuum from instant death, to injuries with immediate manifestation of symptoms, to latent injuries that are initiated at the time of exposure and may manifest over a period of hours, months, or even years.[10] Blast-induced TBI gained the reputation of being the "signature wound" of the recent military actions because of the large number of soldiers acquiring TBI and subsequently developing long-term deficits. This could be explained by the increased number of surviving soldiers due to improved interceptive properties of the currently used body armor providing better protection from penetrating injuries and prompt evacuation of the wounded. Namely, the increased survival rate provides time for neurological deficits and other complications to develop.[11] Indeed, it has been reported that while the majority of actively serving personnel recover from mild TBI, which is the most frequent form of all currently reported military TBIs, in about 15% (estimates range from 10–25%) of cases, physical disabilities and symptoms persist beyond 3 months.[12,13]

Complexity of Injury Scenarios

By definition, blast-induced neurotrauma (BINT) is a TBI caused by a blast generated during an explosion.[14] Blast is one of the products of explosion and represents a region of highly compressed gas that rapidly expands to occupy a volume several times greater than that of the original explosive, the solid residues from the explosive, or its casing together.[15] The effects of explosive blasts on the body are fivefold[11,16]: (1) **primary blast effects** cause injuries (so-called primary blast injuries) solely through the blast wave–body interaction. During the interaction between blast wave and a living body, a fraction of the shock wave is reflected, whereas another fraction of the shock wave energy is absorbed and propagates through the body as a tissue-transmitted shock wave[17]; (2) **secondary blast effects** lead to secondary blast injuries, which can be blunt or penetrating, depending on the interactions between the fragments of debris propelled by the explosion and the body (i.e., whether the fragments damage the integrity of the skull or the skin barrier); (3) **tertiary blast effects** inflict tertiary blast injuries as a consequence of acceleration–deceleration of the body or part of the body[18]; (4) **quaternary blast effects** include the transient but intense heat of the explosion and cause quaternary blast injuries such as flash burns[19]; and (5) **quinary blast effects** that include a broad variety of potentially injurious factors such as the post-detonation environmental contaminants (bacteria and radiation from dirty bombs; and tissue reactions to fuel and metal residues, among others) inducing quinary blast injuries.[20] Every so often, especially in the case of moderate to severe blast injuries, the interplay of the multiple blast effects with the body is simultaneous. In some literature sources, such an injurious environment and related injuries are referred to as "blast plus" scenarios.[21,22]

Individuals who have been exposed to blast describe their experience as "being entirely enveloped by a fast-travelling pressure field." This implies that blast, which generates a loading pressure that varies both spatially and in time due to the combined effects of the static and dynamic pressures of the incident wave,[23] interacts with all body parts and not only with the head. The enveloping effect of blast loading is essential to the type and extent of global displacement of the body as well as to the form of imparted stresses.

Complexity of Clinical Manifestations

The diagnosis of BINT poses special challenges. Symptoms are not immediately visible and may not fully develop for months to years after blast exposure. People with BINT frequently show a constellation of neurological signs, including memory loss for pre- and post-explosion events, confusion, headache,[24,25] impaired sense of reality, reduced attention, impaired decision-making, and lack of social participation. Because BINT is frequently unrecognized, valuable time is often lost for preventive therapy and/or timely rehabilitation.

Taken together, BINT is a unique clinical entity in which the functional and morphological impairments in the brain are coupled with considerable systemic and/or local changes.[26] Hence, the pathobiology of BINT is usually more complex than in blunt, impact-, and/or acceleration-/rotation-induced TBIs.[27] Accordingly, modeling BINT is a considerable challenge due to several generalizable and specific factors.

In this chapter, we discuss two generalizable factors: (1) the basic requirements of injury modeling and (2) the size, geometry, and biological properties of rodents as experimental animals. The factors that are specific to blast modeling are (1) methods of generating militarily and clinically relevant blast conditions, (2) animal holding and positioning in reference to blast conditions that soldiers are exposed to, and (3) alignment of the pathological changes and related symptoms generated in rodent blast models with those seen in humans exposed to blast.

Modeling Requirements for BINT

Generalizable Modeling Requirements and Considerations

The purpose of the experimental models of injuries, including blast injuries, is to replicate certain pathological components or phases of clinical trauma in experimental animals aiming to address pathology and/or treatment. Consequently, the design and choice of the chosen specific model should match the goals of the research.[28] Regardless of the research questions the study addresses, a clinically and militarily relevant blast injury model should fulfill essential general criteria (Table 24.1). In addition to general requirements, the models also should match other BINT-specific particulars, such as position-dependent injury severity and pattern[29–34] and diffuse and not well-demarcated localized functional and/or structural brain damage.[35,36]

Rodents for BINT Modeling

Proper selection of animal species is one of the key elements in planning experiments focusing on BINT. There are numerous species-dependent factors that influence the outcome of blast experiments. It is now known that the level of phylogenetic maturity has a decisive role in the brain's response to a high-pressure environment.[37] Also, the significant anatomical and physiological differences between humans and rodents, especially in circulatory and nervous systems, could limit the utilization of small experimental animals in blast-injury research. Extensive studies conducted in Albuquerque, New Mexico, and confirmed by others demonstrated significant size-dependent interspecies differences in blast tolerance.[31,38,39] The following calculations will serve as a demonstration of the importance of the animal's size in BINT modeling. If we take into account the facts that:

- The overpressure durations for human injury range from 1 to 10 ms, and a low-strength blast wave travels at a little more than 1 foot per millisecond (304.8 m/s);
- One millisecond is roughly the time that it takes for the shock wave to engulf an erect human; thus, the range of durations of military relevance can be defined as the time it takes to engulf the target to 10 times that duration; and
- The approximate dimension of a mouse head is 10% of the dimension of a human head.

Table 24.1:
General criteria for blast injury models

1. The injurious component of the blast should be clearly identified and reproduced in controlled, reproducible, and quantifiable manner.

2. The inflicted injury should be reproducible, quantifiable, and mimic components of human blast injuries.

3. The injury outcome established based on morphological, physiological, biochemical, and/or behavioral parameters should be related to the chosen injurious component of the blast.

4. The mechanical properties (intensity, complexity of blast signature, and/or its duration) of the injurious factor should predict the outcome severity.

All these taken together lead us to the conclusion that the duration of blast overpressure in a militarily relevant experimental setting using mice should be between 0.1 and 1 ms, based on the animal's size. Nevertheless, the majority of currently used rodent shock tubes generate shock waves with durations of more than 10 ms.[23]

In addition to size, the geometry of the animals' body and head also significantly affect blast tolerance.[40] The anatomical differences between human and animal heads, such as bone volume fraction, trabecular separation and number, and connectivity density, among others,[41,42] should be considered as well as the evolutionary and developmental changes in the structure and arrangement of blood vessels.[43] For example, while the internal carotid artery is the main blood supply both in humans and nonhuman primates and in rodents (rats and mice), the lower vertebrates' internal carotid artery directs the blood to the brain parenchyma through the posterior branch without contribution from the basilar artery. In comparison, higher vertebrates have two posterior branches that stem from a single and central branch turning into the branch of the basilar artery.[44] These anatomical differences could significantly influence shock wave propagation through the brain's blood vessels.

Differing lung densities and volumes have also been suggested as a potential factor contributing to interspecies differences in blast tolerance.[45] For example, lung density in larger species, including man, monkey, cat, and dog, is only about half of the lung density of smaller species (e.g., rodents), whereas lung volumes normalized to body mass are three times bigger in large species than in smaller animals.[45] These differences could alter the systemic responses to blast exposure, and, consequently, through changed systemic mechanisms modify the progress and outcome of BINT.

Finally, recent studies showed that, although acute inflammatory stresses from different etiologies result in highly similar genomic responses in humans, the responses in corresponding mouse models correlate poorly with the human conditions and also with one another.[46–48] This questions the extent to which mouse models of BINT can be used to discern inflammatory mechanisms in the brain and other parts of the body triggered by blast exposure.

Rodents remain the most frequently used experimental animals in the BINT research due to their relatively small size and low cost, which allow for repetitive measurements of morphological, biochemical, cellular, and behavioral parameters that require relatively large numbers of animals. This, because of ethical, technical, and/or financial limitations, is less achievable in phylogenetically higher species.[28] Because basic molecular and gene injury-response mechanisms are conserved through evolution, phylogenetically lower species such as rodents can be used to study blast-induced changes at cellular and subcellular levels while bearing in mind the previously discussed caveats.

Blast-Specific Modeling

There are differing opinions about the best approach to TBI modeling. Some researchers state that since injury mechanisms cannot be known with certainty, whereas the neurological dysfunctions are observable (thus, known), the preclinical models should reproduce neurological impairments resulting from the injury rather than faithfully reproducing the relevant biomechanics. This position would imply that the injury models should replicate generalizable manifestations of brain injury such as brain edema, headache, memory deficits, or behavioral impairments, among others. According to the "reproducing signs and symptoms and not source of injuries" approach, any model, for example, that would reproduce brain edema, such as the model using intravenous administration of *Clostridium perfringens* type D-ε toxin to mice to cause severe, generalized, vascular endothelial damage and progressive brain edema[49] could be used to assess blast-induced brain edema and related headache. Nevertheless, accumulating experimental and clinical data suggest a distinct and polyphasic pattern of vascular response mechanisms in the brain after blast,[32,50–52] with blast-induced brain edema showing predilection for certain brain regions such as the cerebellum or brainstem[53] rather than being generalized.

Without any doubt, experimental models that replicate the end mechanisms leading to generalizable injury manifestations might be useful to a certain extent. Nevertheless, we need to understand the biological triggers for the pathological cascades that consist of numerous interwoven mechanisms demonstrating spatial and temporal profiles that are distinctive to BINT. Only then will we be able to leverage the existing knowledge gathered about other TBI types for BINT diagnosis or treatment and for the development of new BINT-specific approaches if needed.

Steps in Planning BINT Experiments

Which Blast Effect to Replicate?

Based on their research question, researchers should clearly define which blast effects they want to reproduce. Namely, if the research study aims at addressing the effects of primary blast injuries, the researchers should pay special attention to prevent any secondary or tertiary blast effects that would potentially interact with the animal's body during the experiment. For example, if the body is allowed to move during the blast exposure, the injury mechanisms would involve both primary and tertiary blast effects, which would make the interpretation of the findings quite complicated.

Open-Field Versus Laboratory Conditions

Experimental studies on primary blast-induced biological responses are performed either in an open environment or laboratory conditions. The open-field studies expose animals to a blast wave that is generated by detonation of an explosive either in a free-field or confined space environment.[54–58] In addition to the shock wave, the open-field explosions also generate acoustic, thermal, optical, and electromagnetic components found in actual blast environments; thus, the injury scenarios are more comparable to in-theater conditions.[59] Nevertheless, the physical characteristics of the shock wave (such as the homogeneity of the pressure field) are less controllable, so a broader range of biologic response should be expected.[59]

Experiments performed in laboratory conditions use either shock tubes (which use compressed air or gas to generate a shock wave) or blast tubes (which use explosive charges).[60,61] Both of them focus the blast wave energy in a linear direction from the source to the subject, thus maximizing the amount of blast energy[62] without the exponential decay of the shock wave's velocity and pressure seen in free-field explosions.[63] The induction system that both the shock and blast tubes routinely use consists of a cylindrical metal tube divided by a plastic or metal diaphragm into two main (driver and driven) sections. The anesthetized animals are fixed individually in special holders designed to prevent any movement of their body in response to the blast. The high pressure in the driver section is generated by either explosive charge or compressed gas, which ruptures the diaphragm when reaching the material's tolerance to pressure. After the diaphragm ruptures, the resultant shock wave travels along the driven section with supersonic velocity and interacts with the animal positioned inside the driven section.[10] The length and/or diameter of the high-pressure chamber directly influences the duration of the overpressure.[63]

Blast tubes use high-energy explosives placed within a heavy-walled, small-diameter driver section (often a gun barrel), expanding into the wider diameter driven (i.e., test) section.[64] The drawbacks to using a blast tube include (1) dispersion of the combustion products and residue in the test section, (2) generation of strong transverse waves either within the driver or in the wider test section caused by the configuration of the charge and the driver, and (3) introduction of additional operating costs and more complex environmental control for safe handling, setting, and firing of the charges.

Shock tubes are widely used devices in laboratory conditions. They use either compressed atmospheric air or another gas to generate a shock wave. The compressed air fails to expand as quickly as would an ideal gas when the membrane is ruptured and also generates a broad range of overpressure peaks. Use of a lighter gas, such as helium, improves the performance of shock tubes because of the increased speed of sound within a helium environment.[63] Moreover, although the features of the positive phase of free-field explosive blast can be replicated by careful adjustment of the driver's length, driver's gas, and the specimen location, the negative phase and recompression shock are often artifacts of the rarefaction from the open end of the tube; thus, the simulated blast wave is incorrect when compared with the signature of the militarily-relevant blast.[64] Because of this, it is recommended that shock tubes be fitted with a reflection-eliminator at their end to eliminate the waves reverberating the length of the tube.

Recently, several experimental devices have been described that use ultrasound[65,66] or other means of generating overpressure such as microwave[67] or laser.[68] Nevertheless, the resulting shock waves do not have the physical properties of a blast (i.e., an explosion-generated shock wave) and do not replicate features of BINT seen in individuals exposed to blast. While bearing in mind the blast physics and the features of the injurious environment, providing information about the shock wave properties is essential for comparing research findings between different laboratories and confirming the clinical and military value of the data. The components of full characterization of the shock wave are shown in Table 24.2.[10,23,69]

Animal Positioning

The biomechanical and biological responses of an animal exposed to the shock wave significantly depend on the animal's location inside the tube[70] as well as on its orientation in relation to the propagating incident shock wave.[32,71,72] The currently existing literature supports the need of placing the specimen inside the shock tube.[70,71] Namely, when the animal is positioned inside the shock tube, it is subjected to a load that is due to the close to pure blast wave, which is comparable to the shock wave generated in free-field conditions. On the other hand, when the animal is positioned at or near the shock tube's exit, there is a sharp decay in pressure after the initial shock front, which is caused

Table 24.2:
The main parameters defining a shock wave

Shock Wave Component	Definition
Static pressure (also known as side-on pressure or overpressure)	Above-ambient pressure generated by compression or heating of the gas. The units are force per unit area or energy per unit volume.
Dynamic pressure (also known as differential pressure or gust)	Generated by the motion of gas and it depends on the gas density (ρ) and gas velocity (U): $P_D = \frac{1}{2} \rho \times U^2$. The units are force per unit area or energy per unit volume.
Stagnation pressure (also known as total pressure, total head pressure, or pitot pressure)	The sum of the static and dynamic pressures, expressed as force per unit experienced by an object in a steady flow environment
Overpressure impulse	In blast physics is a parameter that indicate the total energy in a blast wave. It is defined as the area under the pressure (expressed as force per area) versus time function.
Positive impulse	The integral of the pressure-time trace during the positive phase.
Positive magnitude	The difference between peak positive pressure and ambient pressure
Positive duration	Indicates the time between the moments at which the pressure began to rise above ambient pressure (to) and when the pressure goes below ambient pressure.
Negative magnitude	The difference between ambient and peak negative pressure.

by the expansion wave from the exit of the shock tube eliminating the exponentially decaying blast wave.[70] This phenomenon leads to significant decrease of the positive blast impulse and conversion of most of the blast energy from supersonic blast wave to subsonic jet wind,[73] which has significantly different effects from those generated by a blast wave. Because of the jet wind, the restrained animal is exposed to more severe compression of the head and neck, whereas the thoracic cavity is exposed to a higher pressure of longer positive-phase duration.

During the blast exposure, the animals are safely positioned inside the specimen holders, which are designed to secure the animal in a desired position at assigned location. The choice of the animal holder is another crucial component in shock/blast tube experiments. Namely, if the animal is fixed on a solid platform, the waves reflecting from it will amplify the primary shock wave and increase the complexity and severity of blast injuries. When designing the animal holder, the following mistakes should be avoided (a) using an animal holder that is too large for the shock tube and placed near the shock tube's exit—this could cause unstable flow with probable turbulence caused by more than 30% of blockage and enhanced dynamic pressure; (b) placing the animal inside the animal holder so that only its neck and head are outside of the plexiglas/metal container with neck tightly surrounded by the container's edge—this could increase the probability of compression on the animal's neck caused by the movement of the animal or the

Table 24.3:
Alignment of the pathological changes and related symptoms generated in rodent blast models with those seen in humans exposed to blast

	Humans	Rodents
1. Position-dependent injury patterns & outcome	Blast overpressures can vary significantly depending on the position an orientation of the soldier[74] Body position significantly influences the type and severity of blast injuries[83]	Frontal exposures (torso and head facing blast front) result in increased severity of multi-organ injuries and BINT[32–34,38]
2. Cerebrovascular spasms (CVS) and other vascular changes	Cerebral arterial spasm and intracranial hypertension are frequent and significant complications of moderate to severe BINT Vasospasm can develop early, often within 48 hours of injury, and can also manifest later, typically between 10–14 days postexposure[51,84,85]	CVS is characterized by initial vascular smooth muscle cell (VSMC) hypercontractility, followed by prolonged vessel remodeling and lumen occlusion; traditionally associated with subarachnoid hemorrhage (SAH), but recent results suggest that mechanical injury during bTBI can cause mechano-transduced VSMC hypercontractility and phenotype switching necessary for CVS development, even in the absence of SAH[86,87] Impairments of cerebral vascular endothelium-dependent dilation, potentially a consequence of endothelial dysfunction and/or vascular remodelling in basilar arteries after blast[88] Reduced CBF during the early post-blast period[89] Chronic selective vulnerability of the microvasculature in the brain[90]
3. Impaired electrical activity of the brain	Abnormal low-frequency magnetic activity (MEG: ALFMA, peaked at 1-4Hz)[91] Diminished electroencephalogram (EEG) phase synchrony, poor coordination of frontal neural function[92–95]	Depression of both EEG frequency and amplitude in rats up to 30 min post-blast[96]
4. Metabolic changes in the brain	Lower relative cerebral metabolic rate of glucose (rCMRglc) 15–86 months after blast[36,97] Cerebro-cerebellar hypometabolism 2–5 years post-blast [53,98]	Increased glucose uptake at 1 day post-blast in rats[99] Impaired mitochondrial metabolism[100–103]
5. Contribution of systemic effects to neurological deficits	Oxidative stress[104,105] Systemic inflammation[106–108] Coagulation system; disseminated intravascular coagulation (DIC)[109]	Oxidative stress: ROS, iNOS[110–115] Systemic inflammation[26,50,80,116–118] Coagulation system[119,120]
6. Chronic neurodegeneration	Abnormalities of brain white matter structural integrity[53,121–125]	Increased markers of neuronal cell death (both necrosis and apoptosis) during the early post-blast period[126,127] Impaired cytoskeleton[128,129] Elevated phospho- and cleaved-tau species[130–132] Chronic microglia/macrophage activation[32,50,115,133,134]
7. Endocrine changes	Hypothalamus-pituitary-end organ (thyroid, adrenal, gonadal) deficits[135–137]	Hypothalamus-pituitary-end organ (thyroid, adrenal, gonadal) deficits[138,112]

container during the shock wave propagation; and (c) positioning the holder so that the incident pressure is perpendicular to the animal's neck—this could create a scenario for maximum reflection pressure and forceful head movement with a high probability of a head impact with the container's rim.[10,23]

The animal's orientation toward the shock wave front is especially important since it has been shown that the overpressure load,[38,74] mortality,[32,38] and both the pattern and severity of blast-induced organ damages depend on the orientation of the body toward the shock wave front.[32,38,75,76] Indeed, mice positioned **vertically** (as bipeds) with their torso facing the front of the incoming shock wave had significantly higher mortality than those whose backs faced the shock wave's front[32]; these findings further support the historical data.[29,38] It has been shown that the orientation of the head toward the shock wave front significantly influenced the intracranial pressure (ICP) and possibly other cerebrovascular changes in animals exposed to shock tube–generated blast conditions.[33,34] Moreover, a recent study demonstrated that low-intensity blast exposure produced an impairment of spatial memory that was specific to the orientation of the animal.[77]

Alignment of Pathological Changes

There is a wide range of blast overpressure sustained for various durations in single- or repeated-exposure rodent studies, with a mean peak overpressure of 30–517 kPa (4.35–75 psi) on the nearest surface of the animal's body.[32,78–82] The physical characteristics of the blast conditions vary significantly; thus, a scientifically reliable comparison of the results is almost impossible. Nevertheless, there are several commonalities among experimental findings that also align well with clinical observations (Table 24.3).

References

1. Defense and Veterans Brain Injury Center. DoD worldwide numbers for TBI. http://dvbic. dcoe.mil/sites/default/files/uploads/Worldwide Totals 2000-2014Q1.pdf. Published 2014. Accessed July 2, 2014.

2. Defense Manpower Data Center. *CTS Deployment File Baseline Report*. Washington DC: Armed Force Health Surveillance Center; 2015.

3. Fang R, Markandaya M, DuBose JJ, Cancio LC, Shackelford S, Blackbourne LH. Early in-theater management of combat-related traumatic brain injury: A prospective, observational study to identify opportunities for performance improvement. *J Trauma Acute Care Surg*. 2015;79(4 suppl 2):S181–187.

4. Reid MW, Miller KJ, Lange RT, et al. A multisite study of the relationships between blast exposures and symptom reporting in a post-deployment active duty military population with mild traumatic brain injury. *J Neurotrauma*. 2014;31(23):1899–1906.

5. Carr W, Stone JR, Walilko T, et al. Repeated low-level blast exposure: a descriptive human subjects study. *Mil Med*. 2016;181(5 suppl):28–39.

6. Baker AJ, Topolovec-Vranic J, Michalak A, et al. Controlled blast exposure during forced explosive entry training and mild traumatic brain injury. *J Trauma*. 2011;71(5 suppl 1):S472–477.

7. Karr JE, Areshenkoff CN, Garcia-Barrera MA. The neuropsychological outcomes of concussion: a systematic review of meta-analyses on the cognitive sequelae of mild traumatic brain injury. *Neuropsychology*. 2014;28(3):321–336.

8. Ahmed FA, Kamnaksh A, Kovesdi E, Long JB, Agoston DV. Long-term consequences of single and multiple mild blast exposure n select physiological parameters and blood-based biomarkers. *Electrophoresis.* 2013;34(15):2229–2233.

9. Kaur C, Singh J, Moochhala S, Lim MK, Lu J, Ling EA. Induction of NADPH diaphorase/nitric oxide synthase in the spinal cord motor neurons of rats following a single and multiple non-penetrative blasts. *Histol Histopathol.* 1999;14(2):417–425.

10. Cernak I. Blast injuries and blast-induced neurotrauma—overview of pathophysiology and experimental knowledge: models and findings. In: Kobeissy F, ed. *Brain Neurotrauma: Molecular, Neuropsychological, and Rehabilitation Aspects.* Boca Raton, FL: CRC Press; 2015:629–642.

11. Cernak I, Noble-Haeusslein LJ. Traumatic brain injury: an overview of pathobiology with emphasis on military populations. *J Cereb Blood Flow Metab.* 2010;30(2):255–266.

12. Vasterling JJ, Brailey K, Proctor SP, Kane R, Heeren T, Franz M. Neuropsychological outcomes of mild traumatic brain injury, post-traumatic stress disorder and depression in Iraq-deployed US Army soldiers. *Br J Psychiatry.* 2012;201(3):186–192.

13. DePalma RG. Combat TBI: history, epidemiology, and injury modes. In: Kobeissy KH, ed. *Brain Neurotrauma.* Boca Raton, FL: CRC Press/Taylor & Francis; 2015:5–12.

14. Clemedson CJ. Blast injury. *Physiol Rev.* 1956;36(3):336–354.

15. Cernak I, Noble-Haeusslein L. Pathophysiology of blast injury. In: Institute of Medicine, ed. *Gulf War and Health. Volume 9: Long-Term Effects of Blast Exposures:* National Academies Press; Washington, D.C.; 2014:33–83.

16. DePalma RG, Burris DG, Champion HR, Hodgson MJ. Blast injuries. *N Engl J Med.* 2005;352(13):1335–1342.

17. Clemedson CJ, Jonsson A. Transmission of elastic disturbances caused by air shock waves in a living body. *J Appl Physiol.* 1961;16:426–430.

18. Richmond DR, Bowen IG, White CS. Tertiary blast effects. Effects of impact on mice, rats, guinea pigs and rabbits. *Aerosp Med.* 1961;32:789–805.

19. Mellor SG. The pathogenesis of blast injury and its management. *Br J Hosp Med.* 1988;39(6):536–539.

20. Kluger Y, Nimrod A, Biderman P, Mayo A, Sorkin P. The quinary pattern of blast injury. *Am J Disaster Med.* 2007;2(1):21–25.

21. Moss WC, King MJ, Blackman EG. Skull flexure from blast waves: a mechanism for brain injury with implications for helmet design. *Phys Rev Lett.* 2009;103(10):108702.

22. MacDonald CL, Johnson AM, Nelson EC, et al. Functional status after blast-plus-impact complex concussive traumatic brain injury in evacuated United States military personnel. *J Neurotrauma.* 2014;31(10):889–898.

23. Needham CE, Ritzel D, Rule GT, Wiri S, Young L. Blast testing issues and TBI: experimental models that lead to wrong conclusions. *Front Neurol.* 2015;6:72.

24. Finkel AG, Yerry JA, Klaric JS, Ivins BJ, Scher A, Choi YS. Headache in military service members with a history of mild traumatic brain injury: a cohort study of diagnosis and classification. *Cephalalgia.* 2017 May;37(6):548–559.

25. Eskridge SL, Macera CA, Galarneau MR, et al. Combat blast injuries: Injury severity and posttraumatic stress disorder interaction on career outcomes in male servicemembers. *J Rehabil Res Dev.* 2013;50(1):7–16.

26. Cernak I. The importance of systemic response in the pathobiology of blast-induced neurotrauma. *Front Neurol.* 2010;1:151.

27. Cernak I, Ahmed AF. A comparative analysis of blast-induced neurotrauma and blunt-traumatic brain injury reveals significant differences in injury mechanisms. *Medical Data.* 2010;2(4):297–304.

28. Cernak I. Animal models of head trauma. *NeuroRx.* 2005;2(3):410–422.

29. Bowen IG, Fletcher ER, Richmond D. *Estimate of Man's Tolerance to the Direct Effects of Air Blas.* Washington, DC: US Defense Atomic Support Agency;1968. DA-49-146-XZ-372, DASA-211.

30. Bowen IG, Fletcher ER, Richmond DR, Hirsch FG, White CS. Biophysical mechanisms and scaling procedures applicable in assessing responses of the thorax energized by air-blast overpressures or by nonpenetrating missiles. *Ann NY Acad Sci.* 1968;152(1):122–146.

31. Damon EG, Gaylord CS, Yelverton JT, et al. Effects of ambient pressure on tolerance of mammals to air blast. *Aerosp Med.* 1968;39(10):1039–1047.

32. Cernak I, Merkle AC, Koliatsos VE, et al. The pathobiology of blast injuries and blast-induced neurotrauma as identified using a new experimental model of injury in mice. *Neurobiol Dis.* 2011;41(2):538–551.

33. Chavko M, Watanabe T, Adeeb S, Lankasky J, Ahlers ST, McCarron RM. Relationship between orientation to a blast and pressure wave propagation inside the rat brain. *J Neurosci Methods.* 2011;195(1):61–66.

34. Dal Cengio Leonardi A, Keane NJ, Bir CA, Ryan AG, Xu L, Vandevord PJ. Head orientation affects the intracranial pressure response resulting from shock wave loading in the rat. *J Biomech.* 2012;45(15):2595–2602.

35. Mu W, Catenaccio E, Lipton ML. Neuroimaging in Blast-Related Mild Traumatic Brain Injury. *J Head Trauma Rehabil.* 2017 Jan/Feb;32(1):55–69.

36. Petrie EC, Cross DJ, Yarnykh VL, et al. Neuroimaging, behavioral, and psychological sequelae of repetitive combined blast/impact mild traumatic brain injury in Iraq and Afghanistan war veterans. *J Neurotrauma.* 2014;31(5):425–436.

37. Brauer RW, Mansfield WM, Jr., Beaver RW, Gillen HW. Stages in development of high-pressure neurological syndrome in the mouse. *J Appl Physiol Respir Environ Exerc Physiol.* 1979;46(4):756–765.

38. Richmond DR, Damon EG, Fletcher ER, Bowen IG, White CS. The relationship between selected blast-wave parameters and the response of mammals exposed to air blast. *Ann NY Acad Sci.* 1968;152(1):103–121.

39. Richmond DR, Yelverton JT, Fletcher ER, Phillips YY, Jaeger JJ, Young AJ. *The Biological Effects of Repeated Blasts.* Washington, DC: Defense Nuclear Agency; 1981. DNA 5842F.

40. Bass CR, Panzer MB, Rafaels KA, Wood G, Shridharani J, Capehart B. Brain injuries from blast. *Ann Biomed Eng.* 2012;40(1):185–202.

41. Holzer A, Pietschmann MF, Rosl C, et al. The interrelation of trabecular microstructural parameters of the greater tubercle measured for different species. *J Orthop Res.* 2012;30(3):429–434.

42. Pietschmann MF, Holzer A, Rosl C, et al. What humeri are suitable for comparative testing of suture anchors? An ultrastructural bone analysis and biomechanical study of ovine, bovine and human humeri and four different anchor types. *J Biomech.* 2010;43(6):1125–1130.

43. Vries HD. The evidence of evolution. *Science.* 1904;20(508):395–401.

44. Casals JB, Pieri NC, Feitosa ML, et al. The use of animal models for stroke research: a review. *Comp Med.* 2011;61(4):305–313.

45. White CS, Bowen IG, Richmond DR. Biological tolerance to air blast and related biomedical criteria. CEX-65.4. *CEX Rep Civ Eff Exerc*. 1965:1–239.

46. Seok J, Warren HS, Cuenca AG, Mindrison MN, et al. Genomic responses in mouse models poorly mimic human inflammatory diseases. *Proc Natl Acad Sci U S A*. 2013;110(9):3507–3512.

47. Zschaler J, Schlorke D, Arnhold J. Differences in innate immune response between man and mouse. *Crit Rev Immunol*. 2014;34(5):433–454.

48. Mestas J, Hughes CC. Of mice and not men: differences between mouse and human immunology. *J Immunol*. 2004;172(5):2731–2738.

49. Gardner DE. Brain oedema: an experimental model. *Br J Exp Pathol*. 1974;55(5):453–457.

50. Ahmed F, Cernak I, Plantman S, Agoston DV. The temporal pattern of changes in serum biomarker levels reveal complex and dynamically changing pathologies after exposure to a single low-intensity blast in mice. *Front Neurol*. 2015;6(114):1–13.

51. Armonda RA, Bell RS, Vo AH, et al. Wartime traumatic cerebral vasospasm: recent review of combat casualties. *Neurosurgery*. 2006;59(6):1215–1225; discussion 1225.

52. Vadivelu S, Bell RS, Crandall B, DeGraba T, Armonda RA. Delayed detection of carotid-cavernous fistulas associated with wartime blast-induced craniofacial trauma. *Neurosurg Focus*. 2010;28(5):E6.

53. Meabon JS, Huber BR, Cross DJ, et al. Repetitive blast exposure in mice and combat veterans causes persistent cerebellar dysfunction. *Sci Translat Med*. 2016;8(321):321ra326.

54. Axelsson H, Hjelmqvist H, Medin A, Persson JK, Suneson A. Physiological changes in pigs exposed to a blast wave from a detonating high-explosive charge. *Mil Med*. 2000;165(2):119–126.

55. Rubovitch V, Ten-Bosch M, Zohar O, et al. A mouse model of blast-induced mild traumatic brain injury. *Exp Neurol*. 2011;232(2):280–289.

56. Bauman RA, Ling G, Tong L, et al. An introductory characterization of a combat-casualty-care relevant swine model of closed head injury resulting from exposure to explosive blast. *J Neurotrauma*. 2009;26(6):841–860.

57. Lu J, Ng KC, Ling GS, et al. Effect of blast exposure on the brain structure and cognition in the macaca fascicularis. *J Neurotrauma*. 2011.

58. Savic J, Tatic V, Ignjatovic D, et al. [Pathophysiologic reactions in sheep to blast waves from detonation of aerosol explosives]. *Vojnosanit Pregl*. 1991;48(6):499–506.

59. Ling G, Bandak F, Armonda R, Grant G, Ecklund J. Explosive blast neurotrauma. *J Neurotrauma*. 2009;26(6):815–825.

60. Nishida M. Shock tubes and tunnels: facilities, instrumentation, and techniques. Shock tubes. In: Ben-Dor G, Igra O, Elperin T, eds. *Handbook of Shock Waves*. Vol 1. San Diego, CA: Academic Press; 2001:553–585.

61. Robey R. Shock tubes and tunnels: facilities, instrumentation, and techniques. Blast tubes. In: Ben-Dor G, Igra O, Elperin T, eds. *Handbook of Shock Waves*. Vol 1. San Diego, CA: Academic Press; 2001:623–650.

62. Reneer DV. *Blast-induced Brain Injury: Influence of Shockwave Components*. Lexington: University of Kentucky; 2012.

63. Celander H, Clemedson CJ, Ericsson UA, Hultman HI. A study on the relation between the duration of a shock wave and the severity of the blast injury produced by it. *Acta Physiol Scand*. 1955;33(1):14–18.

64. Ritzel DV, Parks SA, Roseveare J, Rude G, Sawyer TW. Experimental blast simulation for injury studies. Paper presented at: RTO-MP-HFM-2072012; Halifax, Canada.

65. Divani AA, Murphy AJ, Meints J, et al. A novel preclinical model of moderate primary blast-induced traumatic brain injury. *J Neurotrauma*. 2015;32(14):1109–1116.

66. McCabe JT, Moratz C, Liu Y, et al. Application of high-intensity focused ultrasound to the study of mild traumatic brain injury. *Ultrasound Med Biol*. 2014;40(5):965–978.

67. Igarashi Y, Matsuda Y, Fuse A, Ishiwata T, Naito Z, Yokota H. Pathophysiology of microwave-induced traumatic brain injury. *Biomed Rep*. 2015;3(4):468–472.

68. Nakagawa A, Ohtani K, Goda K, et al. Mechanism of traumatic brain injury at distant locations after exposure to blast waves: preliminary results from animal and phantom experiments. *Acta Neurochir Suppl*. 2016;122:3–7.

69. Ngo T, Mendis P, Gupta A, Ramsay J. Blast loading and blast effects on structures—an overview. *Electronic Journal of Structural Engineering*. 2007(Special Issue: Loading on Structures):76–91.

70. Sundaramurthy A, Alai A, Ganpule S, Holmberg A, Plougonven E, Chandra N. Blast-induced biomechanical loading of the rat: an experimental and anatomically accurate computational blast injury model. *J Neurotrauma*. 2012;29(13):2352–2364.

71. Varas JM, Phillipens M, Meijer SR, et al. Physics of IED blast shock tube simulations for mTBI research. *Front Neurol*. 2011;2(58):1–14.

72. Richmond DR, Damon EG, Fletcher ER, Bowen IG, White CS. The relationship between selected blast-wave parameters and the response of mammals exposed to air blast. *Ann NY Acad Sci*. 1968;152(1):103–121.

73. Haselbacher A, Balachandar S, Kieffer SW. Open-ended shock tube flows: Influence of pressure ration and diaphragm position *AIAAA J*. 2007;45:1917–1929.

74. Mathis JT, Clutter JK. Evaluation of orientation and environmental factors on the blast hazards to bomb suit wearers. *Appl Ergon*. 2007;38(5):567–579.

75. Koliatsos VE, Cernak I, Xu L, et al. A mouse model of blast injury to brain: initial pathological, neuropathological, and behavioral characterization. *J Neuropathol Exp Neurol*. 2011;70(5):399–416.

76. Elsayed NM. Toxicology of blast overpressure. *Toxicology*. 1997;121(1):1–15.

77. Ahlers ST, Vasserman-Stokes E, Shaughness MC, et al. Assessment of the effects of acute and repeated exposure to blast overpressure in rodents: toward a greater understanding of blast and the potential ramifications for injury in humans exposed to blast. *Front Neurol*. 2012;3:32.

78. Chavko M, Koller WA, Prusaczyk WK, McCarron RM. Measurement of blast wave by a miniature fiber optic pressure transducer in the rat brain. *J Neurosci Methods*. 2007;159(2):277–281.

79. Zuckerman A, Ram O, Ifergane G, et al. Controlled low-pressure blast-wave exposure causes distinct behavioral and morphological responses modelling mild traumatic brain injury, post-traumatic stress disorder, and comorbid mild traumatic brain injury-post-traumatic stress disorder. *J Neurotrauma*. 2017;34(1):145–164.

80. Simard JM, Pampori A, Keledjian K, et al. Exposure of the thorax to a sublethal blast wave causes a hydrodynamic pulse that leads to perivenular inflammation in the brain. *J Neurotrauma*. 2014;31(14):1292–1304.

81. Reneer DV, Hisel RD, Hoffman JM, Kryscio RJ, Lusk BT, Geddes JW. A multi-mode shock tube for investigation of blast-induced traumatic brain injury. *J Neurotrauma*. 2011;28(1):95–104.

82. Saljo A, Bolouri H, Mayorga M, Svensson B, Hamberger A. Low-level blast raises intracranial pressure and impairs cognitive function in rats: prophylaxis with processed cereal feed. *J Neurotrauma*. 2010;27(2):383–389.

83. Cooper GJ, Maynard RL, Cross NL, Hill JF. Casualties from terrorist bombings. *J Trauma*. 1983;23(11):955–967.

84. Razumovsky A, Tigno T, Hochheimer SM, et al. Cerebral hemodynamic changes after wartime traumatic brain injury. *Acta Neurochir Suppl.* 2013;115:87–90.

85. Bell RS, Ecker RD, Severson MA 3rd, Wanebo JE, Crandall B, Armonda RA. The evolution of the treatment of traumatic cerebrovascular injury during wartime. *Neurosurg Focus.* 2010;28(5):E5.

86. Hald ES, Alford PW. Smooth muscle phenotype switching in blast traumatic brain injury-induced cerebral vasospasm. *Translat Stroke Res.* 2014;5(3):385–393.

87. Alford PW, Dabiri BE, Goss JA, Hemphill MA, Brigham MD, Parker KK. Blast-induced phenotypic switching in cerebral vasospasm. *Proc Natl Acad Sci USA.* 2011;108(31):12705–12710.

88. Toklu HZ, Muller-Delp J, Yang Z, et al. The functional and structural changes in the basilar artery due to overpressure blast injury. *J Cereb Blood Flow Metab.* 2015;35(12):1950–1956.

89. Bir C, Vandevord P, Shen Y, Raza W, Haacke EM. Effects of variable blast pressures on blood flow and oxygen saturation in rat brain as evidenced using MRI. *Magn Reson Imaging.* 2012;30(4):527–534.

90. Gama Sosa MA, De Gasperi R, Janssen PL, et al. Selective vulnerability of the cerebral vasculature to blast injury in a rat model of mild traumatic brain injury. *Acta Neuropathol Commun.* 2014;2:67.

91. Huang M, Risling M, Baker DG. The role of biomarkers and MEG-based imaging markers in the diagnosis of post-traumatic stress disorder and blast-induced mild traumatic brain injury. *Psychoneuroendocrinology.* 2016 Jan;63:398–409.

92. Nasonkin OS. [Effect of air (explosion) injury on the functional activity of the brain]. *Patol Fiziol Eksp Ter.* 1970;14(4):51–55.

93. Cernak I, Savic J, Ignjatovic D, Jevtic M. Blast injury from explosive munitions. *J Trauma.* 1999;47(1):96–103; discussion 103–104.

94. Sponheim SR, McGuire KA, Kang SS, et al. Evidence of disrupted functional connectivity in the brain after combat-related blast injury. *Neuroimage.* 2011;54 Suppl 1:S21–29.

95. Franke LM, Walker WC, Hoke KW, Wares JR. Distinction in EEG slow oscillations between chronic mild traumatic brain injury and PTSD. *Int J Psychophysiol.* 2016;106:21–29.

96. Risling M, Suneson A, Bursell J, Larsson I-L, Persson J. *Evaluation of Diffuse Blastwave Induced Brain Injury using EEG.* Stockholm: Swedish Defence Research Agency; 2002. FOI-R-0757-SE.

97. Stocker RP, Cieply MA, Paul B, et al. Combat-related blast exposure and traumatic brain injury influence brain glucose metabolism during REM sleep in military veterans. *Neuroimage.* 2014.

98. Peskind ER, Petrie EC, Cross DJ, et al. Cerebrocerebellar hypometabolism associated with repetitive blast exposure mild traumatic brain injury in 12 Iraq war Veterans with persistent post-concussive symptoms. *Neuroimage.* 2011;54(suppl 1):S76–82.

99. Awwad HO, Gonzalez LP, Tompkins P, et al. Blast overpressure waves induce transient anxiety and regional changes in cerebral glucose metabolism and delayed hyperarousal in rats. *Front Neurol.* 2015;6:132.

100. Cernak I, Savic J, Malicevic Z, et al. Involvement of the central nervous system in the general response to pulmonary blast injury. *J Trauma.* 1996;40(3 suppl):S100–104.

101. Cernak I, Wang Z, Jiang J, Bian X, Savic J. Cognitive deficits following blast injury-induced neurotrauma: possible involvement of nitric oxide. *Brain Inj.* 2001;15(7):593–612.

102. Arun P, Abu-Taleb R, Oguntayo S, et al. Acute mitochondrial dysfunction after blast exposure: potential role of mitochondrial glutamate oxaloacetate transaminase. *J Neurotrauma*. 2013;30(19):1645–1651.

103. Wang Y, Arun P, Wei Y, et al. Repeated blast exposures cause brain DNA fragmentation in mice. *J Neurotrauma*. 2014;31(5):498–504.

104. Cernak I, Savic VJ, Kotur J, Prokic V, Veljovic M, Grbovic D. Characterization of plasma magnesium concentration and oxidative stress following graded traumatic brain injury in humans. *J Neurotrauma*. 2000;17(1):53–68.

105. Zunic G, Romic P, Vueljic M, Jovanikic O. Very early increase in nitric oxide formation and oxidative cell damage associated with the reduction of tissue oxygenation is a trait of blast casualties. *Vojnosanit Pregl*. 2005;62(4):273–280.

106. Cernak I, Savic J, Zunic G, Pejnovic N, Jovanikic O, Stepic V. Recognizing, scoring, and predicting blast injuries. *World J Surg*. 1999;23(1):44–53.

107. Khil'ko VA, Shulev Iu A, Starchenko AA, et al. [The immunological and biochemical reactions of the cerebrospinal fluid in victims of blast injuries of the skull and brain]. *Vestn Khir Im I I Grek*. 1995;154(4–6):54–55.

108. Khil'ko VA, Shulev Iu A, Zgoda NV, et al. [Cellular immune reactions in the victims of explosive injuries to the skull and brain]. *Vestn Khir Im I I Grek*. 1995;154(1):64–66.

109. Melzer E, Hersch M, Fischer D, Hershko C. Disseminated intravascular coagulation and hypopotassemia associated with blast lung injury. *Chest*. 1986;89(5):690–693.

110. Cernak I, Wang Z, Jiang J, Bian X, Savic J. Ultrastructural and functional characteristics of blast injury-induced neurotrauma. *J Trauma*. 2001;50(4):695–706.

111. Cernak I, Wang ZG, Jiang JX, Bian XW, Savic J. Cognitive deficits following blast injury-induced neurotrauma: possible involvement of nitric oxide. *Brain Injury*. 2001;15(7):593–612.

112. Tumer N, Svetlov S, Whidden M, et al. Overpressure blast-wave induced brain injury elevates oxidative stress in the hypothalamus and catecholamine biosynthesis in the rat adrenal medulla. *Neurosci Lett*. 2013;544:62–67.

113. Du X, Ewert DL, Cheng W, et al. Effects of antioxidant treatment on blast-induced brain injury. *PLoS One*. 2013;8(11):e80138.

114. Abdul-Muneer PM, Schuetz H, Wang F, et al. Induction of oxidative and nitrosative damage leads to cerebrovascular inflammation in an animal model of mild traumatic brain injury induced by primary blast. *Free Radic Biol Med*. 2013;60C:282–291.

115. Readnower RD, Chavko M, Adeeb S, et al. Increase in blood-brain barrier permeability, oxidative stress, and activated microglia in a rat model of blast-induced traumatic brain injury. *J Neurosci Res*. 2010;88(16):3530–3539.

116. Valiyaveettil M, Alamneh Y, Wang Y, et al. Contribution of systemic factors in the pathophysiology of repeated blast-induced neurotrauma. *Neurosci Lett* [28 Jan 2013;539:1–6].

117. Valiyaveettil M, Alamneh YA, Miller SA, et al. Modulation of cholinergic pathways and inflammatory mediators in blast-induced traumatic brain injury. *Chemico-biological interactions*. 2013;203(1):371–375.

118. Gunther M, Plantman S, Gahm C, Sonden A, Risling M, Mathiesen T. Shock wave trauma leads to inflammatory response and morphological activation in macrophage cell lines, but does not induce iNOS or NO synthesis. *Acta Neurochir (Wien)*. 2014;156(12):2365–2378.

119. Prima V, Serebruany VL, Svetlov A, Hayes RL, Svetlov SI. Impact of moderate blast exposures on thrombin biomarkers assessed by calibrated automated thrombography in rats. *J Neurotrauma*. 2013;30(22):1881–1887.

120. Balaban C, Jackson RL, Liu J, Gao W, Hoffer ME. Intracranial venous injury, thrombosis and repair as hallmarks of mild blast traumatic brain injury in rats: lessons from histological and immunohistochemical studies of decalcified sectioned heads and correlative microarray analysis. *J Neurosci Methods*. 2016;272:56–68.

121. Miller DR, Hayes JP, Lafleche G, Salat DH, Verfaellie M. White matter abnormalities are associated with chronic postconcussion symptoms in blast-related mild traumatic brain injury. *Hum Brain Mapp*. 2016;37(1):220–229.

122. Shively SB, Horkayne-Szakaly I, Jones RV, Kelly JP, Armstrong RC, Perl DP. Characterisation of interface astroglial scarring in the human brain after blast exposure: a post-mortem case series. *Lancet Neurol*. 2016;15(9):944–953.

123. Trotter BB, Robinson ME, Milberg WP, McGlinchey RE, Salat DH. Military blast exposure, ageing and white matter integrity. *Brain*. 2015;138(Pt 8):2278–2292.

124. Morey RA, Haswell CC, Selgrade ES, et al. Effects of chronic mild traumatic brain injury on white matter integrity in Iraq and Afghanistan war veterans. *Hum Brain Mapp*. 2013;34(11):2986–2999.

125. Mac Donald C, Johnson A, Cooper D, et al. Cerebellar white matter abnormalities following primary blast injury in US military personnel. *PLoS One*. 2013;8(2):e55823.

126. Sajja VS, Hubbard WB, Hall CS, Ghoddoussi F, Galloway MP, VandeVord PJ. Enduring deficits in memory and neuronal pathology after blast-induced traumatic brain injury. *Sci Rep*. 2015;5:15075.

127. Kamnaksh A, Kwon SK, Kovesdi E, et al. Neurobehavioral, cellular, and molecular consequences of single and multiple mild blast exposure. *Electrophoresis*. 2012;33(24):3680–3692.

128. Valiyaveettil M, Alamneh YA, Wang Y, et al. Cytoskeletal protein alpha-II spectrin degradation in the brain of repeated blast exposed mice. *Brain Res*. 2014;1549:32–41.

129. Saljo A, Bao F, Haglid KG, Hansson HA. Blast exposure causes redistribution of phosphorylated neurofilament subunits in neurons of the adult rat brain. *J Neurotrauma*. 2000;17(8):719–726.

130. Du X, West MB, Cheng W, et al. Ameliorative effects of antioxidants on the hippocampal accumulation of pathologic tau in a rat model of blast-induced traumatic brain injury. *Oxid Med Cell Longev*. 2016;2016:4159357.

131. Huber BR, Meabon JS, Martin TJ, et al. Blast exposure causes early and persistent aberrant phospho- and cleaved-tau expression in a murine model of mild blast-induced traumatic brain injury. *J Alzheimers Dis*. 2013;37(2):309–323.

132. Arun P, Oguntayo S, Albert SV, et al. Acute decrease in alkaline phosphatase after brain injury: A potential mechanism for tauopathy. *Neurosci Lett*. 2015;609:152–158.

133. Huber BR, Meabon JS, Hoffer ZS, et al. Blast exposure causes dynamic microglial/macrophage responses and microdomains of brain microvessel dysfunction. *Neuroscience*. 2016;319:206–220.

134. Kaur C, Singh J, Lim MK, Ng BL, Ling EA. Macrophages/microglia as 'sensors' of injury in the pineal gland of rats following a non-penetrative blast. *Neurosci Res*. 1997;27(4):317–322.

135. Cernak I, Savic VJ, Lazarov A, Joksimovic M, Markovic S. Neuroendocrine responses following graded traumatic brain injury in male adults. *Brain Inj*. 1999;13(12):1005–1015.

136. Wilkinson CW, Pagulayan KF, Petrie EC, et al. High prevalence of chronic pituitary and target-organ hormone abnormalities after blast-related mild traumatic brain injury. *Front Neurol.* 2012;3:11.

137. Baxter D, Sharp DJ, Feeney C, et al. Pituitary dysfunction after blast traumatic brain injury: the UK BIOSAP study. *Ann Neurol.* 2013;74(4):527–536.

138. VandeVord PJ, Sajja VS, Ereifej E, Hermundstad A, Mao S, Hadden TJ. Chronic hormonal imbalance and adipose redistribution is associated with hypothalamic neuropathology following blast exposure. *J Neurotrauma.* 2016;33(1):82–88

Animal Models of Pediatric Traumatic Brain Injury: Lessons Learned

Jimmy W. Huh, Lauren A. Hanlon, and Ramesh Raghupathi

25

Introduction

In the United States, children aged 0–4 have the highest incidence of emergency room visits due to traumatic brain injury (TBI; 1,200 visits per every 100,000 people).[1] The incidence of TBI in this age group consists of both accidental and inflicted or abusive trauma[2,3] as 29% and 43% of TBI-related deaths in children 0–4 are due to motor vehicle accidents and abuse, respectively.[1] Abusive head trauma (AHT) in infants is not just restricted to what has been conventionally defined as "shaken baby syndrome" and now encompasses impact-driven traumas. While it has been historically very difficult to diagnose AHT, the incidence of diagnosis has increased in the past decade.[4–6] The rate of severe and fatal inflicted TBIs, however, drastically decreases after the age of 1 year (3.8/ 100,000).[7] The most common cause of TBI in children over the age of 1 is falls as they are learning to walk and have trouble avoiding obstacles.[3] As children age, motor vehicle accidents and sports accidents become more common causes of injury.[1] The structural and behavioral pathologies in clinical pediatric TBI have been described and form the basis on which combatting the secondary injury processes that may contribute to these pathologies can lead to long-term functional improvement and recovery. Identified therapeutic targets, however, must undergo rigorous preclinical testing in age-appropriate and injury-specific animal models. Despite vast differences between human brains and those of small and large mammals, animal models have by and large successfully modeled the pathology associated with different types and severities of human pediatric TBI. This review focuses on the validation of human pathologies in large and small animal models and the ongoing efforts to develop targeted therapeutic strategies.

Structural Pathology of Pediatric TBI

Tissue pathology following TBI is classified as focal (due to skull fractures and associated contusions) or diffuse (due to tissue tearing and axonal injury)[8]; focal injuries have been attributed to impact forces, whereas diffuse injuries may occur via rotational forces.[9] In the developing brain, traumatic injuries typically result in both pathologies because impact and rotational forces are common mechanisms of injury in both accidental and inflicted trauma. The properties of the infant skull differ from the adult and may further facilitate co-occurrence of these two types of injuries.[10] Margulies and Thibault[11] demonstrated that the decreased thickness and overall pliancy of the infant skull resulted in a decreased ability to absorb energy during the application of an external force and thus greater deformations of the underlying brain resulting in a diffuse pattern of injury. Skull fractures were more common in children who sustained a TBI from accidental causes than from abuse.[12,13] In contrast, a prospective review revealed that subdural hematomas occurred more frequently in children who sustained TBIs due to inflicted (80%) rather than accidental causes (45%), but epidural hematomas were times more likely in children with accidental TBI. Interestingly, the subdural hematomas in brains of infants with inflicted TBI appeared as mixed-density presentations and may be indicative of repetitive brain traumas, whereas accidental trauma resulted in hyperdense subdural hematomas.[14] Evidence of cerebral atrophy and ex-vacuo ventriculomegaly (enlarged ventricular space) has been reported following inflicted or accidental TBI.[12,15,16]

Most impact-based preclinical models of pediatric TBI characterized thus far have utilized impacts to the intact dura following a craniotomy, thereby eliminating a need for evaluating skull fractures[17–23] (Table 25.1). In the models in which impact occurred on the skull surface either via a weight-drop method[24,25] or using a controlled cortical impact device,[26,27] skull fractures, subarachnoid hemorrhage, and subdural hematomas were observed but did not correlate with cavity formation. When the impacts were centered over the parietal cortex of one hemisphere (lateral impact), contusions leading to the formation of a necrotic cavity were observed.[19–23,26,28] In contrast, impact on the midline suture of 17-day-old rats or over the parietal cortex of 11-day-old rats resulted in ex-vacuo ventriculomegaly in the absence of an overt contusion, suggesting that age at injury and/or location of the impact may determine gross tissue pathology.[26,27,29] Rotational-acceleration trauma in piglets resulted in subdural bleeding in the absence of skull fractures suggesting that impact may be necessary to induce vascular damage.[30,31]

White Matter Damage and Axonal Injury Following Pediatric TBI

Damage to the white matter resulting in traumatic axonal injury (TAI) has been identified as the predominant cellular pathology in cases of infant TBI. Whereas imaging modalities have identified overt damage to white matter tracts, neuropathologic studies in postmortem samples have provided evidence of TAI. In the acute period, magnetic resonance imaging (MRI) has revealed evidence of shearing in the corpus callosum of infants who sustained accidental TBIs and evidence of impaired myelination in infants who sustained inflicted injury.[12] In a separate study that investigated the integrity of white matter tracts at least 1 year after injury in early childhood (approximately 3 years old) using diffusion tensor imaging (DTI), reduced fractional anisotropy (FA) was observed in white matter regions including the corpus callosum, internal capsule, and longitudinal fasciculus.[32] In a more recent study, brain-injured young children (aged 6–10) showed a greater decrease in FA compared to brain-injured adolescents (aged 11–15), indicating age-dependency in white matter damage, but both age groups demonstrated similar degrees of change in FA between the 3- and 24-month scans.[33] In postmortem samples, axonal swellings in the subcortical white matter tracts have been visualized with conventional silver staining or β-amyloid precursor protein (β-APP) immunohistochemistry.[34,35] Both impact-based trauma (resulting in skull fractures and cortical lesions) and shaking trauma (no overt skull fractures) lead to axonal injury in the corpus callosum, internal capsule, midbrain, and brainstem.[36–38]

Table 25.1:
Summary of animal models of pediatric traumatic brain injury (TBI)

Model	Species	Age-at-Injury (Days)	Outcomes
Fluid-percussion (parasagittal with craniotomy)	Rat	17–19	Spatial learning and memory, glucose metabolism, calcium flux, cell loss
	Pig	1–5 days; 3–4 weeks	Cortical cerebrovascular reactivity
Weight-drop (parasagittal on intact skull)	Rat	3–30 days	Apoptotic and excitotoxic cell death pathways
Impact-acceleration (midline on intact skull)	Rat	17	Spatial learning and memory, motor function, axonal injury, tissue atrophy
Controlled cortical impact (parasagittal with craniotomy)	Mouse	21	Spatial learning and memory, social communication and recognition, anxiety, hyperactivity, neurodegeneration, microglial reactivity, leukocyte infiltration
	Rat	7, 17	Spatial learning and memory, neurodegeneration
	Rabbit	3–5	Novel object recognition, neurodegeneration, microglial reactivity
	Pig	5, 28	Tissue loss, cerebral blood flow
Closed head impact (parasagittal on intact skull)	Rat	11, 17	Spatial learning and memory, axonal injury, neurodegeneration, apoptotic and excitotoxic cell death pathways, microglial reactivity
Closed head impact (midline on intact skull)	Rat	17	Spatial learning and memory, axonal injury and degeneration, neurodegeneration
Rotational-acceleration (nonimpact)	Pig	5, 28	Exploratory behavior, visual problem solving, axonal injury

White matter damage and TAI in animals have been documented using either MRI[21] or conventional immunostaining techniques with antibodies for β-APP and/or neurofilament. [26,27,29–31,39] As observed in patients, TAI has been reported in multiple white matter tracts such as the corpus callosum, thalamus, and brainstem. In addition to axonal injury and degeneration, a decrease in axonal function (measured using compound action potential in ex vivo preparations) has also been documented.[21,40] Importantly, the data from these preclinical models validate the observations in humans that widespread axonal injury can occur in both the presence and absence of cortical contusions. Proposed secondary mechanisms underlying TAI include ionic dysregulation, calpain-mediated proteolysis, impaired axonal transport, microtubule degradation, and neurofilament compaction.[41] However, a viable treatment strategy for ameliorating white matter damage and functional deficits has not been identified.[39,40]

Cell Death and Inflammation Following Pediatric TBI

Cell loss is apparent in children following TBI through volumetric analysis revealing evidence of tissue atrophy.[15,42,43] Direct indication of cell death in various preclinical models has been facilitated via the use of markers specifically associated with necrosis, apoptosis, and excitotoxicity.[19,25,26,44] High concentrations of glutamate have been reported in the cerebrospinal fluid of children who sustained a severe TBI,[45] suggesting that excitotoxicity leading to either apoptotic or necrotic cell death may occur in the pediatric brain[46,47] and may be identified using activation of caspases and calpains, respectively.[48] Traumatic injury to the 11-day-old or 17-day-old rat revealed evidence of activation of calpains and caspases in multiple brain regions including white matter tracts.[44,49] Similarly, decreased expression of the anti-apoptotic protein Bcl-2 along with activation of the pro-apoptotic protease caspase-3 suggests that apoptotic cascades are activated following injury to the developing brain.[25] Although intervention with glutamate receptor antagonists acutely after trauma to the adult brain provides neuroprotection,[50] the circuitry in the immature brain depends on excitatory neurotransmission for proper development,[51] and, in fact, NMDA receptor antagonists were observed to increase apoptosis in the developing brain following TBI.[52]

Neuronal damage can also be mediated by the posttraumatic activation of microglia, which can release proinflammatory cytokines and other harmful mediators such as nitric oxide.[53,54] Severe TBI in children is associated with an increase in proinflammatory cytokines such as interleukin (IL)-1β, IL-6, and IL-10[55,56]; chemokines IL-8 and MIP-1α, indicating migratory signaling to other immune cells[55]; and significantly higher concentrations of quinolinic acid, indicative of microglia/macrophage activation.[57] Higher concentrations of serum IL-6 have been reported following mild TBI in children and suggest a role for inflammation in a range of injury severities.[58] Impact trauma to the developing animal resulted in microglial activation in multiple brain regions such as the cortex, thalamus, hippocampus, and corpus callosum, which demonstrate evidence of neurodegeneration and axonal injury.[19,22,59,60] Activation of endogenous microglia occurred within a day after injury and continued to be present for at least 3–4 weeks. In addition, infiltration of leukocytes and neutrophils has also been observed.[61] Despite this evidence of neuroinflammation, only a few studies have targeted this cascade for therapeutic purposes.[62] Targeting neutrophil elastase immediately after trauma only reduced acute cell death and had no effect on long-term behavioral outcomes.[63] Short-term minocycline administration within the first week after injury in the neonate rat reduced microglial proliferation and activation and was accompanied by an increase, not a decrease, in the extent of neurodegeneration and no attenuation of spatial learning and memory deficits.[59,60] These observations are suggestive of a differential age-at-injury response because minocycline was found to be neuroprotective in animal models of adult TBI.

Behavioral Deficits Following Pediatric TBI

Cognitive Outcomes

Sustaining an injury in infancy or early childhood has strong implications for the development of cognitive skills. At 3 months following injury, infants and young children who sustained moderate to severe TBIs had significantly decreased Bayley Behavior Rating Scores that take into account age-appropriate behavior and levels of arousal/responsiveness through a series of play activities.[64] Severe TBI in children aged 7–14 years was associated with a lack of improvement in intelligent quotient measures between 6 months and 24 months post-injury, indicating a lack of improvement and developmental arrest.[65] Children with brain trauma also exhibit deficits in verbal working memory, visuospatial memory, and attention.[66–68] Simple cognitive tasks such as spatial learning in the Morris water maze or Novel Object Recognition have been used in animal models of pediatric TBI. A variety of injury models such as lateral fluid-percussion, weight-drop, controlled cortical impact, and rotational-acceleration have identified deficits in these simple cognitive tasks that present in the acute posttraumatic period and, in some cases, were present at months after the trauma.[22,23,28,69–73] A gap in the preclinical literature that needs filling is the utilization of complex cognitive tasks that can be evaluated in adulthood following a traumatic injury during development.

Social and Behavioral Outcomes

Children who sustain brain injuries in early childhood demonstrate decreased social competencies and are at risk of developing psychiatric disorders.[74] In addition, brain-injured children are more likely to exhibit personality changes such as an increase in irritability and aggression associated with disinhibited verbalizations.[75] In the years following injury, children with TBI begin to develop novel depressive and anxiety disorders.[76,77] Limited efforts have gone into identifying these deficits in animal models, although contusive brain trauma in the neonate mouse resulted in prolonged hyperactivity, a decrease in general anxiety-like behavior, and deficits in social behavior weeks to months after the injury.[28,78]

Locomotor Outcomes

Children with severe brain injuries had significantly decreased motor scores at the 6-month time point compared to the mild/moderate injury group[79] and only improved in motor score in the first 6 months following injury.[65] Motor function evaluation in animal models of pediatric TBI have not been extensively evaluated likely because only severe TBI results in deficits in motor activity.[72]

Posttraumatic Seizures

Children who sustain severe injuries demonstrate an increased incidence of seizures in the early stages following injury.[80,81] Both the age at injury and the mechanism of injury appear to be significant risk factors because children under the age of 1 were more likely to demonstrate seizures,[82] and seizure activity was more prevalent following abusive head trauma.[83] Video-electroencephalograph recordings and susceptibility to seizure-inducing agents have been utilized in animal models to demonstrate the incidence of seizure activity in the acute and chronic posttraumatic periods following pediatric TBI.[84,85]

Conclusion

In addition to injury severity, how the immature brain responds to trauma at different ages may help elucidate important age-dependent mechanisms to allow for age-specific therapeutic interventions. Important considerations of preclinical study design include the appropriate age, sex and the type of injury in an animal model to simulate specific populations of pediatric patients. While functional outcomes such as cognition and motor consequences remain important to model the clinical condition, it is becoming clear that psychosocial assessments must also be evaluated. Furthermore, the importance of better understanding the long-term consequences of early pediatric TBI that manifest only in adolescence or young adulthood cannot be overstated. Future research aimed at modulating or protecting against deleterious processes not only during the acute posttraumatic period, but also at the subacute or chronic posttraumatic period may have the potential to promote a "relatively normal" brain development to improve long-term outcomes after early pediatric TBI.

References

1. Faul M, Xu L, Wald MM, Coronado VG. *Traumatic Brain Injury in the United States: Emergency Department Visits, Hospitalizations, and Deaths.* Atlanta, GA: Centers for Disease Control and Prevention, National Center for Injury Prevention and control; 2010.

2. Ewing-Cobbs L, Kramer L, Prasad M, et al. Neuroimaging, physical, and developmental findings after inflicted and noninflicted traumatic brain injury in young children. *Pediatrics.* 1998;102(2 Pt 1):300–307.

3. Keenan HT, Bratton SL. Epidemiology and outcomes of pediatric traumatic brain injury. *Dev Neurosci.* 2006;28(4-5):256–263.

4. Jenny C, Hymel KP, Ritzen A, Reinert SE, Hay TC. Analysis of missed cases of abusive head trauma. *JAMA.* 1999;281(7):621–626.

5. Kelly P, John S, Vincent AL, Reed P. Abusive head trauma and accidental head injury: a 20-year comparative study of referrals to a hospital child protection team. *Arch Dis Child.* 2015;100(12):1123–1130.

6. Narang SK, Estrada C, Greenberg S, Lindberg D. Acceptance of shaken baby syndrome and abusive head trauma as medical diagnoses. *J Pediatr.* 2016;177:273–278.

7. Keenan HT, Runyan DK, Marshall SW, Nocera MA, Merten DF, Sinal SH. A population-based study of inflicted traumatic brain injury in young children. *JAMA.* 2003;290(5):621–626.

8. Andriessen TM, Jacobs B, Vos PE. Clinical characteristics and pathophysiological mechanisms of focal and diffuse traumatic brain injury. *J Cell Mol Med.* 2010;14(10):2381–2392.

9. Johnson VE, Meaney DF, Cullen DK, Smith DH. Animal models of traumatic brain injury. *Handb Clin Neurol.* 2015;127:115–128.

10. Duhaime AC, Gennarelli TA, Thibault LE, Bruce DA, Margulies SS, Wiser R. The shaken baby syndrome. A clinical, pathological, and biomechanical study. *J Neurosurg.* 1987;66(3):409–415.

11. Margulies SS, Thibault KL. Infant skull and suture properties: measurements and implications for mechanisms of pediatric brain injury. *J Biomech Eng.* 2000;122(4):364–371.

12. Ewing-Cobbs L, Prasad M, Kramer L, et al. Acute neuroradiologic findings in young children with inflicted or noninflicted traumatic brain injury. *Childs Nerv Syst.* 2000;16(1):25–33; discussion 34.

13. Keenan HT, Runyan DK, Marshall SW, Nocera MA, Merten DF. A population-based comparison of clinical and outcome characteristics of young children with serious inflicted and noninflicted traumatic brain injury. *Pediatrics.* 2004;114(3):633–639.

14. Tung GA, Kumar M, Richardson RC, Jenny C, Brown WD. Comparison of accidental and nonaccidental traumatic head injury in children on noncontrast computed tomography. *Pediatrics.* 2006;118(2):626–633.

15. Wilde EA, Hunter JV, Newsome MR, et al. Frontal and temporal morphometric findings on MRI in children after moderate to severe traumatic brain injury. *J Neurotrauma.* 2005;22(3):333–344.

16. Ghosh A, Wilde EA, Hunter JV, et al. The relation between Glasgow Coma Scale score and later cerebral atrophy in paediatric traumatic brain injury. *Brain injury.* 2009;23(3):228–233.

17. Prins ML, Lee SM, Cheng CL, Becker DP, Hovda DA. Fluid percussion brain injury in the developing and adult rat: a comparative study of mortality, morphology, intracranial pressure and mean arterial blood pressure. *Brain Res Dev Brain Res.* 1996;95(2):272–282.

18. Armstead WM, Kurth CD. Different cerebral hemodynamic responses following fluid percussion brain injury in the newborn and juvenile pig. *J Neurotrauma.* 1994;11(5):487–497.

19. Tong W, Igarashi T, Ferriero DM, Noble LJ. Traumatic brain injury in the immature mouse brain: characterization of regional vulnerability. *Exp Neurol.* 2002;176(1):105–116.

20. Duhaime AC, Margulies SS, Durham SR, et al. Maturation-dependent response of the piglet brain to scaled cortical impact. *J Neurosurgery.* 2000;93(3):455–462.

21. Ajao DO, Pop V, Kamper JE, et al. Traumatic brain injury in young rats leads to progressive behavioral deficits coincident with altered tissue properties in adulthood. *J Neurotrauma.* 2012;29(11):2060–2074.

22. Zhang Z, Saraswati M, Koehler RC, Robertson C, Kannan S. A new rabbit model of pediatric traumatic brain injury. *J Neurotrauma.* 2015;32(17):1369–1379.

23. Adelson PD, Fellows-Mayle W, Kochanek PM, Dixon CE. Morris water maze function and histologic characterization of two age-at-injury experimental models of controlled cortical impact in the immature rat. *Childs Nerv Syst.* 2013;29(1):43–53.

24. Adelson PD, Robichaud P, Hamilton RL, Kochanek PM. A model of diffuse traumatic brain injury in the immature rat. *J Neurosurgery.* 1996;85(5):877–884.

25. Bittigau P, Sifringer M, Pohl D, et al. Apoptotic neurodegeneration following trauma is markedly enhanced in the immature brain. *Ann Neurol.* 1999;45(6):724–735.

26. Huh JW, Raghupathi R. Chronic cognitive deficits and long-term histopathological alterations following contusive brain injury in the immature rat. *J Neurotrauma.* 2007;24(9):1460–1474.

27. Huh JW, Widing AG, Raghupathi R. Midline brain injury in the immature rat induces sustained cognitive deficits, bihemispheric axonal injury and neurodegeneration. *Exp Neurol.* 2008;213(1):84–92.

28. Pullela R, Raber J, Pfankuch T, et al. Traumatic injury to the immature brain results in progressive neuronal loss, hyperactivity and delayed cognitive impairments. *Dev Neurosci.* 2006;28(4-5):396–409.

29. Adelson PD, Jenkins LW, Hamilton RL, Robichaud P, Tran MP, Kochanek PM. Histopathologic response of the immature rat to diffuse traumatic brain injury. *J Neurotrauma.* 2001;18(10):967–976.

30. Eucker SA, Smith C, Ralston J, Friess SH, Margulies SS. Physiological and histopathological responses following closed rotational head injury depend on direction of head motion. *Exp Neurol.* 2011;227(1):79–88.

31. Raghupathi R, Margulies SS. Traumatic axonal injury after closed head injury in the neonatal pig. *J Neurotrauma.* 2002;19(7):843–853.

32. Yuan W, Holland SK, Schmithorst VJ, et al. Diffusion tensor MR imaging reveals persistent white matter alteration after traumatic brain injury experienced during early childhood. *AJNR. Am J Neuroradiol.* 2007;28(10):1919–1925.

33. Ewing-Cobbs L, Johnson CP, Juranek J, et al. Longitudinal diffusion tensor imaging after pediatric traumatic brain injury: impact of age at injury and time since injury on pathway integrity. *Hum Brain Mapp.* 2016;37(11):3929–3945.

34. Shannon P, Smith CR, Deck J, Ang LC, Ho M, Becker L. Axonal injury and the neuropathology of shaken baby syndrome. *Acta Neuropathol.* 1998;95(6):625–631.

35. Vowles GH, Scholtz CL, Cameron JM. Diffuse axonal injury in early infancy. *J Clin Pathol.* 1987;40(2):185–189.

36. Geddes JF, Hackshaw AK, Vowles GH, Nickols CD, Whitwell HL. Neuropathology of inflicted head injury in children. I. Patterns of brain damage. *Brain.* 2001;124(Pt 7):1290–1298.

37. Geddes JF, Vowles GH, Hackshaw AK, Nickols CD, Scott IS, Whitwell HL. Neuropathology of inflicted head injury in children. II. Microscopic brain injury in infants. *Brain.* 2001;124(Pt 7):1299–1306.

38. Gleckman AM, Bell MD, Evans RJ, Smith TW. Diffuse axonal injury in infants with nonaccidental craniocerebral trauma: enhanced detection by beta-amyloid precursor protein immunohistochemical staining. *Arch Pathol Lab Med.* 1999;123(2):146–151.

39. DiLeonardi AM, Huh JW, Raghupathi R. Impaired axonal transport and neurofilament compaction occur in separate populations of injured axons following diffuse brain injury in the immature rat. *Brain Res.* 2009;1263:174–182.

40. Dileonardi AM, Huh JW, Raghupathi R. Differential effects of FK506 on structural and functional axonal deficits after diffuse brain injury in the immature rat. *J Neuropathol Exp Neurol.* 2012;71(11):959–972.

41. Buki A, Siman R, Trojanowski JQ, Povlishock JT. The role of calpain-mediated spectrin proteolysis in traumatically induced axonal injury. *J Neuropathol Exp Neurol.* 1999;58(4):365–375.

42. Suskauer SJ, Huisman TA. Neuroimaging in pediatric traumatic brain injury: current and future predictors of functional outcome. *Dev Disabil Res Rev.* 2009;15(2):117–123.

43. Verger K, Junque C, Levin HS, et al. Correlation of atrophy measures on MRI with neuropsychological sequelae in children and adolescents with traumatic brain injury. *Brain Inj.* 2001;15(3):211–221.

44. Huh JW, Franklin MA, Widing AG, Raghupathi R. Regionally distinct patterns of calpain activation and traumatic axonal injury following contusive brain injury in immature rats. *Dev Neurosci.* 2006;28(4-5):466–476.

45. Ruppel RA, Kochanek PM, Adelson PD, et al. Excitatory amino acid concentrations in ventricular cerebrospinal fluid after severe traumatic brain injury in infants and children: the role of child abuse. *J Pediatr.* 2001;138(1):18–25.

46. Huh JW, Raghupathi R. New concepts in treatment of pediatric traumatic brain injury. *Anesthesiol Clin.* 2009;27(2):213–240.

47. Portera-Cailliau C, Price DL, Martin LJ. Excitotoxic neuronal death in the immature brain is an apoptosis-necrosis morphological continuum. *J Comp Neurol.* 1997;378(1):70–87.

48. Wang KK. Calpain and caspase: can you tell the difference? *Trends Neurosci.* 2000;23(1):20–26.

49. Schober ME, Requena DF, Davis LJ, et al. Alpha II Spectrin breakdown products in immature Sprague Dawley rat hippocampus and cortex after traumatic brain injury. *Brain Res.* 2014;1574:105–112.

50. Belayev L, Alonso OF, Liu Y, et al. Talampanel, a novel noncompetitive AMPA antagonist, is neuroprotective after traumatic brain injury in rats. *J Neurotrauma.* 2001;18(10):1031–1038.

51. Giza CC, Mink RB, Madikians A. Pediatric traumatic brain injury: not just little adults. *Curr Opin Crit Care.* 2007;13(2):143–152.

52. Pohl D, Bittigau P, Ishimaru MJ, et al. N-Methyl-D-aspartate antagonists and apoptotic cell death triggered by head trauma in developing rat brain. *Proc Nat Acad Sci USA.* 1999;96(5):2508–2513.

53. Woodcock T, Morganti-Kossmann MC. The role of markers of inflammation in traumatic brain injury. *Front Neurol.* 2013;4:18.

54. Loane DJ, Byrnes KR. Role of microglia in neurotrauma. *Neurotherapeutics.* 2010;7(4):366–377.

55. Buttram SD, Wisniewski SR, Jackson EK, et al. Multiplex assessment of cytokine and chemokine levels in cerebrospinal fluid following severe pediatric traumatic brain injury: effects of moderate hypothermia. *J Neurotrauma.* 2007;24(11):1707–1717.

56. Bell MJ, Kochanek PM, Doughty LA, et al. Interleukin-6 and interleukin-10 in cerebrospinal fluid after severe traumatic brain injury in children. *J Neurotrauma.* 1997;14(7):451–457.

57. Berger RP, Heyes MP, Wisniewski SR, Adelson PD, Thomas N, Kochanek PM. Assessment of the macrophage marker quinolinic acid in cerebrospinal fluid after pediatric traumatic brain injury: insight into the timing and severity of injury in child abuse. *J Neurotrauma.* 2004;21(9):1123–1130.

58. Berger RP, Ta'asan S, Rand A, Lokshin A, Kochanek P. Multiplex assessment of serum biomarker concentrations in well-appearing children with inflicted traumatic brain injury. *Pediatr Res.* 2009;65(1):97–102.

59. Chhor V, Moretti R, Le Charpentier T, et al. Role of microglia in a mouse model of paediatric traumatic brain injury. *Brain Behav Immun.* 2017;63:197–209.

60. Hanlon LA, Raghupathi R, Huh JW. Differential effects of minocycline on microglial activation and neurodegeneration following closed head injury in the neonate rat. *Exp Neurol.* 2017;290:1–14.

61. Claus CP, Tsuru-Aoyagi K, Adwanikar H, et al. Age is a determinant of leukocyte infiltration and loss of cortical volume after traumatic brain injury. *Dev Neurosci.* 2010;32(5-6):454–465.

62. Potts MB, Koh SE, Whetstone WD, et al. Traumatic injury to the immature brain: inflammation, oxidative injury, and iron-mediated damage as potential therapeutic targets. *NeuroRx.* 2006;3(2):143–153.

63. Semple BD, Trivedi A, Gimlin K, Noble-Haeusslein LJ. Neutrophil elastase mediates acute pathogenesis and is a determinant of long-term behavioral recovery after traumatic injury to the immature brain. *Neurobiol Dis.* 2015;74:263–280.

64. Ewing-Cobbs L, Prasad M, Kramer L, Landry S. Inflicted traumatic brain injury: relationship of developmental outcome to severity of injury. *Pediatr Neurosurg.* 1999;31(5):251–258.

65. Ewing-Cobbs L, Fletcher JM, Levin HS, Francis DJ, Davidson K, Miner ME. Longitudinal neuropsychological outcome in infants and preschoolers with traumatic brain injury. *J Int Neuropsychol Soc.* 1997;3(6):581–591.

66. Catroppa C, Anderson V. A prospective study of the recovery of attention from acute to 2 years following pediatric traumatic brain injury. *J Int Neuropsychol Soc.* 2005;11(1):84–98.

67. Ewing-Cobbs L, Prasad MR, Swank P, et al. Arrested development and disrupted callosal microstructure following pediatric traumatic brain injury: relation to neurobehavioral outcomes. *NeuroImage.* 2008;42(4):1305–1315.

68. Treble A, Hasan KM, Iftikhar A, et al. Working memory and corpus callosum microstructural integrity after pediatric traumatic brain injury: a diffusion tensor tractography study. *J Neurotrauma.* 2013;30(19):1609–1619.

69. Gurkoff GG, Giza CC, Hovda DA. Lateral fluid percussion injury in the developing rat causes an acute, mild behavioral dysfunction in the absence of significant cell death. *Brain Res.* 2006;1077(1):24–36.

70. Friess SH, Ichord RN, Owens K, et al. Neurobehavioral functional deficits following closed head injury in the neonatal pig. *Exp Neurol.* 2007;204(1):234–243.

71. Adelson PD, Dixon CE, Robichaud P, Kochanek PM. Motor and cognitive functional deficits following diffuse traumatic brain injury in the immature rat. *J Neurotrauma.* 1997;14(2):99–108.

72. Adelson PD, Dixon CE, Kochanek PM. Long-term dysfunction following diffuse traumatic brain injury in the immature rat. *J Neurotrauma.* 2000;17(4):273–282.

73. Raghupathi R, Huh JW. Diffuse brain injury in the immature rat: evidence for an age-at-injury effect on cognitive function and histopathologic damage. *J Neurotrauma.* 2007;24(10):1596–1608.

74. Ewing-Cobbs L, Prasad MR, Mendez D, Barnes MA, Swank P. Social interaction in young children with inflicted and accidental traumatic brain injury: relations with family resources and social outcomes. *J Int Neuropsychol Soc.* 2013;19(5):497–507.

75. Max JE, Robertson BA, Lansing AE. The phenomenology of personality change due to traumatic brain injury in children and adolescents. *J Neuropsych Clin Neurosci.* 2001;13(2):161–170.

76. Max JE, Keatley E, Wilde EA, et al. Depression in children and adolescents in the first 6 months after traumatic brain injury. *Int J Dev Neurosci.* 2012;30(3):239–245.

77. Max JE, Lopez A, Wilde EA, et al. Anxiety disorders in children and adolescents in the second six months after traumatic brain injury. *J Pediatr Rehabil Med.* 2015;8(4):345–355.

78. Semple BD, Canchola SA, Noble-Haeusslein LJ. Deficits in social behavior emerge during development after pediatric traumatic brain injury in mice. *J Neurotrauma.* 2012;29(17):2672–2683.

79. Ewing-Cobbs L, Miner ME, Fletcher JM, Levin HS. Intellectual, motor, and language sequelae following closed head injury in infants and preschoolers. *J Pediatr Psychol.* 1989;14(4):531–547.

80. Annegers JF, Hauser WA, Coan SP, Rocca WA. A population-based study of seizures after traumatic brain injuries. *N Engl J Med.* 1998;338(1):20–24.

81. Liesemer K, Bratton SL, Zebrack CM, Brockmeyer D, Statler KD. Early post-traumatic seizures in moderate to severe pediatric traumatic brain injury: rates, risk factors, and clinical features. *J Neurotrauma.* 2011;28(5):755–762.

82. Arndt DH, Lerner JT, Matsumoto JH, et al. Subclinical early posttraumatic seizures detected by continuous EEG monitoring in a consecutive pediatric cohort. *Epilepsia.* 2013;54(10):1780–1788.

83. Hasbani DM, Topjian AA, Friess SH, et al. Nonconvulsive electrographic seizures are common in children with abusive head trauma. *Pediatr Crit Care Med*. 2013;14(7):709–715.

84. Semple BD, O'Brien TJ, Gimlin K, et al. Interleukin-1 receptor in seizure susceptibility after traumatic injury to the pediatric brain. *J Neurosci*. 2017;37(33):7864–7877.

85. Statler KD, Scheerlinck P, Pouliot W, Hamilton M, White HS, Dudek FE. A potential model of pediatric posttraumatic epilepsy. *Epilepsy Res*. 2009;86(2-3):221–223.

Proteomics-Based Strategies to Define Brain Tissue Biomarkers of Closed Head, Mild Traumatic Brain Injury in Translational Rodent Models

Angela M. Boutté, Joy Guingab-Cagmat, Ahmed Moghieb, Joseph A. Caruso, Paul M. Stemmer, Stephen T. Ahlers, and Kevin K. W. Wang

26

Introduction

Closed head, mild traumatic brain injury (mTBI), commonly known as *concussion*, is caused by a bump or blow to the head and can lead to a disoriented state or loss of consciousness (http://www.cdc.gov/traumaticbraininjury/). MTBI is quite common, affects nearly 4 million people per annum, and has become a significant health concern.[1] mTBI is a well-known risk factor for development of neurodegenerative diseases, specifically chronic traumatic encephalopathy (CTE),[2] as well as a host of psychological, physical, and social disorders.[3,4] Athletes, victims of abuse or accidents, and military personnel constitute a particularly vulnerable subpopulation who are at particularly high risk of attaining an mTBI and suffering from health problems as a result.[5] Treatment and mitigation or prevention of these long-term effects remain challenging, in part due to the complexity and variability of molecular processes that occur in brain tissues due to, not only the initial incident, but also to the complex processes that occur throughout injury progression.[6]

Changes to brain tissue caused by mTBI are often difficult to extrapolate through cognitive assessment alone.[7,8] However, the cellular and molecular effects on the brain may be defined with the use of translational rodent models that are capable of mimicking clinical symptoms or affective states (e.g., impaired consciousness, learning and memory, or balance). MTBI elicits a complex myriad of molecular and pathophysiological responses that may be difficult to pinpoint via predetermined hypotheses that encompass a single gene, protein, process, or pathway. Therefore, proteomics analysis of brain tissues is an increasingly popular method employed to define novel biomarkers and mechanisms associated with, or causative of, both acute responses and long-term neurodegenerative pathology associated with mTBI.

Proteomics analysis is the study of all proteins within a cell, tissue, or organ of interest to define a wide swath of relevant proteins, and has become one of the most sophisticated and sensitive tools used to define differential physiological states. It relies on identifying and quantitating individual peptides and/or proteins followed by genome-wide characterization based on structure, function, co-expression, isoforms, interactions, or pathways. A comprehensive view of these analytes in brain tissues sheds light on key molecular mechanisms that seed the short- and long-term effects of mTBI.

A stringent Web of Science search of titles, abstracts, and keywords for the terms "mild, traumatic brain injury, proteomics, and closed-head injury" yielded several peer-reviewed manuscripts that utilized rodent models. Many publications are well-structured, comprehensive reviews and prospective articles stating the need for the use of proteomics analysis in mTBI research overall. To date, several authors have expressed the necessity of studying the brain proteome in order to define novel biomarkers of injury status or progression. This chapter presents examples of proteomics-based strategies used to determine the effect of mTBI upon the rodent brain (or specific regions reported to be uniquely vulnerable). Due to the plethora of literature available, the focus herein is blast-overpressure (BOP), a well-vetted model that is often used for military-relevant translational research. Several examples are cited, and a comprehensive methodology with results is presented. A relatively new paradigm, direct-impact closed head injury (CHI), and novel proteomics approaches that have yet to be applied to closed head mTBI are also discussed.

Blast Overpressure

BOP exceeds atmospheric pressure as a result of a shock wave caused by an explosion. BOP can cause primary (interaction of the pressure wave and the body), secondary (objects/fragments displaced by the pressure wave and impacting the body), or tertiary (displacement of the body followed by impact upon the body by other objects) injury to tissues and organs. BOP-related injuries affect military personnel as well as civilians who are victims of terrorist attacks or industrial accidents (http://dvbic.dcoe.mil/dod-worldwide-numbers-tbi). BOP is proposed to be a leading factor in mTBI diagnosis,[9] neurodegenerative diseases (e.g., CTE and Alzheimer disease [AD], specifically), and posttraumatic stress disorder (PTSD).[10,11] Rodent models of primary BOP are classified as mild (≤145 kPa or ~21 psi), moderate (146–220 kPa or ~21–32 psi), or high- level/ severe (221–290 kPa or ~32–42 psi).[12] Under each of these conditions, brain tissue proteomics has been used to define several protein biomarkers associated with pathology, behavior, or affective states.

Gel-Based Down-Selection

Two dimensional (2-DE) or differential in-gel (DIGE) electrophoresis relies on detection of protein spots with either dyes (e.g., Commassie blue, Blue Silver, SYPRO Ruby) or fluorescent peptide ligands (cyanine dyes) that bind to lysine or cysteine amino acids. Relative intensities of each protein are detected based on alignment of isoelectric point (pI) and molecular weight (MW) within an x-y plane followed by detection of protein "spots" at specific colorimetric or excitation/emission wavelengths.[13,14] DIGE typically identifies approximately two-fold changes with statistical significance of $p \leq 0.05$ depending on the number of replicate gels utilized.[15,16] Conventionally, this method is coupled to matrix-assisted laser desorption ionization tandem time of flight mass spectrometry (MALDI-TOF/TOF).[17–19] This approach is robust for identification of brain tissue protein abundance across models of varying TBI severity.[20,21]

The rat model of mild, repetitive BOP leads to anterograde impairment and reduced fear conditioning in rats. However, the brain tissue is otherwise normal upon gross histological analysis.[22,23] Two-DE was used to identify specific proteins that were dysregulated as late as four months after repeated, mild injury.[24] Within this study, posterior and anterior cortical regions were pooled prior to analysis by 2D-DIGE. This approach identified 21 differentially abundant proteins, including increased levels of stathmin 1, a cytoskeletal protein involved in regulation of microtubule dynamics. Stathmin 1 levels were confirmed by Western blotting and presented as a link between the long-term effects of BOP-induced mTBI and PTSD-like behaviors in the rat.

Multiplex, Targeted Protein Arrays

A reverse phase protein microarray (RPPM or RPMA), also known as a reverse phase protein array (RPPA), is a sensitive, high-throughput antibody-based method. Similar to a dot blot or an enzyme-linked immunoassay (ELISA), antibodies are fixed to a solid phase (e.g., glass slides). However, this method is unique in that it exploits highly sensitive microarray detection technology that was initially created for genomics. Relative quantification of protein biomarkers is based on antigen binding and fluorophore sensitivity that is then extrapolated as relative concentration.[25,26] This method is much more high-throughput than a single dot-blot or Western blot, yet relies on pre-selection and extensive optimization of antibody–antigen combinations. Therefore, it is ideal for proteomics strategies for which a hypothesis–driven strategy involving a specific pathway or protein class is predefined.

RPPM has been used to indicate up-regulation of the well-known TBI-associated biomarker, glial fibrillary acidic protein (GFAP). Additionally, vascular endothelial growth factor (VEGF) was found to be dysregulated in the amygdala, ventral hippocampus, and prefrontal cortex after mild sound pressure exposure (50 ± 10% dB) in addition to repeated BOP exposure conducted once daily for four consecutive days.[27] As a technical note, the level of mild BOP is listed through a citation as 126–147 kPa (18–21 psi), which may be considered moderate per other models.[28]

The prefrontal cortex and hippocampal tissues were isolated 2 months after rats were exposed to moderate 142 kPa (20.6 psi) of BOP with chronic stress.[29] RPPM analysis indicated that well-known TBI biomarkers, such as of calcium binding protein B (S100β), GFAP, phosphorylated tau, interleukin (IL)-6, tumor necrosis factor-α (TNFα), and VEGF were increased after mild BOP with stress, compared to stress alone. In a closely related study by the same group, an enriched environment mitigated BOP-induced elevation of tau and VEGF in the dorsal hippocampus.[30] Overall, RPPM is sensitive for high-throughput detection of preselected proteins.

Label-Free Dual-Search Proteomics and Pathways Analysis

In a small and thorough study, label-free proteomics and informatics were used to define several proteins and pathways that were increased or suppressed by acute, mild, repeated BOP (rBOP) exposure compared to sham controls exposed to anesthesia alone (repeated (r) Sham) based on a model previously described.[31] Rats were exposed to 74.5 kPa BOP, once a day for three consecutive days. One day after the final BOP exposure, total protein was extracted from the cerebral cortex tissue. Unlike many prior studies, samples derived from each rat were individually analyzed in triplicate using one-dimensional polyacrylamide gel electrophoresis (1D-PAGE) and in-gel tryptic digests, followed by replicate peptide liquid chromatography and tandem mass spectrometry (LC-MS/MS). Protein identification and abundance was determined by peptide spectral counting[32] with two widely used search-assembly platform pairs: MyriMatch with IDPicker (MM-IDP)[33,34] and SEQUEST with Scaffold (SQ-SCF).[35] This methodology also incorporated use of a concatenated forward-decoy database to set thresholds for false positives at the peptide and protein levels.[36] Proteins that (1) could be identified in both search-assembly platforms with the same Uniprot database identifier, (2) met false-positive rate filters (e.g., q value = 2% for peptides, 5% for proteins), and (3) had similar spectral counts after rBOP were considered the "true" dataset representative of proteins affected by acute repeated BOP.

This approach led to identification of thousands of proteins within the cerebral cortex. A key aspect of this strategy confirmed that search-assembly schemas result in variable protein identification, fold change results, and error rates exemplified by true versus decoy (false) identifications. Therefore, use of at least two approaches may be ideal to cross-confirm proteomics data prior to using antibody-based methods, such as Western blots or ELISAs. For instance, MM-IDP identified 3,408 proteins with a 3.13% false discovery rate (FDR) compared to SQ-SCF, which identified 1,292 proteins with a 0.99% FDR. The search-assembly methods also resulted in different numbers of dysregulated proteins. Here, 123 proteins were down-regulated and 131 were up-regulated as defined by MM-IDP. SQ-SCF, however, identified 70 that were down-regulated and 101 were up-regulated after rBOP (Figure 26.1A,B). After comparing the two analyses containing dysregulated proteins, this dataset indicated that 319 proteins were unique to MM-IDP, 156 proteins were identified solely by SQ-SCF, and 31 proteins were common to both platforms (6.1% overlap) (Figure 26.1C). Of these 31 shared proteins, the fold change values generated by MM-IDP and SQ-SCF were highly congruent (Spearman $r = 0.92$, $p \leq 0.05$) (Figure 26.1D).

Rather than focus on individual proteins, data were analyzed using bioinformatics to propose biological processes (BP) and molecular functions (MF) affected by rBOP using WebGestalt.[37] Detailed lists of proteins and their resulting biological processes (Table 26.1) or molecular functions (Table 26.2) are provided for reference. Results are represented by the ratio of enrichment (R) (e.g., processes and functions that are likely up- or down-regulated) with adjusted p-values. A key biological process derived from down-regulated proteins LDH-A and -B was the "lactate metabolic process" (R = 304.24). These data suggest that low-level rBOP may affect a unique subset of proteins that are hubs for lactate metabolism. LDH loss has been shown to occur as a consequence of shearing damage of in vitro cell culture models of blast brain injury.[38,39] Additionally, the lactate-to-pyruvate ratio (an index of LDH loss) is disrupted and associated with chronic brain atrophy among TBI patients.[40]

Gene set enrichment analysis (GSEA) disease mapping of this dataset inferred that rBOP may be linked to neurological diseases (Table 26.3). Upregulated ATPase and calpain-2 were associated with pathways involved in Alzheimer disease and Parkinson disease onset, which are known to be associated with mTBI. Interestingly, these data also mapped to pathways that have not been explicitly associated with brain trauma. Suppressed LDH-A and -B mapped to dystrophin glycoprotein complex signaling and/

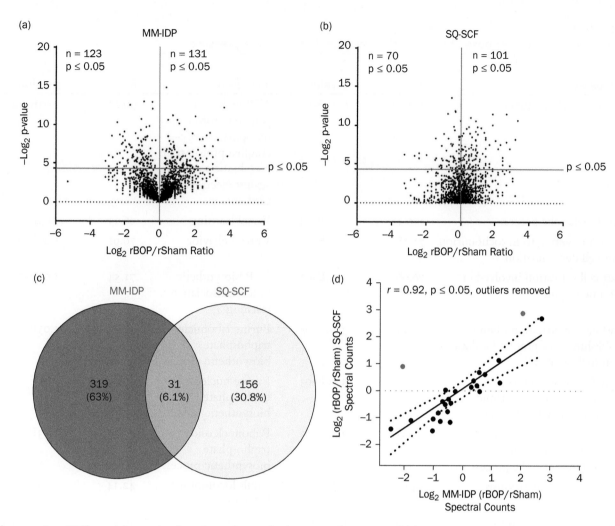

Figure 26.1 Differential protein abundance in cerebral cortex after repeated blast overpressure. (A) MyriMatch with IDPicker (MM-IDP) and (B) SEQUEST with Scaffold (SQ-SCF)–derived volcano plots displaying proteins affected by rBOP compared to rSham. Data are displayed as the Log_2 rBOP/rSham ratio (x-axis) and the $-\text{Log}_2$ p-value derived from 2-tailed t-Tests (y-axis). Red lines represent spectral count ratios with no change in relative spectral count abundance (0, x-axis) and the p-value cutoff ($p \le 0.05$, y-axis). Proteins that were either decreased (upper left quadrant) or increased (upper right quadrant) are shown. (C) Venn diagram of the number of proteins found to be differentially abundant using MM-IDP (left, *blue*) and SQ-SCF (right, *yellow*) platforms. The number of proteins and percentage of overlap are shown. (D) Similarity in the spectral count fold change of proteins affected by rBOP. Scatter plots and $\log_2$ transformed fold change data generated by MM-IDP (x-axis) and SQ-SCF (y-axis). Individual proteins are represented (*black circles*). Proteins that had incongruous fold change values are shown (*red dots*) for reference, but not used for further analysis. The calculated Spearman correlation coefficient (*r*) is displayed.##

or Ca^{2+} overload in the Duchenne muscular dystrophy (DMD) pathway.[41] This complex and its pathways play an important role in blood–brain barrier (BBB) integrity[42] and edema,[43] which are outcomes of mild TBI.[44] Overall, unbiased discovery-based proteomics strategies augmented by two search-discovery platforms have the power to define novel brain tissue biomarkers and associated pathways affected by mild rBOP that could not otherwise be hypothesized based on pathology or behavioral metrics.

Table 26.1:
Biological processes proposed to be affected by repeated blast overpressure

Decreased	R	Adj. p-value	Increased	R	Adj. p-value
Lactate metabolic process	304.24	6.00E-04	ATP hydrolysis-coupled proton transport, energy-coupled proton trans membrane transport, against electrochemical gradient	99.23	1.03E-02
NAD metabolic process	106.48	4.00E-04	Visual learning	96.13	1.03E-02
Protein targeting to mitochondrion mast cell degranulation	78.88	3.40E-03	Visual behavior	76.91	1.03E-02
Mast cell activation involved in immune response	76.06	3.40E-03	ATP biosynthetic process, associative learning	71.54	1.03E-02
Mast cell-mediated immunity establishment of protein localization to mitochondrion	73.44	3.40E-03	Purine ribonucleoside triphosphate biosynthetic process	50.43	1.03E-02
Protein localization to mitochondrion, nicotinamide nucleotide metabolic process	73.44	3.40E-03	Purine nucleoside triphosphate biosynthetic process	49.62	1.03E-02
Pyridine nucleotide metabolic process, pyridine-containing compound metabolic process	66.55	3.70E-03	Ribonucleoside triphosphate biosynthetic process	42.73	1.03E-02
Synaptic vesicle exocytosis	64.54	3.70E-03	Adult locomotory behavior	42.14	1.03E-02
Leukocyte degranulation	60.27	6.00E-04	Nucleoside triphosphate biosynthetic process	40.48	1.03E-02
Oxidoreduction coenzyme metabolic process	60.27	6.00E-04	Single-organism reproductive behavior, proton transport	39.95	1.03E-02
Mast cell activation	54.14	6.00E-04	Hydrogen transport	38.45	1.03E-02
Mitochondrial transport	53.24	4.70E-03	Potassium ion transport	37.51	1.03E-02
Regulated secretory pathway	53.24	4.70E-03	Reproductive behavior	36.62	1.03E-02
Myeloid leukocyte-mediated immunity, myeloid cell activation involved in immune response	50.71	6.00E-04	Learning	36.19	1.03E-02
Glycolysis	50.71	4.70E-03	Purine ribonucleotide biosynthetic process	33.08	1.14E-02
Glucose catabolic process, synaptic vesicle transport	49.91	6.00E-04	Purine nucleoside biosynthetic process, purine ribonucleoside biosynthetic process	31.07	1.14E-02

Table 26.1: Continued

Decreased	R	Adj. p-value	Increased	R	Adj. p-value
Establishment of protein localization to organelle	46.3	5.20E–03	Ribonucleotide biosynthetic process, nucleoside biosynthetic process	30.46	1.14E–02
Hexose catabolic process, monosaccharide catabolic process, neurotransmitter secretion single-organism carbohydrate catabolic process	43.46	5.40E–03	Ribonucleoside biosynthetic process, ribose phosphate biosynthetic process, adult behavior	29.87	1.14E–02
Carbohydrate catabolic process, coenzyme metabolic process, exocytosis	39.44	6.10E–03	Sodium ion transport	29.3	1.14E–02
Cellular carbohydrate metabolic process, hormone transport	36.1	7.50E–03	ATP metabolic process	29.3	1.14E–02
Cofactor metabolic process	29.17	1.01E–02	Locomotory behavior	27.47	1.16E–02
Generation of precursor metabolites and energy	28.78	1.01E–02	Cellular calcium ion homeostasis, calcium ion homeostasis	26.98	1.16E–02
Generation of a signal involved in cell–cell signaling	28.02	1.02E–02	Cellular divalent inorganic cation homeostasis	26.98	1.16E–02
Signal release	27.66	1.04E–02	Divalent inorganic cation homeostasis, cellular metal ion homeostasis	26.75	1.17E–02
Regulation of hormone levels	26.96	1.05E–02	Metal ion homeostasis	25.42	1.23E–02
Carboxylic acid metabolic process, oxoacid metabolic process	22.42	1.41E–02	Cellular cation homeostasis	24.41	1.29E–02
Organic acid metabolic process	20.09	1.64E–02	Cation homeostasis, metal ion transport, cellular ion homeostasis	21.36	1.62E–02
Lactate metabolic process	19.19	1.75E–02	Response to a biotic stimulus	19.85	1.83E–02
NAD metabolic process	16.64	4.70E–03	Small molecule metabolic process	18.46	1.03E–02
Protein targeting to mitochondrion mast cell degranulation	16.22	4.70E–03	ATP hydrolysis-coupled proton transport, energy-coupled proton trans membrane transport, against electrochemical gradient	17.82	1.03E–02

(continued)

Table 26.1: Continued

Decreased	R	Adj. p-value	Increased	R	Adj. p-value
Mast cell activation involved in immune response	16.22	4.70E-03	Visual learning	17.35	1.03E-02
Mast cell-mediated immunity, establishment of protein localization to mitochondrion	15.07	5.40E-03	Visual behavior	16.72	1.03E-02
Protein localization to mitochondrion, nicotinamide nucleotide metabolic process	14.01	6.10E-03	ATP biosynthetic process, associative learning	15.28	1.03E-02
Pyridine nucleotide metabolic process, pyridine-containing compound, metabolic process	11.96	9.20E-03	Purine ribonucleoside triphosphate biosynthetic process	14.24	1.03E-02
Synaptic vesicle exocytosis	9.74	1.32E-02	Purine nucleoside triphosphate biosynthetic process	13.57	1.03E-02
Leukocyte degranulation	9.74	1.32E-02	Ribonucleoside triphosphate biosynthetic process	11.68	1.14E-02
Oxidoreduction coenzyme metabolic process	8.95	1.57E-02	Adult locomotory behavior	9.57	1.35E-02
Mast cell activation	7.83	3.40E-03	Nucleoside triphosphate biosynthetic process	7.78	2.24E-02
Mitochondrial transport	7.38	3.40E-03	Single-organism reproductive behavior, proton transport	6.95	1.14E-02
Regulated secretory pathway	7.23	3.70E-03	Hydrogen transport	4.57	1.16E-02

Webgestalt pathways that mapped to increased or decreased proteins defined by proteomics analysis are indicated. The ratio of enrichment (R) and proteins involved are indicated for each biological process.

Non-Blast Closed Head Injury and Novel Approaches

Advancements in rodent models, computing technology, and biochemical methods for proteomics have grown to encompass a wider array of translational models for which more diverse targets may be detected with a high degree of sensitivity. Novel models include a direct closed head injury (CHI). New approaches, applicable to a number of mTBI models, facilitate deeper analysis of the brain proteome

Isobaric Tagging of Brain Tissue Extracts for Discovery and Quantitation After Closed Head Injury

MTBI may also be caused by direct impact to the head due to blunt force trauma or to falls or accidents in which the head impacts a fixed surface (e.g., a wall or floor). Rodent models such as weight-drop (WD),[45] a modified version of closed cortical impact (CCI),[46,47] and projectile concussive impact (PCI)[48] have been specifically designed

Table 26.2:
Molecular functions proposed to be affected by repeated blast overpressure.

Decreased	R	Adj. p-value	Increased	R	Adj. p-value
L-lactate dehydrogenase activity	741.59	1.87E-05	Sodium:potassium-exchanging ATPase	321.36	5.00E-04
Lactate dehydrogenase activity	741.59	1.87E-05	Potassium-transporting ATPase activity	267.8	5.00E-04
NAD binding	53.83	1.00E-04	Cation-transporting ATPase activity	133.9	5.00E-04
Coenzyme binding	28.23	1.57E-05	ATPase activity, coupled to transmembrane movement of ions,	73.04	1.40E-03
Oxidoreductase activity, acting on the CH-OH group of donors, NAD or NADP as	28.04	5.00E-04	ATPase activity, coupled to transmembrane movement of ions	58.43	1.70E-03
Oxidoreductase activity, acting on CH-OH group of donors	25.67	8.00E-04	ATPase activity, coupled to transmembrane movement of	38.26	3.10E-03
Cofactor binding	20.6	1.87E-05	Hydrolase activity, acting on acid anhydrides, catalyzing transmembrane	37.37	3.10E-03
Synapse	8.8	1.72E-02	ATPase activity, coupled to movement of	37.37	3.10E-03
Protein complex binding	8.16	1.42E-02	P-P-bond-hydrolysis-driven transmembrane transporter activity	33.13	3.80E-03
Cell junction	7.36	1.83E-02	Primary active transmembrane	33.13	3.80E-03
Oxidoreductase activity	6.05	1.02E-02	Amino acid binding	29.48	4.60E-03
Mitochondrion	5.44	4.00E-03	Sodium ion transmembrane transporter	28.69	4.70E-03
Protein binding	2.56	8.00E-04	Potassium ion transmembrane	25.5	5.60E-03
Binding	1.55	1.02E-02	Carboxylic acid binding	16.23	1.26E-02
			ATPase activity, coupled	14.67	1.49E-02
			Active transmembrane transporter	12.17	2.00E-02
			ATPase activity	10.97	2.36E-02
			Monovalent inorganic cation transmembrane transporter activity	10.3	2.59E-02
			Metal ion transmembrane transporter	9.26	3.08E-02

(continued)

Table 26.2: Continued

Decreased	R	Adj. p-value	Increased	R	Adj. p-value
			Adenyl ribonucleotide binding	6.41	1.70E-03
			Adenyl nucleotide binding	6.38	1.70E-03
			Purine ribonucleoside binding	6.26	5.00E-04
			Ribonucleoside binding	6.25	5.00E-04
			Purine nucleoside binding	6.25	5.00E-04
			Nucleoside binding	6.21	5.00E-04
			Purine ribonucleotide binding	6.16	5.00E-04
			Purine nucleotide binding	6.14	5.00E-04
			Ribonucleotide binding	6.1	5.00E-04
			Anion binding	5.44	5.00E-04
			Purine ribonucleoside triphosphate	5.25	3.10E-03
			ATP binding	5.24	9.50E-03
			Nucleoside phosphate binding, nucleotide binding	4.65	1.70E-03
			Small molecule binding ion binding	4.65	1.70E-03
			Sodium:potassium-exchanging ATPase	4.29	2.50E-03
			Potassium-transporting ATPase activity	3.22	5.00E-04
			Cation binding	2.78	3.09E-02
			Catalytic activity	2.29	1.73E-02
			Heterocyclic compound binding	2.22	3.86E-02
			Organic cyclic compound binding	2.2	3.96E-02
			Binding	1.55	3.09E-02

Webgestalt functions that mapped to increased or decreased proteins defined by proteomics analysis are indicated. The ratio of enrichment (R) and proteins involved are indicated for each function.

without a craniotomy component to specifically address this type of injury. Analysis of the brain proteome is likely to reflect the brain's unique response to trauma without the need to consider the impact on other organs.

A model of mouse CHI, also termed as closed skull impact (CSI), is derived from the CCI model and was recently used in an elegant proteomics design, termed microwave and magnetic (M²) proteomics.[49–51] Briefly, a midline incision was made prior to periosteum retraction, and a piston-like device added downward pressure directly

Table 26.3:
Disease-associated pathways derived from proteomics of cerebral cortices affected by repeated blast overpressure

Directionality	Pathway	# of Entities	Overlap	Overlapping Entities	p-value
Decreased	Dystrophin glycoprotein complex signaling in Duchenne muscular dystrophy	67	6	GAPDH;CAPZB;GNAI2;GNAQ;LDHA;LDHB	0.001
	Duchenne muscular dystrophy overview	106	5	GNAQ;GAPDH;GNAI2;LDH	0.001
	FOXA2 signaling in prostate cancer	25	3	GAPDH;LDHA;LDHB	0.003
	Susceptibility genes for Crohn's disease and ulcerative colitis	30	3	GAPDH;LDHA;LDHB	0.004
	Peutz-Jeghers syndrome overview	62	3	GAPDH;LDHA;LDHB	0.033
	Preconditioning ischemia	51	3	GAPDH;LDHA;LDHB	0.061
	Mechanism of cetuximab resistance in colorectal cancer	85	3	GAPDH;LDHA;LDHB	0.085
	Hedgehog signaling in mantle cell lymphoma	16	2	GNAQ;GNAI2	0.002
	WHIM syndrome overview	24	2	GNAQ;GNAI2	0.003
	Model autocrine cytokine/chemokine loops in systemic scleroderma fibroblasts 1	37	2	GNAQ;GNAI2	0.005
	$Ca2^+$ toxicity in lens cells	42	2	CAPN2;ATP2A2	0.003
	Alzheimer disease overview	104	2	CAPN2;ATP2A2	0.019
	$Ca2^+$ overload in Duchenne muscular dystrophy	59	2	CAPN2;ATP2A2	0.023
	$Ca2^+$ toxicity in Alzheimer disease	63	2	CAPN2;ATP2A2	0.035
Increased	Duchenne muscular dystrophy overview	106	2	CAPN2;ATP2A2	0.090
	Proteins involved in pathogenesis of heart dysfunction caused by hypothyroidism	19	1	ATP2A2	0.013
	NO and ADMA signaling in Raynaud disease	21	1	ATP2A2	0.036
	Disease genes identified in syndromic epilepsy	80	1	ATP2A2	0.053
	Neurofibrillary tangle formation in Alzheimer disease	22	1	CAPN2	0.055
	Young-onset SNCA-induced Parkinson disease	24	1	CAPN2	0.061

Webgestalt derived gene set enrichment analysis (GSEA) of diseases that mapped to proteins defined by proteomics analysis are indicated. The ratio of enrichment (R) and proteins involved are indicated for each function.

onto the skull. As reported, this procedure did not result in intracranial bleeds, edema, alterations in brain structure, or high mortality. After the CHI, extracted proteins were subjected to microwave-assisted reduction, alkylation, and digestion. Thereafter, peptides were subjected to isobaric tandem mass tag (TMT) labeling.[52]

TMT tags modify tryptic peptides at the N-terminus and at lysine residues, allowing up to 10 simultaneous comparisons in a high-throughput manner. A key aspect of this work is that it included a normalization strategy, similar to that of 2-DE methods, in which a pooled sample composed of aliquots derived from equal parts of each sample was used as a control. More than 400 proteins were detected in brain tissue lysates isolated at one day through four months after CHI. Of these proteins, myelin basic protein and myelin associated glycoprotein were suppressed over time. Two well-studied TBI-related proteins, α-II spectrin and neurofilament light chain (NF-L), were also decreased at as late as 30 days after CHI.

Novel Targets of the Deeper Proteome

An additional subset of novel targets include posttranslational modifications, such as phosphorylation or deimination (e.g., citrullination) or explicit characterization of peptides generated by proteolysis and enzymatic activity. These methods exploit the power of proteomics analysis at the level of peptides, amino acids, and posttranslational modifications (PTMs). These strategies are robust and often applied to other fields of research (e.g., cancer). These methods are readily applicable to mTBI rodent models.

Analysis of brain tissue collected from swine exposed to mild BOP indicated deimination within several proteins.[53] After 1D-PAGE and immunoblotting, proteins in each gel band were excised and deimination sites were identified at specific arginine residues within specific peptides. Interestingly, this modification was found to occur within GFAP and vimentin, two biomarkers that are well associated with TBI progression.

Lastly, analysis of peptides derived from specific enzymes allows for extrapolation of not only the proteins affected, but of the enzymes that are active as a consequence of mTBI. This functional or activity-based approach has been used with extensive bioinformatics tools to determine that protein fragments of multiple protein targets are generated by calpain and caspase activity, two enzymes that are up-regulated in response to trauma.[54]

Conclusions

MTBI can result in dysregulation of brain tissue proteins, indicated by altered protein levels, peptide generation, and variation of PTMs, which may be used to define novel biomarkers. With translational rodent models of closed head mTBI, identification of these proteins, peptides, and modifications through brain tissue proteomics and informatics is poised to facilitate discovery and validation of individual proteins and of the pathways or mechanisms underlying injury responses. Several methodologies and informatics schema are available, including targeted strategies, such as multiplexed RPPM, or unbiased methods that include electrophoresis and peptide or protein-based mass spectrometry. Labels (or tags) may be used to enhance quantitative capabilities. Identification of novel biomarkers and increased use of bioinformatics may be used to determine the impact that mTBI has on entire pathways or coordinated mechanisms that result in proteolytic or signaling cascades known to result in apoptosis, inflammation, aberrant protein aggregation, and tissue degeneration. Furthermore, these strategies augment our understanding of the full proteomic response and may involve not only analysis of brain tissues or regions, but also concurrent survey of purified cell types (neurons, glia, endothelial cells) and analysis of biological compartments (e.g., the glymphatic, lymphatic, and cerebral spinal fluid) that interact with the brain tissue. Consideration of these aspects may be necessary to fully describe the impact that mTBI has on the brain with appropriate sensitivity and specificity. As such, proteomic technologies are poised to have great impact on closed head, mTBI research.

Acknowledgments

The authors thank David W. Johnson, CPT, US Army; Monmon Myint, SGT, US Army; Vincent Donkor, SPC, US Army; Eric Maudlin-Jeronimo; and Ye Chen, MD, PhD for sample preparation, as well as Arun Peethambaran, Irene Gist, and Joe Long, PhD for technical support.

Disclaimer

The authors have declared no conflict of interest. This material has been reviewed by the Walter Reed Army Institute of Research. There is no objection to its presentation and/or publication. The opinions or assertions contained herein are the private views of the author(s) and are not to be construed either as official or as reflecting true views of the Department of the Army, Department of the Navy, Department of the Defense, Wayne State University, Banyan Biomarkers, or the University of Florida.

Funding Sources

This research was supported by the Combat Casualty Care Research Program (award W81XWH-12-2-0134), the Congressionally Directed Medical Research Program (awards W81XWH-10-2-0091 and -0092), the Military Operational Medicine Research Program, and the US Army Medical Research and Materiel Command. The Wayne State University Proteomics Core is supported through the National Institutes of Health (NIH, Center Grant #P30 ES 020957), the NIH Cancer Center Support Grant (#P30 CA 022453), and the NIH Shared Instrumentation Grant (#S10 OD 010700). The funding sources had no role in the collection, analysis, or interpretation of the data or in the decision to submit for publication.

References

1. Winkler EA, Yue JK, Burke JF, et al. Adult sports-related traumatic brain injury in United States trauma centers. *Neurosurg Focus*. 2016;40(4).
2. Omalu B. Chronic traumatic encephalopathy. *Prog Neurol Surg*. 2014;28:38–49.
3. Walker WC, Franke LM, McDonald SD, Sima AP, Keyser-Marcus L. Prevalence of mental health conditions after military blast exposure, their co-occurrence, and their relation to mild traumatic brain injury. *Brain Inj*. 2015;29(13-14):1581–1588.

4. Chan LG, Feinstein A. Persistent sleep disturbances independently predict poorer functional and social outcomes 1 year after mild traumatic brain injury. *The J Head Traum Rehabil.* 2015;30(6):E67–75.

5. Schwab K, Terrio HP, Brenner LA, et al. Epidemiology and prognosis of mild traumatic brain injury in returning soldiers: a cohort study. *Neurology.* 2017;88(16):1571–1579.

6. Ryan PB, Lee-Wilk T, Kok BC, Wilk JE. Interdisciplinary rehabilitation of mild TBI and PTSD: a case report. *Brain Inj.* 2011;25(10):1019–1025.

7. Yuh EL, Mukherjee P, Lingsma HF, et al. Magnetic resonance imaging improves 3-month outcome prediction in mild traumatic brain injury. *Ann Neurol.* 2013;73(2):224–235.

8. Kushner D. Mild traumatic brain injury—Toward understanding manifestations and treatment. *Arch Intern Med.* 1998;158(15):1617–1624.

9. Benzinger TL, Brody D, Cardin S, et al. Blast-related brain injury: imaging for clinical and research applications: report of the 2008 St. Louis workshop. *J Neurotrauma.* 2009;26(12):2127–2144.

10. Goldstein LE, Fisher AM, Tagge CA, et al. Chronic traumatic encephalopathy in blast-exposed military veterans and a blast neurotrauma mouse model. *Sci Translat Med.* 2012;4(134):134ra160.

11. McKee AC, Robinson ME. Military-related traumatic brain injury and neurodegeneration. *Alzheimers Dement.* 2014;10(3 suppl):S242–253.

12. Mishra V, Skotak M, Schuetz H, Heller A, Haorah J, Chandra N. Primary blast causes mild, moderate, severe and lethal TBI with increasing blast overpressures: experimental rat injury model. *Sci Rep.* 2016;6:26992.

13. Arnold GJ, Frohlich T. 2D DIGE saturation labeling for minute sample amounts. *Methods Mol Biol.* 2012;854:89–112.

14. Viswanathan S, Unlu M, Minden JS. Two-dimensional difference gel electrophoresis. *Nat Protoc.* 2006;1(3):1351–1358.

15. Friedman DB. Assessing signal-to-noise in quantitative proteomics: multivariate statistical analysis in DIGE experiments. *Methods Mol Biol.* 2012;854:31–45.

16. Friedman DB, Lilley KS. Optimizing the difference gel electrophoresis (DIGE) technology. *Methods Mol Biol.* 2008;428:93–124.

17. Bienvenut WV, Deon C, Pasquarello C, et al. Matrix-assisted laser desorption/ionization-tandem mass spectrometry with high resolution and sensitivity for identification and characterization of proteins. *Proteomics.* 2002;2(7):868–876.

18. Gogichaeva NV, Alterman MA. Amino acid analysis by means of MALDI TOF mass spectrometry or MALDI TOF/TOF tandem mass spectrometry. *Methods Mol Biol.* 2012;828:121–135.

19. Suckau D, Resemann A, Schuerenberg M, Hufnagel P, Franzen J, Holle A. A novel MALDI LIFT-TOF/TOF mass spectrometer for proteomics. *Anal Bioanal Chem.* 2003;376(7):952–965.

20. Kobeissy FH, Ottens AK, Zhang Z, et al. Novel differential neuroproteomics analysis of traumatic brain injury in rats. *Mol Cell Proteomics.* 2006;5(10):1887–1898.

21. Ottens AK, Bustamante L, Golden EC, et al. Neuroproteomics: a biochemical means to discriminate the extent and modality of brain injury. *J Neurotrauma.* 2010;27(10):1837–1852.

22. Perez-Garcia G, Gama Sosa MA, De Gasperi R, et al. Chronic post-traumatic stress disorder-related traits in a rat model of low-level blast exposure. *Behav Brain Res.* 2016;340:117–125.

23. Elder GA, Dorr NP, De Gasperi R, et al. Blast exposure induces post-traumatic stress disorder-related traits in a rat model of mild traumatic brain injury. *J Neurotrauma.* 2012;29(16):2564–2575.

24. Ahlers ST, Vasserman-Stokes E, Shaughness MC, et al. Assessment of the effects of acute and repeated exposure to blast overpressure in rodents: toward a greater understanding of blast and the potential ramifications for injury in humans exposed to blast. *Front Neurol.* 2012;3:32.

25. Pierobon M, Vanmeter AJ, Moroni N, Galdi F, Petricoin EF, 3rd. Reverse-phase protein microarrays. *Methods Mol Biol.* 2012;823:215–235.

26. Gyorgy AB, Walker J, Wingo D, et al. Reverse phase protein microarray technology in traumatic brain injury. *J Neurosci Methods.* 2010;192(1):96–101.

27. Kamnaksh A, Kovesdi E, Kwon SK, et al. Factors affecting blast traumatic brain injury. *J Neurotrauma.* 2011;28(10):2145–2153.

28. Long JB, Bentley TL, Wessner KA, Cerone C, Sweeney S, Bauman RA. Blast overpressure in rats: recreating a battlefield injury in the laboratory. *J Neurotrauma.* 2009;26(6):827–840.

29. Kwon SK, Kovesdi E, Gyorgy AB, et al. Stress and traumatic brain injury: a behavioral, proteomics, and histological study. *Front Neurol.* 2011;2:12.

30. Kovesdi E, Gyorgy AB, Kwon SK, et al. The effect of enriched environment on the outcome of traumatic brain injury: a behavioral, proteomics, and histological study. *Front Neurosci.* 2011;5:42.

31. Genovese RF, Simmons LP, Ahlers ST, Maudlin-Jeronimo E, Dave JR, Boutte AM. Effects of mild Tbi from repeated blast overpressure on the expression and extinction of conditioned fear in rats. *Neuroscience.* 2013;254:120–129.

32. Boutte AM, Friedman DB, Bogyo M, Min Y, Yang L, Lin PC. Identification of a myeloid-derived suppressor cell cystatin-like protein that inhibits metastasis. *FASEB J.* 2011;25(8):2626–2637.

33. Holman JD, Ma ZQ, Tabb DL. Identifying proteomic LC-MS/MS data sets with Bumbershoot and IDPicker. *Curr Protoc Bioinformatics.* 2012;Chapter 13:Unit13. 17.

34. Ma ZQ, Dasari S, Chambers MC, et al. IDPicker 2.0: improved protein assembly with high discrimination peptide identification filtering. *J Proteome Res.* 2009;8(8):3872–3881.

35. Tu CJ, Sheng QH, Li J, et al. Optimization of search engines and postprocessing approaches to maximize peptide and protein identification for high-resolution mass data. *J Proteome Res.* 2015;14(11):4662–4673.

36. Feng XD, Ma J, Chang C, Bai MZ, Zhu YP, Shu KX. The application and progress of target-decoy database search strategy in identification and quality control of tandem mass spectrometry data in shotgun proteomics. *Prog Biochem Biophys.* 2016;43(7):661–672.

37. Wang J, Vasaikar S, Shi Z, Greer M, Zhang B. WebGestalt 2017: a more comprehensive, powerful, flexible and interactive gene set enrichment analysis toolkit. *Nucleic Acids Res.* 2017;45(W1):W130–W137.

38. Arun P, Spadaro J, John J, Gharavi RB, Bentley TB, Nambiar MP. Studies on blast traumatic brain injury using in-vitro model with shock tube. *Neuroreport.* 2011;22(8):379–384.

39. LaPlaca MC, Lee VM, Thibault LE. An in vitro model of traumatic neuronal injury: loading rate-dependent changes in acute cytosolic calcium and lactate dehydrogenase release. *J Neurotrauma.* 1997;14(6):355–368.

40. Marcoux J, McArthur DA, Miller C, et al. Persistent metabolic crisis as measured by elevated cerebral microdialysis lactate-pyruvate ratio predicts chronic frontal lobe brain atrophy after traumatic brain injury. *Crit Care Med.* 2008;36(10):2871–2877.

41. Culligan K, Ohlendieck K. Diversity of the brain dystrophin-glycoprotein complex. *J Biomed Biotechnol.* 2002;2(1):31–36.

42. Goodnough CL, Gao Y, Li X, et al. Lack of dystrophin results in abnormal cerebral diffusion and perfusion in vivo. *NeuroImage.* 2014;102:809–816.

43. Vajda Z, Pedersen M, Fuchtbauer EM, et al. Delayed onset of brain edema and mislocalization of aquaporin-4 in dystrophin-null transgenic mice. *P Natl Acad Sci USA.* 2002;99(20):13131–13136.

44. Shetty AK, Mishra V, Kodali M, Hattiangady B. Blood brain barrier dysfunction and delayed neurological deficits in mild traumatic brain injury induced by blast shock waves. *Front Cell Neurosci.* 2014;8:232.

45. Flierl MA, Stahel PF, Beauchamp KM, Morgan SJ, Smith WR, Shohami E. Mouse closed head injury model induced by a weight-drop device. *Nat Protoc.* 2009;4(9):1328–1337.

46. Osier ND, Dixon CE. The controlled cortical impact model: applications, considerations for researchers, and future directions. *Front Neurol.* 2016;7:134.

47. Rubenstein R, Chang BG, Davies P, Wagner AK, Robertson CS, Wang KKW. A novel, ultrasensitive assay for tau: potential for assessing traumatic brain injury in tissues and biofluids. *J Neurotrauma.* 2015;32(5):342–352.

48. Boutte AM, Mountney A, Johnson DW, et al. Delayed consciousness, sensory-motor deficits, and GFAP levels in repeated concussive impact. *J Neurotrauma.* 2014;31(12):A37–A37.

49. Evans TM, Van Remmen H, Purkar A, et al. Microwave & magnetic (M2) proteomics of a mouse model of mild traumatic brain injury. *Transl Proteom.* 2014;3:10–21.

50. Raphael I, Mahesula S, Purkar A, et al. Microwave & magnetic (M2) proteomics reveals CNS-specific protein expression waves that precede clinical symptoms of experimental autoimmune encephalomyelitis. *Sci Rep.* 2014;4:6210.

51. Raphael I, Mahesula S, Kalsaria K, et al. Microwave and magnetic (M(2)) proteomics of the experimental autoimmune encephalomyelitis animal model of multiple sclerosis. *Electrophoresis.* 2012;33(24):3810–3819.

52. O'Brien DP, Timms JF. Employing TMT quantification in a shotgun-MS platform. *Methods Mol Biol.* 2014;1156:187–199.

53. Attilio PJ, Flora M, Kamnaksh A, Bradshaw DJ, Agoston D, Mueller GP. The effects of blast exposure on protein deimination in the brain. *Oxid Med Cell Longev.* 2017;2017:8398072.

54. El-Assaad A, Dawy Z, Nemer G, Kobeissy F. Novel bioinformatics-based approach for proteomic biomarkers prediction of calpain-2 &caspase-3 protease fragmentation: application to betaII-spectrin protein. *Sci Rep.* 2017;7:41039.

Section V

Current and Future Treatments of TBI

Neuroprotection in TBI

Dafin Muresanu, Codruta Birle Barle, Ioana Muresanu,
Cezara Costin, Johannes Vester, Alexandru Rafila,
Olivia Rosu, and Dana Slavoaca

27

General Concepts of Neuroprotection

A brain after a traumatic brain injury (TBI) is a new brain. It is the result of the overlap between the nature of the primary injury and environmental factors, as well as the complexity of the cellular-molecular cascades that lead to secondary injury and the individual characteristics of each patient, such as genetic phenotype, age, gender, comorbidities, and nutritional status.

Neuroprotection in TBI targets the secondary neuronal injury, a multidimensional molecular cascade that includes excitotoxicity, immune response imbalances, oxidative stress, and apoptotic-like processes. These molecular processes lead to dysfunction of the blood–brain barrier (BBB) and alterations of neurotransmitter and hormonal systems. The result is an imbalance of the interplay between endogenous defense activity (EDA) and damage mechanisms (DM).[1] Understanding EDA (Figure 27.1)—neurotrophicity, neuroprotection, neuroplasticity, and neurogenesis—is essential for developing pharmacological neuroprotection. These processes are interconnected and share close molecular pathways with DM. The anticorrelation between EDA and DA, under physiological conditions, maintains the balance between pro-survival signaling and pro-death signaling.

In TBI patients, over the long term, this imbalance between EDA and DM may lead to a neurodegenerative process characterized by a chronic neuroinflammatory process that can continue for years after the injury.[2]

The molecular alterations have direct effects on local circuits and large-scale networks by generating heterogenic phenotypes in which cognitive impairment plays an important role (Figure 27.2).

Due to the complexity of this milieu of interconnected mechanisms, neuroprotection and neurorecovery after TBI represent a challenge and serve as a bridge between evidence-based medicine and personalized medicine.

Pharmacological Neuroprotection in TBI

Recent Lessons from Clinical Studies

There have been 28 phase III randomized clinical trials (RCT) since 1990 without any sustainable positive results.[3] The failure of most RCTs to provide positive clinical

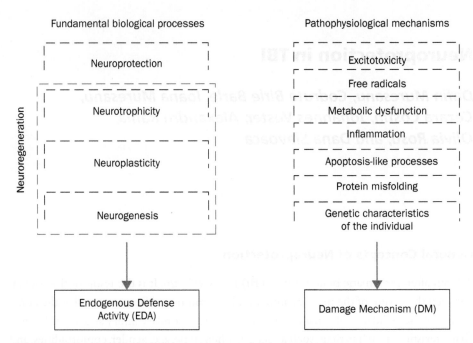

Figure 27.1 Endogenous defense activity and damage mechanism.

data on pharmacological agents generated several observations that could help develop a new way of understanding both neuroprotection and how TBI clinical trials on neuroprotection should be designed:

- Modulatory, pleiotropic, multimodal versus suppressive, monotropic, monomodal mechanism of action
- Short-term versus long-term neuroprotection
- Multidimensional versus unidimensional outcome evaluation

Starting from the observation that the majority of pharmacological agents tested demonstrated a suppressive mechanism of action, with few pleiotropic and unimodal

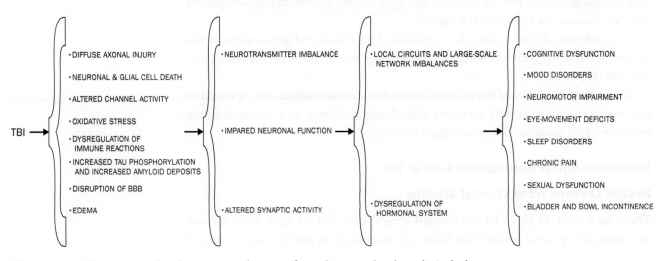

Figure 27.2 The impact of pathogenic mechanisms from the microlevel to clinical phenotypes.

effects (Table 27.1), the emerging idea is to test modulatory, pleiotropic, and multimodal agents.[1] Additionally, it became clear that the heterogeneity of TBI phenotypes is impossible to capture by a single outcome measure. A multidimensional evaluation that includes cognitive aspects assessed over a longer period of time is essential to reach a more complete understanding of the outcome of TBI patients.[4,5]

To date, there are just two such compounds tested in TBI clinical trials: citicoline and Cerebrolysin (CRB). CRB is a parenterally administered multimodal drug consisting of porcine brain-derived peptides that penetrates the BBB after intravenous administration, and it has effects similar to endogenous neurotrophic factors.[6]

Cohort studies[24,25] and a small double-blind placebo-controlled study[23] showed promising results on the Glasgow Outcome Scale (GOS) and GOS-Extended (GOSE) scale, the Mini-Mental State Examination (MMSE), and the Cognitive Abilities Screening Instrument (CASI). These and several other small studies support the idea that CRB is the appropriate option for rehabilitation strategies as it induces a faster recovery and results in an improved long-term outcome not only with respect to motor function but also cognitive abilities. Currently, there is an ongoing RCT, the CAPTAIN trial, with a completely different design, including assessments of long-term neuroprotection, strategies for reducing heterogeneity, and multimodal outcome evaluation.[6] A similar study in stroke patients demonstrated that CRB improves function and global outcome in patients undergoing early rehabilitation.[41] However, the COBRIT trial on citicoline, which was also designed to evaluate more complex functional and cognitive outcomes, failed to show beneficial effects in TBI.[35] A possible explanation could be that, to avoid dichotomization, the authors of this study chose to apply fixed cutoffs,[5] which is in accordance with a more general acceptance, but not with the newest recommendations regarding nonparametric methods [42].

Current Strategies in Experimental Data

Many therapies for TBI are still under development. Modern approaches use a broad range of molecules from traditional to newly developed, including hormones (melatonin, erythropoietin, growth hormone, progesterone),[43–45] peptides and trophic factors ((brain-derived neurotrophic factor [BDNF], nerve growth factor [NGF] vascular endothelial growth factor [VEGF], bradykinin, substance p),[46] antibodies (etanercept, cis p-tau antibody, anti-lysophosphatidic acid antibodies),[47] cannabinoid derivatives,[46,48] nanoparticles (alone or as biological active particle carriers),[49–51] polyphenols (flavonoids, phenolic alcohols, stilbenoids),[45,52] oral antidiabetics (glibenclamide),[8,9,37] antibiotics (minocycline),[45] antioxidants (α-lipoic acid, curcumin, edaravone, luteolin, taurine),[52–55] neurotransmitter modulatory drugs (acetylcholinesterase inhibitors, huperzine A, selective serotonin reuptake inhibitors, imipramine),[45] immunomodulatory drugs (intravenous immunoglobulin G, anakinra),[56] proinflammatory cytokine inhibitors, and other bioactive molecules.[47,57–61]

From delivering oxygen and neurotrophic molecules (including antioxidants and vasogenic agents)[45,46,56] and inhibiting proinflammatory cascades, to obtaining cis-p-tau clearance[45,62,63] to building nanoparticle carriers to deliver drugs to the central nervous system,[13,64] recent studies offer many directions using single active agents or combined therapies to obtain not only structural but also functional improvements in TBI models.

Table 27.1:
Pharmacological agents for neuroprotection in clinical studies on traumatic brain injury (TBI) patients

Pharmacological Agents	Neuroprotective Mechanisms of Action	Suppressive/ Modulatory Activity	Effects on Other Edas	Cognitive Outcome	General Outcome	Adverse Events
Statins (rosuvastatin, atorvastatin)[7-9]	Decrease in apoptosis, antiinflammatory effects by reducing IL-1, TNFα,IL-6, and ICAM-1.	Suppressive	Increase neurogenesis by up-regulating BDNF and VEGF	Slight improvement of amnesia and disorientation related to TBI on Galveston Orientation Amnesia Test (GOAT)	Improved functional outcome after TBI on Disability Rating Score (DRS)	Rhabdomyolysis, myopathy, increased liver and pancreatic enzymes, cognitive decline, increased incidence of diabetes mellitus
Progesterone[8-12]	Decreases apoptosis, decreases glutamate excitotoxicity, reduces membrane lipid peroxidation, limits inflammation	Suppressive	Stimulates the synthesis of BDNF, promotes central and peripheral remyelination, promotes spinogenesis, synaptogenesis, neuronal survival, and dendritic growth	No cognitive outcome assessed	Mixed results on neurological outcome assessed through GOS, mortality, disability rating scale	Headache, muscle and joint pain, gastrointestinal disturbances
Calcium channel blockers (nimodipine)[8,9,13,14]	Reduces calcium-mediated damage	Suppressive	Unknown	No cognitive outcome assessed	No significant effect on neurological outcome	Hypotension, increased liver and pancreatic enzymes
Corticosteroids[8,9]	Reduces brain edema formation, promotes membrane stability and limits free-radical formation	Suppressive	Reduces synaptic plasticity and dendritic spines, impairs hippocampal neurogenesis, and increases synaptic plasticity and dendritic alterations[15,16]	No cognitive outcome assessed	No functional improvement	Increased rate in mortality, hypertension, increased risk of infection, raised intraocular pressure, Cushing's syndrome, peptic ulcer, osteoporosis, myopathy, diabetes mellitus type 2, pancreatitis, sodium and water retention, psychosis, glaucoma, cardiomyopathy

Cyclosporine A [8,9,17,18]	Suppressive	Reduces alteration of mitochondrial function, inhibits lipid peroxidation and free radical oxidative damage	Down-regulation of brain BDNF and TrkB[19]	No improvement in MMSE scores at 3 and 6 months	No functional improvement at 3 and 6 months (GOSE)	Effects on the immune system after prolonged use.
Erythropoietin [8,9,20–21,22]	Suppressive	Limits excitotoxic effects; antioxidative, antiinflammatory effect	Increased neuronal network connectivity	No cognitive outcome assessed	Failed to show improvement of neurological outcome (GOSE)	Increased thromboembolic events, hypertension, hypertensive encephalopathy, seizures
Cerebrolysin [23–34]	Modulatory		Neuroprotective activity, neurotrophic function, increases neuronal survival, promotes neuritic outgrowth and cholinergic fiber regeneration	Improves MMSE, Cognitive Abilities Screening Instrument (CASI), and Short Cognitive Performance Test (SKT); reductions in slow quantitative electroencephalogram (qEEG) activity and an increase in fast frequencies.	Improves functional outcome (GOSE)	Headache, dizziness.
Citicoline [35]	Modulatory	Improves phosphatidylcholine synthesis, increases levels of glutathione, attenuates the release of arachidonic acid, cardiolipin, and sphingomyelin	Enhances neurorecovery (increases dopamine levels)	No improvement TBI-Clinical Trials Network Core Battery (9 scales)	No improvement on GOSE	Headache, insomnia, hypertension
Nitric oxide synthase inhibitor 4 aminotetrahydrobiopten (VAS203) [8,36]	Suppressive	Inhibition of NO-mediated cascade		No cognitive outcome assessed	Improvement of GOSE scores at 6 month	Acute kidney injury

(continued)

Table 27.1: Continued

Pharmacological Agents	Neuroprotective Mechanisms of Action	Suppressive/ Modulatory Activity	Effects on Other Edas	Cognitive Outcome	General Outcome	Adverse Events
Glibenclamide, glyburide[8,9,37]	Reduces edema, inflammation, apoptosis, lesion size, and secondary hemorrhages	Suppressive		No cognitive outcome assessed	No improvement in neurological outcome	Hypoglycemia, jaundice
NNZ-2566, synthetic analog of a peptide derived from insulin-like growth factor-1 (ongoing study)[38]	Inhibits neuroinflammation and proinflammatory cytokine expression	Suppressive	Reduces the level of expression of genes associated with inflammation, necrosis, and apoptosis; inhibits activation of microglia	Cognitive and neuropsychological assessment will be performed	GOSE will be assessed and activities of daily living	
Nerve growth factor (ongoing study)[39]	Increases antioxidant activity and reduces injuries induced by oxygen-free radicals	Modulatory	Promotes neuronal survival and plasticity	Hamilton Anxiety Scale, Hamilton Depression Scale will be assessed	Neurological function will be assessed by GOS, mRS, Barthel Index	Headache, dizziness, gastrointestinal discomfort, pain at site of injection
N-acetylcysteine in combination with probenecid (ongoing study)[40]	Antioxidant activity by increasing glutathione levels and decreasing the oxidative damage; antiinflammatory and anti-apoptotic action	Suppressive	Promotes neuronal survival	No cognitive outcome assessed	Drug safety will be assessed, antioxidant reserve in serum and cerebral spinal fluid	

BDNF, brain-derived neurotrophic factor; GOSE, Glasgow Outcome Scale Extended; ICAM-1, intercellular adhesion molecule; IL-6, interleukin 6; MMSE, Mini-Mental State Examination; TNFα, tumor necrosis factor-α; VEGF, vascular endothelial growth factor.

Chemical and physical agents are being tested alone or in combination (e.g., stem cells combined with nanoparticles, stem cells and flavonoids, polylactide-co-glycolide-labeled nanoparticles associated with neurotrophic agents), and the combinations show more pleiotropic effects than single agents, especially if used with a BBB-permeable carrier.[47,51,52,64]

However, the failure to translate experimental results into clinical studies was alarming and hinted at several potential problems, including the use of simplistic injury models that do not reflect the complexity of secondary injury; the oversight of the genetic, biochemical, and proteomic heterogeneity that normally exists in patients; and the use of outcome measures that do not reflect the multidimensional aspects of TBI outcome in humans.[65]

Other Neuroprotective Therapies

Hyperbaric oxygen could be a promising therapy by acting concomitantly on different pathways, with synergic effects on inflammation, apoptosis, intracranial pressure (ICP), neuroregeneration, and angiogenesis.[66] Additionally, it modulates multiple levels—epigenetic, molecular,[67,68] structural,[69] and functional.[66] However, the results of experimental and clinical trials are conflicting, and there are still questions to answer regarding the therapeutic time window and hyperbaric oxygen administration—length of treatment course, toxic dose, frequency, or the adequate safe pressure.[66,67]

Using stem cells to modulate neurogenesis could be another approach to promote neuroregeneration in TBI. Knowing that there is physiological cell proliferation in the subventricular zone and hippocampal dentate gyrus after TBI, one method boosts this process with the use of growth factors, statins, erythropoietin, or antidepressants.[69] Likewise, transplanted stem cells act through two different mechanisms: by differentiation into new neurons[70] and by secretion of trophic and immunomodulatory factors that promote differentiation of endogenous stem cells.[71] However, the intravenous administration of stem cells showed a preference for migrating to the spleen. As a result, intracerebroventricular transplantation could show better results. In addition, the joint use of stem cells with antiinflammatory substances (minocycline, melatonin), statins,[71] growth factors,[72] or hyperbaric oxygen[73,74] could provide even better outcomes. Currently, there are several ongoing clinical studies showing good preliminary results regarding safety, while the efficacy of these treatments requires more investigation.

Preclinical studies using hypothermia showed significantly beneficial synergic effects in TBI by acting simultaneously at the structural, functional, and molecular levels on ICP, necroptosis, inflammation, or neurogenesis.[75–77] Nevertheless, the clinical trials showed conflicting results. Some single-center trials showed therapeutic hypothermia to have neuroprotective effects in TBI, but several meta-analyses were unable to prove its efficacy in decreasing mortality or unfavorable clinical outcomes, and, moreover, it increased the risk of developing respiratory and cardiac complications.[78–80]

Conclusion

The failure of clinical trials to find an effective neuroprotective therapy changed the old views of the "magic bullet" and "one size fits all" approach. There are many pathological pathways that can be modulated or significantly disturbed by pharmacological approaches, and the lack of their integration into a common pathological integrative "picture" and the difficulty of determining the mechanisms that result in more benefits than the apparent damage keep us on a long road to find a good solution. These include the failure of anti-N-methyl-D-aspartate (NMDA) drugs believed to inhibit excitotoxity while NMDA system activation plays an adaptive and compensatory role in the TBI acute phase; failure of barbiturate-induced coma, although it helped in reducing ICP in 69% of patients; lack of improvement in mortality after mannitol administration, although it showed an increase in brain oxygenation by edema reduction; and failure of dexamethasone use in TBI patients.

The new concept of using pleiotropic multimodal molecules to provide neuroprotection is conforming to the theory of the degeneracy of complex biological systems. Such systems, as the brain is considered to be, are characterized by a nonlinear dynamic behavior, oscillating between plasticity and stability. Degeneracy represents "the ability of elements that are structurally different to perform the same function or yield the same output."[81] This capacity of biological systems to compensate for the failure of one process by substituting other processes that lead to the same result determines robustness. However, under pathological conditions, robustness is responsible for chronic phenotypes.[82] Other characteristics of living systems are the dynamic intercorrelations and interdependencies between subsystems—in our case, between molecular, cellular, and local circuits and large-scale network levels. This view on pathological processes that occur after insults such as TBI improves our understanding of why a therapeutic approach that manipulates only one dysfunctional mechanism is not capable of sustaining neuroprotection. A more feasible approach appears to be a combination therapy, either involving several pharmacological compounds (characterized by pleiotropic, multimodal mechanisms of action), with the potential disadvantage of the accumulation of adverse effects, or an association between different pharmacological and nonpharmacological approaches.

References

1. Muresanu DF, Buzoianu A, Florian SI, von Wild T. Towards a roadmap in brain protection and recovery. *J Cell Mol Med*. 2012;16(12):2861–2871. doi:10.1111/j.1582-4934.2012.01605.x.

2. Faden AI, Wu J, Stoica BA, Loane DJ. Progressive inflammation-mediated neurodegeneration after traumatic brain or spinal cord injury. *Br J Pharmacol*. 2016;173(4):681–691. doi:10.1111/bph.13179.

3. Hawryluk GW, Bullock MR. Past, present, and future of traumatic brain injury research. *Neurosurg Clin N Am*. 2016;27(4):375–396. doi:10.1016/j.nec.2016.05.002.

4. Maas AI, Harrison-Felix CL, Menon D, et al. Common data elements for traumatic brain injury: recommendations from the interagency working group on demographics and clinical assessment. *Archiv Phys Med Rehabil*. 2010;91(11):1641–1649. doi:10.1016/j.apmr.2010.07.232.

5. Bagiella E, Novack TA, Ansel B, et al. Measuring outcome in traumatic brain injury treatment trials: recommendations from the traumatic brain injury clinical trials network. *J Head Trauma Rehabil*. 2010;25(5): 375–382.doi:10.1097/HTR.0b013e3181d27fe3.

6. Poon W, Vos P, Muresanu DF, et al. Cerebrolysin Asian Pacific trial in acute brain injury and neurorecovery: design and methods. *J Neurotrauma*. 2015;32(8):571–580. doi:10.1089/neu.2014.3558.

7. Sanchez-Aguilar M, Tapia-Perez JH, Sanchez-Rodriguez JJ, et al. Effect of rosuvastatin on cytokines after traumatic head injury. *J Neurosurg*. 2013;118(3):669–675. doi:10.3171/2012.12.JNS121084.

8. Gruenbaum SE, Zlotnik A, Gruenbaum BF, et al. Pharmacologic neuroprotection for functional outcomes after traumatic brain injury: a systematic review of the clinical literature. *CNS Drugs*.2016;30:791. doi:10.1007/s40263-016-0355-2.

9. Kabadi SV, Faden AI. Neuroprotective strategies for traumatic brain injury: improving clinical translation. *Int J Mol Sci*. 2014;15(1):1216–1236. doi:10.3390/ijms15011216.

10. Shakeri M, Boustani MR, Mahdkhah A. Effect of progesterone administration on prognosis of patients with diffuse axonal injury due to severe head trauma. *Neurosurg Q*. 2013;24(4):282–5. doi:10.1016/j.clineuro.2013.06.013.

11. Skolnick BE, Maas AI, Narayan RK, et al. A clinical trial of progesterone for severe traumatic brain injury. *N Engl J Med*. 2014;371(26):2467–76. doi:10.1056/NEJMoa1411090.

12. Wright DW, Kellermann AL, Hertzberg VS, Clark PL, Frankel M, Goldstein FC, et al. ProTECT: a randomized clinical trial of progesterone for acute traumatic brain injury. *Ann Emerg Med*. 2007;49(4):391–402 (e1–2). doi:10.1016/j.annemergmed.2006.07.932.

13. Bailey I, Bell A, Gray J, et al. A trial of the effect of nimodipine on outcome after head injury. *Acta Neurochir*.1191;110:97–105. doi:10.1007/bf01400674.

14. Harders A, Kakarieka A, Braakman R. German tSAH Study Group. *J Neurosurg*. 1996;85:82–89. doi:10.3171/jns.1996.85.1.0082.

15. Kim JJ, Diamond DM. The stressed hippocampus, synaptic plasticity and lost memories. *Nat Rev Neurosci*. 2002;3:453–462.

16. Mitra R, Sapolsky RM. Acute corticosterone treatment is sufficient to induce anxiety and amygdaloid dendritic hypertrophy. *Proc Natl Acad Sci USA*. 2008;105:5573–5578.

17. Mazzeo AT, Brophy GM, Gilman CB, et al. Safety and tolerability of cyclosporin A in severe traumatic brain injury patients: results from a prospective randomized trial. *J Neurotrauma*. 2009;26(12):2195–2206. doi:10.1089/neu.2009.1012

18. Aminmansour B, Fard SA, Habibabadi MR, Moein P, Norouzi R, Naderan M. The efficacy of cyclosporine-A on diffuse axonal injury after traumatic brain injury. *Adv Biomed Res*. 2014;3:35. doi:10.4103/2277-9175.125031.

19. Chen CC, Hsu LW, Huang LT, Huang TL. Chronic administration of cyclosporine A changes expression of BDNF and TrkB in rat hippocampus and midbrain. *Neurochem Res*. 2010;35(7):1098–1104. doi:10.1007/s11064-010-0160-0.

20. Robertson CS, Hannay HJ, Yamal JM, et al. Effect of erythropoietin and transfusion threshold on neurological recovery after traumatic brain injury: a randomized clinical trial. *JAMA*. 2014;312(1):36–47. doi:10.1001/jama.2014.6490.

21. Aloizos S, Evodia E, Gourgiotis S, Isaia EC, Seretis C, Baltopoulos GJ. Neuroprotective effects of erythropoietin in patients with severe closed brain injury. *Turk Neurosurg*. 2015;25(4):552–558. doi:10.5137/1019-5149.JTN.9685-14.4.

22. Nichol A, French C, Little L, et al. Erythropoietin in traumatic brain injury (EPO-TBI): a double-blind randomised controlled trial. *Lancet*. 2015;386(10012):2499–2506. doi:10.1016/S0140-6736(15)00386-4.

23. Chen CC, Wei ST, Tsaia SC, Chen XX, Cho DY. Cerebrolysin enhances cognitive recovery of mild traumatic brain injury patients: double-blind, placebo-controlled, randomized study. *Br J Neurosurgery*. 2013 Dec;27(6):803–7. doi:10.3109/02688697.2013.793287.

24. Muresanu DF, Ciurea AV, Gorgan RM, et al. A retrospective, multi-center cohort study evaluating the severity- related effects of cerebrolysin treatment on clinical outcomes in traumatic brain injury. *CNS Neurol Disord Drug Target.* 2015;14(5):587–599.

25. Wong GK, Zhu XL, Poon WS. Beneficial effect of cerebrolysin on moderate and severe head injury patients: result of a cohort study. *Acta Neurochir Suppl.* 2005;95:59–60.

26. Khalili h, Niakan A, Ghaffar PF. Effects of cerebrolysin on functional recovery in patients with severe disability after traumatic brain injury: a historical cohort study. *Clin Neurol Neurosurg.* 2017;152:34–38. doi:10.1016/j.clineuro.2016.11.011.

27. König P, Waanders R, Witzmann, A, et al. Cerebrolysin in traumatic brain injury. A pilot study of a neurotrophic and neurogenic agent in the treatment of acute traumatic brain injury. *J Neurol Neurochir Psychiatr.* 2006;7(3):12–20.

28. Wang M, Liu S, Xie C. The effect observation of head injury treated with Cerebrolysin. *J Xian Med Univ.* 1998;19(4):2–4.

29. Fei Z, Shenyui YI. Changes of free radicals in the plasma of patients with craniocerebral trauma and therapeutic effect of Cerebrolysin. *Chinese J Nerv Mental Dis.*1992;18:6.

30. Zhou D, Yang S. Effect of Cerebrolysin on acute brain injury patients. *Zhong Hua Chuang Shang.* 1993;9:289–290.

31. Duma ST, Mutz N. Efficacy of a peptide dextran combination (CEREDEX) in the treatment of brain injuries. *Neuropsychiatrie.* 1990;4(2):69–72.

32. Onose G, Mureşanu DF, Ciurea AV, et al. Neuroprotective and consequent neurorehabilitative clinical outcomes, in patients treated with the pleiotropic drug cerebrolysin. *J Med Life.* 2009;2(4):350–360.

33. Alvarez XA, Sampedro C, Pérez P, et al. Positive effects of cerebrolysin on electroencephalogram slowing, cognition and clinical outcome in patients with postacute traumatic brain injury: an exploratory study. *Int Clin Psychopharmacol.* 2003;18(5):271–278.

34. Alvarez XA, Sampedro C, Figueroa J, et al. Reductions in qEEG slowing over 1 year and after treatment with Cerebrolysin in patients with moderate-severe traumatic brain injury. *J Neural Transm (Vienna).* 2008;115(5):683–692. doi:10.1007/s00702-008-0024-9.

35. Zafonte RD, Bagiella E, Ansel BM, et al. Effect of citicoline on functional and cognitive status among patients with traumatic brain injury: Citicoline Brain Injury Treatment Trial (COBRIT). *JAMA.* 2012;308(19):1993–2000. doi:10.1001/jama.2012.13256.

36. Stover JF, Belli A, Boret H, et al. Nitric oxide synthase inhibition with the antipterin VAS203 improves outcome in moderate and severe traumatic brain injury: a placebo-controlled randomized phase II trial (NOSTRA). *J Neurotrauma.* 2014;31(19):1599–1606 (October 1, 2014). doi:10.1089/neu.2014.3344.

37. Ding J, Yuan F, Guo JY, Chen H, Tian HL. Influence of glibenclamide on outcome in patients with type 2 diabetes and traumatic brain injury. *Clin Neurol Neurosurg.* 2013;115(10):2166–2169. doi:10.1016/j.clineuro.2013.08.010.

38. Xiong Y, Zhang Y, Mahmood A, Chopp M. Investigational agents for treatment of traumatic brain injury. *Exp Opin Invest Drugs.* 2015;24(6):743–760. doi:10.1517/13543784.2015.1021919.

39. Zhao M, Li X, Xu C, Zou L. Efficacy and safety of nerve growth factor for the treatment of neurological diseases: a meta-analysis of 64 randomized controlled trials involving 6,297 patients. *Neural Regen Res.* 2015;10(5):819–828. doi:10.4103/1673-5374.156989.

40. Kochanek PM, Jackson TC, Ferguson NM, et al. Emerging therapies in traumatic brain injury. *Semin Neurol.* 2015;35(1):83–100. doi:10.1055/s-0035-1544237.

41. Muresanu DF, Heiss WD, Hoemberg V, et al. Cerebrolysin and Recovery After Stroke (CARS): a randomized, placebo-controlled, double-blind, multicenter trial. *Stroke*. 2016;47(1):151–159. doi:10.1161/STROKEAHA.115.009416.

42. Rothmann MD, Wiens BL, Chan ISF. *Design and Analysis of Non-Inferiority Trials*. Chapman and Hall/ CRC Press, Taylor & Francis Group; 2011.

43. Simon D, McGeachy M, Bayir H, Clark R, Loane D, Kochanek P. The far reaching neuroinflammation after traumatic brain injury. *Nat Rev Neurol*. 2017;13(3):171–191. doi:10.1038/nrneurol.2017.13.

44. Wang L, Wang X, Su H, et al. Recombinant human erythropoietin improves the neurofunctional recovery of rats following traumatic brain injury via increase in circulating endothelial progenitor cells. *Transl Stroke Res*. 2013;6(1):50–59. doi:10.1007/s12975-014-0362-x.

45. Diaz- Arrastia R, Kochanek P, Bergold P, et al. Pharmacotherapy of traumatic brain injury: state of the science and the road forward: report of the Department of Defense Neurotrauma Pharmacology Workgroup. *J Neurotrauma*. 2014;31(2):135–158. doi:10.1089/neu.2013.3019.

46. Álvarez XA, Figueroa J, Muresanu DF. Peptidergic drugs for the treatment of traumatic brain injury. *Future Neurol*. 2013;8(2):175–192. doi:10.2217/fnl.12.95.

47. Tobinik E. Author's reply to Page "Selective TNF inhibition for chronic stroke and traumatic brain injury: an observational study involving 629 consecutive patients treated with perispinal etanercept." *CNS Drugs*. 2013;27(5):399–402. doi:10.1007/s40263-012-0013-2.

48. Nguyen BM, Kim D, Bricker S, et al. Effect of marijuana use on outcomes in traumatic brain injury. *Am Surg*. 2014;80(10):979–983.

49. Lopez-Rodriguez A, Acaz-Fonseca E, Viveros M, Garcia-Segura L. Changes in cannabinoid receptors, aquaporin 4 and vimentin expression after traumatic brain injury in adolescent male mic3. Association with edema and neurological deficit. *Plos One*. 2015;10(6):012872. doi:10.1371/journal.pone.0128782.

50. Johnson BN, Palmer CP, Bourgeois EB, Elkind JA, Putnam BJ, Cohen AS. Augmented inhibition from cannabinoid-sensitive interneurons diminishes CA1 output after traumatic brain injury. *Front Cell Neurosci*. 2014;8:435. doi:10.3389/fncel.2014.00435.

51. Li X, Tzeng S, Liu X, et al. Nanoparticle-mediated transcriptional modification enhances neuronal differentiation of human neural stem cells following transplantation in rat brain. *Biomaterials*. 2016;84:157–166. doi:10.1016/j.biomaterials.2016.01.037.

52. Ullah F, Liang A, Rangel A, Gyengesi E, Niedermayer G, Münch G. High bioavailability curcumin: an anti-inflammatory and neurosupportive bioactive nutrient for neurodegenerative diseases characterized by chronic neuroinflammation [published online ahead of print, February 15, 2017]. *Arch Toxicol*. doi:10.1007/s00204-017-1939-4.

53. Toklu HZ, Hakan T, Biber N, Solakoğlu S, Oğünç AV, Sener G. The protective effect of alpha lipoic acid against traumatic brain injury in rats. *Free Radic Res*. 2009;43(7):658–667. doi:10.1080/10715760902988843.

54. Y. Su, W. Fan, Z. Ma, et al. Taurine improves functional and histological outcomes and reduces inflammation in traumatic brain injury. *Neuroscience*. 2014;266:56–65. doi:10.1016/j.

55. Ohta M, Higashi Y, Yawata T, Kitahara M, Nobumoto A, Ishida E. Attenuation of axonal injury and oxidative stress by ederavone protects against cognitive impairments after traumatic brain injury. *Brain Res*. 2013;1490:184–192. doi:10.1016/j.brainres.2012.09.011.

56. Jeong S, Lei B, Wang H, Dawson H, James M. Intravenous immunoglobulin G improves neurobehavioral and histological outcomes after traumatic brain injury in mice. *J Neuroimmunol.* 2014;276(1-2):112–118. doi:10.1016/j.jneuroim.2014.08.626.

57. Crack P, Zhang M, Morganti-Kossmann M. Anti-lysophosphatodic acid antibodies improve traumatic brain injury outcomes. *J Neuroinflammation.* 2014;11(1):37. doi:10.1186/1742-2094-11-37.

58. Shenaq M, Kassem H, Peng C. Neuronal damage and functional deficits re ameliorated by inhibition of aquaporin and H1F1α after traumatic brain injury (TBI). *J Neurol Sci.* 2012;323(1-2): 134–140. doi:10.1016/j.jns.2012.08.036.

59. Russo MV, McGavern DB: Inflammatory neuroprotection following traumatic brain injury. *Science.* 2016;353(6301):783–785. doi:10.1126/science.aaf6260.

60. Sun W, Liu J, Huan Y, Zhang C. Intracranial injection of recombinant stromal-derived factor-1 alpha (SDF-1 α) attenuates traumatic brain injury in rats. *Inflamm Res.* 2013;63(4):287–297. doi:10.1007/s00011-013-0699-8.

61. Okuma Y, Date I, Nishibori M. Anti-high mobility group box-1 antibody therapy for traumatic brain injury. *Yakugaru Zasshi.* 2014;134(6): 701–705. doi:10.1248/yakushi.13-00255-2.

62. Maas A, Rozenbeek B, Manley G. Clinical trials in traumatic brain injury: past experience and current developments. *Neurotherapeutics.* 2010;7(1):115–126. doi:10.1016/j.nurt.2009.10.022.

63. De RiveroVaccari JP, Lotocki G, Alonso OF, Bramlett HM, Dietrich WD, Keane RW. Therapeutic neutralization of the NLRP1 inflammasome reduces the innate immune response and improves histopathology after traumatic brain injury. *J Cereb Blood Flow Metab.* 2009;29(7):1251–1261. doi:10.1038/jcbfm.2009.46.

64. Ruozi B, Belletti D, Sharma HS, Sharma A, Muresanu DF, et al. PLGA nanoparticles loaded cerebrolysin: studies on their preparation and investigation of the effect of storage and serum stability with reference to traumatic brain injury. *Mol Neurobiol.* 2015;52:899–912. doi:10.1007/s12035-015-9235-x.

65. Loane DJ, Stoica BA, Faden AI. Neuroprotection for traumatic brain injury. *Handb Clin Neurol.* 2015;127:343–366. doi:10.1016/B978-0-444-52892-6.00022-2.

66. Hu Q, Manaenko A, Xu T, Guo ZN, Tang JP, Zhang JH. Hyperbaric oxygen therapy for traumatic brain injury: bench-to-bedside. *Med Gas Res.* 2016;6(2):102–110. doi:10.4103/2045-9912.184720.

67. Harch PG. Hyperbaric oxygen in chronic traumatic brain injury: oxygen, pressure, and gene therapy. *Med Gas Res.* 2015;5:9. doi:10.1186/s13618-015-0030-6.

68. Meng XE, Zhang Y, Li N, et al. Effects of hyperbaric oxygen on the Nrf2 signaling pathway in secondary injury following traumatic brain injury. *Genet Mol Res.* 2016;15(1). doi:10.4238/gmr.15016933.

69. Sun D. Endogenous neurogenic cell response in the mature mammalian brain following traumatic injury. *Exp Neurol.* 2016;275(03):405–410. doi:10.1016/j,expneurol.2015.04.

70. Maskouri S, Crowley MG, Liska MG, Corey S, Borlongan CV. Utilizing pharmacotherapy and mesenchymal stem cell therapy to reduce inflammation following traumatic brain injury. *Neural Regen Res.* 2016;11(9):1379–1384. doi:10.4103/1673-5374.191197.

71. Dori I, Petrakis S, Giannakopoulou A, et al. Seven days post-injury fate and effects of genetically labelled adipose-derived mesenchymal cells on a rat traumatic brain injury experimental model. *Histol Histopathol.* 2016;32(10):1041–1055. doi:10.14670/HH-11-864.

72. Duan H, Li X, Wang C, et al. Functional hyaluronate collagen scaffolds induce NSCs differentiation into functional neurons in repairing the traumatic brain injury. *Acta Biomater.* 2016;45:182–195. doi:10.1016/j.actbio.2016.08.043.

73. Eve DJ, Steele MR, Sanberg PR, Borlongan CV. Hyperbaric oxygen therapy as a potential treatment for post-traumatic stress disorder associated with traumatic brain injury. *Neuropsychiatr Dis Treat.* 2016;12:2689–2705. doi:10.2147/NDT.S110126.

74. Zhou H-X, Liu Z-G, Liu X-J, Chen Q-X. Umbilical cord-derived mesenchymal stem cell transplantation combined with hyperbaric oxygen treatment for repair of traumatic brain injury. *Neural Regen Res.* 2016;11(1):107–113. doi:10.4103/1673-5374.175054.

75. Hirst TC, Watzlawick R, Rhodes JK, Macleod MR, Andrews PJD. Study protocol—a systematic review and meta-analysis of hypothermia in experimental traumatic brain injury: why have promising animal studies not been replicated in pragmatic clinical trials? *Evid Based Preclin Med.* 2016;3(2):e00020. doi:10.1002/ebm2.20.

76. Liu T, Zhao D, Cui H, et al. Therapeutic hypothermia attenuates tissue damage and cytokine expression after traumatic brain injury by inhibiting necroptosis in the rat. *Sci Rep.* 2016;6:24547. doi:10.1038/srep24547.

77. Chen C, Ma TZ, Wang LN, et al. Mild hypothermia facilitates the long-term survival of newborn cells in the dentate gyrus after traumatic brain injury by diminishing a pro-apoptotic microenvironment. *Neuroscience.* 2016;335:114–121. doi:10.1016/j.neuroscience.2016.08.038.

78. Zhu Y, Yin H, Zhang R, Ye X, Wei J. Therapeutic hypothermia versus normothermia in adult patients with traumatic brain injury: a meta-analysis. *Springerplus.* 2016;5:801. doi:10.1186/s40064-016-2391-2.

79. Yokobori S, Yokota H. Targeted temperature management in traumatic brain injury. *J Intens Care.* 2016;4:28. doi:10.1186/s40560-016-0137-4.

80. Dunkley S, Mcleod A. Therapeutic hypothermia in patients following traumatic brain injury: a systematic review. *Nurs Crit Care.* 2016;doi:10.1111/nicc.12242.

81. Edelman GM, Gally JA. Degeneracy and complexity in biological systems. *Proc Natl Acad Sci USA.* 2001;98:13763–13768. doi:10.1073/pnas.231499798.

82. Ratté S, Prescott SA. Afferent hyperexcitability in neuropathic pain and the inconvenient truth about its degeneracy. *Curr Opin Neurobiol.* 2016;36:31–37. doi:10.1016/j.conb.2015.08.007.

Bioengineering in Brain Trauma Research

Michelle C. LaPlaca

28

Role of Bioengineering in Neurotrauma

Bioengineering (and *biomedical engineering*) can broadly be defined as the application of engineering principles to biological and medical problems in order to understand, interact with, and/or influence function. In the early days of bioengineering, the brain was largely considered a black box, meaning that engineers focused on failure modes rather than correlating forces with brain function. Since that time, not only have engineering and computational science evolved, but biology and medicine have also intertwined with engineering principles to a point where modern bioengineers are truly interdisciplinary. Today, bioengineering has helped to inform basic scientists and clinicians about injury tolerances, interactions of secondary mechanisms, and measurement of brain function. Many bioengineers who study the nervous system consider themselves neuroengineers.

Bioengineering and neuroengineering are both very multidisciplinary, incorporating several engineering and bioscience domains. *Bioengineering subdisciplines* that pertain to neurotrauma research and clinical translation are electrical engineering, biomechanics and biotransport, material science, and physiology and neuroscience.

- *Electrical engineering*: Electrical engineering was a major influence on the evolution of bioengineering, specifically in biosignal detection and processing. Using neurobiology, which has a rich history in discovery of the electrical nature of the nervous system,[1] electrical engineers developed ways to detect signals from the brain and neurons. Medical imaging and biomedical optics also emerged from electrical engineering and involve techniques and approaches for indirect analysis of neural function.
- *Biomechanics and biotransport*: In 1943, Holbourn reported that brain rotation produced the shear strain in brain tissue that caused injury,[2] beginning the modern period of brain injury biomechanics. Measurement instruments and computational methods have become more sophisticated, making injury biomechanics a cornerstone of neurotrauma research. Biomechanical approaches are used to develop injury tolerance criteria spanning from molecular to macroscopic scales. Biotransport (i.e., mass transport and fluid mechanics) is a subdiscipline closely related to biomechanics that is critical for studying blood flow in the brain, molecular flux across barriers, edema, and drug delivery.
- *Material science*: Brain is a very complex living material, presenting an interesting challenge, especially in the large-deformation, high-loading rate scenarios of traumatic

brain injury (TBI). Material science is important in studying material properties of the brain as well as in the development of biomaterials for brain interfacing (e.g., electrodes) and regenerative scaffolds.[3] In addition, material science includes aspects of applied neurotrauma research such as safety engineering and sports engineering.

- *Physiology and neuroscience*: Physiology is a core pillar in bioengineering, and the term is used loosely here to encompass molecular and cell biology as well as systems physiology. It is important to consider how TBI affects other organs given the interdependence among body systems. Neuroscience, in particular, is a central discipline in neurotrauma research and spans from molecular to systems neuroscience. Most bioengineers who study TBI also have training in neuroscience.

Bioengineering approaches in neurotrauma research and clinical applications can be divided into observation, measurement, and simulation of real-world injury situations (e.g., video analysis, football helmet sensors, reconstruction using anthropomorphic test dummies, computer simulation), the development and validation of scaled injury surrogates (e.g., preclinical cell and animal models, computer simulation), the development of research and clinical tools and technologies (e.g., preclinical drug testing, optogenetics, diagnostics, monitoring tools), investigations of injury mechanisms and reparative strategies (e.g., pharmacologic, regenerative, therapeutic), and data science and bioinformatics applied to both research and clinical data.

The study of TBI requires a multimodal approach to confront the associated complexity and heterogeneity (Figure 28.1). We will take into account these bioengineering principles and approaches as we address some of the challenges facing the neurotrauma field through the following topics: (1) a material description of the brain, (2) biomechanics of neurotrauma, (3) human surrogates for neurotrauma research, and (4) emerging bioengineering concepts and technologies for neurotrauma research.

A Material Description of the Brain

Brain is a multiphasic material, meaning that it has both solid and fluid components, with unique electrochemical, electrophysiological, and material properties.[4] Additionally, brain is a soft porous tissue that is approximately the density of water and composed of cells, fluids, and extracellular matrix (ECM). Brain cells have different material properties depending on the tissue density, number and length of processes, degree of myelination, and orientation. These differences can contribute to stress and strain incongruities at interfaces such as gray and white matter. The ECM within brain tissue is mostly nonfibrillar glycosaminoglycans, which is in contrast to the fibrillary matrix in peripheral soft tissues, contributing to the relatively low elastic modulus and high compliance of brain (i.e., its "softness").[5,6]

The fluid portion of the brain is divided among the interstitial fluid (ISF), cerebrospinal fluid (CSF), and the blood, with controlled movement between compartments. Fluid dynamics and molecular flux between compartments can be mathematically described using compartmental models. Interestingly, the selective permeability of the blood–brain barrier (BBB) limits hydrostatically driven bulk flow from the capillaries to the brain, making oncotic forces dominant, unlike other capillary beds.[7] Furthermore, the fixed charge density of the tissue favors water influx. Following TBI, cell damage

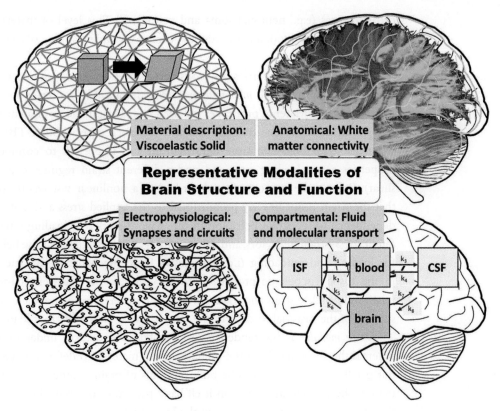

Figure 28.1 The brain can be modeled in many different ways depending on the information needed. Representative modalities include a nonlinear viscoelastic solid (*top left*), where material properties are assigned and then the stress and strain patterns can be computed. Anatomic heterogeneity is important for examining features like connectivity of white matter (as shown in the diffusion tensor image, *top right*) or evolving lesions. Electrophysiological representations can use neuron- to network-level analysis (*bottom left*). Electrochemical and biotransport descriptions are useful to describe molecular flux and water movement following traumatic brain injury (*bottom right*).

From DTI by Creative Commons Attribution 2.0 Generic license.

https://commons.wikimedia.org/wiki/File:Connectome.jpg; Author: jgmarcelino from New castle upon Tyne, UK; FE mesh by Oleg Alexandrov, self-made, with en:Matlab, Public Domain, https://commons.wikimedia.org/w/index.php?curid=2245302

exposes negatively charged proteins, which, together with increased permeability of the BBB, can exacerbate water flux and contribute to edema.[7]

Overall, brain is nonhomogeneous and anisotropic (i.e., its properties depend on orientation), qualities that are important for describing how a material responds to loading. The gray matter contains mostly cell bodies and forms the cerebral cortex and underlying nuclei, while the white matter consists of highly aligned, mostly myelinated axons. Not only is the brain visually anatomically nonhomogeneous, but the material properties also are variable (or heterogeneous) across the brain. White matter is highly oriented and therefore has higher anisotropy compared to gray matter and different material properties. In addition to the degree of anisotropy, material properties vary with specific brain region, species, and age.[8,9] On a smaller scale, there are differences in material properties between cells types (e.g., neurons and astrocytes) and even within cell structures (e.g., neuronal soma and process).[4,10] This level of material complexity requires multiscale modeling in order to advance an understanding of the brain response to loading.[11]

When material properties are considered in the context of mechanical loading conditions, they are called *mechanical properties*, though the two terms are regularly used interchangeably. Material properties are used in analytical and computational models of TBI to understand force transduction and tolerance criteria. Since TBI is most often associated with high-rate large deformation, it is important to consider mechanical properties across loading rates and under different strain regimes (e.g., compression, shear). Brain tissue is most often described as a nonlinear viscoelastic solid, meaning that the strain is not linearly proportional to the applied stress and that there is a time dependence to the strain behavior. In other words, different loading rates result in different stress–strain behaviors, and dampening is exhibited such that the behavior changes for loading and unloading (i.e., hysteresis). Fluid mechanical properties are captured in the tissue viscoelastic properties, contributing to the rate sensitivity. Constitutive relationships relate stress and strain through the material moduli, which measure the resistance of the material to deform (i.e., the stiffness) under different loading conditions. The *bulk modulus* is the tendency for a material to deform under uniform loading, whereas the *shear modulus* is the tendency for a material to deform when two opposite but parallel forces act on it. The bulk modulus of brain is orders of magnitude higher than its shear modulus. The brain itself has a pre-stress (or residual stress), which means that there is a non-zero stress state in the brain under normal conditions,[12] an important consideration for ex vivo measurements of material properties. In addition, injured tissue changes mechanical properties, providing a basis for reduced thresholds and vulnerability in repeated loading.[13]

Material properties vary with physiologic (species, age, disease state) and anatomic factors (e.g., gray vs. white matter, cortex versus hippocampus).[9,14–18] The type of mechanical testing (e.g., compression, shear), residual stress, and loading conditions (e.g., strain rate, frequency) is also important when comparing mechanical properties. Test conditions during mechanical property testing such as postmortem time, temperature, hydration, and anisotropy also can introduce additional variables.[16] It is especially important to determine mechanical properties at rates representative of TBI.[19]

Biomechanics of Neurotrauma

Biomechanics relates the forces on the head to the movement of the head and resulting stress and strain in the tissue (Figure 28.2). Biomechanics is critical to developing tolerance criteria for safety engineering and a better understanding of force transduction to the brain. A conceptual understanding of injury biomechanics is helpful when measuring real-world injury scenarios, using animal models or computer simulations of TBI, or developing preventative and protective measures; other authors have provided more extensive coverage of injury biomechanics.[20–22]

Loading conditions refer to the parameters of the physical insult and include type of force, force magnitude, loading rate, area and direction of loading, and duration. The loading conditions associated with any particular TBI, however, are most often not known, and, when they are measured (e.g., helmet sensors) there are inherent

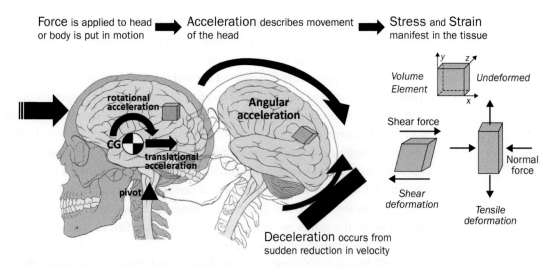

Figure 28.2 Traumatic brain injury is initiated by forces, or loads, to the head that surpass the structural and functional thresholds. Unless there is rigid support, the head will rotate, with the neck as a pivot. The movement can be expressed as velocity, or acceleration, followed by deceleration when the head is stopped. Angular acceleration is a combination of linear and pure rotational acceleration. The mechanical response of the tissue is the stress and strain. Shown is a volume element of the brain with shear stress and normal stress resulting in shear strain and tensile/compression strain, respectively.

From https://commons.wikimedia.org/wiki/File:Skull_and_brain_normal_human.svg]

limitations.[23,24] In addition, the loading conditions for each injury situation are unique and, when considered with heterogeneous factors among individuals, make generalizability difficult.

Loads to the head occur because of collision between the head and an obstruction (or an object striking the head; contact force) or a force to the body that causes the head to move (inertial force), or a combination of contact and inertial loading. Inertial force usually involves an impact that stops the movement; inertial-only loading is far less common. The energy in a collision is either released to the environment, transferred to the contacting object (e.g., ground, dashboard), stored or dissipated (e.g., helmet padding, airbag, skull), or transferred to the brain. The brain is softer than the skull; therefore, the brain continues to move (i.e., deform) longer than does the skull following an impact.

The initiating impact or jolt of the head will cause acceleration, whereas an impact that stops movement corresponds to deceleration. Translational acceleration occurs when the force vector travels straight through the center of gravity (CG). Pure rotational acceleration occurs when force causes the object to rotate about the CG. Angular acceleration is a combination of translational (or linear) and rotational acceleration when the force vector does not travel directly through the CG. The terms *angular* and *rotational* are routinely used interchangeably in TBI literature, with both typically referring to angular movement.

For a TBI to occur, the external load to the head must be transduced to the brain tissue. The insult level at which structural and functional compromise or failure takes place is an injury threshold and described by tolerance criteria. The mechanical response is the stress and strain in the tissue that results from load propagation. Stress represents the force distributed over an area, and the strain is a measure of the material deformation of that area. Stress and strain are determined by the force magnitude and loading rate, degree of force dissipation, the direction of applied force with respect to the geometry and orientation of the head and intracranial tissue, and the material properties of the tissue.

A volume element of the brain (usually a cube at the tissue scale) is used during mechanical analysis to remove some of the anatomical complexities and calculate the mechanical response for particular loading conditions and material properties. This concept is important for understanding finite element analysis, which is a common computational tool in injury biomechanics. For a three-dimensional volume element, the x-, y-, and z-axes are defined and geometrical planes are designated (e.g., x-y plane). Stresses and strains on the planes are described as vector quantities, such as principal stress and strain and maximum shear stress and strain.

In TBI, because of the nature of the loading and the soft brain tissue, the strains are large, or finite (as opposed to small, infinitesimal), and governed by finite strain theory. Furthermore, the anisotropy of the brain will cause complex strain patterns to emerge (i.e., combinations of positive normal tensile strain, negative normal compressive strain, and shear strain). Since the shear modulus of brain is higher than the bulk modulus, the brain will easier to deform in shear.

Primary damage may manifest in neurons, glial cells, and vascular cells as axonal stretching, membrane disruption, ion imbalance, interruption in normal conduction and synaptic transmission, and glial damage (nano- and microscale). At the tissue and organ level (meso- and macroscale), structural failure of the brain includes contusion, hemorrhage, and tears. Development of functional tolerance criteria requires understanding of the relationship among traumatic insult, mechanical response of the brain tissue, and the resulting injury cascades and neuropathology. While there are no simple threshold values to describe TBI, injury tolerance curves for translational contact loading have been established, with recent indices proposed to consider more complex loading scenarios.[25–27]

Human Surrogates for Neurotrauma Research

TBI models include human (volunteers, cadaver, anthropomorphic), animal, cell and tissue, and computational (e.g., finite element model [FEM]).[28] Using surrogates to study human TBI has the underlying premise that the surrogate, or model, will represent the human mechanically and pathophysiologically (for live surrogates), and, ideally, the findings should be model-independent. Human volunteers can inform the mechanical response to low-magnitude, low-rate head movements with anatomical appropriateness, yet the response is not easily extrapolated to traumatic levels due to the nonlinear properties of brain.[29] Traumatic loading can be applied to cadavers to study macroscale biomechanics on human tissue.[30,31] Model skulls can also be used for tracking motion and instrumented to physically measure strain and strain rate.[32,33] Anthropomorphic test dummies (e.g., Hybrid III, THOR) have been made for many different sized humans and are critical for motor vehicle safety testing and head impact studies.[34] While all of these methods capture the size and geometry of human anatomy, in order to assess the mechanics of living tissue under high-rate loading and the physiology associated with TBI, animals and cell models must be used.[35–39]

One of the significant advantages to using animal surrogates and computational modeling is the ability to control the loading conditions. The species and injury method should be chosen based on the type of injury (e.g., direct impact and/or inertial loading) and the question at hand.[40] For example, if large deformations are desired, it may be necessary to use a model with a craniectomy, while diffuse, mild injuries may be better represented by closed head injury models. The scaling of human injury to animals is far from linear and consideration should be given to brain mass, head-to-body mass ratio, mechanical properties, anatomy, quadrupedalism, gyrencephalic versus lissencephalic brains, and the physiologic differences.[41] Outcome measures should considered in the context of human deficits to facilitate translation.[40] In addition, the heterogeneity in preclinical animal models necessitates larger multilaboratory investigations and data sharing efforts.[42]

In vitro models of neurotrauma involve cell or slice preparations of brain that are cultured and subject to stretch, compression, or shear deformation.[43,44] Cell-level models allow simplification and control of the environment and can provide real-time sampling and monitoring as well as investigations of injury mechanisms.[45,46] Cell and tissue models are critical for determining cell-level tolerances.[47,48]

Computer modeling of TBI using FEM is a useful technique to link vary loading scenarios with tissue-level mechanical tolerances.[49,50] Anatomical structures such as the skull, intracranial membranes, and ventricles can be incorporated, as well as subregions and topological features like cortical sulci.[51] FEM are built using the concept of volume elements, where elements fill the geometrically defined brain and are assigned material properties. Loads can be applied to the model and the stresses and strains calculated and correlated with injury patterns.[52] It is critical to validate FEM[22] and compare across models as tolerance criteria are formed.[53] Recent advances in FEM modeling include using precomputed models to decrease time in calculations, potentially opening up the possibility of using results clinically.[54] In addition, multiscale details like axonal anisotropy or white matter microstructure can bridge FEM with axonal-level injury criteria and connectome-based network analyses.[11,55]

Emerging Bioengineering Concepts and Technologies

Bidirectional translational neurotrauma involves bioengineering at all levels, from moving laboratory discoveries to the clinic and using clinical findings as feedback to drive innovation. The eventual goal of translational research is to integrate diagnostics and treatments into clinical practice and to bring about effective health policy change at the community level. While many preclinical candidate treatments have failed,[56,57] these lessons drive investigators to delve into potential reasons for failure such as heterogeneity and surrogate model fidelity.

One of the challenges with positively impacting clinical practice is the inherent heterogeneity of TBI, from the biomechanics of the insult to the injury response. The diversity seen in the injury response is evident across both time scales and length scales (Figure 28.3). A data-driven approach is essential to understanding these dynamic and complex responses and in developing evidence-based clinical guidelines[58,59] to facilitate a personalized medicine approach to neurotrauma care. Traumanomics is a systems approach that entails combining individual characteristics and premorbid factors with

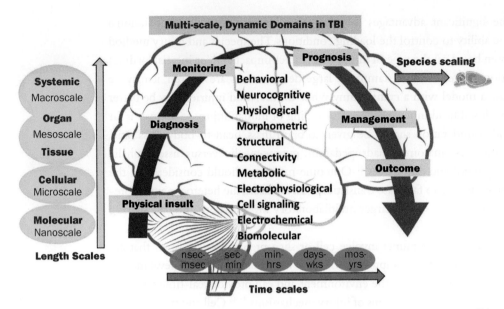

Figure 28.3 Both length and time scales are important to neurotrauma investigations. Functions at all levels contribute to overall outcome. Lengths scale range from nanoscale (molecules) to the macroscale, which involves the entire body. Traumatic loading occurs on the order of milliseconds to tens of milliseconds, with higher loading rates being more damaging than lower rates. The traumatic brain injury (TBI) response is very dynamic over time as both electrical and molecular signals change, affecting connectivity and overall metabolic and physiologic function. The stages of clinical TBI, from the insult to the outcome, involve complex dynamics across cellular and neurological domains that require a systems approach rather than linear examination of single metrics. All of this must also be taken into account when scaling from human to animals.

Rat brain from Creative Commons Zero 1.0 Public Domain License; Human brain and circuit.

injury variables, biomechanics, and outcome measures to create probabilistic models and drive new hypotheses. Data analytics methods such as machine learning can be used to analyze different types of data across time, rather than relying on a few separate metrics to guide diagnosis and clinical management.[60–62]

Data science approaches are needed to integrate multiple diagnosis tools and identify TBI subphenotypes. Fluid biomarkers and imaging both show promise in providing critical information, especially when combined with symptoms and other clinical measures. Particular challenges to fluid biomarkers are the sensitivity and specificity to TBI[63–65]; however, emerging technologies such as nanoprobes, multibiomarker panels, and better signal detection could be used to improve biomarker utility. Numerous advances in imaging have been made recently[66,60] and can be incorporated into a multifaceted diagnostic approach.

In summary, bioengineering is a broad engineering discipline that is a cornerstone of neurotrauma research. Bioengineering approaches to TBI traditionally have focused on biomechanics, including characterization of material properties, development of surrogate models, and determination of tolerance criteria. Engineering also influences diagnostic, monitoring, and reparative strategies in TBI research and clinical applications. These efforts continuously make use of improved technological and computational tools and will undoubtedly continue to have a positive impact on TBI research. And, finally, while heterogeneity is perhaps the biggest challenge the neurotrauma field faces, the incorporation of data science and informatics analyses provides an exciting opportunity to begin to unravel some of the complexity around TBI.

References

1. Yuste R. From the neuron doctrine to neural networks. *Nat Rev Neurosci.* 2015;16(8):487–497.
2. Holbourn AHS. Mechanics of head injury. *Lancet.* 1943;2:438–441.
3. Addington CP, Roussas A, Dutta D, Stabenfeldt SE. Endogenous repair signaling after brain injury and complementary bioengineering approaches to enhance neural regeneration. *Biomark Insights.* 2015(suppl 1):43.
4. Goriely A, Budday S, Kuhl E. Chapter two-neuromechanics: from neurons to brain. *Adv Appl Mech.* 2015;48:79–139.
5. Novak U, Kaye AH. Extracellular matrix and the brain: components and function. *J Clin Neurosci.* 2000;7(4):280–290.
6. Barnes JM, Przybyla L, Weaver VM. Tissue mechanics regulate brain development, homeostasis and disease. *J Cell Sci.* 2017;130(1):71–82.
7. Goriely A, Geers MG, Holzapfel GA, et al. Mechanics of the brain: perspectives, challenges, and opportunities. *Biomech Model Mechanobiol.* 2015;14(5):931–965.
8. Prange MT, Margulies SS. Regional, directional, and age-dependent properties of the brain undergoing large deformation. *J Biomed Eng.* 2002;124:244–252.
9. Jin X, Zhu F, Mao H, Shen M, Yang KH. A comprehensive experimental study on material properties of human brain tissue. *J Biomechanics.* 2013;46(16):2795–2801.
10. Franze K, Janmey PA, Guck J. Mechanics in neuronal development and repair. *Annu Rev Biomed Eng.* 2013;15:227–251.
11. Cloots RJ, van Dommelen JA, Kleiven S, Geers MG. Multi-scale mechanics of traumatic brain injury: predicting axonal strains from head loads. *Biomech Model Mechanobiol.* 2013;12(1):1–14.
12. Xu G, Bayly PV, Taber LA. Residual stress in the adult mouse brain. *Biomech Model Mechanobiol.* 2009;8(4):253–262.
13. Alfasi AM, Shulyakov AV, Del Bigio MR. Intracranial biomechanics following cortical contusion in live rats: Laboratory investigation. *J Neurosurg.* 2013;119(5):1255–1262.
14. Gefen A, Margulies SS. Are in vivo and in situ brain tissues mechanically similar? *J Biomech.* 2004;37(9):1339–1352.
15. Prange MT, Margulies SS. Regional, directional, and age-dependent properties of the brain undergoing large deformation. *J Biomech Eng.* 2002;124(2):244–252.
16. Hrapko M, Van Dommelen J, Peters G, Wismans J. The influence of test conditions on characterization of the mechanical properties of brain tissue. *J Biomech Eng.* 2008;130(3):031003.
17. Rashid B, Destrade M, Gilchrist MD. Mechanical characterization of brain tissue in simple shear at dynamic strain rates. *J Mech Behav Biomed Mater.* 2013;28:71–85.
18. Budday S, Nay R, de Rooij R, et al. Mechanical properties of gray and white matter brain tissue by indentation. *J Mech Behav Biomed Mater.* 2015;46:318–330.
19. Rashid B, Destrade M, Gilchrist MD. Mechanical characterization of brain tissue in tension at dynamic strain rates. *J Mech Behav Biomed Mater.* 2014;33:43–54.
20. McLean A, Anderson RW. Biomechanics of closed head injury. *Head Inj.* 1997:25–37.

21. Goldsmith W. The state of head injury biomechanics: past, present, and future: part 1. *Crit Rev Biomed Eng.* 2001;29(5&6):441–600.

22. Meaney DF, Morrison B, Bass CD. The mechanics of traumatic brain injury: a review of what we know and what we need to know for reducing its societal burden. *J Biomech Eng.* 2014;136(2):021008.

23. Beckwith JG, Greenwald RM, Chu JJ. Measuring head kinematics in football: correlation between the head impact telemetry system and Hybrid III headform. *Ann Biomed Eng.* 2012;40(1):237–248.

24. Jadischke R, Viano DC, Dau N, King AI, McCarthy J. On the accuracy of the Head Impact Telemetry (HIT) system used in football helmets. *J Biomech.* 2013;46(13):2310–2315.

25. Newman JA, Shewchenko N, Welbourne E. A proposed new biomechanical head injury assessment function-the maximum power index. *Stapp Car Crash J.* 2000;44:215–247.

26. Kleiven S. Evaluation of head injury criteria using a finite element model validated against experiments on localized brain motion, intracerebral acceleration, and intracranial pressure. *Int J Crashworthiness.* 2006;11(1):65–79.

27. Takhounts EG, Craig MJ, Moorhouse K, McFadden J, Hasija V. Development of brain injury criteria (BrIC). *Stapp Car Crash J.* 2013;57:243.

28. Crandall JR, Bose D, Forman J, et al. Human surrogates for injury biomechanics research. *Clin Anat.* 2011;24(3):362–371.

29. Badachhape AA, Okamoto RJ, Durham RS, et al. The relationship of three-dimensional human skull motion to brain tissue deformation in magnetic resonance elastography studies. *J Biomech Eng.* 2017;139(5):051002.

30. King AI. Fundamentals of impact biomechanics: part I-biomechanics of the head, neck, and thorax. *Annu Rev Biomed Eng.* 2000;2(1):55–81.

31. Ommaya A, Goldsmith W, Thibault L. Biomechanics and neuropathology of adult and paediatric head injury. *Br J Neurosurg.* 2002;16(3):220–242.

32. Margulies SS, Thibault LE, Gennarelli TA. Physical model simulations of brain injury in the primate. *J Biomech.* 1990;23(8):823–836.

33. Viano D, Aldman B, Pape K, Hoof Jv, Holst Hv. Brain kinematics in physical model tests with translational and rotational acceleration. *Int J Crashworthiness.* 1997;2(2):191–206.

34. Mertz HJ, Irwin AL. Anthropomorphic test devices and injury risk assessments. In: Yoganandan N, Nahum AM, Melvin JW, eds. *Accidental Injury.* New York: Springer; 2015:83–112.

35. Morales D, Marklund N, Lebold D, et al. Experimental models of traumatic brain injury: do we really need to build a better mousetrap? *Neuroscience.* 2005;136(4):971–989.

36. Goldsmith W, Monson KL. The state of head injury biomechanics: past, present, and future part 2: physical experimentation. *Crit Rev Biomed Eng.* 2005;33(2).

37. DeWitt DS, Perez-Polo R, Hulsebosch CE, Dash PK, Robertson CS. Challenges in the development of rodent models of mild traumatic brain injury. *J Neurotrauma.* 2013;30:688–701.

38. Namjoshi DR, Good C, Cheng WH, et al. Towards clinical management of traumatic brain injury: a review of models and mechanisms from a biomechanical perspective. *Dis Model Mech.* 2013;6(6):1325–1338.

39. Xiong Y, Mahmood A, Chopp M. Animal models of traumatic brain injury. *Nat Rev Neurosci.* 2013;14(2):128–142.

40. Shultz SR, McDonald SJ, Haar CV, et al. The potential for animal models to provide insight into mild traumatic brain injury: translational challenges and strategies. *Neurosci Biobehav Rev.* 2016;76:396–414.

41. Panzer MB, Wood GW, Bass CR. Scaling in neurotrauma: how do we apply animal experiments to people? *Exp Neurol.* 2014;261:120–126.

42. Kochanek PM, Bramlett HM, Dixon CE, et al. Operation brain trauma therapy: approach to modeling, therapy evaluation, drug selection, and biomarker assessments, for a multi-center pre-clinical drug screening consortium for acute therapies in severe traumatic brain injury. *J Neurotrauma.* 2015;522:513–522.

43. Kumaria A, Tolias C. In vitro models of neurotrauma. *Br J Neurosurg.* 2008;22(2):200–206.

44. Morrison B III, Elkin BS, Dollé J-P, Yarmush ML. In vitro models of traumatic brain injury. *Annu Rev Biomed Eng.* 2011;13:91–126.

45. LaPlaca MC, Prado GR. Neural mechanobiology and neuronal vulnerability to traumatic loading. *J Biomech.* 2010;43(1):71–78.

46. Kang WH, Morrison B. Predicting changes in cortical electrophysiological function after in vitro traumatic brain injury. *Biomech Model Mechanobiol.* 2015;14(5):1033–1044.

47. Wright RM, Ramesh K. An axonal strain injury criterion for traumatic brain injury. *Biomech Model Mechanobiol.* 2012;11(1-2):245.

48. Kang WH, Morrison B. Functional tolerance to mechanical deformation developed from organotypic hippocampal slice cultures. *Biomech Model Mechanobiol.* 2015;14(3):561–575.

49. Tse KM, Lim SP, Tan VBC, Lee HP. A review of head injury and finite element head models. *Am J Eng Technol Soc.* 2014;1(5):28–52.

50. Dixit P, Liu G. A review on recent development of finite element models for head injury simulations. *Arch Comput Methods Eng.* 2016:1–53.

51. Ghajari M, Hellyer PJ, Sharp DJ. Computational modelling of traumatic brain injury predicts the location of chronic traumatic encephalopathy pathology. *Brain.* 2016;140(2):333–343.

52. Fahlstedt M, Depreitere B, Halldin P, Vander Sloten J, Kleiven S. Correlation between injury pattern and finite element analysis in biomechanical reconstructions of traumatic brain injuries. *J Biomech.* 2015;48(7):1331–1335.

53. Ji S, Ghadyani H, Bolander RP, et al. Parametric comparisons of intracranial mechanical responses from three validated finite element models of the human head. *Ann Biomed Eng.* 2014;42(1):11–24.

54. Ji S, Zhao W. A pre-computed brain response atlas for instantaneous strain estimation in contact sports. *Ann Biomed Eng.* 2015;43(8):1877–1895.

55. Kraft RH, Mckee PJ, Dagro AM, Grafton ST. Combining the finite element method with structural connectome-based analysis for modeling neurotrauma: connectome neurotrauma mechanics. *PLoS Comput Biol.* 2012;8(8):e1002619.

56. Menon DK, Maas AI. Traumatic brain injury in 2014: Progress, failures and new approaches for TBI research. *Nat Rev Neurol.* 2015;11(2):71–72.

57. Bragge P, Synnot A, Maas AI, et al. A state-of-the-science overview of randomized controlled trials evaluating acute management of moderate-to-severe traumatic brain injury. *J Neurotrauma.* 2016;33(16):1461–1478.

58. Manley GT, Maas AI. Traumatic brain injury: an international knowledge-based approach. *JAMA.* 2013;310(5):473–474.

59. Maas A. Traumatic brain injury: changing concepts and approaches. *Chin J Traumatol.* 2016;19(1):3–6.

60. Bigler ED. Systems biology, neuroimaging, neuropsychology, neuroconnectivity and traumatic brain injury. *Front Syst Neurosci.* 2016;10(55):1–23.

61. Kurowski BG, Treble-Barna A, Pitzer AJ, et al. Applying systems biology methodology to identify genetic factors possibly associated with recovery after traumatic brain injury. *J Neurotrauma*. 2017;34(14):2280–2290.

62. Nielson JL, Cooper SR, Yue JK, et al. Uncovering precision phenotype-biomarker associations in traumatic brain injury using topological data analysis. *PloS One*. 2017;12(3):e0169490.

63. Yokobori S, Hosein K, Burks S, Sharma I, Gajavelli S, Bullock R. Biomarkers for the clinical differential diagnosis in traumatic brain injury—a systematic review. *CNS Neurosci Ther*. 2013;19(8):556–565.

64. Boutte A, Kobeissy F, Wang KK, et al. Protein biomarkers in traumatic brain injury: an omics approach. *Biomark Brain Inj Neurol Disord*. 2014:42.

65. Kawata K, Liu CY, Merkel SF, Ramirez SH, Tierney RT, Langford D. Blood biomarkers for brain injury: what are we measuring? *Neurosci Biobehav Rev*. 2016;68:460–473.

66. Kou Z, VandeVord PJ. Traumatic white matter injury and glial activation: from basic science to clinics. *Glia*. 2014;62(11):1831–1855.

Neuroregenerative Medicine in TBI

Jinhui Chen, Xiaoting Wang, and Xiang Gao

29

Traumatic Brain Injury Causes Cell Loss in the Hippocampus

Traumatic brain injury (TBI) is a complicated disease process encompassing primary injury by initial insult and prolonged secondary injury by diffused and progressive impacts to a much larger region other than solely the focal site.[1] Among several cortical and subcortical regions showing diffuse cell loss, hippocampus is one of the most vulnerable structures. In 1989, Cortez and colleagues examined neuronal alterations by histochemical marker, acid fuchsin, and staining and observed rapid neuronal abnormality in the ipsilateral hippocampus, specifically neuron count reduction in the CA2–CA3 region, within 24 hours after experimental TBI induced by a lateral fluid percussion (FPI) model. The effects prolonged to at least 4 weeks later and were displayed as less residual neurons in the injured hippocampus.[2] Later, in 1992, Lowenstein and colleagues detected selective hilar neuron death as well by the same model and recorded consequent granule neuron hyperactivity.[3] In 1993, the same group reported positive correlation between hilar neuron survival and Morris water maze performance after FPI and first associated neuronal loss in the hippocampus after TBI with cognitive deficits.[4] Other groups then described the temporal and spatial profiles of neuronal loss in the hippocampus.[5,6]

Although these studies used induced brain trauma representing different aspects of human clinical settings through the FPI model, research using the controlled cortical impact (CCI) model displayed similar cell loss pattern in the hippocampus. The CCI model was first customized for study in mouse in 1995 by the McIntosh group, and they reported injured neurons in CA2–CA3, CA3, and the dentate gyrus of the hippocampus at 48 hours after injury.[7] Correspondingly, memory deficits were observed. Later, more groups expanded the research to a larger temporal profile of up to 4 weeks post-trauma, described neuronal injury as dystrophy, and characterized both necrotic and apoptotic features in damaged dentate gyrus granule neurons.[8–12] Our own group also distinguished predominant immature but not mature neuronal death in the dentate gyrus and reported necrotic rather than apoptotic death of those immature neurons rapidly and intensively within 24 hours after initial injury in a CCI model at moderate settings.[13,14]

Enormous efforts have been made in the development of neuroprotective reagents, and this has led to about 30 clinical trials. Although none of them has yet been successful, there is still reason for hope. In that vein, Kabadi and Faden reviewed most of the recent neuroprotection strategies and discussed those efforts that they believed would produce translatable results in clinical trials in the future.[15] In addition to neuroprotection, some groups turned to regenerative medicine for help and applied cell therapy—specifically stem cell therapy—as an alternative. Most current cell-based therapies focus on cell transplantation and show encouraging results by improving motor function and/or learning capacity in rodent models. However, the appropriate route of cell delivery, proper cell dose for transplantation, ideal stem cell type, and in vitro expansion to harvest adequate amounts of cells are all obstacles restricting the translation of these therapies from animal studies to clinical trials.[16] To bypass those barriers for cell therapy, interventions based on endogenous neuronal stem cells (NSCs) seem to be a shortcut to neural repair, at least for restoring the injured hippocampus.

Neuronal Stem Cells and Adult Neurogenesis in Normal Conditions

Traditionally, neurogenesis was thought to only occur during embryonic and postnatal development, and the nervous system was considered to be nonregenerative once mature. However, in the early 1960s, Smart first reported cell proliferation in the adult mouse brain by [H³]-thymidine labeling and radioautography.[17] Then Altman and colleagues reported a series of results displaying generation of new neurons in adult rat brain by the same technique.[18–20] However, only after the functional relevance of adult neurogenesis was proved to be involved in the learning capacity of songbirds by substantial works from the Nottebohm group was the significance of adult neurogenesis eventually recognized.[21] Later, extensive investigations were done on the isolation of adult NSCs, the characterization of specific markers for NSCs, the description of the adult neurogenesis process, and the determination of key factors regulating NSCs activity and subsequent adult neurogenesis, as well as the functions and dysfunctions of adult neurogenesis. Several experts in the NSC and adult neurogenesis field have published a few comprehensive and excellent reviews covering these topics[22–25]; here, we will simply highlight some main conclusions and important indications relevant to the study of NSC proliferation and neurogenesis after TBI.

Studies in the past two decades have confirmed the wide existence of NSCs in adult canaries,[26] rodents,[27] primates,[28] and human beings.[29,30] In addition, it has been demonstrated that adult neurogenesis specifically occurs in two neurogenic niches: the subventricular zone (SVZ) of the lateral ventricle and the subgranular zone (SGZ) of the hippocampal dentate gyrus. In the adult SVZ, NSCs continuously give rise to immature precursors, and then precursors differentiate to neuroblasts, which further migrate through a rostral migratory stream and become interneurons in the olfactory bulb (OB) (Figure 29.1).[23,31] In the adult SGZ, NSCs give birth to precursors, subsequently generate immature neurons, migrate a very small distance to the granule cell layer (GCL), become mature granule neurons, develop an extensive dendritic morphology, and integrate into preexisting network.[23,32–34] The function of adult neurogenesis has also been studied intensively from the focus of either stimulatory or inhibitory factors. In the SVZ, focal irradiation, antimitotic agents, and genetic models were applied to inhibit adult neurogenesis in individual studies, and deficits in odor discrimination, short-term olfactory memory, and long-term olfactory memory were reported.[35–37] By contrast, using an odor enrichment experiment, Rochefort and colleagues related enhanced neurogenesis in the adult OB to promoted odor memory.[38] Recently, using optogenetics, specific activation of adult-born neurons in OB was shown to facilitate learning and

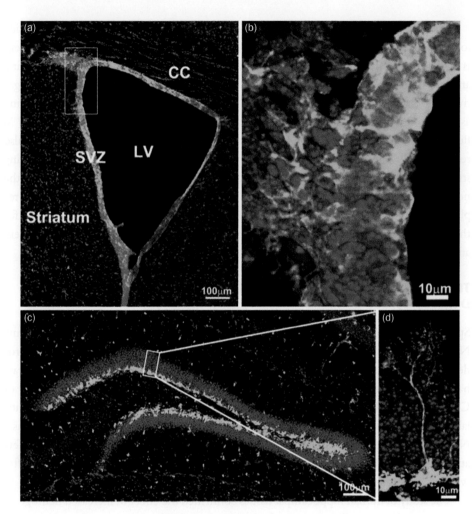

Figure 29.1 Neural stem cells in the adult brain.

memory in odor discrimination in mouse. Taken together, it is proposed that adult neurogenesis in the SVZ is mainly related to olfactory-associative functions. In the SGZ, adult neurogenesis is considered to support life-long learning and memory capacity since the function of hippocampus in this area has long been confirmed. Enriched environment again enhances neurogenesis in the SGZ as well, and the promotion correlates with improved spatial memory performance in Morris water maze tests.[39,40] Deficits in hippocampal neurogenesis by a transgenic mouse model displayed dysfunction of trace memory formation.[41] Similar studies ablated adult neurogenesis by focal irradiation or transgenic neural precursor elimination, observed impaired contextual fear conditioning but not spatial memory, and also found that neurogenesis modulates the duration of hippocampus dependency before a piece of fear memory is stored in cortical structures.[42,43] Other groups have also reported involvement of adult hippocampal neurogenesis in clearance instead of formation of memory as a novel function. A transgenic mouse model and pharmacological tools were used in these experimental settings.[44,45] To summarize, neurogenesis in the hippocampus plays important roles in learning and memory potential in adulthood.

Over the course of a lifetime, adult neurogenesis is modulated by many physiological and pathological circumstances. As mentioned earlier, enriched environment is a common condition that can positively regulate neurogenesis, just as can learning and physical exercises like running.[38–40,46,47] On the contrary, other factors can negatively modulate neurogenesis levels, such as aging and stress.[48,49] These factors, occurring as common events in daily life, dynamically alter neurogenesis levels and result in fluctuations of functional outcomes. Meanwhile, some pathological conditions are also relevant to the neurogenesis level. It has been reported that brain injuries, including stroke, epilepsy, and TBI, can stimulate NSC proliferation and subsequently alter the neurogenesis level.[50–59] This phenomenon indicates that NSC-mediated neuronal replacement and neuroplasticity, as innate repair machinery, is an appropriate target for therapeutic intervention and holds great promise for functional outcome improvement after brain injuries.

TBI Reshapes Adult Neurogenesis in the Hippocampal Dentate Gyrus

Specifically in the case of TBI, it is widely observed that cell proliferation, including NSC proliferation, is increased after initial injury, especially in the hippocampus in rodent experiment models (Figure 29.2).[54–58,60–62] An increase in NPC proliferation rate has been shown to occur in dentate gyrus injured through fluid percussion[55,57,62,63] or CCI[54,58,60,61,64] and through air-compression cortical contusion trauma.[56] Experimental labeling with 5-bromo-2'-deoxyuridine (BrdU) generally suggests that TBI increases NPC proliferation in the hippocampus.[54–58,60–64] Further analysis has shown that proliferation begins to increase 24 hours after CCI and remains elevated for up to 1 week, after which it is restored back to control level.[58]

The study of human hippocampal tissues confirmed the effect of increased neurogenic precursor proliferation.[65] Our group further confirmed that it is the quiescent NSCs that have mainly been activated by the injury.[59] This phenomenon indicates that an NSC-mediated innate repair mechanism is activated for neuronal replacement in the injured adult hippocampus. However, NSC proliferation is just the very first step of neurogenesis. Therefore, increased NSC proliferation is not necessarily related to increased neurogenesis; namely, neuronal replacement. Indeed, there is a discrepancy in the results of how

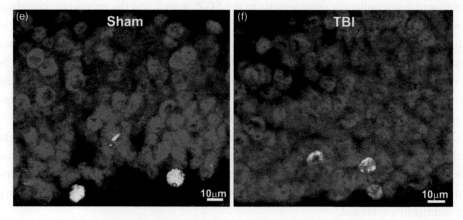

Figure 29.2 Neurogenesis in the adult hippocampus.

TBI affects the production of mature neurons. In evaluating different data, increased, unchanged, and decreased neurogenesis have all been reported.[54–56,58,61–63,66,67] Furthermore, although it is generally agreed that TBI enhances NPC proliferation, the effect of TBI on neurogenesis is still controversial, with reports that neurogenesis in the dentate gyrus decreases,[56,61] is unchanged,[55,57] and increases.[62,63] Our recent work has shown that injury severity is one of the factors that may vary in previous studies and thus partially contributes to this divergence (Table 29.1). We demonstrated that TBI severity induced by the CCI model positively correlates with the NSC proliferation level, while only severe but not mild or moderate TBI can lead to increased production of post-injury–born mature neurons.[68] In addition to injury severity, different injury models used and different time points studied may also lead to the varied conclusions. To better understand the effects of TBI on neurogenesis, it is necessary to carefully evaluate the status of every step during neurogenesis since injury environment may also affect newborn neuron survival, migration, maturation, and morphology development, as well as functional integration.

Under normal conditions, more than 75% adult-born neurons die in the first 3 weeks after birth.[24,69,70] It is still unclear how the injured environment influences survival of post-injury–born neurons. Our previous study reported selectively dramatic loss of doublecortin protein-expressing immature neurons in the dentate gyrus within 24 hours in a moderate CCI setting, while the number of immature neurons returned to sham levels 2 weeks later, roughly the time needed for injury-activated NSCs to differentiate to postmitotic immature neurons.[13,68] Although increased NSC proliferation

Table 29.1:
Summary of major studies on neurogenesis after TBI.

Result on neurogenesis	Injury model	Injury parameters	Species	Cell birthdate label	Evaluation time	Neurogenesis criteria	Authors
No clear conclusion	CCI	4.4m/s, 1.0mm deformation	mouse	BrdU labeled for 1 week after injury	60 days post-injury	BrdU/ Calbindin	Kernie et al, 2001[29]
		6m/s, 2.75mm deformation	rat	BrdU labeled for 9 days after injury	30 days post-injury	BrdU/ Calbindin	Dash et al, 2001[28]
	weight drop	20g, 9cm		not labeled	7 days post-injury	βIII tubulin	Braun et al, 2002[93]
Increase	FPI	2.1 ± 0.08 atm	rat	BrdU labeled at 2 days after injury	4 weeks post-injury	BrdU/NeuN	Sun et al, 2005[33]
		2.2 ± 0.02 atm		BrdU labeled from 2 days to 5 days after injury	10 weeks post-injury	BrdU/ FluoroGold	Sun et al, 2007[34]
Unchanged	FPI	2.16 ± 0.06 atm	rat	BrdU labeled at 18h and 20h after injury	15 days post-injury	BrdU/βIII tubulin	Rice et al, 2003[31]
	CCI	3.0m/s, 1.0mm deformation	mouse	BrdU labeled for 1 week after injury	5 weeks post-injury	BrdU/NeuN	Gao et al, 2013[37]
	weight drop	450g, 2m, 3.6m/s	rat	BrdU labled from 24h to 4days after injury	8 weeks post-injury	BrdU/NeuN	Bye et al, 2013[95]
Decreased	CCI	4.5m/s, 1mm deformation	mouse	BrdU labeled for 1 week after injury	4 weeks post-injury	BrdU/NeuN	Rola et al, 2006[32]

is a resource for amending cell loss, no evidence illustrates whether or not the survival rate of post-injury–born neurons is changed and contributes to the repair. A few studies quantified proliferated cell survival by BrdU incorporation and observed unchanged BrdU-positive cell survival in the SGZ 14 days after TBI.[55,67] Because they are lacking neuronal marker specification, the identities of those surviving BrdU-positive cells are questionable, and it needs more investigations to clearly address the survival rate of newborn neurons after TBI. Other than survival, rapid migration from the SGZ to the GCL is also an important event for newborn neurons to properly mature and integrate into local circuits. A recently published study displayed aberrant localization of neurons born around 5 days after injury, indicating ectopic migration under injury circumstances.[71] Our own unpublished data also support the migration problem in moderate and severe CCI. We observed an increased proportion of newborn neurons migrate from SGZ to outer GCL or even further, to the border between GCL and molecular layer. Since adult-born neurons normally locate in the inner GCL, the abnormal location of new neurons may lead to circuit disorganization, suggesting a potential contributor for posttraumatic epilepsy.[72] Despite abnormal migration, surviving post-injury–born neurons also suffer altered morphological development. Neurons born after CCI showed more proximal branches but fewer distal branches from their somas, as well as more widespread morphologies of their dendritic arborizations. This morphology may contribute to a shift from connections with distal inputs to proximal inputs, thus disrupting original information flow. However, their electrophysiological properties are relatively comparable to neurons in sham animals.[71] Moreover, the post-injury–born neurons have been proved to successfully integrate into neurocircuitries by forming synapses with upstream prefrontal paths and downstream CA3 pyramidal neurons, and they are able to uptake transsynaptic tracers from postsynaptic CA3 neurons and evoke action potentials to upstream prefrontal path stimulation.[63,71,73] Taken together, post-injury–born neurons have both similarities and differences compared with normal neurons. Since no clear evidence directly supports beneficial or maladaptive effects of specific post-injury–born neuron activation on behavioral outcomes, when considering endogenous neurogenesis as a therapeutic treatment for TBI, more attentions should be paid to the functional relevance of post-injury neurons on the network and behavioral levels.

The morphological and electrophysiological studies just discussed elucidated the functional properties of adult-born neurons generated post-trauma on the individual cell level; however, on the population level, determining how the production of mature neurons is affected by TBI is still controversial. As mentioned earlier, increased, unchanged, and decreased neurogenesis have all been reported by different groups.[54–56,58,61–63,66,67] By carefully analyzing how individual groups evaluated neurogenesis in their specific circumstances, we found a few variations that might cause the current discrepancies. The first few reports of neurogenesis after TBI came from Kernie et al. and Dash et al. In 2001, Kernie and colleagues evaluated neurogenesis after TBI in adult mice by a CCI model. They labeled proliferated cells by BrdU in the first week after injury and identified progeny cell types at 60 days after injury. Their data showed a fivefold increase in BrdU-positive cells in the injured hippocampus, and some of the BrdU-positive cells were co-labeled with the mature neuron marker calbindin. The results indicated that TBI stimulated NSC proliferation, which can give birth to mature neurons.[54] At almost the same time, Dash et al. conducted TBI by a CCI model in adult rats and labeled cell proliferation for 9 days post-trauma. In their work, BrdU-positive cells were assessed at 10 days after TBI and also displayed dramatic increases in the dentate gyrus. BrdU-positive cell fates were identified at 3 weeks after the last BrdU injection in injured animals, and co-labeling with calbindin was also detected, indicating production of post-injury–born mature neurons.[58] Kernie et al. and Dash et al. demonstrated similar results on NSC proliferation and neurogenesis induced by TBI; however, without quantification and comparison of BrdU and calbindin double-positive cells in injured and sham animals, how TBI reshapes neurogenesis is still elusive. Later, in 2002, Braun and colleagues conducted a study in adult rats by a weight-drop model and evaluated βIII-tubulin–expressing cells. They found increased numbers of these neurogenic cells in the dentate gyrus at 3 and 7 days after TBI, implicating involvement of neurogenesis in repair post-trauma.[56] Collectively, these early investigations brought about consensus on TBI-enhanced NSC proliferation and that these proliferated NSCs can give birth to mature neurons, although the question of to what degree TBI reshapes neurogenesis is still left to be answered. To address this question, more studies have been conducted by different groups. Sun's study in adult rats by FPI model reported increased neurogenesis by injecting BrdU at 2 days after TBI and assessing BrdU and neuronal nuclei (NeuN) double-positive cells in the GCL at 4 weeks after TBI.[62] Their following work further confirmed the result in a long-term manner at 10 weeks after TBI.[63] By contrast, Rola et al. reported the opposite result in adult mice by CCI model. Using BrdU injection for the first week after TBI and counting BrdU and NeuN double-positive cells, Rola reported decreased neurogenesis in the SGZ at 4 weeks post-trauma.[61] However, using a similar strategy, our group labeled cell proliferation in the first week and quantified BrdU and NeuN double-positive cells at 5 weeks after TBI. In the setting of moderate CCI in adult mice, we detected unchanged neurogenesis following trauma instead.[66] Bye and colleagues also observed unchanged BrdU and NeuN double-positive cells at 8 weeks after TBI in a traumatic axonal injury (TAI) model in adult rats by labeling cell proliferation in the first 5 days.[67] Rice et al. induced TBI in adult rats by FPI model and labeled cell proliferation by BrdU injection at 18 hours and 20 hours after injury. Co-labeling of BrdU and βIII-ubulin was quantified 15 days later, and, similarly, no obvious difference was detected in the SGZ between sham and injured animals, while an increased number of double-positive cells was observed in the SVZ.[55] Collectively, some key variables in different groups included the evaluation of diverse injury models, individual injury settings, different species, varying label strategy, and dynamic time course. Each of the variables in itself or in combination might be the reason for the existing discrepancies. Our recent work teased out injury severity as one of the variables that can affect neurogenesis following trauma. We illustrated that NSC proliferation positively correlates to injury severity, while only severe but not mild or moderate TBI can increase neurogenesis in a CCI model in adult mice.[68] Further investigations are needed to evaluate other possible factors affecting the results and to help depict a profile of how TBI reshapes neurogenesis.

TBI is always more likely to occur as a sudden accident rather than as a progressive-onset disease, and it is not as simple and consistent as what researchers are studying in animal models. Although several animal models mimic different pathogenic perspectives of human TBI (e.g., diffusive or focal, closed head or penetrating), some other factors complicating TBI consequences still need to be considered. In addition to the injury itself, another element that confounds the case is the age at which injury initially occurred. In clinical observation, young children are more susceptible to neurological complications after TBI.[74,75] An aged population tends to have poor functional outcomes in similar injury conditions.[76] Although age-dependent pathological changes, like apoptosis level, oxidative degree, and inflammatory range, contribute to the difference, the capacity of repair may be an alternative reason why age makes a difference.[77–79] As mentioned in the prior section, age on its own affects neurogenesis. Juvenile animals have higher basal neurogenesis levels than adults, while neurogenesis declines in aging animals.[62,80] However, most studies regarding neurogenesis after TBI were done in adult animals, and few focused on neurogenesis in pediatric TBI or after TBI in aging animals. TBI in childhood causes detrimental issues other than simply neuronal loss: it also disrupts the development of the immature brain and results in more complicated neurological and cognitive dysfunctions in later life. Thus, it is important to strengthen investigations on neurogenesis after TBI in pediatric settings to facilitate specific repair strategies aimed at development rescue. A study done in rodents compared SVZ neurogenesis after pediatric TBI at different developmental stages and found that the cell proliferation in SVZ after TBI is increased in immature animals, but the effect declines with increased age from postnatal day 6 to 10 and 21.[81] Sun and colleagues have also observed a higher cell proliferation enhancement in the SGZ after TBI in juvenile rats than in adults in a moderate FPI model.[62] Likewise, the Nobel-Haeusslein group observed deceased cell proliferation in the SGZ and neuronal differentiation in the GCL at relatively the same juvenile age, but in the subacute phase after injury.[82] According to current data, immature brains tend to respond more strongly to TBI in the acute phase, but may sustain impaired neurogenesis later on, indicating a potential mechanism for the profound impairments after pediatric TBI. Although prevalence of TBI in the elderly population is concerning, how NSCs respond to TBI in aged brain is still elusive. In other brain injury models, like stroke, NSC proliferation has been reported to be increased even in aging patients.[83] It is likely that TBI may also trigger NSC proliferation in aging subjects, although the injury mechanisms might be different. More attention should be paid to NSC proliferation after TBI in the aging group, as well as neuronal differentiation and survival of generated neurons. By carefully screening for the effect of age on neurogenesis after TBI in different age cohorts, more specific strategies of neural repair can be set up under individual situations, thus moving us closer to personalized medicine in the future.

Function of Adult Neurogenesis After TBI

Sustained neurogenesis over the course of a lifetime is responsible for learning and memory capacity, which is always defective after TBI due to neuronal loss and neurocircuitry disconnection in the damaged hippocampus. Both humans and rodents have spontaneous recovery to some degree, showing intrinsic neuroplasticity after injury.[84,85] Neurogenesis after TBI is considered to be one of the mechanisms that mediates this neuroplasticity by replacing dead neurons and rewiring damaged connections. In animal experiments, increased neurogenesis after TBI by administration of various neurotrophic factors has shown positive correlation with cognitive function improvement.[86–91] Other studies validated the involvement of neurogenesis in functional recovery by inhibiting neurogenesis post-injury via transgenic ablation of neurogenic cells or the systemic administration of cell proliferation inhibitor and observing the elimination of spontaneous recovery.[92,93] Moreover, detailed investigations on newly generated neurons post-injury also proved their integration into local circuitries, providing one more piece of evidence for the connection between injury-induced neurogenesis and functional improvements.[63,71,73] However, without direct functional evaluation specifically on the neurons born after injury, the beneficial effect of neurogenesis is still questionable. By contrast, aberrant neurogenesis is also proposed to contribute to posttraumatic epilepsy, and abnormal migration as well as disrupted dendritic arborization has already been reported in post-injury–born neurons.[71] Moreover, although integration of newborn neurons was proved, the exact identities of the presynaptic and postsynaptic neurons they made connections with are elusive. It is uncertain whether the newly formed connections follow intrinsic patterns or disturb the original organization. The recently developed DREADD (designed receptors exclusively activated by designed drugs) technique is a promising tool for specifically investigating newly generated neurons.[94] By exclusively activating or silencing post-injury–born neurons and examining the resulting cognitive function outcomes, the question of whether injury-induced neurogenesis is beneficial or maladaptive can be answered. Additionally, by combining transgenic reporter line and transsynaptic virus infection, it is possible to trace rewired networks and further support functional evaluation of neurogenesis after TBI. Only if a positive influence of post-injury neurogenesis is confirmed can interventions using endogenous NSCs and neurogenesis be potentially translated to clinical trials.

Future Directions

TBI is a complex disease process, and combinational therapy will be the optimal strategy over any single operation. By achieving a complete understanding of the pathophysiology of TBI, a comprehensive profile of events occurring after TBI may guide the development of a series of sequential therapeutic interventions. For example, to be effective, neuroprotective drugs should be applied immediately to prevent cell death and protect dendrites and axons from degeneration, together with agents to protect against hemorrhage and intracranial pressure increases and to supply energy within hours of initial injury. Later, neurogenic and/or angiogenic reagents may be introduced within the first few days to enhance tissue restoration and neurovascular structure repair. Additionally, neurotrophic drugs would be administered to help newborn neurons survive, develop, mature, and properly function to replenish damaged networks.

We still have a long way to go to reach an effective cure for TBI and achieve full recovery in human patients; however, by using intensive studies in animal models, we are gradually approaching that destination, step by step. Only if we better understand the mechanisms behind the pathophysiology can better strategies be developed to target the issue, solve the problem, and eventually rescue the functional deficits.

References

1. McIntosh TK, Saatman KE, Raghupathi R, et al. The Dorothy Russell Memorial Lecture. The molecular and cellular sequelae of experimental traumatic brain injury: pathogenetic mechanisms. *Neuropathol Appl Neurobiol*. 1998;24(4):251–267.

2. Cortez SC, McIntosh TK, Noble LJ. Experimental fluid percussion brain injury: vascular disruption and neuronal and glial alterations. *Brain Res.* 1989;482(2):271–282.

3. Lowenstein DH, Thomas MJ, Smith DH, McIntosh TK. Selective vulnerability of dentate hilar neurons following traumatic brain injury: a potential mechanistic link between head trauma and disorders of the hippocampus. *J Neurosci.* 1992;12(12):4846–4853.

4. Hicks RR, Smith DH, Lowenstein DH, Saint Marie R, McIntosh TK. Mild experimental brain injury in the rat induces cognitive deficits associated with regional neuronal loss in the hippocampus. *J Neurotrauma.* 1993;10(4):405–414.

5. Hicks R, Soares H, Smith D, McIntosh T. Temporal and spatial characterization of neuronal injury following lateral fluid-percussion brain injury in the rat. *Acta Neuropathol.* 1996;91(3):236–246.

6. Sato M, Chang E, Igarashi T, Noble LJ. Neuronal injury and loss after traumatic brain injury: time course and regional variability. *Brain Res.* 2001;917(1):45–54.

7. Smith DH, Soares HD, Pierce JS, et al. A model of parasagittal controlled cortical impact in the mouse: cognitive and histopathologic effects. *J Neurotrauma.* 1995;12(2):169–178.

8. Colicos MA, Dixon CE, Dash PK. Delayed, selective neuronal death following experimental cortical impact injury in rats: possible role in memory deficits. *Brain Res.* 1996;739(1-2):111–119.

9. Chen S, Pickard JD, Harris NG. Time course of cellular pathology after controlled cortical impact injury. *Exp Neurol.* 2003;182(1):87–102.

10. Hall ED, Sullivan PG, Gibson TR, Pavel KM, Thompson BM, Scheff SW. Spatial and temporal characteristics of neurodegeneration after controlled cortical impact in mice: more than a focal brain injury. *J Neurotrauma.* 2005;22(2):252–265.

11. Hall ED, Bryant YD, Cho W, Sullivan PG. Evolution of post-traumatic neurodegeneration after controlled cortical impact traumatic brain injury in mice and rats as assessed by the de Olmos silver and fluorojade staining methods. *J Neurotrauma.* 2008;25(3):235–247.

12. Colicos MA, Dash PK. Apoptotic morphology of dentate gyrus granule cells following experimental cortical impact injury in rats: possible role in spatial memory deficits. *Brain Res.* 1996;739(1-2):120–131.

13. Gao X, Deng-Bryant Y, Cho W, Carrico KM, Hall ED, Chen J. Selective death of newborn neurons in hippocampal dentate gyrus following moderate experimental traumatic brain injury. *J Neurosci Res.* 2008;86(10):2258–2270.

14. Zhou H, Chen L, Gao X, Luo B, Chen J. Moderate traumatic brain injury triggers rapid necrotic death of immature neurons in the hippocampus. *J Neuropathol Exp Neurol.* 2012;71(4):348–359.

15. Kabadi SV, Faden AI. Neuroprotective strategies for traumatic brain injury: improving clinical translation. *Int J Mol Sci.* 2014;15(1):1216–1236.

16. Gennai S, Monsel A, Hao Q, et al. Cell-based therapy for traumatic brain injury. *Br J Anaesth.* 2015;115(2):203–212.

17. Smart I. The subependymal layer of the mouse brain and its cell production as shown by autography after [H3]-thymidine injection. *J Comp Neurol.* 1961;116:325–327.

18. Altman J, Das GD. Autoradiographic and histological evidence of postnatal hippocampal neurogenesis in rats. *J Comp Neurol.* 1965;124(3):319–335.

19. Altman J, Das GD. Autoradiographic and histological studies of postnatal neurogenesis. I. A longitudinal investigation of the kinetics, migration and transformation of cells

incorporating tritiated thymidine in neonate rats, with special reference to postnatal neurogenesis in some brain regions. *J Comp Neurol.* 1966;126(3):337–389.

20. Altman J. Autoradiographic and histological studies of postnatal neurogenesis. IV. Cell proliferation and migration in the anterior forebrain, with special reference to persisting neurogenesis in the olfactory bulb. *J Comp Neurol.* 1969;137(4):433–457.

21. Nottebohm F. Neuronal replacement in adult brain. *Brain Res Bull.* 2002;57(6):737–749.

22. Kempermann G, Gage FH. Neurogenesis in the adult hippocampus. *Novartis Found Symp.* 2000;231:220–235; discussion 235–241, 302–6.

23. Ming GL, Song H. Adult neurogenesis in the mammalian central nervous system. *Annu Rev Neurosci.* 2005;28:223–250.

24. Christian KM, Song H, Ming GL. Functions and dysfunctions of adult hippocampal neurogenesis. *Annu Rev Neurosci.* 2014;37:243–262.

25. Faigle R, Song H. Signaling mechanisms regulating adult neural stem cells and neurogenesis. *Biochimica Biophysica Acta.* 2013;1830(2):2435–2448.

26. Alvarez-Buylla A, Garcia-Verdugo JM, Mateo AS, Merchant-Larios H. Primary neural precursors and intermitotic nuclear migration in the ventricular zone of adult canaries. *J Neurosci.* 1998;18(3):1020–1037.

27. Reynolds BA, Weiss S. Generation of neurons and astrocytes from isolated cells of the adult mammalian central nervous system. *Science.* 1992;255(5052):1707–1710.

28. Kornack DR, Rakic P. Continuation of neurogenesis in the hippocampus of the adult macaque monkey. *Proc Nat Acad Sci USA.* 1999;96(10):5768–5773.

29. Kukekov VG, Laywell ED, Suslov O, et al. Multipotent stem/progenitor cells with similar properties arise from two neurogenic regions of adult human brain. *Exp Neurol.* 1999;156(2):333–344.

30. Roy NS, Wang S, Jiang L, et al. In vitro neurogenesis by progenitor cells isolated from the adult human hippocampus. *Nat Med.* 2000;6(3):271–277.

31. Doetsch F, Caille I, Lim DA, Garcia-Verdugo JM, Alvarez-Buylla A. Subventricular zone astrocytes are neural stem cells in the adult mammalian brain. *Cell.* 1999;97(6):703–716.

32. Zhao C, Teng EM, Summers RG Jr, Ming GL, Gage FH. Distinct morphological stages of dentate granule neuron maturation in the adult mouse hippocampus. *J Neurosci.* 2006;26(1):3–11.

33. van Praag H, Schinder AF, Christie BR, Toni N, Palmer TD, Gage FH. Functional neurogenesis in the adult hippocampus. *Nature.* 2002;415(6875):1030–1034.

34. Cameron HA, McKay RD. Adult neurogenesis produces a large pool of new granule cells in the dentate gyrus. *J Comp Neurol.* 2001;435(4):406–417.

35. Gheusi G, Cremer H, McLean H, Chazal G, Vincent JD, Lledo PM. Importance of newly generated neurons in the adult olfactory bulb for odor discrimination. *Proc Nat Acad Sci USA.* 2000;97(4):1823–1828.

36. Breton-Provencher V, Lemasson M, Peralta MR 3rd, Saghatelyan A. Interneurons produced in adulthood are required for the normal functioning of the olfactory bulb network and for the execution of selected olfactory behaviors. *J Neurosci.* 2009;29(48):15245–15257.

37. Arruda-Carvalho M, Akers KG, Guskjolen A, Sakaguchi M, Josselyn SA, Frankland PW. Posttraining ablation of adult-generated olfactory granule cells degrades odor-reward memories. *J Neurosci.* 2014;34(47):15793–15803.

38. Rochefort C, Gheusi G, Vincent JD, Lledo PM. Enriched odor exposure increases the number of newborn neurons in the adult olfactory bulb and improves odor memory. *J Neurosci.* 2002;22(7):2679–2689.

39. Kempermann G, Kuhn HG, Gage FH. More hippocampal neurons in adult mice living in an enriched environment. *Nature.* 1997;386(6624):493–495.

40. Nilsson M, Perfilieva E, Johansson U, Orwar O, Eriksson PS. Enriched environment increases neurogenesis in the adult rat dentate gyrus and improves spatial memory. *J Neurobiol.* 1999;39(4):569–578.

41. Shors TJ, Miesegaes G, Beylin A, Zhao M, Rydel T, Gould E. Neurogenesis in the adult is involved in the formation of trace memories. *Nature.* 2001;410(6826):372–376.

42. Saxe MD, Battaglia F, Wang JW, et al. Ablation of hippocampal neurogenesis impairs contextual fear conditioning and synaptic plasticity in the dentate gyrus. *Proc Nat Acad Sci USA.* 2006;103(46):17501–17506.

43. Kitamura T, Saitoh Y, Takashima N, et al. Adult neurogenesis modulates the hippocampus-dependent period of associative fear memory. *Cell.* 2009;139(4):814–827.

44. Feng R, Rampon C, Tang YP, et al. Deficient neurogenesis in forebrain-specific presenilin-1 knockout mice is associated with reduced clearance of hippocampal memory traces. *Neuron.* 2001;32(5):911–926.

45. Akers KG, Martinez-Canabal A, Restivo L, et al. Hippocampal neurogenesis regulates forgetting during adulthood and infancy. *Science.* 2014;344(6184):598–602.

46. Gould E, Beylin A, Tanapat P, Reeves A, Shors TJ. Learning enhances adult neurogenesis in the hippocampal formation. *Nat Neurosci.* 1999;2(3):260–265.

47. van Praag H, Kempermann G, Gage FH. Running increases cell proliferation and neurogenesis in the adult mouse dentate gyrus. *Nat Neurosci.* 1999;2(3):266–270.

48. Kuhn HG, Dickinson-Anson H, Gage FH. Neurogenesis in the dentate gyrus of the adult rat: age-related decrease of neuronal progenitor proliferation. *J Neurosci.* 1996;16(6):2027–2033.

49. Gould E, McEwen BS, Tanapat P, Galea LA, Fuchs E. Neurogenesis in the dentate gyrus of the adult tree shrew is regulated by psychosocial stress and NMDA receptor activation. *J Neurosci.* 1997;17(7):2492–2498.

50. Parent JM, Yu TW, Leibowitz RT, Geschwind DH, Sloviter RS, Lowenstein DH. Dentate granule cell neurogenesis is increased by seizures and contributes to aberrant network reorganization in the adult rat hippocampus. *J Neurosci.* 1997;17(10):3727–3738.

51. Yagita Y, Kitagawa K, Ohtsuki T, et al. Neurogenesis by progenitor cells in the ischemic adult rat hippocampus. *Stroke.* 2001;32(8):1890–1896.

52. Parent JM, Valentin VV, Lowenstein DH. Prolonged seizures increase proliferating neuroblasts in the adult rat subventricular zone-olfactory bulb pathway. *J Neurosci.* 2002;22(8):3174–3188.

53. Yamashita T, Ninomiya M, Hernandez Acosta P, et al. Subventricular zone-derived neuroblasts migrate and differentiate into mature neurons in the post-stroke adult striatum. *J Neurosci.* 2006;26(24):6627–6636.

54. Kernie SG, Erwin TM, Parada LF. Brain remodeling due to neuronal and astrocytic proliferation after controlled cortical injury in mice. *J Neurosci Res.* 2001;66(3):317–326.

55. Rice AC, Khaldi A, Harvey HB, et al. Proliferation and neuronal differentiation of mitotically active cells following traumatic brain injury. *Exp Neurol.* 2003;183(2):406–417.

56. Braun H, Schafer K, Hollt V. BetaIII tubulin-expressing neurons reveal enhanced neurogenesis in hippocampal and cortical structures after a contusion trauma in rats. *J Neurotrauma.* 2002;19(8):975–983.

57. Chirumamilla S, Sun D, Bullock MR, Colello RJ. Traumatic brain injury induced cell proliferation in the adult mammalian central nervous system. *J Neurotrauma.* 2002;19(6):693–703.

58. Dash PK, Mach SA, Moore AN. Enhanced neurogenesis in the rodent hippocampus following traumatic brain injury. *J Neurosci Res*. 2001;63(4):313–319.

59. Gao X, Enikolopov G, Chen J. Moderate traumatic brain injury promotes proliferation of quiescent neural progenitors in the adult hippocampus. *Exp Neurol*. 2009;219(2):516–523.

60. Ramaswamy S, Goings GE, Soderstrom KE, Szele FG, Kozlowski DA. Cellular proliferation and migration following a controlled cortical impact in the mouse. *Brain Res*. 2005;1053(1-2):38–53.

61. Rola R, Mizumatsu S, Otsuka S, et al. Alterations in hippocampal neurogenesis following traumatic brain injury in mice. *Exp Neurol*. 2006;202(1):189–199.

62. Sun D, Colello RJ, Daugherty WP, et al. Cell proliferation and neuronal differentiation in the dentate gyrus in juvenile and adult rats following traumatic brain injury. *J Neurotrauma*. 2005;22(1):95–105.

63. Sun D, McGinn MJ, Zhou Z, Harvey HB, Bullock MR, Colello RJ. Anatomical integration of newly generated dentate granule neurons following traumatic brain injury in adult rats and its association to cognitive recovery. *Exp Neurol*. 2007;204(1):264–272.

64. Yoshimura S, Teramoto T, Whalen MJ, et al. FGF-2 regulates neurogenesis and degeneration in the dentate gyrus after traumatic brain injury in mice. *J Clin Invest*. 2003;112(8):1202–1210.

65. Zheng W, ZhuGe Q, Zhong M, et al. Neurogenesis in adult human brain after traumatic brain injury. *J Neurotrauma*. 2013;30(22):1872–1880.

66. Gao X, Chen J. Moderate traumatic brain injury promotes neural precursor proliferation without increasing neurogenesis in the adult hippocampus. *Exp Neurol*. 2013;239:38–48.

67. Bye N, Carron S, Han X, et al. Neurogenesis and glial proliferation are stimulated following diffuse traumatic brain injury in adult rats. *J Neurosci Res*. 2011;89(7):986–1000.

68. Wang X, Gao X, Michalski S, Zhao S, Chen J. Traumatic brain injury severity affects neurogenesis in adult mouse hippocampus. *J Neurotrauma*. 2015;33(8):721–733.

69. Sierra A, Encinas JM, Deudero JJ, et al. Microglia shape adult hippocampal neurogenesis through apoptosis-coupled phagocytosis. *Cell Stem Cell*. 2010;7(4):483–495.

70. Tashiro A, Sandler VM, Toni N, Zhao C, Gage FH. NMDA-receptor-mediated, cell-specific integration of new neurons in adult dentate gyrus. *Nature*. 2006;442(7105):929–933.

71. Villasana LE, Kim KN, Westbrook GL, Schnell E. Functional integration of adult-born hippocampal neurons after traumatic brain injury (1,2,3). *eNeuro*. 2015;2(5).

72. Hunt RF, Boychuk JA, Smith BN. Neural circuit mechanisms of post-traumatic epilepsy. *Front Cell Neurosci*. 2013;7:89.

73. Emery DL, Fulp CT, Saatman KE, Schutz C, Neugebauer E, McIntosh TK. Newly born granule cells in the dentate gyrus rapidly extend axons into the hippocampal CA3 region following experimental brain injury. *J Neurotrauma*. 2005;22(9):978–988.

74. Giza CC, Prins ML. Is being plastic fantastic? Mechanisms of altered plasticity after developmental traumatic brain injury. *Dev Neurosci*. 2006;28(4-5):364–379.

75. Maxwell WL. Traumatic brain injury in the neonate, child and adolescent human: an overview of pathology. *Int J Dev Neurosci*. 2012;30(3):167–183.

76. Stocchetti N, Paterno R, Citerio G, Beretta L, Colombo A. Traumatic brain injury in an aging population. *J Neurotrauma*. 2012;29(6):1119–1125.

77. Fan P, Yamauchi T, Noble LJ, Ferriero DM. Age-dependent differences in glutathione peroxidase activity after traumatic brain injury. *J Neurotrauma*. 2003;20(5):437–445.

78. Timaru-Kast R, Luh C, Gotthardt P, et al. Influence of age on brain edema formation, secondary brain damage and inflammatory response after brain trauma in mice. *PloS One.* 2012;7(8):e43829.

79. Sun D, McGinn M, Hankins JE, Mays KM, Rolfe A, Colello RJ. Aging- and injury-related differential apoptotic response in the dentate gyrus of the hippocampus in rats following brain trauma. *Front Aging Neurosci.* 2013;5:95.

80. Jinno S. Decline in adult neurogenesis during aging follows a topographic pattern in the mouse hippocampus. *J Comp Neurol.* 2011;519(3):451–466.

81. Covey MV, Jiang Y, Alli VV, Yang Z, Levison SW. Defining the critical period for neocortical neurogenesis after pediatric brain injury. *Dev Neurosci.* 2010;32(5-6):488–498.

82. Potts MB, Rola R, Claus CP, Ferriero DM, Fike JR, Noble-Haeusslein LJ. Glutathione peroxidase overexpression does not rescue impaired neurogenesis in the injured immature brain. *J Neurosci Res.* 2009;87(8):1848–1857.

83. Macas J, Nern C, Plate KH, Momma S. Increased generation of neuronal progenitors after ischemic injury in the aged adult human forebrain. *J Neurosci.* 2006;26(50):13114–13119.

84. Schmidt RH, Scholten KJ, Maughan PH. Time course for recovery of water maze performance and central cholinergic innervation after fluid percussion injury. *J Neurotrauma.* 1999;16(12):1139–1147.

85. Prigatano GP. Recovery and cognitive retraining after craniocerebral trauma. *J Learn Disabil.* 1987;20(10):603–613.

86. Kleindienst A, McGinn MJ, Harvey HB, Colello RJ, Hamm RJ, Bullock MR. Enhanced hippocampal neurogenesis by intraventricular S100B infusion is associated with improved cognitive recovery after traumatic brain injury. *J Neurotrauma.* 2005;22(6):645–655.

87. Lu D, Mahmood A, Qu C, Goussev A, Schallert T, Chopp M. Erythropoietin enhances neurogenesis and restores spatial memory in rats after traumatic brain injury. *J Neurotrauma.* 2005;22(9):1011–1017.

88. Lu D, Mahmood A, Zhang R, Copp M. Upregulation of neurogenesis and reduction in functional deficits following administration of DEtA/NONOate, a nitric oxide donor, after traumatic brain injury in rats. *J Neurosurg.* 2003;99(2):351–361.

89. Wu H, Lu D, Jiang H, et al. Simvastatin-mediated upregulation of VEGF and BDNF, activation of the PI3K/Akt pathway, and increase of neurogenesis are associated with therapeutic improvement after traumatic brain injury. *J Neurotrauma.* 2008;25(2):130–139.

90. Lu D, Qu C, Goussev A, et al. Statins increase neurogenesis in the dentate gyrus, reduce delayed neuronal death in the hippocampal CA3 region, and improve spatial learning in rat after traumatic brain injury. *J Neurotrauma.* 2007;24(7):1132–1146.

91. Sun D, Bullock MR, McGinn MJ, et al. Basic fibroblast growth factor-enhanced neurogenesis contributes to cognitive recovery in rats following traumatic brain injury. *Exp Neurol.* 2009;216(1):56–65.

92. Blaiss CA, Yu TS, Zhang G, et al. Temporally specified genetic ablation of neurogenesis impairs cognitive recovery after traumatic brain injury. *J Neurosci.* 2011;31(13):4906–4916.

93. Sun D, Daniels TE, Rolfe A, Waters M, Hamm R. Inhibition of injury-induced cell proliferation in the dentate gyrus of the hippocampus impairs spontaneous cognitive recovery after traumatic brain injury. *J Neurotrauma.* 2015;32(7):495–505.

94. Lee HM, Giguere PM, Roth BL. DREADDs: novel tools for drug discovery and development. *Drug Discov Today.* 2014;19(4):469–473.

Stem Cell Studies in Traumatic Brain Injury

Dong Sun

30

Introduction

Traumatic brain injury (TBI) is a global public health concern, with limited treatment options available. In the United States alone, between 3.2 and 5.3 million people suffer long-term cognitive impairments as a result of TBI.[1] While there have been significant advancements in TBI-related mortality in the past 10 years, approximately 80,000 individuals in the United States annually sustain TBIs that result in significant long-term disability. These impairments involve both sensory motor and memory functions and can result in a total vegetative state. TBI is characterized by both neuronal and white matter loss with resultant brain atrophy and functional neurological impairment. To date, there is no effective treatment for TBI. Current therapies are mostly focused on reducing secondary injuries. Strategies targeting regeneration and repair are limited. Recent identification of functional neural stem cells (NSCs) in the mature mammalian brain and advances in techniques for generating NSCs in culture have raised the possibility of developing stem cell–based therapies to enhance the repair and regeneration of injured brain following TBI. Two approaches—modulating endogenous NSCs or utilizing exogenous stem cells—are gaining increasing attention in the field of neural regeneration. This chapter reviews recent progress in experimental TBI therapeutic development with endogenous neurogenesis and neural transplantation.

Endogenous Neural Stem Cell Study

Endogenous Neurogenesis in the Normal Mature Mammalian Brain

NSCs are multipotent, self-renewing cells that generate both neurons and glia in the nervous system. One of the leading discoveries in neuroscience research in recent years is the identification of adult NSCs in the mature mammalian brain. It is now well established that new neurons are constantly generated throughout life in the mature mammalian brain from NSCs residing in the neurogenic regions of the subventricular zone (SVZ) and the dentate gyrus (DG) of the hippocampus.[2,3] NSCs in the SVZ give rise to olfactory interneurons, whereas NSCs in the DG generate dentate granular neurons.[4,5] In rodent brains, adult NSCs are capable of generating large numbers of new neurons throughout life. However, in normal adult rodent brains under normal housing conditions, approximately half of the newly generated neurons in the DG and olfactory-bound SVZ cells have a transient existence of 2 weeks or less.[6–9] Those surviving adult-generated new neurons send out axon projections to their targeted areas and form synapses within the local neural circuitry, thus becoming functional neurons.

In the DG, adult NSC-derived new neurons play important roles in hippocampal-dependent learning and memory functions,[10–12] whereas the SVZ-derived new olfactory interneurons are required for the normal functioning of the olfactory bulb network and some selected olfactory behaviors.[13–15]

In rodent brains, the degree of adult neurogenesis declines with increasing age and is affected by many factors. Biochemical factors such as growth factors and steroids tightly regulate the proliferation and differentiation of the NSCs.[16–18] Other factors such as exercise, enriched environment, or stress can also affect the level of neurogenesis.[19–21] Studies have also shown that TBI induces an up-regulation of neurogenesis in varying types of TBI models.[22]

Endogenous Neural Stem Cell Response Following TBI

It is now well recognized that TBI results in an increased proliferation of NSCs and the generation of new neurons within the SVZ and hippocampus. TBI-induced activation of NSCs has been observed in multiple types of experimental TBI models including fluid percussive injury (FPI),[23,24] controlled cortical impact injury (CCI),[25,26] closed head weight-drop injury,[27] and acceleration-impact injury.[28] Common to all reported TBI models, the most prominent endogenous cell response in both the DG and SVZ following TBI is an increase in cell proliferation. This injury-enhanced cell proliferation is relatively transient and is observed during the first week post-injury, with a peak time at 2 days in the DG in both rat FPI and mouse CCI models.[29,30] Increased generation of new neurons resulting from the TBI-enhanced NSC proliferation was also observed particularly in the hippocampus in these models.[27,31] It was also noted that an increased hippocampal neurogenesis in both cell proliferation and generation of new neurons was only observed in the more severely injured animals.[27] These studies clearly demonstrated that TBI stimulates activation of endogenous NSCs in the neurogenic regions of the mature rodent brain and that the response of NSCs to the injury signal is time- and severity-dependent. Further studies have found that injury-induced newly generated granular cells integrate into the existing hippocampal circuitry,[31,32] and this injury-enhanced endogenous NSC response is directly associated with the innate cognitive recovery observed following TBI in rodents.[33,34]

Compared to rodent brains, the degree and function of adult neurogenesis in the human brain is less clear. Similar to rodent brains, the SVZ and the hippocampus in human brains are the active neurogenic regions.[35,36] Proliferating NSCs have been found in these areas from autopsy brain samples. However, the degree of neurogenesis in the SVZ and the subsequent migration of newly generated neurons from SVZ to the neocortex and olfactory bulbs are rather limited and are only observed in early childhood.[37–39] However, a recent study has reported a substantial degree of hippocampal neurogenesis in human brains and that the rate of neurogenesis is comparable between middle-aged humans and mice.[40] Thus far, clear evidence of TBI-induced generation of new neurons in humans is lacking due to difficulties in obtaining human brain samples, as well as technical challenges to birth-dating NSCs. Nevertheless, neurons expressing immature neuronal markers were reported in human brains in regions around lesions of focal infarction,[41] TBI,[42] and subarachnoid hemorrhage.[43]

Treatment Targeting Endogenous Neural Stem Cells for TBI

Although TBI enhances endogenous NSC response, the capacity of this self-repair is rather limited. To achieve the goal of regeneration, recent experimental studies have explored many therapeutic strategies to further enhance post-TBI NSC response. These strategies have shown varying degrees of beneficial effects in improving sensory-motor and cognitive functional recovery in injured animals, and these beneficial effects are related to increased mobilization of endogenous stem cell pools, including NSC proliferation, neuronal differentiation, and survival.

Growth Factors, Small Molecules, or Peptides Imitating Growth or Neurotrophic Factors

Growth factors are essential for cell proliferation, differentiation, and survival. Studies have shown that direct supplementation via intraventricular infusion of growth factors such as basic fibroblast growth factor,[44] epidermal growth factor,[45] vascular endothelial growth factor,[46,47] or calcium binding protein B (S100β), a neurotropic protein secreted by astrocytes,[48] can significantly enhance TBI-induced NSC proliferation in the hippocampus and the SVZ and improve cognitive functional recovery in injured animals (Figures 30.1 and 30.2).

Direct application of growth factor for clinical use is limited due to the invasive delivery method. Small molecules, which act as agonist-mimicking growth factor functions, could be more applicable to clinical use, with better peneration through the blood–brain barrier and with a longer half-life. Studies have reported beneficial effects of 7,8-dihydroxyflavone, a synthetic neurotrophin TrkB receptor agonist that imitates brain-derived neurotrophic factor[49,50]; LM11A-31, a small-molecule p75NTR signaling modulator[51]; cerebrolysin, a pharmacologically prepared low-molecular-weight neuropeptide derived from purified porcine brain proteins which has pharmacodynamic properties similar to endogenous neurotrophic factors[52]; and peptide 6, a small molecule that corresponds to an active region of human ciliary neurotrophic factor (CNTF).[53] Cerebrolysin has been shown to enhance cognitive improvements in mild TBI patients in a clinical trial.[54]

Drugs with Clinical Use and Other Pharmacological Agents

Therapies that can be readily translated into clinical application include those drugs that are approved by the US Food and Drug Administration (FDA) or drugs that are already in clinical use. Thus far, several FDA-approved drugs used in the treatment of TBI include statins, a class of hydroxymethylglutaryl-coenzyme A reductase inhibitors for treating hyperlipidemia; tissue plasminogen activator (tPA), the drug for early stroke treatment; selective serotonin reuptake inhibitors imipramine and fluoxetine; NeuroAid (MLC901), a traditional Chinese medicine used for stroke; and angiotensin II receptor type 2 (AT2) agonists, which have been tested in animal studies in varying TBI models.[55–61]

Apart from these drugs, several pharmacologic agents have been identified with functions stimulating endogenous NSC response and improving cognitive recovery of injured animals following TBI. These agents include erythropoietin (EPO), a hormone that regulates production of red blood cells[62,63]; thymosin β4, a small peptide G-actin sequestering molecule[64]; and the P7C3 class of aminopropyl carbazole agents.[65]

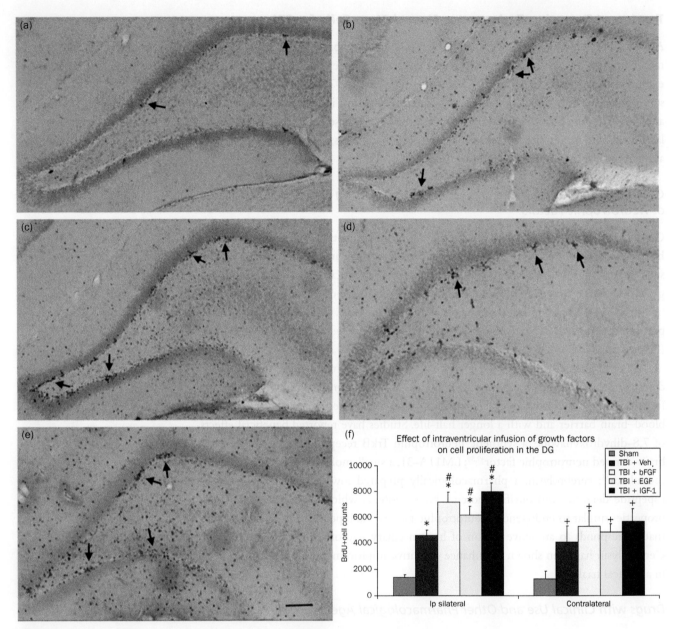

Figure 30.1 Growth factor infusion enhances cell proliferation in the DG. Coronal sections of the ipsilateral dentate gyrus (DG) taken from the following animals at 7 days post-injury: (A) sham with vehicle infusion; (B) injured with vehicle infusion; (C) injured with bFGF infusion; (D) injured with EGF infusion; and (E) injured with IGF-1 infusion. Increased numbers of proliferating neural stem cells (NSCs) labeled with thymidine analog BrdU were observed in the injured animals with either vehicle or growth factor infusions compared to the sham (*brown dots indicated by arrows*). NSCs labeled with bromodeoxyuridine (BrdU) in the DG were clustered and mainly located in the subgranular zone. Bar = 100 μm. (F) Quantification analysis of the degree of cell proliferation in the DG. Compared to sham, injured animals with vehicle or growth infusion had significantly higher numbers of proliferating cells in the granular zone in both ipsilateral (*$p < 0.05$) and contralateral side (+$p < 0.05$), n = 5 per group. Compared to injured with vehicle infusion, injured animals which received basic fibroblast growth factor (bFGF), epidermal growth factor (EGF), or insulin–like growth factor (IGF-1) had significantly higher numbers of BrdU-positive cells in the ipsilateral granular zone (#$p < 0.05$).

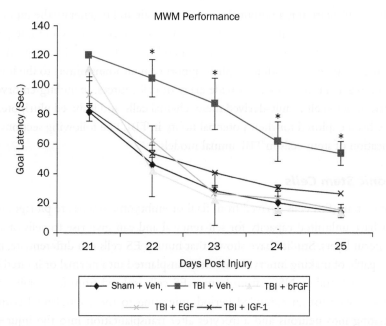

Figure 30.2 Growth factor infusion improves cognitive recovery following traumatic brain injury (TBI). Graph compares Morris water maze performance of injured rats infused with either basic fibroblast growth factor (bFGF), epidermal growth factor (EGF), insulin-like growth factor (IGF-1), or vehicle, to sham animals infused with vehicle alone. Injured rats infused with bFGF, EGF, or IGF-1 showed a significant improvement of cognitive recovery as compared to injured rats with vehicle (★$p<0.01$, n = 10/group). This cognitive recovery, as characterized by shorter goal latency in the water maze performance, reached similar levels to that observed in sham animals through days 21–25 following injury.

Physical or Other Radical Approaches

Under homeostatic condition, increased hippocampal neurogenesis is observed in response to several physiological stimuli such as physical exercise and environmental enrichment.[21,66] Studies have reported that environmental enrichment or physical exercise applied to injured animals at appropriate times following TBI can further increase generation of new neurons in the hippocampus and improve cognitive recovery.[67–69] Similar positive results were also observed following a transcranial low-light laser therapy.[67]

Summary

Overall, these strategies have shown promising effects for TBI treatment by enhancing NSC proliferation, neuronal differentiation, and survival of newly generated neurons. In addition, they may offer neural protective effects to improve the recovery of functions in injured animals. These studies have demonstrated the potential of targeting endogenous repair mechanisms via NSCs for neural regeneration following TBI.

Stem Cell Transplantation for Brain Repair and Regeneration

Following TBI, injury-induced neural tissue loss is permanent. Currently, there is no effective treatment to improve neural structural and functional recovery in patients.

Stem cell transplantation is a potential strategy to repair and regenerate the injured brain because transplanted cells may differentiate into region-specific cells and integrate into the host tissue to replace lost cells in the injured brain. Alternatively, transplanted cells could acting as carriers, providing trophic support or neurotransmitters to the host tissue to facilitate regeneration. To date, a wide array of cell sources, including embryonic or adult-derived stem cells, adult-derived mesenchymal cells, and induced pluripotent stem cells, have been explored for their potential utility in TBI. The following sections discuss the application of stem cells in TBI animal models.

Embryonic Stem Cells

Embryonic stem (ES) cells derived from fetal or embryonic brains are pluripotent stem cells that have unlimited capacity for self-renewal and can give rise to cells of all three primary germ layers. Studies have shown that human ES cells can differentiate, migrate, and are capable of making innervations after transplanted into normal or injured brain.[70] In experimental studies, NSCs from human ES cells isolated from fetal brain were capable of surviving for an extended period, migrating to the contralateral cortex, and differentiating into neurons and astrocytes after transplantation into the injured brain following a focal brain injury.[71] It is reported that transplanted NSCs from human ES cells can differentiate into mature neurons and release growth factors that improve cognitive functional recovery in the injured host.[72] Long-term survival (up to 1 year) of grafted NSCs derived from mice fetal brains is reported, with extensive migration in the injured brain and maturation into neurons or glial cells accompanied by improved motor and spatial learning functions in the host.[73–75] Additionally, in vitro modified ES cells either predifferentiated into mature neurons expressing neurotransmitters or overexpressing growth factors can significantly promote graft survival and neuronal differentiation and also improve the motor and cognitive functional recovery of injured recipients.[76–79]

Adult Neural Stem Cells

As mentioned earlier, mature mammalian CNS harbors multipotent NSCs capable of differentiating into mature neurons and glia.[80,81] These adult-derived NSCs are capable of becoming region-specific cells when transplanted into the normal adult rodent brain.[82–84] After transplantation into the injured brain following TBI, these cells can survive for a long period and become region-specific functional cells.[85] Apart from the neurogenic regions, neural stem/progenitor-like cells can also be isolated from various regions of the adult human brain using neurosurgical resection tissues and can become mature neurons and glia in culture.[86–93] Because of their adult origin, these cells may possibly be used as autologous cell sources for neural transplantation therapies to regenerate the injured CNS, as demonstrated in a study that grafted adult human-derived NSCs into the demyelinated rat spinal cord.[94] However, due to their adult origin, these cells have less plasticity compared to ES cells. To date, very few studies have reported the outcome of these adult human-derived NSCs in the injured mature CNS. Olstorn and colleagues reported that a small portion (4% ± 1%) of adult human NSCs can survive for 16 weeks after transplantation into the posterior periventricular region in normal adult rats or rats with hippocampal CA1 ischemic injury.[95]

Induced Pluripotent Stem Cells

Recent developments in cell reprogramming techniques have generated *induced pluripotent stem cells* (iPSCs) from somatic cells, which provides prospects for novel stem cell replacement strategies. iPSCs can provide large quantities of pluripotent cells with high plasticity.

Human iPSCs possess properties of unlimited self-renewal and the pluripotent potential to differentiate into multilineage cells, including neurons. More importantly, iPSCs can be derived from patients themselves and have potential for autologous transplantation, thus avoiding ethical and graft rejection concerns. These unique properties of iPSCs have raised hope that many neurological diseases, including TBI, might be cured or treated. Thus far, rapid progress has been made in the field of reprogramming, but the optimal source of somatic cells used for applications in neurological disorders has not yet been identified. Thus far, limited studies have explored iPSCs as a neural transplantation cell source following stroke[96–99] and spinal cord injury.[100,101] In TBI models, only two publications found in PubMed explored the feasibility of using iPSCs for post-TBI transplantation, with rather limited information about the function, survival, and integration rate of iPSCs in the injured brain.[102,103]

Mesenchymal-Derived Cells

Recently, adult-derived mesenchymal cells, including bone marrow stromal cells (BMSCs), human amnion-derived multipotent progenitor cells, human adipose-derived stem cells, human umbilical cord blood, and peripheral blood derived MSCs, have been tested as treatment for TBI in both animal studies and clinic trials.[104–110] These mesenchymal-derived cells are undifferentiated cells with a mixed cell population that includes stem and progenitor cells. In culture conditions, they can be induced to differentiate into neuronal phenotypes. These cells produce high levels of growth factors, cytokines, and extracellular matrix molecules that could have potential neurotrophic or neuroprotective effects in the injured brain.[111,112]

The potential of BMSCs for treating TBI has been extensively assessed in experimental TBI models. Cells were delivered either focally to the injured brain or systemically through intravenous or intraarterial injections during the acute or subacute phase after TBI, and a significant reduction in neurological deficits, including motor and cognitive deficits, was reported.[109,113,114] The effect of BMSCs in improving sensorimotor function in injured animals was reported even when delivered at 2 months following TBI.[110] Further studies have demonstrated that the beneficial effect of these mesenchymal cells is due primarily to the bioactive factors they produce to facilitate the endogenous plasticity and remodeling of the host brain, rather than direct neural replacement because direct neuronal differentiation and long-term survival were rarely observed.[111]

Conclusion

Extensive studies have demonstrated the possibility of stem cell therapy for brain repair and regeneration. Considerable progress has been made in stem cell–based neural regeneration in stroke and neurodegenerative diseases in both experimental and clinical settings. However for post-TBI neural regeneration of injured brain, we still have a long way to go from experimental studies to clinical application due to the complexity and diversity of brain trauma. To successfully repair and regenerate the injured brain with stem cells, many challenges must be overcome. In the case of endogenous neurogenesis, strategies that can promote long-term survival and guide newly generated cells to migrate to the injury site are needed. In neural transplantation, the fate of transplanted cells is determined by the intrinsic properties of the grafted cells and local environmental cues in the host. To achieve successful neural transplantation, it is necessary to improve both aspects. These challenges must be overcome in experimental TBI studies before stem cell therapies can have clinical application.

References

1. Coronado VG, McGuire LC, Sarmiento K, et al. Trends in Traumatic Brain Injury in the US and the public health response: 1995–2009. *J Safety Res.* 2012;43(4):299–307.

2. Altman J, Das GD. Autoradiographic and histological evidence of postnatal hippocampal neurogenesis in rats. *J Comp Neurol.* 1965;124(3):319–335.

3. Lois C, Alvarez-Buylla A. Proliferating subventricular zone cells in the adult mammalian forebrain can differentiate into neurons and glia. *Proc Natl Acad Sci USA.* 1993;90(5):2074–2077.

4. Gritti A, Bonfanti L, Doetsch F, et al. Multipotent neural stem cells reside into the rostral extension and olfactory bulb of adult rodents. *J Neurosci.* 2002;22(2):437–445.

5. Kempermann G, Gast D, Kronenberg G, Yamaguchi M, Gage FH. Early determination and long-term persistence of adult-generated new neurons in the hippocampus of mice. *Development.* 2003;130(2):391–399.

6. Gould E, Vail N, Wagers, M, Gross CG. Adult-generated hippocampal and neocortical neurons in macaques have a transient existence. *Proc Nat Acad Sci USA.* 2001;98(19):10910–10917.

7. Mouret A, Gheusi, G, Gabellec MM, de Chaumont F, Olivo-Marin JC, Lledo PM. Learning and survival of newly generated neurons: when time matters. *J Neurosci.* 2008;28(45):11511–11516.

8. Sultan S, Rey N, Sacquet J, Mandairon N, Didier A. Newborn neurons in the olfactory bulb selected for long-term survival through olfactory learning are prematurely suppressed when the olfactory memory is erased. *J Neurosci.* 2011;31(42):14893–14898.

9. Dayer AG, Ford AA, Cleaver KM, Yassaee M, Cameron HA. Short-term and long-term survival of new neurons in the rat dentate gyrus. *J Comp Neurol.* 2003;460(4):563–572.

10. Deng W, Saxe MD, Gallina IS, Gage FH. Adult-born hippocampal dentate granule cells undergoing maturation modulate learning and memory in the brain. *J Neurosci.* 2009;29(43):13532–13542.

11. Clelland CD, Choi M, Romberg C, et al. A functional role for adult hippocampal neurogenesis in spatial pattern separation. *Science.* 2009;325(5937):210–213.

12. Aimone JB, Li Y, Lee SW, Clemenson GD, Deng W, Gage, FH. Regulation and function of adult neurogenesis: from genes to cognition. *Physiol Rev.* 2014;94(4):991–1026.

13. Moreno MM, Linster C, Escanilla O, Sacquet J, Didier A, Mandairon N. Olfactory perceptual learning requires adult neurogenesis. *Proc Nat Acad Sci USA.* 2009;106(42):17980–17985.

14. Breton-Provencher V, Lemasson M, Peralta MR III, Saghatelyan A. Interneurons produced in adulthood are required for the normal functioning of the olfactory bulb network and for the execution of selected olfactory behaviors. *J Neurosci.* 2009;29(48):15245–15257.

15. Sakamoto M, Kageyama R, Imayoshi I. The functional significance of newly born neurons integrated into olfactory bulb circuits. *Front Neurosci.* 2014;8: 121.

16. Tanapat P, Hastings NB, Reeves AJ, Gould E. Estrogen stimulates a transient increase in the number of new neurons in the dentate gyrus of the adult female rat. *J Neurosci.* 1999;19(14):5792–5801.

17. Cameron HA, Gould E. Adult neurogenesis is regulated by adrenal steroids in the dentate gyrus. *Neuroscience.* 1994;61(2):203–209.

18. Kuhn HG, Winkler J, Kempermann G, Thal LJ, Gage FH. Epidermal growth factor and fibroblast growth factor-2 have different effects on neural progenitors in the adult rat brain. *J Neurosci.* 1997;17(15):5820–5829.

19. Gould E, Tanapat P. Stress and hippocampal neurogenesis. *Biol Psychiatry.* 1999;46(11):1472–1479.

20. Kempermann G, van Praag H, Gage FH. Activity-dependent regulation of neuronal plasticity and self repair. *Prog Brain Res.* 2000;127:35–48.

21. van Praag H, Kempermann G, Gage FH. Running increases cell proliferation and neurogenesis in the adult mouse dentate gyrus. *Nat Neurosci.* 1999;2(3):266–270.

22. Sun D. Endogenous neurogenic cell response in the mature mammalian brain following traumatic injury. *Exp Neurol.* 2016;275(Pt 3):405–410.

23. Chirumamilla S, Sun D, Bullock MR, Colello RJ. Traumatic brain injury induced cell proliferation in the adult mammalian central nervous system. *J Neurotrauma.* 2002;19(6):693–703.

24. Rice AC, Khaldi A, Harvey HB, et al. Proliferation and neuronal differentiation of mitotically active cells following traumatic brain injury. *Exp Neurol.* 2003;183(2):406–417.

25. Dash PK, Mach SA, Moore AN. Enhanced neurogenesis in the rodent hippocampus following traumatic brain injury. *J Neurosci Res.* 2001;63(4):313–319.

26. Gao X, Enikolopov G, Chen J. Moderate traumatic brain injury promotes proliferation of quiescent neural progenitors in the adult hippocampus. *Exp Neurol.* 2009;219(2):516–523.

27. Villasana LE, Westbrook GL, Schnell E. Neurologic impairment following closed head injury predicts post-traumatic neurogenesis. *Exp Neurol.* 2014;261:156–162.

28. Bye N, Carron S, Han X, et al. Neurogenesis and glial proliferation are stimulated following diffuse traumatic brain injury in adult rats. *J Neurosci Res.* 2011;89(7):986–1000.

29. Sun D, Colello RJ, Daugherty WP, et al. Cell proliferation and neuronal differentiation in the dentate gyrus in juvenile and adult rats following traumatic brain injury. *J Neurotrauma.* 2005;22(1):95–105.

30. Gao X, Chen J. Moderate traumatic brain injury promotes neural precursor proliferation without increasing neurogenesis in the adult hippocampus. *Exp Neurol.* 2013;239:38–48.

31. Sun D, McGinn MJ, Zhou Z, Harvey HB, Bullock MR, Colello RJ. Anatomical integration of newly generated dentate granule neurons following traumatic brain injury in adult rats and its association to cognitive recovery. *Exp Neurol.* 2007;204(1):264–272.

32. Emery DL, Fulp CT, Saatman KE, Schutz C, Neugebauer E, McIntosh TK. Newly born granule cells in the dentate gyrus rapidly extend axons into the hippocampal CA3 region following experimental brain injury. *J Neurotrauma.* 2005;22(9):978–988.

33. Blaiss CA, Yu TS, Zhang G, et al. Temporally specified genetic ablation of neurogenesis impairs cognitive recovery after traumatic brain injury. *J Neurosci.* 2011;31(13):4906–4916.

34. Sun D, Daniels TE, Rolfe A, Waters M, Hamm R. Inhibition of injury-induced cell proliferation in the dentate gyrus of the hippocampus impairs spontaneous cognitive recovery after traumatic brain injury. *J Neurotrauma* 2015;32(7):495–505.

35. Eriksson PS, Perfilieva E, Bjork-Eriksson T, et al. Neurogenesis in the adult human hippocampus. *Nat Med.* 1998;4(11):1313–1317.

36. Sanai N, Tramontin AD, Quinones-Hinojosa A, et al. Unique astrocyte ribbon in adult human brain contains neural stem cells but lacks chain migration. *Nature.* 2004;427(6976):740–744.

37. Bhardwaj RD, Curtis MA, Spalding KL, et al. Neocortical neurogenesis in humans is restricted to development. *Proc Nat Acad Sci USA.* 2006;103(33):12564–12568.

38. Sanai N, Nguyen T, Ihrie RA, et al. Corridors of migrating neurons in the human brain and their decline during infancy. *Nature.* 2011;478(7369):382–386.

39. Bergmann O, Liebl J, Bernard S, et al. The age of olfactory bulb neurons in humans. *Neuron.* 2012;74(4):634–639.

40. Spalding KL, Bergmann O, Alkass K, et al. Dynamics of hippocampal neurogenesis in adult humans. *Cell.* 2013;153(6):1219–1227.

41. Taylor SR, Smith C, Harris BT, Costine BA, Duhaime AC. Maturation-dependent response of neurogenesis after traumatic brain injury in children. *J Neurosurg Pediatr.* 2013;12(6):545–554.

42. Zheng W, Zhuge Q, Zhong M, et al. Neurogenesis in adult human brain after traumatic brain injury. *J Neurotrauma.* 2013;30(22):1872–1880.

43. Sgubin D, Aztiria E, Perin A, Longatti P, Leanza G. Activation of endogenous neural stem cells in the adult human brain following subarachnoid hemorrhage. *J Neurosci Res.* 2007;85(8):1647–1655.

44. Sun D, Bullock MR, McGinn MJ, et al. Basic fibroblast growth factor-enhanced neurogenesis contributes to cognitive recovery in rats following traumatic brain injury. *Exp Neurol.* 2009;216(1):56–65.

45. Sun D, Bullock MR, Altememi N, et al. The effect of epidermal growth factor in the injured brain after trauma in rats. *J Neurotrauma.* 2010;27(5):923–938.

46. Lee C, Agoston DV. Vascular endothelial growth factor is involved in mediating increased de novo hippocampal neurogenesis in response to traumatic brain injury. *J Neurotrauma.* 2010;27(3):541–553.

47. Thau-Zuchman O, Shohami E, Alexandrovich AG, Leker RR. Vascular endothelial growth factor increases neurogenesis after traumatic brain injury. *J Cereb Blood Flow Metab.* 2010;30(5):1008–1016.

48. Kleindienst A, McGinn MJ, Harvey HB, Colello RJ, Hamm RJ, Bullock MR. Enhanced hippocampal neurogenesis by intraventricular S100B infusion is associated with improved cognitive recovery after traumatic brain injury. *J Neurotrauma* 2005;22(6):645–655.

49. Chen, L, Gao, X, Zhao, S, Hu, W, Chen, J. The small-molecule TrkB agonist 7, 8-dihydroxyflavone decreases hippocampal newborn neuron death after traumatic brain injury. *J Neuropathol Exp Neurol.* 2015;74(6):557–567.

50. Zhao S, Yu A, Wang X, Gao X, Chen J. Post-injury treatment of 7,8-dihydroxyflavone promotes neurogenesis in the hippocampus of the adult mouse. *J Neurotrauma.* 2016;33(22):2055–2064.

51. Shi J, Longo FM, Massa SM. A small molecule p75(NTR) ligand protects neurogenesis after traumatic brain injury. *Stem Cells.* 2013;31(11):2561–2574.

52. Zhang Y, Chopp M, Meng Y, et al. Cerebrolysin improves cognitive performance in rats after mild traumatic brain injury. *J Neurosurg.* 2015;122(4):843–855.

53. Chohan MO, Bragina O, Kazim SF, et al. Enhancement of neurogenesis and memory by a neurotrophic peptide in mild to moderate traumatic brain injury. *Neurosurgery.* 2015;76(2): 201–214.

54. Chen CC, Wei ST, Tsaia SC, Chen XX, Cho DY. Cerebrolysin enhances cognitive recovery of mild traumatic brain injury patients: double-blind, placebo-controlled, randomized study. *Br J Neurosurg.* 2013;27(6):803–807.

55. Lu D, Qu C, Goussev A, et al. Statins increase neurogenesis in the dentate gyrus, reduce delayed neuronal death in the hippocampal CA3 region, and improve spatial learning in rat after traumatic brain injury. *J Neurotrauma* 2007;24(7):1132–1146.

56. Han X, Tong J, Zhang J, et al. Imipramine treatment improves cognitive outcome associated with enhanced hippocampal neurogenesis after traumatic brain injury in mice. *J Neurotrauma.* 2011;28(6):995–1007.

57. Wang Y, Neumann M, Hansen K, et al. Fluoxetine increases hippocampal neurogenesis and induces epigenetic factors but does not improve functional recovery after traumatic brain injury. *J Neurotrauma.* 2011;28(2):259–268.

58. Umschweif G, Liraz-Zaltsman S, Shabashov D, et al. Angiotensin receptor type 2 activation induces neuroprotection and neurogenesis after traumatic brain injury. *Neurotherapeutics.* 2014;11(3):665–678.

59. Xie C, Cong D, Wang X, et al. The effect of simvastatin treatment on proliferation and differentiation of neural stem cells after traumatic brain injury. *Brain Res.* 2015;1602:1–8.

60. Meng Y, Chopp M, Zhang Y, et al. Subacute intranasal administration of tissue plasminogen activator promotes neuroplasticity and improves functional recovery following traumatic brain injury in rats. *PLoS One.* 2014;9(9):e106238.

61. Quintard H, Lorivel T, Gandin C, Lazdunski M, Heurteaux C. MLC901, a traditional chinese medicine induces neuroprotective and neuroregenerative benefits after traumatic brain injury in rats. *Neuroscience.* 2014;277:72–86.

62. Xiong Y, Mahmood A, Meng Y, et al. Delayed administration of erythropoietin reducing hippocampal cell loss, enhancing angiogenesis and neurogenesis, and improving functional outcome following traumatic brain injury in rats: comparison of treatment with single and triple dose. *J Neurosurg.* 2010;113(3):598–608.

63. Zhang Y, Chopp M, Mahmood A, Meng Y, Qu C, Xiong Y. Impact of inhibition of erythropoietin treatment-mediated neurogenesis in the dentate gyrus of the hippocampus on restoration of spatial learning after traumatic brain injury. *Exp Neurol.* 2012;235(1):336–344.

64. Xiong Y, Mahmood A, Meng Y, et al. Neuroprotective and neurorestorative effects of thymosin beta4 treatment following experimental traumatic brain injury. *Ann NY Acad Sci.* 2012;1270:51–58.

65. Blaya MO, Bramlett HM, Naidoo J, Pieper AA, Dietrich WD. Neuroprotective efficacy of a proneurogenic compound after traumatic brain injury. *J Neurotrauma.* 2014;31(5):476–486.

66. Kempermann G, Kuhn HG, Gage FH. More hippocampal neurons in adult mice living in an enriched environment. *Nature.* 1997;386(6624):493–495.

67. Xuan W, Vatansever F, Huang L, Hamblin MR. Transcranial low-level laser therapy enhances learning, memory, and neuroprogenitor cells after traumatic brain injury in mice. *J Biomed Opt.* 2014;19(10):108003.

68. Gaulke LJ, Horner PJ, Fink AJ, McNamara CL, Hicks RR. Environmental enrichment increases progenitor cell survival in the dentate gyrus following lateral fluid percussion injury. *Brain Res Mol Brain Res.* 2005;141(2):138–150.

69. Piao CS, Stoica BA, Wu J, et al. Late exercise reduces neuroinflammation and cognitive dysfunction after traumatic brain injury. *Neurobiol Dis.* 2013;54, 252–263.

70. Hentze H, Graichen R, Colman A. Cell therapy and the safety of embryonic stem cell-derived grafts. *Trends Biotechnol.* 2007;25(1):24–32.

71. Wennersten A, Meier X, Holmin S, Wahlberg L, Mathiesen T. Proliferation, migration, and differentiation of human neural stem/progenitor cells after transplantation into a rat model of traumatic brain injury. *J Neurosurg.* 2004;100(1):88–96.

72. Gao J, Prough DS, McAdoo DJ, et al. Transplantation of primed human fetal neural stem cells improves cognitive function in rats after traumatic brain injury. *Exp Neurol.* 2006;201(2):281–292.

73. Shear DA, Tate MC, Archer DR, et al. Neural progenitor cell transplants promote long-term functional recovery after traumatic brain injury. *Brain Res.* 2004;1026(1):11–22.

74. Riess P, Zhang C, Saatman KE, et al. Transplanted neural stem cells survive, differentiate, and improve neurological motor function after experimental traumatic brain injury. *Neurosurgery.* 2002;51(4):1043–1052.

75. Boockvar JA, Schouten J, Royo N, et al. Experimental traumatic brain injury modulates the survival, migration, and terminal phenotype of transplanted epidermal growth factor receptor-activated neural stem cells. *Neurosurgery.* 2005;56(1):163–171.

76. Becerra GD, Tatko LM, Pak ES, Murashov AK, Hoane MR. Transplantation of GABAergic neurons but not astrocytes induces recovery of sensorimotor function in the traumatically injured brain. *Behav Brain Res.* 2007;179(1):118–125.

77. Bakshi A, Shimizu S, Keck CA, et al. Neural progenitor cells engineered to secrete GDNF show enhanced survival, neuronal differentiation and improve cognitive function following traumatic brain injury. *Eur J Neurosci.* 2006;23(8):2119–2134.

78. Ma H, Yu B, Kong L, Zhang Y, Shi Y. Neural stem cells over-expressing brain-derived neurotrophic factor (BDNF) stimulate synaptic protein expression and promote functional recovery following transplantation in rat model of traumatic brain injury. *Neurochem Res.* 2012;37(1):69–83.

79. Blaya MO, Tsoulfas P, Bramlett HM, Dietrich WD. Neural progenitor cell transplantation promotes neuroprotection, enhances hippocampal neurogenesis, and improves cognitive outcomes after traumatic brain injury. *Exp Neurol.* 2015;264, 67–81.

80. Lois C, Alvarez-Buylla A. Proliferating subventricular zone cells in the adult mammalian forebrain can differentiate into neurons and glia. *Proc Nat Acad Sci USA.* 1993;90(5):2074–2077.

81. Gage FH, Kempermann G, Palmer TD, Peterson DA, Ray J. Multipotent progenitor cells in the adult dentate gyrus. *J Neurobiol.* 1998;36(2):249–266.

82. Gage FH, Coates PW, Palmer TD, et al. Survival and differentiation of adult neuronal progenitor cells transplanted to the adult brain. *Proc Nat Acad Sci USA.* 1995;92(25):11879–11883.

83. Richardson RM, Broaddus WC, Holloway KL, Sun D, Bullock MR, Fillmore HL. Heterotypic neuronal differentiation of adult subependymal zone neuronal progenitor cells transplanted to the adult hippocampus. *Mol Cell Neurosci.* 2005;28(4):674–682.

84. Zhang RL, Zhang L, Zhang ZG, et al. Migration and differentiation of adult rat subventricular zone progenitor cells transplanted into the adult rat striatum. *Neuroscience* 2003;116(2):373–382.

85. Sun D, Gugliotta M, Rolfe A, et al. Sustained survival and maturation of adult neural stem/progenitor cells after transplantation into the injured brain. *J Neurotrauma.* 2011;28(6):961–972.

86. Kukekov VG, Laywell ED, Suslov O, et al. Multipotent stem/progenitor cells with similar properties arise from two neurogenic regions of adult human brain. *Exp Neurol.* 1999;156(2):333–344.

87. Arsenijevic Y, Villemure JG, Brunet JF, et al. Isolation of multipotent neural precursors residing in the cortex of the adult human brain. *Exp Neurol.* 2001;170(1):48–62.

88. Brunet JF, Pellerin L, Arsenijevic Y, Magistretti P, Villemure JG. A novel method for in vitro production of human glial-like cells from neurosurgical resection tissue. *Lab Invest.* 2002;82(6):809–812.

89. Brunet JF, Pellerin L, Magistretti P, Villemure JG. Cryopreservation of human brain tissue allowing timely production of viable adult human brain cells for autologous transplantation. *Cryobiology.* 2003;47(2):179–183.

90. Roy NS, Benraiss A, Wang S, et al. Promoter-targeted selection and isolation of neural progenitor cells from the adult human ventricular zone. *J Neurosci Res.* 2000;59(3):321–331.

91. Nunes MC, Roy NS, Keyoung HM, et al. Identification and isolation of multipotential neural progenitor cells from the subcortical white matter of the adult human brain. *Nat Med.* 2003;9(4):439–447.

92. Windrem MS, Roy NS, Wang J, et al. Progenitor cells derived from the adult human subcortical white matter disperse and differentiate as oligodendrocytes within demyelinated lesions of the rat brain. *J Neurosci Res.* 2002;69(6):966–975.

93. Richardson RM, Holloway KL, Bullock MR, Broaddus WC, Fillmore HL. Isolation of neuronal progenitor cells from the adult human neocortex. *Acta Neurochir (Wien).* 2006;148(7):773–777.

94. Akiyama Y, Honmou O, Kato T, Uede T, Hashi K, Kocsis JD. Transplantation of clonal neural precursor cells derived from adult human brain establishes functional peripheral myelin in the rat spinal cord. *Exp Neurol.* 2001;167(1):27–39.

95. Olstorn H, Moe MC, Roste GK, Bueters T, Langmoen IA. Transplantation of stem cells from the adult human brain to the adult rat brain. *Neurosurgery.* 2007;60(6):1089–1098.

96. Jensen MB, Yan H, Krishnaney-Davison R, Al Sawaf A, Zhang SC. Survival and differentiation of transplanted neural stem cells derived from human induced pluripotent stem cells in a rat stroke model. *J Stroke Cerebrovasc Dis.* 2013;22(4):304–308.

97. Chau MJ, Deveau TC, Song M, Gu X, Chen D, Wei L. iPSC Transplantation increases regeneration and functional recovery after ischemic stroke in neonatal rats. *Stem Cells.* 2014;32(12):3075–3087.

98. Yuan T, Liao W, Feng NH, et al. Human induced pluripotent stem cell-derived neural stem cells survive, migrate, differentiate, and improve neurological function in a rat model of middle cerebral artery occlusion. *Stem Cell Res Ther.* 2013;4(3):73.

99. Tatarishvili J, Oki K, Monni E, et al. Human induced pluripotent stem cells improve recovery in stroke-injured aged rats. *Restor Neurol Neurosci.* 2014;32(4):547–558.

100. Lu P, Woodruff G, Wang Y, et al. Long-distance axonal growth from human induced pluripotent stem cells after spinal cord injury. *Neuron.* 2014;83(4):789–796.

101. Salewski RP, Mitchell RA, Li L, et al. Transplantation of induced pluripotent stem cell-derived neural stem cells mediate functional recovery following thoracic spinal cord injury through remyelination of axons. *Stem Cells Transl Med.* 2015;4(7):743–754.

102. Dunkerson J, Moritz KE, Young J, et al. Combining enriched environment and induced pluripotent stem cell therapy results in improved cognitive and motor function following traumatic brain injury. *Restor Neurol Neurosci.* 2014;32(5):675–687.

103. Tang H, Sha H, Sun H, et al. Tracking induced pluripotent stem cells-derived neural stem cells in the central nervous system of rats and monkeys. *Cell Reprogram.* 2013;15(5):435–442.

104. Chen Z, Tortella FC, Dave JR, et al. Human amnion-derived multipotent progenitor cell treatment alleviates traumatic brain injury-induced axonal degeneration. *J Neurotrauma.* 2009;26(11):1987–1997.

105. Yan ZJ, Zhang P, Hu YQ, et al. Neural stem-like cells derived from human amnion tissue are effective in treating traumatic brain injury in rat. *Neurochem Res.* 2013;38(5):1022–1033.

106. Nichols JE, Niles JA, DeWitt D, et al. Neurogenic and neuro-protective potential of a novel subpopulation of peripheral blood-derived CD133+ ABCG2+CXCR4+ mesenchymal stem cells: development of autologous cell-based therapeutics for traumatic brain injury. *Stem Cell Res Ther.* 2013;4(1):3.

107. Tajiri N, Acosta SA, Shahaduzzaman M, et al. Intravenous transplants of human adipose-derived stem cell protect the brain from traumatic brain injury-induced neurodegeneration and motor and cognitive impairments: cell graft biodistribution and soluble factors in young and aged rats. *J Neurosci.* 2014;34(1):313–326.

108. Lu D, Mahmood A, Wang L, Li Y, Lu M, Chopp M. Adult bone marrow stromal cells administered intravenously to rats after traumatic brain injury migrate into brain and improve neurological outcome. *Neuroreport.* 2001;12(3):559–563.

109. Mahmood A, Lu D, Yi L, Chen JL, Chopp M. Intracranial bone marrow transplantation after traumatic brain injury improving functional outcome in adult rats. *J Neurosurg.* 2001;94(4):589–595.

110. Bonilla C, Zurita M, Otero L, Aguayo C, Vaquero J. Delayed intralesional transplantation of bone marrow stromal cells increases endogenous neurogenesis and promotes functional recovery after severe traumatic brain injury. *Brain Inj.* 2009;23(9):760–769.

111. Li Y, Chopp M. Marrow stromal cell transplantation in stroke and traumatic brain injury. *Neurosci Lett.* 2009;456(3):120–123.

112. Zhang R, Liu Y, Yan K, et al. Anti-inflammatory and immunomodulatory mechanisms of mesenchymal stem cell transplantation in experimental traumatic brain injury. *J Neuroinflammation.* 2013;10(1):106.

113. Lu D, Mahmood A, Wang L, Li Y, Lu M, Chopp M. Adult bone marrow stromal cells administered intravenously to rats after traumatic brain injury migrate into brain and improve neurological outcome. *Neuroreport.* 2001;12(3):559–563.

114. Mahmood A, Lu D, Lu M, Chopp M. Treatment of traumatic brain injury in adult rats with intravenous administration of human bone marrow stromal cells. *Neurosurgery* 2003;53(3):697–702.

Section VI

Spinal Cord Injury

Spinal Cord Injury: Neurointensive Care and Surgical Intervention

John Paul G. Kolcun, Peng-Yuan Chang, and Michael Y. Wang

31

Introduction

Traumatic spinal cord injury (SCI) is a severe condition which requires immediate medical treatment, often including surgical repair and stabilization. Historically, the prognosis for victims of SCI was grim at best. As early as 2500 BCE, the author of the famed Edwin Smith surgical papyrus referred to SCI chillingly as ". . . an ailment not to be treated." Outcomes for these patients did not improve for millennia: during World War I, American neurosurgeon Harvey Cushing reported from France that up to 80% of SCI patients died within the first weeks following injury.[1]

Advancements in the natural and clinical sciences have greatly reduced mortality for contemporary SCI patients. These modern tools of medicine have allowed physicians to develop several therapies for the acute and chronic treatment of SCI.

The key aspects of successfully managing acute SCI patients include a rapid and accurate assessment of the injury, stabilizing the patient, initiating an ongoing treatment protocol, and prophylaxis against complications common to SCI and bedridden patients. Assessment and stabilization truly begin with first responders to the scene of injury, but ongoing care—with more subtle diagnostics—typically occurs in an intensive care unit (ICU) setting or a specialized spine care unit.

Etiology and Epidemiology

There are an estimated 12,500 new cases of SCI annually, predominately occurring among men (~80%), with an average age of 42 years at the time of injury. The leading cause of SCI in the United States is vehicular accident (38%), predominately automobile. Together with falls (30%), these are the major contributors to SCI prevalence. Other causes include violence (primarily gunshot injury), sport-related injury, and medical/surgical injury (Figure 31.1).[2,3]

As mortality has declined, outcomes are by no means ideal for SCI patients, as less than 1% will reach full neurological recovery at the time of hospital discharge. Most patients will leave the hospital with incomplete tetraplegia (45%) or incomplete paraplegia (21%).[3]

While quality of life following SCI has proved difficult to assess, the primary complaint among patients following injury is social disadvantage.[4] The monetary cost of SCI is more easily measured, reaching hundreds of thousands of dollars in the first year after injury, with continued costs in subsequent years of life.[2]

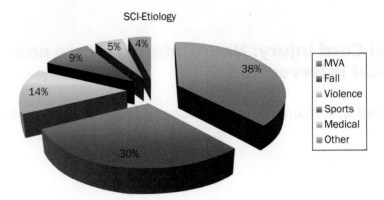

SCI-Etiology

- MVA
- Fall
- Violence
- Sports
- Medical
- Other

Figure 31.1 Etiology of spinal cord injury.

Assessment and Diagnosis

Physical Exam

Upon encountering a victim of SCI, a detailed history must be obtained from the patient (if conscious) and any bystanders or witnesses to the injury. The patient may require immediate stabilization—including respiratory or hemodynamic support—depending on the nature and severity of the injury. If the patient is unconscious, injury to the cervical and thoracic spinal cord must be assumed until proved otherwise and considered in transporting and handling the patient. As some 39% of SCI patients present with another associated injury, attention must be given to the head and vital organs for signs of trauma and emergent wounds dealt with swiftly.[2] When the patient is stable and a thorough history has been taken, both a general and neurological assessment should be carried out to assess the extent of damage.

General examination should include palpation of the entire spine, with attention to the cervical and lumbar lordoses, deformity of spinous processes, and vertebral tenderness. Consideration of the patient's vital signs in this phase of examination can yield insight into possible complications; for example, respiratory irregularities may suggest damage to the cervical spine because spinal nerves C3–C5 supply the diaphragm.

Neurologic Exam

Neurological assessment includes the following criteria: touch sensation, pain sensation, voluntary muscle control, reflexive muscle function, and cranial nerve function.[5-9] The level of injury may be determined by assessing these various parameters and isolating the spinal level beneath which function is absent (complete SCI) or impaired (incomplete SCI). The American Spinal Injury Association (ASIA) has defined *incomplete spinal injury* as the preservation of some degree of function—sensory or motor—beneath the level of injury.[9] ASIA provides assessment guidelines, complete with a standardized form for use by the physician, in which particular muscle groups are used to infer the condition of the spinal cord at each segment (Figure 31.2). The selected muscles are not only reliably innervated by particular spinal segments, but their motions are easily assessed in the bedridden patient (Table 31.1). The Functional Independence Measure (FIM) is also recommended as a tool to assess the patient's level of rehabilitation and ability to carry out the tasks of daily living.[5,10]

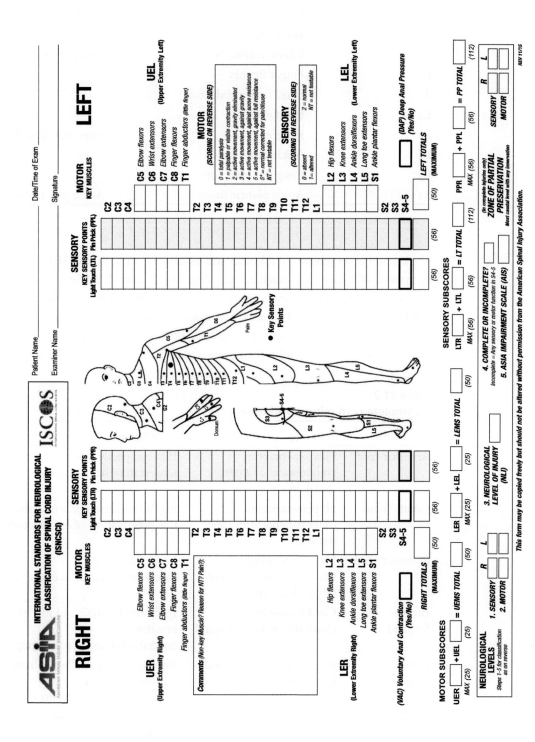

Figure 31.2 American Spinal Cord Injury (ASIA) exam sheet.

Table 31.1:
Muscle/reflex assessment

Spinal Level	Muscles Tested	Reflexes
C5	Elbow flexors	Biceps jerk
C6	Wrist extensors	
C7	Elbow extensors	Triceps jerk
C8	Finger flexors	
T1	Small finger abductors	
L2	Hip flexors	
L3	Knee extensors	Knee jerk (patellar)
L4	Ankle dorsiflexion	
L5	Long toe extensors	
S1	Ankle plantar flexors	Ankle jerk (Achilles)

A number of known syndromes are associated with partial SCI, the signs and symptoms of which may misdirect the diagnosis (Table 31.2). Familiarity with these syndromes' manifestations and vigilance in examination will prevent the physician from misdiagnosing a victim of trauma. Examples include anterior, central, and posterior cord syndromes; Brown-Séquard syndrome (often resulting from stab injuries or lateral fractures); conus medullaris syndrome (affecting the sacral cord); and cauda equina

Table 31.2:
Incomplete cord injury syndromes

Syndrome	Etiology	Symptoms
Anterior cord	Flexion-rotation; compression of anterior spinal artery	Bilateral paralysis with loss of pain/temperature below injury
Central cord	Hyperextension; older patients with canal stenosis	Flaccid weakness of arms/hands, relative preservation of leg function
Posterior cord	Hyperextension; fracture of posterior vertebral elements	Loss of sensation; ataxia due to proprioceptive deficit
Brown-Sequard	Cord hemi-section; classically by knife-wound	Ipsilateral paralysis and loss of sensation, contralateral loss of pain/temperature
Conus medullaris	Injury to sacral cord and lumbar roots	Bowel/bladder and lower limb dysfunction, mixed upper/lower neuron signs
Cauda equina	Injury to lumbosacral roots	Bowel/bladder and lower limb dysfunction, lower neuron signs
Spinal shock	Spinal concussion	Motor paralysis and loss of sensation; initial areflexia with gradual return, final hyperreflexia

syndrome (affecting the lumbosacral roots). Again, a thorough history will aid the physician in understanding the nature, vector, and intensity of the trauma, which may suggest particular mechanical disruptions to the spine and particular regions of partial injury.

Radiographic Evaluation

Following examination, radiographs may be obtained to both confirm physical findings and uncover any abnormalities which are not apparent on exam. In cervical injuries, x–ray imaging should be obtained only in symptomatic patients.[11–13] A three-view series of images is ideal, including lateral, anteroposterior, and odontoid views. The lateral is by far the most important view and should be taken first, as it can be obtained from a supine patient. This view should encompass the entire cervical spine, including the upper portion of the first thoracic vertebra, so as to not exclude lower cervical injuries.[14,15] The anteroposterior view should be taken at 20 degrees from the normal angle, with an inferosuperior orientation. Odontoid views are obtained at a normal angle through the patient's opened mouth, in order to assess the odontoid process of the atlas, C2. In thoracic or lumbar SCI, anteroposterior and lateral views are sufficient on x-ray, but computed tomography (CT) or magnetic resonance imaging (MRI) is usually required to demonstrate greater detail (Figure 31.3). In interpreting spinal radiographs, the reading physician should examine the vertebral bodies for alignment and structural integrity and inspect the intervertebral disc space for signs of abnormality. Signs of secondary damage—such as hematoma—may also be apparent in the soft tissues surrounding the spine. In general, radiography is not recommended in awake, alert patients who lack typical signs or symptoms of SCI.[16,17]

Finally, the possibility of spinal cord injury without radiographic abnormality (SCIWORA) must be considered. Is this condition, objective signs of SCI are observed but there is no evidence of damage on plain radiographs or tomography. SCIWORA is often seen in children due to the vulnerability of the still-developing spine.[18,19] Current guidelines recommend plain film, CT, and MR imaging of the suspected area of injury

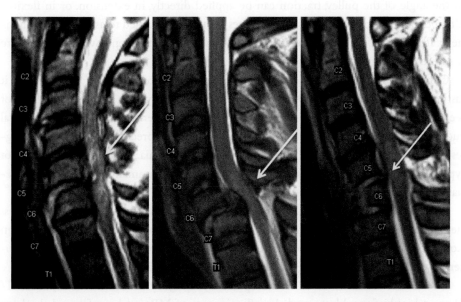

Figure 31.3. Magnetic resonance imaging (MRI) of cervical spinal cord injury.

to garner as much information as possible and exclude possible diagnoses.[20] In some case, plain films of the entire spine may prove useful.

Treatment

Nonsurgical Therapy

The primary aims of SCI treatment in an ICU setting are maintaining optimal conditions for the spine to recover from trauma, preventing any complications which could further injure the cord, and managing the patient's pain and nutrition during recovery.

The reduction of spinal fractures can be accomplished in the ICU by traction or external immobilization (bracing). In cervical injuries, traction can be applied with skull calipers or a halo. The use of halo traction allows transfer to a halo brace, with the potential of early patient mobilization. The majority of cervical injury classes can be managed entirely in the ICU, but surgical intervention may be required in specific cases of vertebral damage or joint dislocation. Injuries well-treated by external immobilization include fractures of the occipital condyle, some varieties of isolated atlas (C2) fracture, the so-called *hangman's fracture* of the axis (C1), and the majority of C1–C2 combination fractures.[21–25] Surgical intervention is recommended for more severe cases of these injuries and in dislocations of the atlanto-occipital joint.[26,27] Thoracic and lumbar injuries are typically treated conservatively, with prolonged bed rest followed by cautious mobilization with external bracing.

Halo traction can be administered at the bedside.[28] The patient is placed in a head-neutral position, and the halo ring sized at approximately 1cm greater than the head circumference. Four sites are chosen to place the halo pins: two anterior and two posterior. After treatment at these sites with sterile preparation and a local anesthetic, the pins are placed and hand-tightened to just contact the skin. Now in position, the pins can be tightened with a screwdriver and finally locked into the halo frame with locking nuts. The halo vest is then placed on the patient and stabilized to the halo with rods. For traction, the patient should be in a bed with a pulley system and weights at the head. Based on the angle of the pulley, traction can be applied directly, in extension, or in flexion. When traction is applied, lateral x-ray images should be obtained to assure proper alignment. It should be noted that traction is contraindicated in patients with skull fracture or severe osteoporosis.

Controlled hypothermia is a therapy of growing interest in SCI.[29–31] Although it has been used for well over 50 years in central nervous system disease, there has not been proportionate success and widespread use of hypothermia in SCI. While clinical studies to date have been largely inconclusive, numerous preclinical experiments suggest improved outcomes in SCI with moderate hypothermia. Proposed mechanisms of hypothermia's therapeutic effect include reductions of inflammation, tissue oxygen demand, and hemorrhage.

Pharmacologic treatment of SCI has been investigated as a possible means to suppress the devastating effects to the cord that follow the initial trauma.[32–37] Two drugs have been most extensively studied and controversy continues to surround their use: the corticosteroid methylprednisolone (MP), and GM-1 ganglioside (GM1).

The results of the National Acute Spinal Cord Injury Study (NASCIS) trials II/III were highly favorable toward the effectiveness of MP and have formed the basis for contemporary use of MP in a clinical setting.[33,34] However, numerous subsequent studies have questioned the validity of the NASCIS trials, both in methodology and analysis, and have shown multiple and severe side effects to MP use, often over-shadowing any clinical benefit.[35,36] MP remains a tool at the physician's disposal, but it must be used with the knowledge of its seemingly limited efficacy and possible extensive harm.

GM1 has been explored as an adjunct therapy in SCI patients who were administered MP. Initial studies seemed favorable, and researchers speculated that GM1 treatment recovered strength in paralyzed muscles. Following these early findings, more and larger studies have shown no significant benefit conferred by GM1 therapy in SCI mortality or neurologic outcome, although there is still some suggestion of potential clinical effect.[32,37] GM1 remains an option in current practice that requires still further investigation.

Finally, consideration must be given to the patient's general condition, including pain and nutritional management.[38] Typical narcotic analgesics can be used with SCI patients, but those with respiratory suppression must be closely monitored, and naloxone should be on hand in case of inadvertent overdose. Blood electrolytes should be closely monitored, with special attention paid to sodium and calcium levels. In particular, calcium may be released from bone during prolonged bed rest, leading to symptomatic hypercalcemia.[39]

Surgical Procedures

Surgery may be indicated for severe injuries. As the preceding therapies are intended to optimize the physiologic conditions for cord recovery, the goal of surgery in SCI is to resolve any mechanical barrier to healing via decompression and reconstruction.

Atlanto-occipital injury may require fusion at the atlanto-occipital or atlanto-axial levels.[27] Severe subaxial cervical fractures can be managed with anterior cervical disc-ectomy and fusion (ACDF) or posterior fixation. Thoracolumbar injuries are typically treated with posterior laminectomy and fusion, two levels above and below the fracture.[40] In general, surgical strategy should be tailored to the specific pathology and radiographic findings in each patient.

Finally, the timing of surgery following SCI must be considered. There has been long controversy over the benefits of immediate (within 25 hours of injury) versus delayed surgery (200 hours after surgery). While past analyses found no significant difference in outcomes between early or late operation,[41,42] more recent data suggest that early surgery both improves patient outcomes and is more cost-effective.[43,44]

Complications

Spinal shock in SCI is characterized by decreased or absent reflexes inferior to the level of injury, followed by the gradual return of reflexes and, finally, hyperreflexia. While this condition has been recognized for more than two centuries, a new model of understanding spinal shock was proposed in 2004.[45] It describes four phases of disease, which parallel the physiologic process of injury and healing, as well as the degree of reflexes that can be elicited clinically. These phases span from the day of injury to 1 year post-injury and may suggest optimal times for certain therapies based on the patient and nature of injury.

Autonomic dysreflexia (AD) is seen in up to 90% of patients with mid-thoracic or higher level SCI. This condition is characterized by episodes of hypertension and bradycardia triggered by seemingly innocuous peripheral stimulation (e.g., bladder distension or mild foot compression). AD is thought to result from the disruption of normal parasympathetic inhibitory signals from the brain, as well as an increased sensitivity of peripheral receptors.[46] In acute episodes, the patient should be seated upright with any restrictive clothing loosened. Blood pressure should be monitored and a short-acting antihypertensive administered if the systolic pressure remains above 150 mm Hg.[47]

Respiratory and cardiovascular complications can greatly impair cord healing by reducing the oxygen available to the site of injury. Respiratory insufficiency is seen most frequently in cervical spine injuries, and the physician should closely monitor these patients for respiratory function, impaired cough, or abnormal blood gases. The most common cardiovascular complication is hypovolemic shock (due to blood loss during the initial trauma) or neurogenic shock (due to disruption of autonomic tracts in the cord). Blood pressure should be routinely monitored, and hypotension (systolic pressure under 90 mm Hg) should be avoided.[48] In selecting a pressor, phenylephrine should be avoided because it is noninotropic and may lead to reflex bradycardia. Bradycardic patients may require atropine to bring the heart rate to desired levels.

Risk of thromboembolism must also be considered in SCI patients because they are bedridden for considerable periods of time and may persist in a pro-coagulant state following trauma. Low-molecular-weight heparins are a current first-line prophylaxis, especially in victims of cervical cord injuries. In addition to anticoagulation therapy, these patients should be monitored during and after their time in the ICU for signs of deep venous thrombosis or pulmonary embolism.[49]

Conclusion

Leading causes of SCI include vehicular collisions and falls, and many SCI patients have associated injuries. A thorough history from the patient and any witnesses to the trauma can greatly aid the diagnosis.

ASIA classification of injury is the standard for neurologic assessment following SCI; FIM is also a useful tool. Radiographs are indicated for all symptomatic victims of spinal trauma and are usually supplemented with CT and MR imaging.

In the ICU, major therapies include traction or bracing to accomplish the closed reduction of spinal fractures; other controversial treatments, such as hypothermia or methylprednisolone, require further investigation.

Major complications of SCI seen during treatment include spinal shock, respiratory insufficiency, thrombosis, and autonomic dysreflexia.

References

1. Donovan WH. Donald Munro Lecture. Spinal cord injury: past, present, and future. *J Spinal Cord Med*. 2007;30(2):85–100.

2. National Spinal Cord Injury Statistical Center. *2014 Annual Statistical Report for the Spinal Cord Injury Model Systems Public Version*. University of Alabama at Birmingham: Birmingham, Alabama. 2014.

3. National Spinal Cord Injury Statistical Center. *Facts and Figures at a Glance*. University of Alabama at Birmingham: Birmingham, Alabama. 2015.

4. Hammell KW. Exploring quality of life following high spinal cord injury: a review and critique. *Spinal Cord*. 2004;42(9):491–502.

5. Clinical assessment after acute cervical spinal cord injury. *Neurosurgery*. 2002;50(3 suppl):S21–29.

6. Cohen ME, Ditunno JF Jr, Donovan WH, Maynard FM Jr. A test of the 1992 International Standards for Neurological and Functional Classification of Spinal Cord Injury. *Spinal Cord*. 1998;36(8):554–560.

7. El Masry WS, Tsubo M, Katoh S, El Miligui YH, Khan A. Validation of the American Spinal Injury Association (ASIA) motor score and the National Acute Spinal Cord Injury Study (NASCIS) motor score. *Spine (Phila Pa 1976)*. 1996;21(5):614–619.

8. Kalsi-Ryan S, Wilson J, Yang JM, Fehlings MG. Neurological grading in traumatic spinal cord injury. *World Neurosurg*. 2014;82(3-4):509–518.

9. American Spinal Injury Association/International Medical Society of Paraplegia. International standards for neurological and functional classification of spinal cord injury, revised. American Spinal Injury Association, Chicago, IL. 1996.

10. Ditunno JF Jr. Functional assessment measures in CNS trauma. *J Neurotrauma*. 1992;9(suppl 1):S301–305.

11. Radiographic assessment of the cervical spine in symptomatic trauma patients. *Neurosurgery*. 2002;50(3 suppl):S36–43.

12. Ajani AE, Cooper DJ, Scheinkestel CD, Laidlaw J, Tuxen DV. Optimal assessment of cervical spine trauma in critically ill patients: a prospective evaluation. *Anaesth Intensive Care*. 1998;26(5):487–491.

13. MacDonald RL, Schwartz ML, Mirich D, Sharkey PW, Nelson WR. Diagnosis of cervical spine injury in motor vehicle crash victims: how many X-rays are enough? *J Trauma*. 1990;30(4):392–397.

14. Davis JW, Phreaner DL, Hoyt DB, Mackersie RC. The etiology of missed cervical spine injuries. *J Trauma*. 1993;34(3):342–346.

15. Reid DC, Henderson R, Saboe L, Miller JD. Etiology and clinical course of missed spine fractures. *J Trauma*. 1987;27(9):980–986.

16. Radiographic assessment of the cervical spine in asymptomatic trauma patients. *Neurosurgery*. 2002;50(3 suppl):S30–35.

17. Hoffman JR, Mower WR, Wolfson AB, Todd KH, Zucker MI. Validity of a set of clinical criteria to rule out injury to the cervical spine in patients with blunt trauma. National Emergency X-Radiography Utilization Study Group. *N Engl J Med*. 2000;343(2):94–99.

18. Pang D, Wilberger JE Jr. Spinal cord injury without radiographic abnormalities in children. *J Neurosurg*. 1982;57(1):114–129.

19. Pang D, Pollack IF. Spinal cord injury without radiographic abnormality in children: the SCIWORA syndrome. *J Trauma*. 1989;29(5):654–664.

20. Rozzelle CJ, Aarabi B, Dhall SS, et al. Spinal cord injury without radiographic abnormality (SCIWORA). *Neurosurgery*. 2013;72(suppl 2):227–233.

21. Gelb DE, Hadley MN, Aarabi B, et al. Initial closed reduction of cervical spinal fracture-dislocation injuries. *Neurosurgery*. 2013;72(suppl 2):73–83.

22. Karam YR, Traynelis VC. Occipital condyle fractures. *Neurosurgery*. 2010;66(3 suppl):56–59.

23. Ryken TC, Aarabi B, Dhall SS, et al. Management of isolated fractures of the atlas in adults. *Neurosurgery*. 2013;72(suppl 2):127–131.

24. Ryken TC, Hadley MN, Aarabi B, et al. Management of acute combination fractures of the atlas and axis in adults. *Neurosurgery*. 2013;72(suppl 2):151–158.

25. Gelb DE, Aarabi B, Dhall SS, et al. Treatment of subaxial cervical spinal injuries. *Neurosurgery*. 2013;72(suppl 2):187–194.

26. Aarabi B, Hadley MN, Dhall SS, et al. Management of acute traumatic central cord syndrome (ATCCS). *Neurosurgery*. 2013;72(suppl 2):195–204.

27. Theodore N, Aarabi B, Dhall SS, et al. The diagnosis and management of traumatic atlanto-occipital dislocation injuries. *Neurosurgery*. 2013;72(suppl 2):114–126.

28. Lu DC. Bedside procedures. In: Baaj AA, Mummaneni PV, Uribe JS, Vaccaro AR, Greenberg MS, eds. *Handbook of Spine Surgery*. New York: Thieme Medical Publishers; 2012:76–82.

29. Ahmad FU, Wang MY, Levi AD. Hypothermia for acute spinal cord injury: a review. *World Neurosurg*. 2014;82(1–2):207–214.

30. Hansebout RR, Hansebout CR. Local cooling for traumatic spinal cord injury: outcomes in 20 patients and review of the literature. *J Neurosurg Spine*. 2014;20(5):550–561.

31. O'Toole JE, Wang MC, Kaiser MG. *Hypothermia and human spinal cord injury: updated position statement and evidence-based recommendations from the AANS/CNS Joint Section on Disorders of the Spine and Peripheral Nerves*. AANS/CNS Joint Section on Disorders of the Spine and Peripheral Nerves;2014.

32. Chappell ET. Pharmacological therapy after acute cervical spinal cord injury. *Neurosurgery*. 2002;51(3):855–856; author reply 856.

33. Bracken MB, Shepard MJ, Hellenbrand KG, et al. Methylprednisolone and neurological function 1 year after spinal cord injury. Results of the National Acute Spinal Cord Injury Study. *J Neurosurg*. 1985;63(5):704–713.

34. Bracken MB, Shepard MJ, Collins WF Jr, et al. Methylprednisolone or naloxone treatment after acute spinal cord injury: 1-year follow-up data. Results of the second National Acute Spinal Cord Injury Study. *J Neurosurg*. 1992;76(1):23–31.

35. Bydon M, Lin J, Macki M, Gokaslan ZL, Bydon A. The current role of steroids in acute spinal cord injury. *World Neurosurg*. 2014;82(5):848–854.

36. Hurlbert RJ. Methylprednisolone for acute spinal cord injury: an inappropriate standard of care. *J Neurosurg*. 2000;93(1 suppl):1–7.

37. Geisler FH, Coleman WP, Grieco G, Poonian D, Sygen Study G. The Sygen multicenter acute spinal cord injury study. *Spine (Phila Pa 1976)*. 2001;26(24 suppl):S87–98.

38. Dhall SS, Hadley MN, Aarabi B, et al. Nutritional support after spinal cord injury. *Neurosurgery*. 2013;72(suppl 2):255–259.

39. Management of acute spinal cord injuries in an intensive care unit or other monitored setting. *Neurosurgery*. 2002;50(3 suppl):S51–57.

40. Ponnappan RK. Trauma. In: Baaj AA, Mummaneni PV, Uribe JS, Vaccaro AR, Greenberg MS, eds. *Handbook of Spine Surgery*. New York: Thieme Medical Publishers; 2012:114–126.

41. Belanger E, Levi AD. The acute and chronic management of spinal cord injury. *J Am Coll Surg*. 2000;190(5):603–618.

42. Fehlings MG, Tator CH. An evidence-based review of decompressive surgery in acute spinal cord injury: rationale, indications, and timing based on experimental and clinical studies. *J Neurosurg*. 1999;91(1 suppl):1–11.

43. Furlan JC, Craven BC, Massicotte EM, Fehlings MG. Early versus delayed surgical decompression of spinal cord after traumatic cervical spinal cord injury: a cost-utility analysis. *World Neurosurg.* 2016 Apr;88:166–174.

44. Liu JM, Long XH, Zhou Y, Peng HW, Liu ZL, Huang SH. Is urgent decompression superior to delayed surgery for traumatic spinal cord injury? A meta-analysis. *World Neurosurg.* 2016;87:124–131.

45. Ditunno JF, Little JW, Tessler A, Burns AS. Spinal shock revisited: a four-phase model. *Spinal Cord.* 2004;42(7):383–395.

46. Wan D, Krassioukov AV. Life-threatening outcomes associated with autonomic dysreflexia: a clinical review. *J Spinal Cord Med.* 2014;37(1):2–10.

47. Consortium for Spinal Cord Medicine. Acute management of autonomic dysreflexia: individuals with spinal cord injury presenting to health-care facilities. *J Spinal Cord Med.* 2002;25(suppl 1):S67–88.

48. Levi L, Wolf A, Belzberg H. Hemodynamic parameters in patients with acute cervical cord trauma: description, intervention, and prediction of outcome. *Neurosurgery.* 1993 Dec;33(6):1007–16; discussion 1016–7.

49. Dhall SS, Hadley MN, Aarabi B, et al. Deep venous thrombosis and thromboembolism in patients with cervical spinal cord injuries. *Neurosurgery.* 2013;72(suppl 2):244–254.

Animal Models of Spinal Cord Injury

Candace L. Floyd

32

Spinal Cord Injury Incidence

The global spinal cord injury (SCI) incidence as estimated by the World Health Organization and the International Spinal Cord Society is 40–80 new cases per million population per year, or between 250,000 to 500,000 people newly injured each year.[1] The National Spinal Cord Injury Statistical Center (NSCIS) estimated that approximately 17,000 new cases of SCI occur each year in the United States.[2] This results in an estimated 282,000 persons living with SCI in the United States in 2016. With relation to etiology, the NSCIS reports that, in the United States, vehicle crashes are currently the leading cause (38%) of SCI, followed by falls (30%), and acts of violence (13%), which primarily includes gunshot wounds. When the neurological level and extent of the SCI lesion are classified, the NSCIS data show that persons with incomplete tetraplegia comprise the greatest population (45%), followed by incomplete paraplegia (21%), and then persons with complete paraplegia (20%). Persons with complete tetraplegia comprise the smallest population, accounting for 13%. Fewer than 1% of persons experience a complete neurological recovery by hospital discharge,[2] thus SCI is a life event which leads to lasting, often substantial, alterations in the health and well-being of the patient. As the average age of incurrence of a SCI is 34.9 years,[3] these changes affect the patient throughout his or her entire lifetime. Eighty percent of persons with SCI are male,[3] as reported in the NSCIS[3] and WHO data.[1]

Clearly, the personal and economic costs of SCI are staggering, and this has prompted research with the goal of understanding the pathological processes of SCI to develop effective therapeutic strategies. SCI pathology is described in two components, primary and secondary injury. In general terms, primary injury refers to the damage to the spinal cord that is sustained at the initial trauma. This includes the mechanical injury components to the fragile tissue, such as shearing and compression. Secondary injury refers to the extensive biochemical and cellular cascade that is initiated by the primary injury and can last for days, weeks, and months after the initial insult. The secondary injury cascade is thought to be the main pathological process that exacerbates injury and inhibits repair and healing. However, the secondary injury cascade is also viewed as a critical window of opportunity for therapeutic interventions that protect the injured spinal cord tissues and promote repair and recovery. Thus, modeling of SCI in animal models is critical to understanding these complex injury mechanisms as well as to developing efficacious therapeutic interventions.

Classification of Spinal Cord Injury Based on Pathology

There are several methodologies and structures for classifications for SCI, with the most prevalent clinical classification system for clinical symptoms being that of the American Spinal Injury Association (ASIA). The ASIA system is based on sensory and motor examinations and a classification framework of impairment that ranges from grade A (functionally complete) to grade E (sensory and motor functions are normal) (see ASIA-Spinalinjury.org). Although extremely useful for classification in the clinical arena, this system is based on functional characteristics and does not delineate underlying pathology. Thus, the ASIA system is not optimal as a guide for animal modeling based on pathology. Alternatively, pioneering work by Bunge and colleagues[4] established a classification system based on spinal cord pathology. This system includes four classification categories and is based on gross morphology, imaging, and histology assessment, as summarized in Table 32.1. As a pathology-based system, the Bunge classification provides a useful infrastructure for clinically relevant animal modeling.

The first of these classifications, *solid cord injury*, is characterized by a spinal cord that grossly appears normal without discoloration, softening, or cyst formation. However, upon histological analysis, dorsal column demyelination and motor neuron loss can be observed.[4] Injuries belonging to this category are rarely observed clinically (10% of patients), and currently there are no animal models in use to study this type of injury.

The second category is that of *laceration*, which is most commonly observed clinically due to penetrating objects or sharp bone fragments.[4] Injuries of this type are characterized by disruption of the meninges resulting in widespread systemic cell infiltration and a connective tissue scar formed at the lesion epicenter that often adheres

Table 32.1:
Features of spinal cord injury types and corresponding animal models

Injury Type	Clinical Features		Clinical Frequency	Animal Models	Typical Research Question
	Gross features	Histological Features			
Solid cord injury	Normal	Demyelination, motor neuron loss	10%	None	N/A
Laceration	Meningeal disruption, connective tissue scar	Fiber disruption across the lesion, systemic cell infiltration	20%	Full or hemi-transection, selective tract ablation	Regeneration or repair of injured axons, tissue grafting
Maceration (compression)	Loss of cord topography	Fiber disruption across the lesion	20%	Aneurysm clip, epi- or subdural balloon, forceps	Protection, particularly with ischemic component
Contusion	Fluid-filled cyst, rim of spared tissue surrounding epicenter	Hemorrhage, necrosis, glial scar	50%	Full or unilateral contusion	Protection in highly clinically relevant model

to the overlying dura.[4,5] Animal models of lacerating injury include bilateral or hemi-transection of the spinal cord in which the cord is exposed and tissue severed with a sharp object. Alternatively, suction may be applied to selectively ablate motor or sensory tracts. This injury type, however, is observed relatively rarely clinically (21% of cases), and, as such, laceration models do not reflect the majority of human SCIs. Transection models of SCI are most commonly used when the research question centers on regeneration or repair of injured axons. Indeed, a recent Preferred Reporting Items for Systematic Reviews and Meta-analysis (PRISMA)-guided systematic review of 2,209 articles on animal models of SCI illustrated that 717 manuscripts used some type of transection model, mostly focusing on the effects of strategies for repair and regeneration.[6] It is important to note that transection models are also commonly used to study pathophysiology, particularly related to damage to axons or myelin.[6] The selection of the appropriate transection model is of particular importance when axonal regeneration is an outcome measure because transection models limit the misinterpretation of "the spared axon conundrum." This conundrum is the identification of axons as "regenerated" when these axons are actually "spared." Spared axons are less likely with a transection model in which the spinal cord tissue is cut. This concept is more fully discussed by Steward and colleagues.[7]

The third category of SCI is that of *cord maceration* or *compression*. This injury results from massive compression of the cord resulting in large disruption of the spinal cord anatomy such that cord topography is lost.[4,5] Very few fibers are observed crossing the length of the lesion, distinguishing this injury type from that of contusion. About 20% of clinical cases fall into the compression category. Compression injury is modeled in animals most commonly by using aneurysm clips and epidural or subdural balloons resulting in prolonged disruption of blood flow to cord tissue. Other models that are less frequently used involve the use of a screw or spacer to compress the spinal cord. The recent PRISMA-guided systematic review indicated that, of the recently published articles on animals models of SCI, approximately 20% of these used compression models.[6] Compression models are often used to evaluate spinal cord pathology and associated therapeutic strategies for protection, particularly when the pathological component of spinal cord ischemia is considered critical.

The fourth SCI category is that of *contusion*, characterized by contusive injury to the spinal cord resulting in areas of hemorrhage and necrosis that ultimately give rise to a fluid-filled cyst at the lesion epicenter with a rim of spared (although generally dysmyelinated) tissue at the pial surface of the cord.[4] The meninges remain intact, resulting in less systemic cell infiltrate and a scar surrounding the lesion consisting of virtually no connective tissue components, distinguishing this injury type from laceration injury. The majority of clinical cases of SCI (70%) are contusive type injuries with some degree of compression, acute or chronic, resulting from fracture/dislocation of the spinal column and subsequent compression of the cord. As such, there are many animal models of this type of SCI that have been shown to have pathophysiological elements comparable to those observed in human cases of SCI. Accordingly, the majority (41%) of recent articles as highlighted in the PRISMA-guided systematic review employ contusion models.[6] Similar to compression models and owing largely to the pathological similarity to the clinical pathology, contusion models are most often used to assess spinal cord pathophysiology and related protective therapeutic interventions. It is also important to note that some models add a compression component to a contusion model such that the contusion impact is then followed by an extended dwell time or continued weight compression as this type of model is thought to be highly clinically relevant. Due to the prevalence of contusion models, the more widely used animal models of contusive SCI are discussed herein in both rodent and large animal species.

Selection of Level of Injury in Animal Models

Recently, Nowrouzi and colleagues[8] reviewed the most-cited publications on SCI. They found the topic of those manuscripts with the greatest annual and lifetime citations was either treatment (40%) or pathology (40%). Additionally, they found that 50% of the publications with the greatest annual and lifetime citation discussed SCI research using animal models.[8] These data suggest that the use of animal models in SCI research remains an important and prevalent component of research and advancement of knowledge, particularly as related to understanding the pathobiology of SCI and in the development of novel treatment strategies. As described earlier, there are three main categories of SCI models used in animals, namely transection, compression, and contusion. The selection of the model is critically important and should be based on the question to be evaluated.

A second key consideration in modeling SCI is the spinal level at which the SCI occurs in the clinical population as related to the spinal level at which the injury is induced in the animal model. The level of injury is defined as the vertebral level at which the epicenter of the injury occurs. Figures 32.1 and 32.2 illustrate the spinal cord innervation targets from the cervical (C1–C8), thoracic (T1–T12), lumbar (L1–L5), and sacral regions (S1–S5) and the typical neurological level of SCI at discharge. Both in the clinic and in the laboratory, the level of injury predicts the degree of functional impairment because typically function is impaired at that level and for all levels below the SCI lesion. For example, a SCI in the high cervical region (C1–C4) results in the most severe impairment and results in paralysis of the upper and lower limbs as well as the respiratory centers, termed *ventilator-dependent tetraplegia*. In contrast, a SCI at the lower thoracic region (T7–T12) will involve innervation to the trunk and lower limbs, resulting in paraplegia. The National SCI Statistical Center data[2] indicate that the majority of patients are injured in the cervical levels, with injuries at the lower cervical (C5–C8) being most common. The next most common spinal level of SCI is at the thoracolumbar region. Interestingly, the early models of contusive SCI were performed in the mid-thoracic region of the spinal cord resulting in hindlimb deficits while allowing the animal to ambulate to some extent via preserved function of the forelimbs. The mid-thoracic injury model has been used throughout the past century and has increased our understanding of SCI pathophysiology and progression substantially, leading to characterization of widely used quantitative analyses of hindlimb motor and sensory function. The mid-thoracic injury models remain highly clinically relevant and prominently used.[6]

However, it is important to consider that more than 50% of clinical cases of SCI occur in the mid-cervical region, as indicated in Figure 32.2. Several key anatomical differences between these two regions also emphasize that the selection of the most appropriate region for the SCI model is of critical importance. The first of these is the

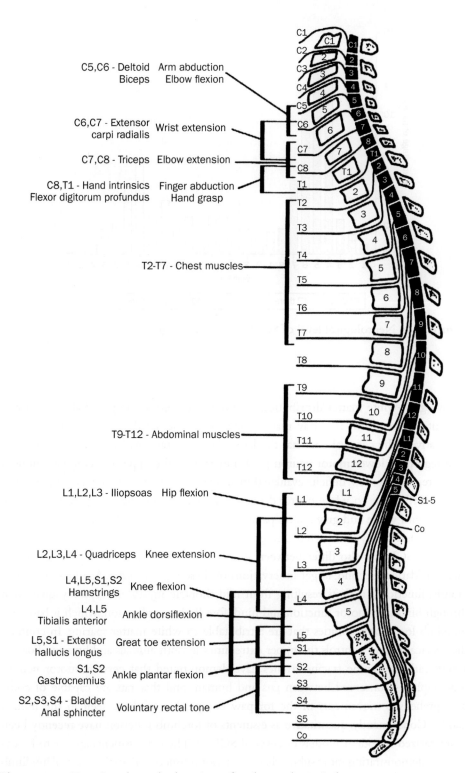

Figure 32.1 Drawing show the location of each vertebrate in human.

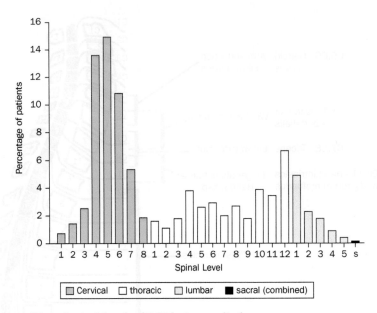

Figure 32.2 Neurological level of SCI lesion at discharge.

relative gray–white matter distribution. The thoracic cord is composed almost entirely of white matter, with the gray matter innervating the small intercostal musculature. Alternatively, the cervical cord has the largest gray matter area by volume of all spinal cord regions as lower motor neuron pools innervating the upper extremity are housed in this region. As such, deficits evaluated in animal models of mid-thoracic SCI are primarily attributable to white matter damage,[9] whereas deficits following cervical injury include both white and gray matter pathology.[10–12] As the physical properties, metabolic demands, and cell types of white and gray matter differ, it is likely the pathophysiology following SCI may also differ between spinal cord regions, but this idea requires further elucidation. Second, target innervations of these regions differ. As mentioned previously, functional deficits resulting from mid-thoracic injury are typically quantified through hindlimb motor function and hind–fore limb coordination, which is based on hindlimb locomotor abilities that are attributable to white matter sparing. In contrast, the cervical region controls the upper extremities in both animals and humans. For example, carbanocyanine tracing studies have demonstrated that cervical motor neuron topography is conserved between rats and humans and that rats are capable of complex prehensile movements of the forepaw comparable to those seen in the human hand.[13] Consequently, quantitative assessments of forelimb function have recently been characterized in rodent models of cervical SCI.[10–15] These assessments appear to be capable of demonstrating more subtle changes in motor function than the classical hindlimb function assessments, which may reveal subtle effects of potential therapeutics that may be missed if employed in a mid-thoracic injury model. As cervical spinal cord lesions result in fore- and hindlimb dysfunction, cervical hemicontusion[10–15] or hemisection[16,17] models have been developed to ensure mobility and health of the animal. The motor and sensory deficits observed following this type of injury reflect those observed in the clinical example of Brown-Sequard syndrome, a unilateral injury of the spinal cord.[18,19]

Contusion Models

Various mechanisms to induce contusion injuries to the spinal cord have been employed for almost a century and have evolved from simple weight-drop techniques to sophisticated computer-controlled devices capable of controlling precise injury parameters. These advances have resulted in animal injury models that have been well characterized, are reproducible, and produce models with a high degree of relevance to human SCI pathophysiology.[4]

The earliest contusion model was that described by Allen in 1911, in which weights were dropped onto canine spinal cords exposed by laminectomy.[20] By dropping weights from different distances gravity is employed to apply differing forces and result in differing compression of the spinal cord. Others later applied this model to make seminal discoveries related to histological changes,[21] vasculature impairments,[22] myelin breakdown, and edema[23,24] following SCI.

In 1975, force transducers were added to the weight-drop model to quantify the force of impact in primate models.[25] Subsequently, canine, feline, and primate models were used to describe progressive tissue damage processes in finer detail as well as the effects of putative therapeutics in SCI.[26,27] Metabolic dysfunction, myelin breakdown, free radical production, respiratory function, ionic shifts, blood–brain barrier breakdown, cellular immunity, glutamate release, and the roles of necrotic and apoptotic cell death were described as reviewed by a pioneer in the field, Dr. Wise Young.[28] This gave rise to the current understanding of a biphasic injury process in which primary mechanical tissue trauma causes complex, interacting biochemical processes resulting in secondary progressive tissue damage.[29,30]

The elucidation of these delayed secondary injury mechanisms formed the rationale for using therapeutics targeting these processes to limit motor deficit. In 1985, a weight-drop contusion device similar to those described previously for large animals was used in a rat model.[31–33] Use of contusion SCI models in the rat has led to major advances in SCI research, including quantitative assessments of injury-induced alterations in ascending and descending fiber tracts, neurons and neuronal networks, gliosis, and motor and sensory functional deficits/recovery.[34]

In terms of species used to model SCI, a recent PRISMA-guided systematic review indicated that rodents comprise the most widely used model, with approximately 72% of recently surveyed studies being conducted in rats and 16% being conducted in mice. With regard to animal models based on the use of large animals, rabbits, cats, dogs, pigs, and nonhuman primates accounted for approximately 2% of the total each. However, there is growing interest in the use of non-rodent models for SCI research, perhaps as a translational intermediary between discovery research in rodents and first-in-human clinical trials.[35,36] Some of the new emphasis on large animal models of SCI arises from comparative neuroanatomy in that the central nervous system of larger animals includes a gyrencephalic brain and anatomical organizational structure of the spinal cord that is more similar to human than are rodent systems.[37]

References

1. World Health Organization (edited by Jerome Bickenbach). *International Perspectives on Spinal Cord Injury*. Malta: International Spinal Cord Society; 2013:1–250. http://apps.who.int/iris/bitstream/handle/10665/94190/9789241564663_eng.pdf?sequence=1; accessed 7-18-2018

2. National Spinal Cord Injury Statistical Center and the Model Systems Knowledge Translation Center. Spinal Cord Injury (SCI) Facts and Figures at a Glance. 2016. https://www.nscisc.uab.edu/Public/Facts%20and%20Figures%20-%202018.pdf; accessed 7-18-2018.

3. National Spinal Cord Injury Statistical Center. 2015 Annual statistical report—complete public version. Published 2015. https://www.nscisc.uab.edu/PublicDocuments/reports/pdf/2015%20NSCISC%20Annual%20Statistical%20Report%20Complete%20Public%20Version.pdf; accessed 7-18-2018.

4. Bunge RP, Puckett WR, Becerra JL, Marcillo A, Quencer RM. Observations on the pathology of human spinal cord injury. A review and classification of 22 new cases with details from a case of chronic cord compression with extensive focal demyelination. *AdvNeurol*. 1993;59:75–89.

5. Norenberg MD, Smith J, Marcillo A. The pathology of human spinal cord injury: defining the problems. *J Neurotrauma*. 2004;21(4):429–440.

6. Sharif-Alhoseini M, Khormali M, Rezaei M, et al. Animal models of spinal cord injury: a systematic review. *Spinal Cord*. 2017;55(8):714–721.

7. Steward O, Zheng B, Tessier-Lavigne M. False resurrections: distinguishing regenerated from spared axons in the injured central nervous system. *J Comp Neurol*. 2003;459(1):1–8.

8. Nowrouzi B, Assan-Lebbe A, Sharma B, Casole J, Nowrouzi-Kia B. Spinal cord injury: a review of the most-cited publications. *Eur Spine J*. 2016;26(1):28–39.

9. Basso DM. Neuroanatomical substrates of functional recovery after experimental spinal cord injury: implications of basic science research for human spinal cord injury. *Phys Ther*. 2000;80(8):808–817.

10. Dunham KA, Siriphorn A, Chompoopong S, Floyd CL. Characterization of a graded cervical hemicontusion spinal cord injury model in adult male rats. *J Neurotrauma*. 2010;27(11):2091–2106.

11. Gensel JC, Tovar CA, Hamers FP, Deibert RJ, Beattie MS, Bresnahan JC. Behavioral and histological characterization of unilateral cervical spinal cord contusion injury in rats. *J Neurotrauma*. 2006;23(1):36–54.

12. Soblosky JS, Song JH, Dinh DH. Graded unilateral cervical spinal cord injury in the rat: evaluation of forelimb recovery and histological effects. *Behav Brain Res*. 2001;119(1):1–13.

13. McKenna JE, Prusky GT, Whishaw IQ. Cervical motoneuron topography reflects the proximodistal organization of muscles and movements of the rat forelimb: a retrograde carbocyanine dye analysis. *J Comp Neurol*. 2000;419(3):286–296.

14. Anderson KD, Sharp KG, Hofstadter M, Irvine KA, Murray M, Steward O. Forelimb locomotor assessment scale (FLAS): novel assessment of forelimb dysfunction after cervical spinal cord injury. *Exp Neurol*. 2009;220(1):23–33.

15. Irvine KA, Ferguson AR, Mitchell KD, et al. The Irvine, Beatties, and Bresnahan (IBB) Forelimb Recovery Scale: an assessment of reliability and validity. *Front Neurol*. 2014;5:116.

16. Gill LC, Ross HH, Lee KZ, et al. Rapid diaphragm atrophy following cervical spinal cord hemisection. *Respir Physiol Neurobiol*. 2014;192:66–73.

17. Gonzalez-Rothi EJ, Armstrong GT, Cerreta AJ, et al. Forelimb muscle plasticity following unilateral cervical spinal cord injury. *Muscle Nerve*. 2016;53(3):475–478.

18. Rumana CS, Baskin DS. Brown-Sequard syndrome produced by cervical disc herniation: case report and literature review. *Surg Neurol*. 1996;45(4):359–361.

19. Porto GB, Tan LA, Kasliwal MK, Traynelis VC. Progressive Brown-Sequard syndrome: a rare manifestation of cervical disc herniation. *J Clin Neurosci*. 2016;29:196–198.

20. Allen AR. Surgery of experimental lesion of spinal cord equivalent to crush injury of fracture dislocation of spinal column: a preliminary report. *JAMA*. 1911(57):878–880.

21. Guth LRK, Baker CA, Baker JH. Neurohistological and enzyme histochemical staining of adjacent sections in series cut from normal and traumatized spinal cords. *Exp Neurol*. 1977;57(1):179–191.

22. Ducker TB, Assenmacher DR. Microvascular response to experimental spinal cord trauma. *Surg Forum*. 1969;20:428–430.

23. Wullenweber R, Ebhardt G, Collmann H, Duisberg R. Spinal cord blood flow after experimental trauma in the dog. I. Morphological findings after standardized trauma. *Adv Neurol*. 1978;20:407–414.

24. Collmann H, Wullenweber R, Sprung C, Duisberg R. Spinal cord blood flow after experimental trauma in the dog. II. Early changes of spinal cord blood flow in the surrounding area of a traumatic lesion. *Adv Neurol*. 1978;20:443–450.

25. Daniell HB, Francis WW, Lee WA, Ducker TB. A method of quantitating injury inflicted in acute spinal cord studies. *Paraplegia*. 1975;13(3):137–142.

26. Parker AJ, Smith CW. Functional recovery from spinal cord trauma following dexamethazone and chlorpromazine therapy in dogs. *Res Vet Sci*. 1976;21(2):246–247.

27. Goodkin R, Campbell JB. Sequential pathologic changes in spinal cord injury: a preliminary report. *Surg Forum*. 1969;20:430–432.

28. Young W. Spinal cord contusion models. *Prog Brain Res*. 2002;137:231–255.

29. Witiw CD, Fehlings MG. Acute spinal cord injury. *J Spinal Disord Tech*. 2015;28(6):202–210.

30. Rowland JW, Hawryluk GW, Kwon B, Fehlings MG. Current status of acute spinal cord injury pathophysiology and emerging therapies: promise on the horizon. *Neurosurg Focus*. 2008;25(5):E2.

31. Noble LJ, Wrathall JR. Spinal cord contusion in the rat: morphometric analyses of alterations in the spinal cord. *Exp Neurol*. 1985;88(1):135–149.

32. Gale K, Kerasidis H, Wrathall JR. Spinal cord contusion in the rat: behavioral analysis of functional neurologic impairment. *Exp Neurol*. 1985;88(1):123–134.

33. Wrathall JR, Pettegrew RK, Harvey F. Spinal cord contusion in the rat: production of graded, reproducible, injury groups. *Exp Neurol*. 1985;88(1):108–122.

34. Kjell J, Olson L. Rat models of spinal cord injury: from pathology to potential therapies. *Dis Model Mech*. 2016;9(10):1125–1137.

35. Kwon BK, Streijger F, Hill CE, et al. Large animal and primate models of spinal cord injury for the testing of novel therapies. *Exp Neurol*. 2015;269:154–168.

36. Kwon BK, Hillyer J, Tetzlaff W. Translational research in spinal cord injury: a survey of opinion from the SCI community. *J Neurotrauma*. 2010;27(1):21–33.

37. Leonard AV MJ, Pat BM, Hadley MN, Floyd CL. Localization of the corticospinal tract within the porcine spinal cord: Implications for experimental modeling of traumatic spinal cord injury. *Neurosci Lett*. 2017;648:1–7.

Why Do We Not Have a Drug to Treat Acute Spinal Cord Injury?

James W. Geddes

33

A major goal of spinal cord injury (SCI) research has been the development of a neuroprotective drug that improves functional and neuropathological outcomes when administered after the injury. Unfortunately, we do not yet have such a drug or combination of drugs. Numerous proposed treatment strategies for acute SCI appear promising in preclinical studies, but none has translated successfully in clinical trials to date.[1–6] Methylprednisolone initially showed promise, with subsequent studies questioning its efficacy and safety profile.[7–11] What are we doing wrong? Possible reasons for the failure in translation are the focus of this chapter.

Reproducibility Crisis

At present, the US National Institutes of Health are funding 486 studies on SCI at an annual cost of $142 million. Additional funding is provided by similar government agencies in other countries and by several private and nonprofit organizations. This support has resulted in more than 5,000 papers on acute SCI and possible treatments and approximately 146 clinical trials for acute SCI. Despite this support and these efforts, there are no drugs approved by the US Food and Drug Administration (FDA) for the treatment of acute SCI.

The lack of success in identifying neuroprotective drugs is not restricted to SCI. Promising preclinical results for neuroprotective therapeutics for stroke, traumatic brain injury (TBI), amyotrophic lateral sclerosis, and other disorders have largely failed in clinical trials.[12–18] In addition to neuroprotective preclinical efficacy not translating to the bedside, replication of published preclinical SCI studies often fails to reproduce the significant findings.[19] As with clinical trials, this issue is not restricted to SCI or neuroscience but is a concern across the life sciences.[20,21] Preclinical cancer papers in high-impact journals could not be reproduced, in some cases, even by the original investigators.[22,23] This has created a crisis in confidence in preclinical research findings.[24–26]

Multiple factors have been identified that contribute to the crisis in confidence and reproducibility of preclinical studies, with major contributors being bias and inappropriate statistical analysis—particularly small sample sizes and an overreliance on the *p* value.[24,27–29] Meta-analysis of selected preclinical SCI studies revealed bias that may contribute to inflated effect sizes, and analysis of preclinical TBI studies has identified inappropriate statistical procedures that increase significant effects.[30–32] Proposed remedies include greater attention to blinding, randomization, transparency in the presentation of all results, inclusion of positive and negative controls, validation of key reagents, and use and reporting of appropriate statistical tests including confidence intervals.[33–36] For preclinical stroke research, a recent development is the use of preclinical randomized multicenter trials to overcome some of the problems just described.[37–39] This is clearly worthy of consideration for SCI.

Animal Models

Experimental SCI models are essential for investigation of potential treatment strategies. The modern era of SCI research began in the early 1900s with the studies of Alfred Reginald Allen, a neurologist from Pennsylvania.[40] Dr. Allen developed a weight-drop instrument for graded impact to the spinal cord, used to study contusive spinal trauma in dogs.[41,42] The protocol was similar to current studies and included anesthesia, laminectomy in the lower thoracic region, and dropping a weight from various heights via a guide tube to produce graded, reproducible injuries to the spinal cord. The weight-drop model has since been adapted to rats, mice, cats, miniature pigs, and nonhuman primates.[43–49] Subsequent models utilize electromechanical and electromagnetic devices for contusion injuries to rodent spinal cords.[50–55] Many of the injury devices can be used for thoracic, cervical, or sacral injuries. In addition to the widely used contusion injury models, rat models are also available for compression, laceration, dislocation, and distraction spinal cord injuries.[56,57] For a more detailed review and discussion of SCI models, see the relevant literature listed herein.[52,58–60]

The suitability of animal models for therapeutic evaluation depends on their accurate representation of the human condition. Preclinical injury models are reproducible by design in terms of injury severity, location, age, sex, and weight of the animal, as well as pre- and post-injury treatment and conditions. As a result of this consistency, relatively small improvements can be detected using functional outcome measures.[61–65] Most animal experiments involve dorsal injuries to the thoracic spine. Contusion injury to the thoracic rat spinal cord is validated to model several characteristics of human SCI, including alterations in spinal cord morphology, electrophysiology, and neurological function, with greater lesion sizes resulting in more pronounced deficits.[66]

In contrast to the animal models, spinal cord injuries suffered as a result of motor vehicle accidents, falls, gunshot wounds, sport/recreational injuries, and other causes vary considerably in severity, location, patient age, gender, weight, and the presence or absence of other injuries.[67] The most frequent human injuries are anterior injuries to the cervical cord.[68,69] This variability in injury location can influence the resultant pathology and outcomes due to nature of the vascular supply to the cord as well as the location of descending and ascending tracts.[60,70,71] Additionally, laminectomy is performed prior to animal injuries, which may facilitate recovery due to decompression, and animals are anesthetized during the injury procedure which may influence physiological responses. Choice of anesthetics and postoperative analgesics also influence outcomes,[72–75] as well as pre-injury alcohol and/or drug use in human cases. Human SCIs are often accompanied by avulsion or traction injuries of the spinal roots along with fracture dislocations.[76,77] Traumatic brain injuries occur in approximately half of individuals with SCI.[67,78] This variability of injury conditions presents challenges in identifying improvements resulting from drug treatment.[79–83] It is not feasible to model all of the variables in animal models.

However, concomitant brain and spinal cord injuries are being investigated,[67] and a dislocation model of anterior SCI has been developed although not fully characterized.[56]

Therapeutic Targets: Revisiting Allen's Hypothesis

In his pioneering studies using the weight-drop SCI model in dogs, Dr. Allen introduced the concept of secondary injury mechanisms, and the recognition that such mechanisms should be the target of therapeutics is the underpinning of virtually all strategies for treating acute SCI.[84–87]

> Either there is a destruction of axis cylinders directly consequent to the impact, or else, owing to the impact, there is an edematous and hemorrhagic outpouring into the cord tissue, by which its pressure and chemical activity inhibits temporarily all conduction function, or destroys permanently the "spinal cord". . . direct injury to the axis cylinder by the impact is beyond our reach, at that we should better confine our attention to the amelioration of the heightened intramedullary pressure.[41(p. 878)]

Most investigations have focused on a single target or mechanism based on damaging intracellular cascades. Specific pharmacologic inhibitors are often preferred to "dirty drugs" that hit multiple targets. However, there is increasing recognition that a single "magic bullet" is unlikely to be a successful intervention. Combinational therapies against two or more targets may be necessary.[88]

Perhaps we have overlooked some obvious targets. In stroke, neuroprotection strategies have largely failed while pharmacologic or mechanical interventions to restore blood flow have been successful under appropriate conditions.[89] For TBI, intracranial pressure monitoring and management is standard care,[90–92] yet intraspinal pressure (ISP) monitoring is rarely performed following SCI.

Allen hypothesized that the hemorrhagic lesion and elevated intramedullary pressure were major contributors to neurodegeneration and spinal cord dysfunction.[41] The contribution of hemorrhage to spinal cord damage and dysfunction has been investigated in several subsequent studies.[93–99] The initial intraparenchymal hemorrhage is predominantly localized to central gray matter due to the nature of the compressive forces, with the hemorrhagic lesions later expanding to white matter.[96,97,100] The distribution of the hemorrhage largely coincides with the subsequent cavity.[97] The damage to the microvasculature and release of blood into the parenchyma results in impaired perfusion and ischemic damage, along with inflammation and other consequences of intraparenchymal hemorrhage.[97] Much of our knowledge on such effects and underlying mechanisms is extrapolated from intracerebral hemorrhage studies where the damage is thought to result from inflammatory signaling pathways, thrombin formation, red cell lysis, iron toxicity, edema, and oxidative stress.[101–103]

To directly examine the consequences of intraspinal hemorrhage in the absence of severe mechanical insult, a recent study used a collagenase microinjection model.[99] The collagenase-induced hemorrhagic lesion in the rat spinal cord resulted in neuron death, extended axonal damage, disruption of the blood–spinal cord barrier, leukocyte recruitment, and neutrophil mobilization, along with locomotor deficits. Thus, hemorrhage alone is an important contributor to both the pathological and functional outcomes of SCI.

Another potential contributor to damage following SCI is the elevation in ISP, also first noted by Allen.[41] Previously, it was assumed that the anatomy of the spinal cord allows for substantial swelling without damaging the spinal tissue. However, data from mice, rats, dogs, and humans demonstrate a two- to threefold elevation in ISP following moderate to severe SCI, which persists for approximately 1 week post-injury.[104,105] Intracranial pressure is carefully managed following TBI to maintain brain tissue perfusion and oxygenation.[90,92,106] In contrast, ISP is typically not monitored following SCI. This presents an opportunity for treatment as greater elevations in ISP correspond to worse neurological outcomes.[104,107] In animal models, perioperative hypertension predicts worse outcomes.[108]

Consistent with the original observations of Allen, these findings support contributions of intraspinal hemorrhage and elevated ISP to the secondary injury cascade following SCI. To treat both, Allen proposed early laminectomy and myelotomy "to drain the injured tissue of the products of edema and hemorrhage."[41] A full-depth myelotomy, performed 6 hours following experimental weight-drop injury to the dog spinal cord, improved histologic outcomes although only descriptive results were reported.[42] Myelotomy has been explored in several subsequent experimental studies, each with positive outcomes.[109–115] Allen also performed myelotomy on three individuals following SCI, with inconclusive results.[42] There do not appear to have been subsequent clinical attempts, other than myelotomy associated with the insertion of bioscaffolds or transplanted cells into the injured spinal cord.[116–118]

It should be noted that for intracerebral hemorrhage, hematoma evacuation was not shown to improve outcomes as compared to medical management.[119–121] However, a pharmacologic approach to reduce hemorrhage, glibenclamide, is beneficial in experimental models of cervical SCI.[122,123]

A less drastic surgical option than myelotomy to treat elevated ISP is durotomy/duraplasty or peotomy, with laminectomy alone being insufficient.[124–126] In a rat cervical spine injury model, durotomy followed by duraplasty reduced cavitation, scar formation, and lesion volume and improved grip strength as compared to durotomy alone.[115] In a human SCI study with a small sample size, laminectomy plus duraplasty was more effective than laminectomy alone in reducing ISP, improving spinal cord perfusion, and improving spinal vascular reactivity.[125]

Together, these results suggest that treatments targeting hemorrhage and management of elevations in ISP are promising targets for the treatment of acute SCI and that attention to these targets may allow for greater efficacy of additional neuroprotective strategies. Similar to hemorrhagic stroke, hemorrhagic lesions following SCI likely contribute significantly to the cellular damage. Elevations in ISP may further exacerbate pathology by reducing perfusion to the injured cord. These targets were identified by Allen more than 100 years ago and remain relevant today.

References

1. Siddiqui AM, Khazaei M, Fehlings MG. Translating mechanisms of neuroprotection, regeneration, and repair to treatment of spinal cord injury. *Prog Brain Res.* 2015;218:15–54.

2. Silva NA, Sousa N, Reis RL, Salgado AJ. From basics to clinical: a comprehensive review on spinal cord injury. *Prog Neurobiol*. 2014;114:25–57.

3. Estrada V, Muller HW. Spinal cord injury—there is not just one way of treating it. *F1000Prime Rep*. 2014;6:84.

4. Varma AK, Das A, Wallace GT, et al. Spinal cord injury: a review of current therapy, future treatments, and basic science frontiers. *Neurochem Res*. 2013;38(5):895–905.

5. Tator CH, Hashimoto R, Raich A, et al. Translational potential of preclinical trials of neuroprotection through pharmacotherapy for spinal cord injury. *J Neurosurg Spine*. 2012;17(1 suppl):157–229.

6. Kwon BK, Okon E, Hillyer J, et al. A systematic review of non-invasive pharmacologic neuroprotective treatments for acute spinal cord injury. *J Neurotrauma*. 2011;28(8):1545–1588.

7. Bracken MB, Shepard MJ, Collins WF, et al. A randomized, controlled trial of methylprednisolone or naloxone in the treatment of acute spinal-cord injury. Results of the Second National Acute Spinal Cord Injury Study. *N Engl J Med*. 1990;322(20):1405–1411.

8. Evaniew N, Belley-Cote EP, Fallah N, Noonan VK, Rivers CS, Dvorak MF. Methylprednisolone for the treatment of patients with acute spinal cord injuries: a systematic review and meta-analysis. *J Neurotrauma*. 2016;33(5):468–481.

9. Hurlbert RJ, Hamilton MG. Methylprednisolone for acute spinal cord injury: 5-year practice reversal. *Can J Neurol Sci*. 2008;35(1):41–45.

10. Coleman WP, Benzel D, Cahill DW, et al. A critical appraisal of the reporting of the National Acute Spinal Cord Injury Studies (II and III) of methylprednisolone in acute spinal cord injury. *J Spinal Disord*. 2000;13(3):185–199.

11. Hurlbert RJ. Methylprednisolone for acute spinal cord injury: an inappropriate standard of care. *J Neurosurg*. 2000;93(1 suppl):1–7.

12. Savitz SI, Fisher M. Future of neuroprotection for acute stroke: in the aftermath of the SAINT trials. *Ann Neurol*. 2007;61(5):396–402.

13. O'Collins VE, Macleod MR, Donnan GA, Horky LL, van der Worp BH, Howells DW. 1,026 experimental treatments in acute stroke. *Ann Neurol*. 2006;59(3):467–477.

14. Howells DW, Sena ES, O'Collins V, Macleod MR. Improving the efficiency of the development of drugs for stroke. *Int J Stroke*. 2012;7(5):371–377.

15. Mitsumoto H, Brooks BR, Silani V. Clinical trials in amyotrophic lateral sclerosis: why so many negative trials and how can trials be improved? *Lancet Neurol*. 2014;13(11):1127–1138.

16. Loane DJ, Stoica BA, Faden AI. Neuroprotection for traumatic brain injury. *Handb Clin Neurol*. 2015;127:343–366.

17. Contestabile A. Amyotrophic lateral sclerosis: from research to therapeutic attempts and therapeutic perspectives. *Curr Med Chem*. 2011;18(36):5655–5665.

18. Menon DK, Maas AI. Traumatic brain injury in 2014. Progress, failures and new approaches for TBI research. *Nat Rev Neurol*. 2015;11(2):71–72.

19. Steward O, Popovich PG, Dietrich WD, Kleitman N. Replication and reproducibility in spinal cord injury research. *Exp Neurol*. 2012;233(2):597–605.

20. Frye SV, Arkin MR, Arrowsmith CH, et al. Tackling reproducibility in academic preclinical drug discovery. *Nat Rev Drug Discov*. 2015;14(11):733–734.

21. Pusztai L, Hatzis C, Andre F. Reproducibility of research and preclinical validation: problems and solutions. *Nat Rev Clin Oncol*. 2013;10(12):720–724.

22. Begley CG, Ellis LM. Drug development: Raise standards for preclinical cancer research. *Nature*. 2012;483(7391):531–533.

23. Prinz F, Schlange T, Asadullah K. Believe it or not: how much can we rely on published data on potential drug targets? *Nat Rev Drug Discov*. 2011;10(9):712.

24. Ioannidis JP. Why most published research findings are false. *PLoS Med*. 2005;2(8):e124.

25. Baker M. 1,500 scientists lift the lid on reproducibility. *Nature*. 2016;533(7604):452–454.

26. Voelkl B, Wurbel H. Reproducibility crisis: are we ignoring reaction norms? *Trends Pharmacol Sci*. 2016;37(7):509–510.

27. Button KS, Ioannidis JP, Mokrysz C, et al. Empirical evidence for low reproducibility indicates low pre-study odds. *Nat Rev Neurosci*. 2013;14(12):877.

28. Button KS, Ioannidis JP, Mokrysz C, et al. Confidence and precision increase with high statistical power. *Nat Rev Neurosci*. 2013;14(8):585–586.

29. Button KS, Ioannidis JP, Mokrysz C, et al. Power failure: why small sample size undermines the reliability of neuroscience. *Nat Rev Neurosci*. 2013;14(5):365–376.

30. Burke DA, Whittemore SR, Magnuson DS. Consequences of common data analysis inaccuracies in CNS trauma injury basic research. *J Neurotrauma*. 2013;30(10):797–805.

31. Watzlawick R, Sena ES, Dirnagl U, et al. Effect and reporting bias of RhoA/ROCK-blockade intervention on locomotor recovery after spinal cord injury: a systematic review and meta-analysis. *JAMA Neurol*. 2014;71(1):91–99.

32. Akhtar AZ, Pippin JJ, Sandusky CB. Animal studies in spinal cord injury: a systematic review of methylprednisolone. *Altern Lab Anim*. 2009;37(1):43–62.

33. Begley CG, Ioannidis JP. Reproducibility in science: improving the standard for basic and preclinical research. *Circ Res*. 2015;116(1):116–126.

34. Landis SC, Amara SG, Asadullah K, et al. A call for transparent reporting to optimize the predictive value of preclinical research. *Nature*. 2012;490(7419):187–191.

35. Ioannidis JP. How to make more published research true. *PLoS Med*. 2014;11(10):e1001747.

36. Kilkenny C, Browne W, Cuthill IC, Emerson M, Altman DG; Group NCRRGW. Animal research: reporting in vivo experiments: the ARRIVE guidelines. *Br J Pharmacol*. 2010;160(7):1577–1579.

37. Llovera G, Hofmann K, Roth S, et al. Results of a preclinical randomized controlled multicenter trial (pRCT): anti-CD49d treatment for acute brain ischemia. *Sci Transl Med*. 2015;7(299):299ra121.

38. Balduini W, Carloni S, Cimino M. Preclinical randomized controlled multicenter trials (pRCT) in stroke research: a new and valid approach to improve translation? *Ann Transl Med*. 2016;4(24):549.

39. Llovera G, Liesz A. The next step in translational research: lessons learned from the first preclinical randomized controlled trial. *J Neurochem*. 2016;139(suppl 2):271–279.

40. Schlesinger EB. Alfred Reginald Allen: the mythic career of a gifted neuroscientist. *Surg Neurol*. 1991;36(3):229–233.

41. Allen A. Surgery of experimental lesion of spinal cord equivalent to crush injury of fracture dislocation of spinal column: a preliminary report. *JAMA*. 1911;LVII(11):878–880.

42. Allen AR. Remarks on the histopathological changes in the spinal cord due to impact: an experimental study. *J Nerv Ment Dis*. 1914;41(3):141–147.

43. Wrathall JR, Pettegrew RK, Harvey F. Spinal cord contusion in the rat: production of graded, reproducible, injury groups. *Exp Neurol*. 1985;88(1):108–122.

44. Noble LJ, Wrathall JR. An inexpensive apparatus for producing graded spinal cord contusive injury in the rat. *Exp Neurol*. 1987;95(2):530–533.

45. Kuhn PL, Wrathall JR. A mouse model of graded contusive spinal cord injury. *J Neurotrauma*. 1998;15(2):125–140.

46. Lee JH, Jones CF, Okon EB, et al. A novel porcine model of traumatic thoracic spinal cord injury. *J Neurotrauma*. 2013;30(3):142–159.

47. Nout YS, Rosenzweig ES, Brock JH, et al. Animal models of neurologic disorders: a non-human primate model of spinal cord injury. *Neurotherapeutics*. 2012;9(2):380–392.

48. Arunkumar MJ, Srinivasa Babu K, Chandy MJ. Motor and somatosensory evoked potentials in a primate model of experimental spinal cord injury. *Neurol India*. 2001;49(3):219–224.

49. Ford RW. A reproducible spinal cord injury model in the cat. *J Neurosurg*. 1983;59(2):268–275.

50. Noyes DH. Electromechanical impactor for producing experimental spinal cord injury in animals. *Med Biol Eng Comput*. 1987;25(3):335–340.

51. Gruner JA. A monitored contusion model of spinal cord injury in the rat. *J Neurotrauma*. 1992;9(y2):123–126; discussion 126–128.

52. Young W. Spinal cord contusion models. *Prog Brain Res*. 2002;137:231–255.

53. Stokes BT, Jakeman LB. Experimental modelling of human spinal cord injury: a model that crosses the species barrier and mimics the spectrum of human cytopathology. *Spinal Cord*. 2002;40(3):101–109.

54. Scheff SW, Rabchevsky AG, Fugaccia I, Main JA, Lumpp JE, Jr. Experimental modeling of spinal cord injury: characterization of a force-defined injury device. *J Neurotrauma*. 2003;20(2):179–193.

55. Rabchevsky AG, Fugaccia I, Sullivan PG, Blades DA, Scheff SW. Efficacy of methylprednisolone therapy for the injured rat spinal cord. *J Neurosci Res*. 2002;68(1):7–18.

56. Choo AM, Liu J, Liu Z, Dvorak M, Tetzlaff W, Oxland TR. Modeling spinal cord contusion, dislocation, and distraction: characterization of vertebral clamps, injury severities, and node of Ranvier deformations. *J Neurosci Methods*. 2009;181(1):6–17.

57. Pearse DD, Lo TP Jr, Cho KS, et al. Histopathological and behavioral characterization of a novel cervical spinal cord displacement contusion injury in the rat. *J Neurotrauma*. 2005;22(6):680–702.

58. Onifer SM, Rabchevsky AG, Scheff SW. Rat models of traumatic spinal cord injury to assess motor recovery. *ILAR J*. 2007;48(4):385–395.

59. Cheriyan T, Ryan DJ, Weinreb JH, et al. Spinal cord injury models: a review. *Spinal Cord*. 2014;52(8):588–595.

60. Kjell J, Olson L. Rat models of spinal cord injury: from pathology to potential therapies. *Dis Model Mech*. 2016;9(10):1125–1137.

61. Fouad K, Hurd C, Magnuson DS. Functional testing in animal models of spinal cord injury: not as straight forward as one would think. *Front Integr Neurosci*. 2013;7:85.

62. Basso DM, Beattie MS, Bresnahan JC. A sensitive and reliable locomotor rating scale for open field testing in rats. *J Neurotrauma*. 1995;12(1):1–21.

63. Basso DM, Beattie MS, Bresnahan JC. Graded histological and locomotor outcomes after spinal cord contusion using the NYU weight-drop device versus transection. *Exp Neurol*. 1996;139(2):244–256.

64. Basso DM, Fisher LC, Anderson AJ, Jakeman LB, McTigue DM, Popovich PG. Basso Mouse Scale for locomotion detects differences in recovery after spinal cord injury in five common mouse strains. *J Neurotrauma*. 2006;23(5):635–659.

65. Kwon BK, Okon EB, Tsai E, et al. A grading system to evaluate objectively the strength of pre-clinical data of acute neuroprotective therapies for clinical translation in spinal cord injury. *J Neurotrauma*. 2011;28(8):1525–1543.

66. Metz GA, Curt A, van de Meent H, Klusman I, Schwab ME, Dietz V. Validation of the weight-drop contusion model in rats: a comparative study of human spinal cord injury. *J Neurotrauma*. 2000;17(1):1–17.

67. Inoue T, Lin A, Ma X, et al. Combined SCI and TBI: recovery of forelimb function after unilateral cervical spinal cord injury (SCI) is retarded by contralateral traumatic brain injury (TBI), and ipsilateral TBI balances the effects of SCI on paw placement. *Exp Neurol*. 2013;248:136–147.

68. Norenberg MD, Smith J, Marcillo A. The pathology of human spinal cord injury: defining the problems. *J Neurotrauma*. 2004;21(4):429–440.

69. Sekhon LH, Fehlings MG. Epidemiology, demographics, and pathophysiology of acute spinal cord injury. *Spine (Phila Pa 1976)*. 2001;26(24 suppl):S2–12.

70. Akhtar AZ, Pippin JJ, Sandusky CB. Animal models in spinal cord injury: a review. *Rev Neurosci*. 2008;19(1):47–60.

71. Friedli L, Rosenzweig ES, Barraud Q, et al. Pronounced species divergence in corticospinal tract reorganization and functional recovery after lateralized spinal cord injury favors primates. *Sci Transl Med*. 2015;7(302):302ra134.

72. Aceves M, Mathai BB, Hook MA. Evaluation of the effects of specific opioid receptor agonists in a rodent model of spinal cord injury. *Spinal Cord*. 2016;54(10):767–777.

73. Nout YS, Beattie MS, Bresnahan JC. Severity of locomotor and cardiovascular derangements after experimental high-thoracic spinal cord injury is anesthesia dependent in rats. *J Neurotrauma*. 2012;29(5):990–999.

74. Grissom TE, Mitzel HC, Bunegin L, Albin MS. The effect of anesthetics on neurologic outcome during the recovery period of spinal cord injury in rats. *Anesth Analg*. 1994;79(1):66–74.

75. Redfors B, Shao Y, Omerovic E. Influence of anesthetic agent, depth of anesthesia and body temperature on cardiovascular functional parameters in the rat. *Lab Anim*. 2014;48(1):6–14.

76. de la Torre JC. Spinal cord injury. Review of basic and applied research. *Spine (Phila Pa 1976)*. 1981;6(4):315–335.

77. Rosenzweig ES, McDonald JW. Rodent models for treatment of spinal cord injury: research trends and progress toward useful repair. *Curr Opin Neurol*. 2004;17(2):121–131.

78. Hagen EM, Eide GE, Rekand T, Gilhus NE, Gronning M. Traumatic spinal cord injury and concomitant brain injury: a cohort study. *Acta Neurol Scand Suppl*. 2010(190):51–57.

79. Wu X, Liu J, Tanadini LG, et al. Challenges for defining minimal clinically important difference (MCID) after spinal cord injury. *Spinal Cord*. 2015;53(2):84–91.

80. Alexander MS, Anderson KD, Biering-Sorensen F, et al. Outcome measures in spinal cord injury: recent assessments and recommendations for future directions. *Spinal Cord*. 2009;47(8):582–591.

81. Steeves JD. Bench to bedside: challenges of clinical translation. *Prog Brain Res*. 2015;218:227–239.

82. Steeves JD, Lammertse D, Curt A, et al. Guidelines for the conduct of clinical trials for spinal cord injury (SCI) as developed by the ICCP panel: clinical trial outcome measures. *Spinal Cord*. 2007;45(3):206–221.

83. Reier PJ, Lane MA, Hall ED, Teng YD, Howland DR. Translational spinal cord injury research: preclinical guidelines and challenges. *Handb Clin Neurol*. 2012;109:411–433.

84. Choo AM, Liu J, Dvorak M, Tetzlaff W, Oxland TR. Secondary pathology following contusion, dislocation, and distraction spinal cord injuries. *Exp Neurol.* 2008;212(2):490–506.

85. Tator CH, Fehlings MG. Review of the secondary injury theory of acute spinal cord trauma with emphasis on vascular mechanisms. *J Neurosurg.* 1991;75(1):15–26.

86. Dumont RJ, Okonkwo DO, Verma S, et al. Acute spinal cord injury, part I: pathophysiologic mechanisms. *Clin Neuropharmacol.* 2001;24(5):254–264.

87. Young W. Secondary injury mechanisms in acute spinal cord injury. *J Emerg Med.* 1993;11(suppl 1):13–22.

88. Bunge MB. Novel combination strategies to repair the injured mammalian spinal cord. *J Spinal Cord Med.* 2008;31(3):262–269.

89. Prabhakaran S, Ruff I, Bernstein RA. Acute stroke intervention: a systematic review. *JAMA.* 2015;313(14):1451–1462.

90. Le Roux P. Intracranial pressure monitoring and management. In: Laskowitz D, Grant G, eds. *Translational Research in Traumatic Brain Injury.* Boca Raton, FL: CRC Press/Taylor and Francis Group; 2016. https://www.ncbi.nlm.nih.gov/books/NBK326713/

91. Sheth KN, Stein DM, Aarabi B, et al. Intracranial pressure dose and outcome in traumatic brain injury. *Neurocrit Care.* 2013;18(1):26–32.

92. Romner B, Grande PO. Traumatic brain injury: Intracranial pressure monitoring in traumatic brain injury. *Nat Rev Neurol.* 2013;9(4):185–186.

93. Nelson E, Gertz SD, Rennels ML, Ducker TB, Blaumanis OR. Spinal cord injury. The role of vascular damage in the pathogenesis of central hemorrhagic necrosis. *Arch Neurol.* 1977;34(6):332–333.

94. Balentine JD. Pathology of experimental spinal cord trauma. I. The necrotic lesion as a function of vascular injury. *Lab Invest.* 1978;39(3):236–253.

95. Wallace MC, Tator CH, Frazee P. Relationship between posttraumatic ischemia and hemorrhage in the injured rat spinal cord as shown by colloidal carbon angiography. *Neurosurgery.* 1986;18(4):433–439.

96. Tator CH, Koyanagi I. Vascular mechanisms in the pathophysiology of human spinal cord injury. *J Neurosurg.* 1997;86(3):483–492.

97. Mautes AE, Weinzierl MR, Donovan F, Noble LJ. Vascular events after spinal cord injury: contribution to secondary pathogenesis. *Phys Ther.* 2000;80(7):673–687.

98. Sinescu C, Popa F, Grigorean VT, et al. Molecular basis of vascular events following spinal cord injury. *J Med Life.* 2010;3(3):254–261.

99. Losey P, Young C, Krimholtz E, Bordet R, Anthony DC. The role of hemorrhage following spinal-cord injury. *Brain Res.* 2014;1569:9–18.

100. Alshareef M, Krishna V, Ferdous J, et al. Effect of spinal cord compression on local vascular blood flow and perfusion capacity. *PLoS One.* 2014;9(9):e108820.

101. Keep RF, Hua Y, Xi G. Intracerebral haemorrhage: mechanisms of injury and therapeutic targets. *Lancet Neurol.* 2012;11(8):720–731.

102. Zhou Y, Wang Y, Wang J, Anne Stetler R, Yang QW. Inflammation in intracerebral hemorrhage: from mechanisms to clinical translation. *Prog Neurobiol.* 2014;115:25–44.

103. Hua Y, Keep RF, Hoff JT, Xi G. Brain injury after intracerebral hemorrhage: the role of thrombin and iron. *Stroke.* 2007;38(2 suppl):759–762.

104. Werndle MC, Saadoun S, Phang I, et al. Monitoring of spinal cord perfusion pressure in acute spinal cord injury: initial findings of the injured spinal cord pressure evaluation study. *Crit Care Med.* 2014;42(3):646–655.

105. Khaing ZZ, Cates LN, Fischedick AE, McClintic AM, Mourad PD, Hofstetter CP. Temporal and spatial evolution of raised intraspinal pressure after traumatic spinal cord injury. *J Neurotrauma*. 2017;34(3):645–651.

106. Brain Trauma F, American Association of Neurological S, Congress of Neurological S, et al. Guidelines for the management of severe traumatic brain injury. VI. Indications for intracranial pressure monitoring. *J Neurotrauma*. 2007;24(suppl 1):S37–44.

107. Saadoun S, Chen S, Papadopoulos MC. Intraspinal pressure and spinal cord perfusion pressure predict neurological outcome after traumatic spinal cord injury. *J Neurol Neurosurg Psychiatry*. 2016; 88(5):451–453.

108. Nielson JL, Paquette J, Liu AW, et al. Topological data analysis for discovery in preclinical spinal cord injury and traumatic brain injury. *Nat Commun*. 2015;6:8581.

109. Freeman LW, Wright TW. Experimental observations of concussion and contusion of the spinal cord. *Ann Surg*. 1953;137(4):433–443.

110. Rivlin AS, Tator CH. Effect of vasodilators and myelotomy on recovery after acute spinal cord injury in rats. *J Neurosurg*. 1979;50(3):349–352.

111. Kalderon N, Muruganandham M, Koutcher JA, Potuzak M. Therapeutic strategy for acute spinal cord contusion injury: cell elimination combined with microsurgical intervention. *PLoS One*. 2007;2(6):e565.

112. Yang DG, Li JJ, Gu R, et al. Optimal time window of myelotomy in rats with acute traumatic spinal cord injury: a preliminary study. *Spinal Cord*. 2013;51(9):673–678.

113. Hu AM, Li JJ, Sun W, et al. Myelotomy reduces spinal cord edema and inhibits aquaporin-4 and aquaporin-9 expression in rats with spinal cord injury. *Spinal Cord*. 2015;53(2):98–102.

114. Gu R, Zhang X, Yang DG, et al. Protective effect of dorsal longitudinal myelotomy at 72 Hours after spinal cord injury in rat model. *Neurol Asia*. 2012;17(2):141–146.

115. Smith JS, Anderson R, Pham T, Bhatia N, Steward O, Gupta R. Role of early surgical decompression of the intradural space after cervical spinal cord injury in an animal model. *J Bone Joint Surg Am*. 2010;92(5):1206–1214.

116. Lima C, Pratas-Vital J, Escada P, Hasse-Ferreira A, Capucho C, Peduzzi JD. Olfactory mucosa autografts in human spinal cord injury: a pilot clinical study. *J Spinal Cord Med*. 2006;29(3):191–203; discussion 204–6.

117. Lima C, Escada P, Pratas-Vital J, et al. Olfactory mucosal autografts and rehabilitation for chronic traumatic spinal cord injury. *Neurorehabil Neural Repair*. 2010;24(1):10–22.

118. Theodore N, Hlubek R, Danielson J, et al. First human implantation of a bioresorbable polymer scaffold for acute traumatic spinal cord injury: a clinical pilot study for safety and feasibility. *Neurosurgery*. 2016;79(2):E305–312.

119. Mendelow AD, Gregson BA, Fernandes HM, et al. Early surgery versus initial conservative treatment in patients with spontaneous supratentorial intracerebral haematomas in the International Surgical Trial in Intracerebral Haemorrhage (STICH): a randomised trial. *Lancet*. 2005;365(9457):387–397.

120. Mendelow AD, Gregson BA, Rowan EN, et al. Early surgery versus initial conservative treatment in patients with spontaneous supratentorial lobar intracerebral haematomas (STICH II): a randomised trial. *Lancet*. 2013;382(9890):397–408.

121. Morotti A, Goldstein JN. Diagnosis and management of acute intracerebral hemorrhage. *Emerg Med Clin North Am*. 2016;34(4):883–899.

122. Simard JM, Tsymbalyuk O, Ivanov A, et al. Endothelial sulfonylurea receptor 1-regulated NC Ca-ATP channels mediate progressive hemorrhagic necrosis following spinal cord injury. *J Clin Invest.* 2007;117(8):2105–2113.

123. Popovich PG, Lemeshow S, Gensel JC, Tovar CA. Independent evaluation of the effects of glibenclamide on reducing progressive hemorrhagic necrosis after cervical spinal cord injury. *Exp Neurol.* 2012;233(2):615–622.

124. Harwell DM, Gibson JL, Fessler RD, Holtz J, Pettigrew DB, Kuntz Ct. Pia mater significantly contributes to spinal cord intraparenchymal pressure in a simulated model of edema. *Spine (Phila Pa 1976).* 2016;41(9):E524–529.

125. Phang I, Werndle MC, Saadoun S, et al. Expansion duroplasty improves intraspinal pressure, spinal cord perfusion pressure, and vascular pressure reactivity index in patients with traumatic spinal cord injury: injured spinal cord pressure evaluation study. *J Neurotrauma.* 2015;32(12):865–874.

126. Saadoun S, Werndle MC, Lopez de Heredia L, Papadopoulos MC. The dura causes spinal cord compression after spinal cord injury. *Br J Neurosurg.* 2016;30(5):582–584.

Recent Developments in Regenerative Strategies to Treat Spinal Cord Injuries

Wenjing Sun, Andrea Tedeschi, and Riyi Shi

34

Introduction

Injuries to the adult spinal cord cause long-term sensory and motor disabilities due to interruption of axonal pathways and their failure to spontaneously regenerate. Research over the past three decades has demonstrated that the presence of a nonpermissive environment and the poor intrinsic growth ability of most central nervous system (CNS) neurons account for regeneration failure and lack of functional recovery in the adult.[1-4] To maximize any potential for functional regeneration, simultaneously overcoming extrinsic and intrinsic barriers may be necessary. Thus, one single strategy is unlikely to fully repair the damaged CNS.

Early during development, axons grow rapidly to reach target areas.[5] At later stages of development, as well as in adulthood, mechanisms controlling intrinsic axon growth ability are securely switched off to allow for synapse formation, neuronal function, and consolidation of neural circuits.[6-9] As the body continues to grow, the expansion of the nervous system is controlled by the stretch growth of integrated axonal tracts.[10] Promoting long-distance axon regeneration and connectivity represents the ultimate goal to fully repair the injured spinal cord. It is important to note that early during development, growing axons need to travel a relatively short distance to reach appropriate targets. After injury in the adult, however, such distances can be several meters long in large animals, representing a tremendous challenge for regeneration-based strategies. Nonetheless, recent developments in genetic and tissue engineering have created several possibilities to foster long-distance regeneration and functional recovery after SCI.

Genetic Engineering Strategies

The correct development of the nervous system relies on spatially and temporally controlled gene expression. While a considerable amount of regenerative strategies aim at recapitulating developmental processes, it is important to note that the environment in which adult axons reside is very different from the one found early during development.[11]

Increasing evidence suggests that the ability to regenerate body parts, including the nervous system, is encoded within the genome.[8,12,13] In contrast to the adult mammalian CNS, nervous system regeneration spontaneously occurs in a number of animal lineages including invertebrates, fish, amphibians, and reptiles.[14] Expanding the repertoire of genetic and computational tools available to study signaling pathways controlling axon growth and regeneration has identified several candidate genes whose manipulation has proved effective in promoting axon regeneration in a variety of model systems, including the adult CNS.[1]

By utilizing nine genetically diverse inbred mouse strains, Omura et al. has recently determined the contribution of genetic variation on CNS repair and regeneration after stroke, optic nerve injury, and SCI.[12] In particular, a greater level of regeneration in CAST/Ei mice correlates with the expression of a core set of genes including Activin and transforming growth factor beta (TGFβ) superfamily members.[12]

Several classes of genes appear to be differentially regulated in model systems where regeneration takes place.[8] Manipulation of a few genes is unlikely to fully repair the injured CNS. By controlling the expression of several targets, transcription factors orchestrate a plethora of biological processes. Recent studies have demonstrated that manipulation of several transcription factors including KLF, ATF3, c-Jun, STAT3, and Sox11 among others is sufficient to activate a robust regenerative response in the adult.[15–23] Other than transcription factors, gene expression is also controlled via changes in chromatin status, DNA methylation, and nucleosome positioning and dynamics. In this regard, alteration of the epigenetic landscape has been shown to shift the balance between regeneration incompetent and competent neuronal states.[24–26] When development is completed, a number of evolutionarily conserved pathways and genes, including phosphatase and tensin homolog (*Pten*) and retinoblastoma protein (*Rb*), prevent excessive cellular growth and size. Given that these genes are expressed in mature neurons, He and colleagues have hypothesized that these genes may play a crucial role in restraining axon growth in the adult CNS. Indeed, deletion of *Pten* has became one of the most powerful strategies to promote axon regeneration in the central and peripheral nervous systems in acute and chronic injury models.[27–31] More importantly, deletion of *Pten* synergizes with other strategies in promoting more robust axon regeneration and functional recovery after CNS injury,[32–37] providing confirmation that multitarget strategies are more likely to repair the traumatically injured CNS.

With the development of novel screening approaches and revolutionary tools for transcriptomics,[38] the number of potential candidates that could promote nervous system repair and regeneration continues to expand.[8,16,39–44]

In the future, combinatorial optimization may suggest more effective ways to synergistically combine several strategies with the goal to improve outcome measures. In addition, the development of genetic tools that allow us to localize and fine-tune gene expression over a discrete period of time may foster the development of personalized protocols that could be adapted to a variety of SCI types, locations, and severities.

Tissue Engineering Strategies

While intrinsic axon growth and repair capacity decline over time,[29] adult CNS axons regenerate when provided with a permissive substrate.[45] Thus, the CNS environment can be manipulated to regain regeneration competence in the adult.[46–48]

Tissue loss after SCI often results in formation of fluid-filled cavities surrounded by the glial scar, creating an additional physical barrier to axon regeneration and CNS repair.[49,50] By filling the cavity using implantable biomaterial scaffolds with adjustable mechanical properties, several strategies aim at creating a more permissive microenvironment to promote axon regeneration and tissue repair after CNS injury. While providing scaffolding, biomaterials have the potential to modulate gene delivery approaches. Several biomaterials are compatible with the host extracellular environment and adapt with many different shapes and compositions to meet the needs of the system of interest. Thus far, naturally derived biomaterials such as fibrin, collagen, hyaluronic acid, and Matrigel, as well as synthetic ones like poly-L-lactic acid and polyethylene glycol among others, have been utilized for SCI repair.[51,52]

Transplantation of genetically engineered multipotent neural progenitor cells capable of releasing trophic factors represents a promising strategy to bridge severe SCI by creating neuronal relays.[53] Along this line, Lu et al. embedded neural stem cells (NSCs) from rodent and human sources within a fibrin matrix containing a mixture of growth factors and grafted them into the site of a complete spinal cord transection in rats.[54] Transplanted cells that differentiated into neurons were able to send out numerous axons extending over long distances. Three-dimensional scaffolds made by biodegradable fibrin offer several advantages including high adhesion, compatibility with host extracellular matrix, and the ability to completely fill the cavity at the injury site without causing an inflammatory response. The addition of a growth factor cocktail in the fibrin matrix is pivotal, as the neural relays between host and grafted neurons cannot form in the absence of trophic factors.[54,55] The need for immunosuppression clearly represents a limitation for cell-based strategies; especially considering that SCI patients are immunodeficient and thus, highly susceptible to infection.[56–58] Recruitment of resident NSCs in the adult spinal cord may be an alternative approach to consider.[59] Nonetheless, recent observation suggests that alternative cell sources are equally effective in promoting robust axonal growth and CNS repair with no need for immunosuppression regimens.[60] Despite the fact that numerous axons originating from the graft are able to form new synapses and integrate into spinal circuits, functional recovery in these animals is relatively modest, suggesting that additional barriers need to be overcome to maximize recovery after severe SCI. Nonetheless, the work by Lu et al. represents a major step forward in tissue engineering and regenerative medicine. A more recent study has demonstrated that replacing the site of injury with homologous NSCs embedded in a fibrin matrix containing a growth factor cocktail promotes exuberant regeneration of corticospinal (CST) axons beyond the injury site.[61] Interestingly, direct contact with grafted cells seems necessary to trigger CST axon regeneration, suggesting that the cell graft may secrete active and diffusible molecules that contribute to the observed phenotype.

Several studies have demonstrated the importance of other cellular sources, such as Schwann cells, in fostering axon regeneration and recovery in experimental models of SCI.[62–64] Transplantation of an engineered Schwann cell graft capable of secreting neurotrophin and chondroitinase has been shown to promote axon regeneration, remyelination, and functional recovery in rats following a contusion lesion of the spinal cord.[65] Fluid bridges of Schwann cells and Matrigel have been shown to promote regeneration of brainstem axons.[63] A Schwann cell graft creates a more permissive interface with the spinal cord by recruiting host cells and allowing astrocytic processes to extend into the graft. Regenerating axons are visualized in close association with astrocytic processes within the Schwann cell bridge.[63] Interestingly, several studies in which CNS regeneration has been documented have reported the presence of glial bridges within the injury epicenter.[30,66,67] A Matrigel-embedded three-dimensional culture of Schwann cells shows a significant increase in cell survival, as well as graft vascularization, after implantation into the injured spinal cord of rats.[68] Among other approaches, the use of Matrigel for Schwann cell–seeded matrices has clear advantages due to its structural and adhesive properties that allow fine control of injection parameters and cell attachment, respectively.

Over the past three decades, tissue engineering has continued to evolve.[69,70] In combination with genetic approaches, the development of three-dimensional scaffold materials that allow homogeneous seeding of cells and controlled delivery of trophic factors has provided enormous possibilities to restore, replace, or regenerate the injured spinal cord.

Conclusion

Despite the complexity of SCI pathophysiology, recent developments in genetic and tissue engineering have offered possibilities to foster long-distance regeneration and functional recovery. However, inducing a sufficient number of axons to grow substantial distances still represents a major challenge. In addition, axon regeneration is only one of the first steps needed to restore function. Axon regeneration, synapse formation, remyelination, and refinement of neural networks through physical rehabilitation are temporally distinct cellular programs.[71] Therefore, each step needs to be spatially and temporally controlled to maximize any chance of functional recovery. Alternative strategies that include structural plasticity of spared neuronal circuits and axonal pathways should be also considered. Thus far, the majority of genetic targeting approaches include deletion or overexpression mutants. Rapid genetic screens in lower organisms such as *Drosophila* and *C. elegans* have offered novel targets for potential treatments.[72,73] The development of novel genetic tools that control gene expression on demand with inducible and tunable regulatory elements that recognize exogenous signals and differentially control protein abundance clearly represents an incredible source of opportunities for repair and regenerative strategies. Each of the cellular programs detailed in this chapter likely engages integration of different extracellular signals. In this regard, engineering biomaterials with controlled physical, chemical, and biological properties capable of releasing bioactive signaling molecules with temporal and spatial resolution may facilitate the transition from one cellular program to another. In fact, being able to accurately release biomolecules at the right time and in close proximity to the target would not only increase specificity in their action, but would also minimize side effects. Engineering spinal cord tissues that mimic the structural and biological properties of the native tissue[74] may be useful to screen libraries for compounds that could promote tissue repair and regeneration. Finally, by utilizing genetic models that more closely reproduce neurobehavioral and neuropathological features of human SCI, highly promising findings may easily translate to large animals and nonhuman primates prior to embarking on clinical trials.

Disclaimer

Riyi Shi is the co-founder of NeuroVigor, a start-up company with business interests in developing effective therapies for CNS neurodegenerative diseases and trauma.

The other authors declare that the research was conducted in the absence of any commercial or financial relationships that could be construed as a potential conflict of interest.

References

1. He Z, Jin Y. Intrinsic control of axon regeneration. *Neuron.* 2016;90(3):437–451.

2. Liu K, Tedeschi A, Park KK, He Z. Neuronal intrinsic mechanisms of axon regeneration. *Annu Rev Neurosci.* 2011;34:131–152.

3. Schwab ME, Strittmatter SM. Nogo limits neural plasticity and recovery from injury. *Curr Opin Neurobiol.* 2014;27:53–60.

4. Silver J, Schwab ME, Popovich PG. Central nervous system regenerative failure: role of oligodendrocytes, astrocytes, and microglia. *Cold Spring Harb Perspect Biol.* 2014;7(3):a020602.

5. Goldberg JL. How does an axon grow? *Genes Dev.* 2003;17(8):941–958.

6. Lorenzana AO, Lee JK, Mui M, Chang A, Zheng B. A surviving intact branch stabilizes remaining axon architecture after injury as revealed by in vivo imaging in the mouse spinal cord. *Neuron.* 2015;86(4):947–954.

7. Shewan D, Berry M, Cohen J. Extensive regeneration in vitro by early embryonic neurons on immature and adult CNS tissue. *J Neurosci.* 1995;15(3 Pt 1):2057–2062.

8. Tedeschi A, Dupraz S, Laskowski CJ, et al. The calcium channel subunit Alpha2delta2 suppresses axon regeneration in the adult CNS. *Neuron.* 2016;92(2):419–434.

9. Wu Z, Ghosh-Roy A, Yanik MF, Zhang JZ, Jin Y, Chisholm AD. Caenorhabditis elegans neuronal regeneration is influenced by life stage, ephrin signaling, and synaptic branching. *Proc Natl Acad Sci USA.* 2007;104(38):15132–15137.

10. Smith DH. Stretch growth of integrated axon tracts: extremes and exploitations. *Prog Neurobiol.* 2009;89(3):231–239.

11. Crair MC, Mason CA. Reconnecting eye to brain. *J Neurosci.* 2016;36(42):10707–10722.

12. Omura T, Omura K, Tedeschi A, et al. Robust axonal regeneration occurs in the injured CAST/Ei mouse CNS. *Neuron.* 2015;86(5):1215–1227.

13. Wasik K, Gurtowski J, Zhou X, et al. Genome and transcriptome of the regeneration-competent flatworm, Macrostomum lignano. *Proc Natl Acad Sci USA.* 2015;112(40):12462–12467.

14. Tanaka EM, Ferretti P. Considering the evolution of regeneration in the central nervous system. *Nat Rev Neurosci.* 2009;10(10):713–723.

15. Blackmore MG, Wang Z, Lerch JK, et al. Kruppel-like Factor 7 engineered for transcriptional activation promotes axon regeneration in the adult corticospinal tract. *Proc Natl Acad Sci USA.* 2012;109(19):7517–7522.

16. Chandran V, Coppola G, Nawabi H, et al. A Systems-level analysis of the peripheral nerve intrinsic axonal growth program. *Neuron.* 2016;89(5):956–970.

17. Cho Y, Shin JE, Ewan EE, Oh YM, Pita-Thomas W, Cavalli V. Activating injury-responsive genes with hypoxia enhances axon regeneration through neuronal HIF-1alpha. *Neuron.* 2015;88(4):720–734.

18. Luo X, Ribeiro M, Bray ER, et al. Enhanced transcriptional activity and mitochondrial localization of STAT3 Co-induce axon regrowth in the adult central nervous system. *Cell Rep.* 2016;15(2):398–410.

19. Moore DL, Blackmore MG, Hu Y, et al. KLF family members regulate intrinsic axon regeneration ability. *Science.* 2009;326(5950):298–301.

20. Niemi JP, DeFrancesco-Lisowitz A, Cregg JM, Howarth M, Zigmond RE. Overexpression of the monocyte chemokine CCL2 in dorsal root ganglion neurons causes a conditioning-like increase in neurite outgrowth and does so via a STAT3 dependent mechanism. *Exp Neurol.* 2016;275(Pt 1):25–37.

21. Stern S, Haverkamp S, Sinske D, et al. The transcription factor serum response factor stimulates axon regeneration through cytoplasmic localization and cofilin interaction. *J Neurosci.* 2013;33(48):18836–18848.

22. Tedeschi A. Tuning the orchestra: transcriptional pathways controlling axon regeneration. *Front Mol Neurosci.* 2011;4:60.

23. Wang Z, Reynolds A, Kirry A, Nienhaus C, Blackmore MG. Overexpression of Sox11 promotes corticospinal tract regeneration after spinal injury while interfering with functional recovery. *J Neurosci.* 2015;35(7):3139–3145.

24. Cho Y, Sloutsky R, Naegle KM, Cavalli V. Injury-induced HDAC5 nuclear export is essential for axon regeneration. *Cell.* 2013;155(4):894–908.

25. Finelli MJ, Wong JK, Zou H. Epigenetic regulation of sensory axon regeneration after spinal cord injury. *J Neurosci.* 2013;33(50):19664–19676.

26. Puttagunta R, Tedeschi A, Soria MG, et al. PCAF-dependent epigenetic changes promote axonal regeneration in the central nervous system. *Nat Commun.* 2014;5:3527.

27. Christie KJ, Webber CA, Martinez JA, Singh B, Zochodne DW. PTEN inhibition to facilitate intrinsic regenerative outgrowth of adult peripheral axons. *J Neurosci.* 2010;30(27):9306–9315.

28. Du K, Zheng S, Zhang Q, et al. Pten deletion promotes regrowth of corticospinal tract axons 1 year after spinal cord injury. *J Neurosci.* 2015;35(26):9754–9763.

29. Geoffroy CG, Hilton BJ, Tetzlaff W, Zheng B. Evidence for an age-dependent decline in axon regeneration in the adult mammalian central nervous system. *Cell Rep.* 2016;15(2):238–246.

30. Liu K, Lu Y, Lee JK, et al. PTEN deletion enhances the regenerative ability of adult corticospinal neurons. *Nat Neurosci.* 2010;13(9):1075–1081.

31. Park KK, Liu K, Hu Y, et al. Promoting axon regeneration in the adult CNS by modulation of the PTEN/mTOR pathway. *Science.* 2008;322(5903):963–966.

32. Bei F, Lee HH, Liu X, et al. Restoration of visual function by enhancing conduction in regenerated axons. *Cell.* 2016;164(1-2):219–232.

33. de Lima S, Koriyama Y, Kurimoto T, et al. Full-length axon regeneration in the adult mouse optic nerve and partial recovery of simple visual behaviors. *Proc Natl Acad Sci USA.* 2012;109(23):9149–9154.

34. Jin D, Liu Y, Sun F, Wang X, Liu X, He Z. Restoration of skilled locomotion by sprouting corticospinal axons induced by co-deletion of PTEN and SOCS3. *Nat Commun.* 2015;6:8074.

35. Lewandowski G, Steward O. AAVshRNA-mediated suppression of PTEN in adult rats in combination with salmon fibrin administration enables regenerative growth of corticospinal axons and enhances recovery of voluntary motor function after cervical spinal cord injury. *J Neurosci.* 2014;34(30):9951–9962.

36. Li S, He Q, Wang H, et al. Injured adult retinal axons with Pten and Socs3 co-deletion reform active synapses with suprachiasmatic neurons. *Neurobiol Dis.* 2015;73:366–376.

37. Marin MA, de Lima S, Gilbert HY, Giger RJ, Benowitz L, Rasband MN. Reassembly of excitable domains after CNS axon regeneration. *J Neurosci.* 2016;36(35):9148–9160.

38. Wang Z, Gerstein M, Snyder M. RNA-Seq: a revolutionary tool for transcriptomics. *Nat Rev Genet.* 2009;10(1):57–63.

39. Chen L, Wang Z, Ghosh-Roy A, et al. Axon regeneration pathways identified by systematic genetic screening in C. elegans. *Neuron.* 2011;71(6):1043–1057.

40. Duan X, Qiao M, Bei F, Kim IJ, He Z, Sanes JR. Subtype-specific regeneration of retinal ganglion cells following axotomy: effects of osteopontin and mTOR signaling. *Neuron.* 2015;85(6):1244–1256.

41. Hammarlund M, Nix P, Hauth L, Jorgensen EM, Bastiani M. Axon regeneration requires a conserved MAP kinase pathway. *Science.* 2009;323(5915):802–806.

42. Mokalled MH, Patra C, Dickson AL, Endo T, Stainier DY, Poss KD. Injury-induced ctgfa directs glial bridging and spinal cord regeneration in zebrafish. *Science.* 2016;354(6312):630–634.

43. Nix P, Hammarlund M, Hauth L, Lachnit M, Jorgensen EM, Bastiani M. Axon regeneration genes identified by RNAi screening in C. elegans. *J Neurosci.* 2014;34(2):629–645.

44. O'Donovan KJ, Ma K, Guo H, et al. B-RAF kinase drives developmental axon growth and promotes axon regeneration in the injured mature CNS. *J Exp Med.* 2014;211(5):801–814.

45. David S, Aguayo AJ. Axonal elongation into peripheral nervous system "bridges" after central nervous system injury in adult rats. *Science.* 1981;214(4523):931–933.

46. Houle JD, Tom VJ, Mayes D, Wagoner G, Phillips N, Silver J. Combining an autologous peripheral nervous system "bridge" and matrix modification by chondroitinase allows robust, functional regeneration beyond a hemisection lesion of the adult rat spinal cord. *J Neurosci.* 2006;26(28):7405–7415.

47. Kalinski AL, Sachdeva R, Gomes C, et al. mRNAs and protein synthetic machinery localize into regenerating spinal cord axons when they are provided a substrate that supports growth. *J Neurosci.* 2015;35(28):10357–10370.

48. Paveliev M, Fenrich KK, Kislin M, et al. HB-GAM (pleiotrophin) reverses inhibition of neural regeneration by the CNS extracellular matrix. *Sci Rep.* 2016;6:33916.

49. Basso DM, Beattie MS, Bresnahan JC. Graded histological and locomotor outcomes after spinal cord contusion using the NYU weight-drop device versus transection. *Exp Neurol.* 1996;139(2):244–256.

50. Beattie MS, Bresnahan JC, Komon J, et al. Endogenous repair after spinal cord contusion injuries in the rat. *Exp Neurol.* 1997;148(2):453–463.

51. Gunther MI, Weidner N, Muller R, Blesch A. Cell-seeded alginate hydrogel scaffolds promote directed linear axonal regeneration in the injured rat spinal cord. *Acta Biomater.* 2015;27:140–150.

52. Hurtado A, Cregg JM, Wang HB, et al. Robust CNS regeneration after complete spinal cord transection using aligned poly-L-lactic acid microfibers. *Biomaterials.* 2011;32(26):6068–6079.

53. Tetzlaff W, Okon EB, Karimi-Abdolrezaee S, et al. A systematic review of cellular transplantation therapies for spinal cord injury. *J Neurotrauma.* 2011;28(8):1611–1682.

54. Lu P, Wang Y, Graham L, et al. Long-distance growth and connectivity of neural stem cells after severe spinal cord injury. *Cell.* 2012;150(6):1264–1273.

55. Lu P, Kadoya K, Tuszynski MH. Axonal growth and connectivity from neural stem cell grafts in models of spinal cord injury. *Curr Opin Neurobiol.* 2014;27:103–109.

56. Brommer B, Engel O, Kopp MA, et al. Spinal cord injury-induced immune deficiency syndrome enhances infection susceptibility dependent on lesion level. *Brain.* 2016;139(Pt 3):692–707.

57. Ueno M, Ueno-Nakamura Y, Niehaus J, Popovich PG, Yoshida Y. Silencing spinal interneurons inhibits immune suppressive autonomic reflexes caused by spinal cord injury. *Nat Neurosci.* 2016;19(6):784–787.

58. Zhang Y, Guan Z, Reader B, et al. Autonomic dysreflexia causes chronic immune suppression after spinal cord injury. *J Neurosci.* 2013;33(32):12970–12981.

59. Barnabe-Heider F, Frisen J. Stem cells for spinal cord repair. *Cell Stem Cell.* 2008;3(1):16–24.

60. Lu P, Woodruff G, Wang Y, et al. Long-distance axonal growth from human induced pluripotent stem cells after spinal cord injury. *Neuron.* 2014;83(4):789–796.

61. Kadoya K, Lu P, Nguyen K, et al. Spinal cord reconstitution with homologous neural grafts enables robust corticospinal regeneration. *Nat Med.* 2016;22(5):479–487.

62. Fouad K, Schnell L, Bunge MB, Schwab ME, Liebscher T, Pearse DD. Combining Schwann cell bridges and olfactory-ensheathing glia grafts with chondroitinase promotes locomotor recovery after complete transection of the spinal cord. *J Neurosci.* 2005;25(5):1169–1178.

63. Williams RR, Henao M, Pearse DD, Bunge MB. Permissive Schwann cell graft/spinal cord interfaces for axon regeneration. *Cell Transplant.* 2015;24(1):115–131.

64. Xu XM, Chen A, Guenard V, Kleitman N, Bunge MB. Bridging Schwann cell transplants promote axonal regeneration from both the rostral and caudal stumps of transected adult rat spinal cord. *J Neurocytol.* 1997;26(1):1–16.

65. Kanno H, Pressman Y, Moody A, et al. Combination of engineered Schwann cell grafts to secrete neurotrophin and chondroitinase promotes axonal regeneration and locomotion after spinal cord injury. *J Neurosci.* 2014;34(5):1838–1855.

66. Goldshmit Y, Sztal TE, Jusuf PR, Hall TE, Nguyen-Chi M, Currie PD. Fgf-dependent glial cell bridges facilitate spinal cord regeneration in zebrafish. *J Neurosci.* 2012;32(22):7477–7492.

67. Lee JK, Geoffroy CG, Chan AF, et al. Assessing spinal axon regeneration and sprouting in Nogo-, MAG-, and OMgp-deficient mice. *Neuron.* 2010;66(5):663–670.

68. Patel V, Joseph G, Patel A, et al. Suspension matrices for improved Schwann-cell survival after implantation into the injured rat spinal cord. *J Neurotrauma.* 2010;27(5):789–801.

69. Chan BP, Leong KW. Scaffolding in tissue engineering: general approaches and tissue-specific considerations. *Eur Spine J.* 2008;17(suppl 4):467–479.

70. Madigan NN, McMahon S, O'Brien T, Yaszemski MJ, Windebank AJ. Current tissue engineering and novel therapeutic approaches to axonal regeneration following spinal cord injury using polymer scaffolds. *Respir Physiol Neurobiol.* 2009;169(2):183–199.

71. Wahl AS, Omlor W, Rubio JC, et al. Neuronal repair. Asynchronous therapy restores motor control by rewiring of the rat corticospinal tract after stroke. *Science.* 2014;344(6189):1250–1255.

72. Jorgensen EM, Mango SE. The art and design of genetic screens: Caenorhabditis elegans. *Nat Rev Genet.* 2002;3(5):356–369.

73. St Johnston D. The art and design of genetic screens: drosophila melanogaster. *Nat Rev Genet.* 2002;3(3):176–188.

74. Dvir T, Timko BP, Kohane DS, Langer R. Nanotechnological strategies for engineering complex tissues. *Nat Nanotechnol.* 2011;6(1):13–22.

Stem Cell Therapy for Spinal Cord Injury

Ping Wu, Mingliang Yang, Yan Hao, Shiqing Feng,
and Jianjun Li

35

Introduction

Traumatic spinal cord injury (SCI) causes structural and functional damage to the spinal cord, characterized by the loss of motor, sensory, and other functions below the level of the lesion. A recent survey shows an incidence ranging from 10.4 to 83 (average of 29.5) cases per million per year and a prevalence of 223–755 (average of 485) per million.[1] In spite of remarkable progress made in basic research, clinical intervention and rehabilitation, the neurological recovery, especially for complete SCI, is still extremely poor.

Stem cells have the characteristics of both self-renewal and differentiation into specific types of cells. Theoretically, stem cell–based interventions for nervous system disorders may promote neural functional recovery via (1) differentiating into neurons to construct new neural networks and rebuild circuits, (2) differentiating into oligodendrocytes to provide remyelination, and (3) secreting various regulatory and neurotrophic factors to modify the microenvironment of the injured spinal cord and promote neural regeneration. An increasing body of preclinical evidence in the past decades suggests the safety and efficacy of stem cell–based therapies for neural regeneration and repair,[2–5] which has led to a considerable number of clinical trials of stem cell transplantation to treat SCI. This chapter provides the current view of stem cells as a new therapeutic strategy for SCI, particularly focusing on the types of stem cells being used in preclinical experiments and clinical trials.

Preclinical Studies of Stem Cell–Based Therapy for SCI

Stem cells are classified into three major categories based on their potential to generate specified cell types: *totipotent*, *pluripotent*, and *multipotent* (http://www.isscr.org/visitor-types/public/stem-cell-glossary). *Totipotent stem cells* refer to fertilized eggs that have the potential to generate both embryonic and extraembryonic cell types that form a whole organism. Compared to the totipotent cells, *pluripotent* and *multipotent stem cells* have a reduced differentiation potential but are the focus of this review because they are the most commonly used stem cells in preclinical and clinical studies for SCI.

Multipotent stem cells are unspecified cells that reside in the developing or developed tissues or organs. They can self-renew for long periods of time and have the potential to differentiate into multiple types of cells with specific functions. Three major types of multipotent stem cells have so far been tested for their potential of transplantation to promote recovery from SCI: mesenchymal stem cells, neural stem cells, and hematopoietic stem cells.

Pluripotent stem cells are "master cells" that can generate any type of human cells. They can be maintained in culture dishes for indefinite self-renewal and proliferation to give rise to an enormous number of cells. Two types of stem cells with demonstrated pluripotency have been used in preclinical studies and/or clinical trials for SCI regeneration: embryonic stem cells and induced pluripotent stem cells.[6,7]

Transplantation of Exogenous Stem Cells

Most preclinical studies use the transplantation approach to evaluate stem cell therapy in animal SCI models. The vast majority of these stem cell transplantations were conducted in rodents,[8,9] with only a few done in large animals, including canine, porcine, and nonhuman primates.[10–15] To date, most of these preclinical studies using a variety of stem cells or stem cell–derived cells (listed below) suggest that stem cell–based cell transplantation is a promising strategy for neural restoration after SCI.

Mesenchymal stem cells, also referred to as mesenchymal stromal cells, are multipotent cells that can differentiate into myocytes (muscle cells), osteoblasts (bone cells), chondrocytes (cartilage cells), adipocytes (fat cells), and fibroblasts (in skin, tendon, and other tissues).[16] They can be isolated from bone marrow,[17–19] adipose tissue,[20,21] umbilical cord,[22–24] and many other tissues.[25] The presence of these cells in many adult tissues makes their isolation easier and allows autologous transplantation without immune rejection and ethical concerns.[26] In a systematic review and meta-analysis of more than 150 preclinical studies using stem cell transplantation to treat SCI in rodents, nearly half of the studies used mesenchymal stem cells.[27] More importantly, treatment with mesenchymal stem cells resulted in a substantial beneficial effect on motor function recovery after SCI.[28] Potential mechanisms appear to be indirect, such as providing a neuroprotective effect, regulating the inflammatory response, providing substrates for axonal remodeling, or promoting the expression of growth factors to enhance neoangiogenesis for the creation of a favorable environment.[29–37]

Neural stem cells (NSCs) are also called neural progenitor or precursor cells, or neuroepithelial cells during development.[38–40] Starting in the late 1980s, scientists successfully isolated and cultured NSCs without genetic modification, initially from the rodent brain[41–43] and later from discarded human brain tissues.[44,45] Cultivation of NSCs from spinal cord has also been well documented.[46,47] NSCs populate the nervous system by differentiating into three neural lineages, including neurons, astrocytes, and oligodendrocytes. With these unique properties, NSCs can be used to replace neural cells lost after SCI.[48–53] In fact they are the other major type of stem cells being tested in animal studies. A systematic review and meta-analysis of 74 preclinical animal studies confirmed that NSC transplantation improves motor function recovery after SCI and suggests that the efficacy of transplantation depended mainly on injury model, intervention phase, cell number, and immunosuppression.[54] Greater improvement was seen in the transection SCI model, with a larger number of cells grafted in the acute phase of injury, whereas immunosuppression negatively affect the motor recovery. One of the mechanisms for functional recovery may be that grafted NSCs differentiate into neurons, which mainly act as relays to rewire the spinal cord.[55–58] Although the injured spinal cord is usually unfavorable to neuronal differentiation,[59] special manipulations of cells before transplantation seem to foster the capability of NSCs to become neurons in the injured cord.[53,60–63] Another mechanism of NSC-mediated functional improvement is that these cells generate new oligodendrocytes to remyelinate surviving axons.[62,64,65] The newborn neurons send axons that extend to long distances and are myelinated and integrated into host circuitry.[61] Finally, grafted NSCs or their differentiated immature astrocytes produce neurotrophic factors and reduce inflammation.[51,55,62]

Hematopoietic stem cells are multipotent cells that give rise to all blood cells such as red blood cells, white blood cells, and platelets, as well as immune cells such as lymphocytes and macrophages.[66] The primary source of hematopoietic stem cells is bone marrow. However, peripheral blood and umbilical cord blood also contain many hematopoietic stem cells. Significantly fewer preclinical studies have been done by transplanting hematopoietic stem cells from peripheral or umbilical cord blood and from bone marrow. Most of these studies reported a beneficial effect to improve motor function after SCI in rodents.[67–71] Mechanisms include trophic support for host neurons and oligodendrocytes, reduction in cell death and demyelination, and promoting angiogenesis and antiinflammation.[67,68,72]

Embryonic stem cells and induced pluripotent stem cells . Embryonic stem cells were first isolated from the human embryo by Thomson et al. two decades ago.[73] They are derived from the inner cell mass of a blastocyst at about 5–7 days after fertilization. The pluripotent capacity of these cells to generate any types of cells, including neural cells, has attracted great public attention, but also generated ethical and moral concerns. In seeking alternatives, Yamanaka et al. created a new type of pluripotent cells, named *induced pluripotent stem cells*. These genetically reprogrammed cells have the capacities of embryonic stem cells, and they are generated by forcing adult cells (e.g., skin fibroblasts) to express genes that are unique to embryonic stem cells.[74,75] The autologous property of the induced pluripotent stem cells from a patient's own cells is particularly attractive since it offers a strategy to avoid ethical concerns and immune rejection.[7,76–78]

Several preclinical studies first differentiated embryonic or induced pluripotent stem cells to become NSCs or oligodendrocytes and then grafted these cells into injured spinal cord in animal models. Such regimens significantly improved motor function in rodents and nonhuman primates.[61,79–83] Mechanisms underlying the benefits of these cells are suggested to be replacing lost neurons to form new circuits, improving myelin repair and axon regeneration, providing neurotrophic factors, and reducing inflammation.[50,60,82,84,85] A recent meta-analysis indicates variations in motor function recovery and that the efficacy of induced pluripotent stem cell–derived NSC transplantation varies and seems to be related to the age of the somatic cell donor (embryonic or adult).[54] Despite the advantages of these cells, the genetic/epigenetic abnormalities and tumorigenesis associated with the artificial reprogramming of these cells requires careful quality control and further development of better technologies.[79]

Combination cell therapy . In order to improve the functional efficacy of stem cell transplantation, a number of animal studies have used various approaches of combining stem cell transplantation with other cell types, bioengineering materials, pharmacological reagents, or rehabilitation.[55,86] Such combination strategies appear to enhance grafted cell survival and thus their function.[87] A meta-analysis of NSC transplantation suggested that scaffold use in transplantation effectively enhanced motor functional recovery in rodents.[54] Stem cell transplantation combined with immune modulation and rehabilitation also promoted a synergistic functional benefit.[9,79] In terms of other cell types, Schwann cells appear to be promising since these peripheral myelin-forming cells can integrate into the host spinal cord and served as scaffold to promote axon regeneration.[88–91] Several preclinical studies showed a synergistic effect to promote motor function recovery after co-transplantation of Schwann cells and several stem cell types such as mesenchymal or NSCs.[92]

Potential of Endogenous Cell–Mediated Repair

The presence of NSCs in the adult spinal cord raises the possibility that modulation of these endogenous cells may offer an alternative strategy to cell transplantation.[47,93,94] For example, mobilizing endogenous NSCs is a noninvasive autologous cell therapy that could circumvent many of the limitations and risks of transplantation.[95] In adult spinal cord, endogenous NSCs are mainly located in the ependymal layer of the central canal. They stay quiescent in the intact spinal cord but are rapidly activated following SCI.[96] After injury, most spinal NSCs differentiate into astrocytes, which contribute to glia scar formation; a few become oligodendrocytes, but rarely neurons.[97] Several studies have indicated that it is possible to modulate endogenous stem cells; for example, intracerebroventricular infusion of growth factors significantly increased their proliferation.[98] However, it remains unknown how to manipulate endogenous NSCs to efficiently generate the desired cell types (i.e., neurons and oligodendrocytes) after SCI.

In addition to spinal cord NSCs, scientists are working to reprogram astrocytes in brain and spinal cord and turn them into functional neurons.[99,100] The rationale behind turning astrocytes into neurons is that astrocytes reactivate and become the dominant cell type after injury to form glial scars; reprogramming these astrocytes into neurons could theoretically reduce glial scar formation and replace lost neurons. Zhang and colleagues have reported a proof-of-concept study confirming the possibility of converting astrocytes into neurons in the rodent spinal cord after injury.[100] However, it remains to be seen whether such a manipulation could lead to functional recovery after SCI.

Clinical Studies of Stem Cell–Based Therapy for SCI

There are mainly four types of stem cells being investigated in clinical trials for spinal cord repair. Table 35.1 lists clinical trials selected based on the status of their authorized registration for rigorous evaluation of treatment safety and efficacy.

Types of Stem Cells in Clinical Trials

Mesenchymal stem cells. Similar to preclinical studies, the majority of clinical trials also used mesenchymal stem cells from bone marrow. The autologous cells were either directly transplanted into the injury site or administrated through intrathecal or intravenous routes. The commonly reported improvements include increased sensory and motor functions and the transition from a complete to incomplete SCI.[101,102] In a trial grafting mesenchymal stem cells subacutely into the injury site and combined with granulocyte-macrophage colony stimulating factor, Park et al.[103] reported that 4 out of 6 patients

Table 35.1:
Selected clinical trials of stem cell therapy registered or approved by US Food and Drug Administration for treatment of spinal cord injury

Disease	Cell Type	Sponsor	Trial Type	Start Date	Current Status
SCI	BMSC (i.thec)	TCA Cellular Therapy	Phase I	Jul. 2010	ongoing
SCI in children	BMPC (i.v.)	Hermann/TIRR	Phase I	Apr. 2011	recruiting
SCI	BMSC (i.thec)	International Stemcell Services limited	Phase I/II	Jan. 2008	completed
Chronic SCI	BM transplant	Cairo Univ. (Egypt)	Phase I/II	Dec. 2008	completed
SCI	HuCNS-SC (i.med)	StemCells Inc	phase I/II	Mar. 2011	Phase I completed
SCI	HuSP-SC (i.med)	Neuralstem Inc	phase I	2013	ongoing
SCI	ESC-OPC (i.med)	Geron Co.	Phase I	Oct. 2010	ceased

BMSC, bone marrow stem cell; BMPC, bone marrow progenitor cell; BM, bone marrow; HuCNS-SC, human central nervous system–derived stem cell; HuSP-SC, human spinal cord–derived stem cell; ESC-OPC, embryonic stem cell–derived oligodendrocyte progenitor cell; i.thec, intrathecal; i.v, intravenous; i.med, intramedullary; SCI, spinal cord injury.

gained significant function recovery with the American Spinal Injury Association (ASIA) Impairment Scale, moving from grade A to C. Significant improvements in motor and sensory scores were also reported in one trial of chronic SCI patients.[104] However, most studies reported only limited neurological improvement for chronic SCI.[105,106] Generally, the clinical trials suggested that mesenchymal stem cell transplantation in acute and sub-acute SCI patients seems to be more effective than in chronic patients.[107]

Neural stem cells. Two sources of NSCs, human fetal brain[108] and spinal cord,[109] have been used in clinical trials for treatment of SCI. The human fetal brain–derived stem cells were investigated in a phase I/II clinical trial (sponsored by StemCells, Inc., Table 35.1). In phase I, 12 chronic thoracic SCI patients received stem cells directly grafted into the spinal lesion with a 12-month follow-up to monitor safety and efficacy. The company reported positive outcomes, including motor improvement.[110] Later, another phase II trial was initiated to include cervical SCI patients but was recently terminated due to business decisions. The human fetal spinal cord–derived stem cells were also approved by the FDA for treating chronic SCI patients. A phase I study planned to recruit eight chronic patients with complete thoracic SCI to evaluate the safety, survival, and effectiveness of the grafts. The sponsor (Neuralstem, Inc.) announced the phase I safety trial in January 2013. Recently, they reported a promising finding from 4 patients who received NSC grafts for 1.5–2.3 years.[111] All patients tolerated the transplantation well without serious adverse events, and two of them showed some neurological improvements.

Hematopoietic stem cells . These cells, with their advantage of autologous treatment for SCI, can be readily isolated from bone marrow or peripheral blood. One study reported improvement in motor and sensory functions in all nine patients with chronic complete SCI after the transplantation of autologous bone marrow–derived hematopoietic stem cells.[112] Another study also confirmed the safety and efficacy of these stem cells to improve the life quality of patients.[113] In this retrospective study including 202 patients, cells were intrathecally administered every 3 month for 3–5 years, and the restoration of neurologic deficit was proved stable and evident in 57.4% of all cases. Another recent study combining transplantation of umbilical cord blood mononuclear cells with locomotor training showed beneficial effects in chronic complete SCI patients.[114,115]

Embryonic stem cells . The first approved clinical trial of human embryonic stem cells for SCI was GRNOPC1 therapy.[76,116] GRNOPC1, containing embryonic stem cell–derived oligodendrocyte progenitor cells, is developed by Geron Corporation to treat specific forms of SCI through a mechanism of demyelination of damaged axons.[85,117] The trial was initiated to determine its safety and efficacy in chronic SCI patients by directly injecting cells into the injury site of the spinal cord. Results from four patients enrolled in the trial were released in October 2011 and indicated no serious adverse events occurred following GRNOPC1. However, the trial was discontinued in November 2011 due to lack of funding and complicated regulatory procedures.[110,118] Currently, there are no other FDA-approved clinical trials of embryonic stem cells for human SCI.

Procedure and Evaluation of Stem Cell Transplantation

Several administration routes have been used to deliver cells. Intramedullary transplantation allows cells to be directly delivered into the injured site. The procedure requires a spinal surgery to adequately explore the lesion or a puncture through a spinous gap into the injured cord using the stereotactic injection method. A single injection in one site is limited to less than 30 μL and must be given slowly to avoid additional damage. For patients with complete or chronic SCI, transplantation of 10^7–10^8 cells seems to be more beneficial.[116] Other routes, such as intrathecal, intravenous, and intraarterial injections have also been tested. These routes are easier to operate, allow more cell delivery, and cause no further damage to the cord. The suggested quantity of cells to be delivered by these routes vary from 10^6 to 10^9 cells.[2,106]

Neurological improvements include a decline of sensory level (or increase of sensitivity), increase of muscle power, and the transition from a complete to an incomplete SCI. Other changes include spasm relief, improved sexual function, and increased bowel sensations and sweating. In a systematic review and meta-analysis of 275 patients, the ASIA improvement rate was in favor of bone marrow mesenchymal stem cells.[116] Another review reported that 43% of 328 patients had improved ASIA scale scores 1 year after stem cell treatments.[119] However, the designs of these trials raised some issues, and the contribution of spontaneous recovery following injury could not be ruled out. Thus the actual effect of stem cell transplantation still remains uncertain for human SCI.

The potential adverse effects directly to the spinal cord were the abnormal growth of grafts, additional damage due to needle penetration, and infection. Tumors developed from the transplanted stem cells were rarely reported in clinical studies. The immune response of human spinal cord to transplanted stem cells is unclear. Some studies reported a slightly higher occurrence of neuropathic pain following transplantation.[107] However, since there is a high incidence of pain following SCI, no proof has been documented attributing pain to cell implantation. Fever and headache due to the intrathecal injection was frequently reported, but often resolved with time.

Conclusion

Remarkable progress has been made by scientists and clinicians over the past two decades to test the potential of stem cell–based therapy to treat SCI. Transplanting a variety of stem cells or stem cell–derived cells in numerous preclinical animal studies showed some beneficial effects to promote sensory and motor function recovery, which led to a number of clinical trials. The outcomes of some trials suggested that stem cell transplantation in general is safe and feasible for SCI patients. However, the exact efficacy of cell therapy remains to be fully validated.

While the best type of stem cells for SCI repair is yet to be determined, mesenchymal and neural stem cells have been serving as the predominant sources for both preclinical and clinical studies.[110] As summarized in Figure 35.1, these and hematopoietic stem cells are all able to provide neurotrophic and antiinflammatory effects to promote survival of neurons and oligodendrocytes as well as axon regeneration and remyelination.[33,120] In addition, NSCs originating from different sources such as fetal tissues, embryonic stem cells, or induced pluripotent stem cells may be ideal to provide the desired neurons, oligodendrocytes, and astrocytes. On the other hand, mesenchymal and hematopoietic stem cells are appealing since they allow autologous transplantation that avoids both immune rejection and ethical and moral concerns. Obviously both positive efficacy and adverse consequences should be carefully weighed.

Previous preclinical studies have heavily relied on rodent models. The recent failure to demonstrate efficacy of clinical-grade NSCs (HuCNS-SC) in SCI rodents underlines the need to improve cell product characterization and to establish potency assays to reduce variation among different cell lots.[121,122] It also calls for unbiased interpretation of rodent data from various injury models[27,28,54] and emphasizes the need to use large

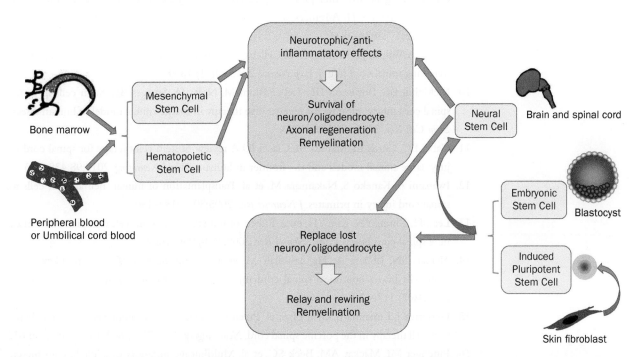

Figure 35.1 Main mechanisms underlying stem cell–mediated beneficial effects to promote recovery from spinal cord injury.

animals for their close similarity to humans prior to clinical trials.[10,11,123] Furthermore, long-term studies are absolutely necessary to monitor issues related to immunogenicity, tumorigenicity, and gender-dependent responses to cell transplantation.[27] Manipulating endogenous NSCs offers another attractive approach that deserves further exploration to aid spinal cord recovery. Finally, many studies suggested that any single therapeutic approach may not be sufficient to sustain a significant functional recovery after SCI. The need for combination therapy is increasingly acknowledged.[3,124]

References

1. Wyndaele M, Wyndaele JJ. Incidence, prevalence and epidemiology of spinal cord injury: what learns a worldwide literature survey? *Spinal Cord.* 2006;44(9):523–529.

2. Li XC, Zhong CF, Deng GB, Liang RW, Huang CM. Efficacy and safety of bone marrow-derived cell transplantation for spinal cord injury: a systematic review and meta-analysis of clinical trials. *Clin Transplant.* 2015;29(9):786–795.

3. Tetzlaff W, Okon EB, Karimi-Abdolrezaee S, et al. A systematic review of cellular transplantation therapies for spinal cord injury. *J Neurotrauma.* 2011;28(8):1611–1682.

4. Harrop JS, Hashimoto R, Norvell D, et al. Evaluation of clinical experience using cell-based therapies in patients with spinal cord injury: a systematic review. *J Neurosurg Spine.* 2012;17(1 suppl):230–246.

5. Zietlow R, Lane EL, Dunnett SB, Rosser AE. Human stem cells for CNS repair. *Cell Tissue Res.* 2008;331(1):301–322.

6. Ilic D, Devito L, Miere C, Codognotto S. Human embryonic and induced pluripotent stem cells in clinical trials. *Br Med Bull.* 2015;116:19–27.

7. Salewski RP, Eftekharpour E, Fehlings MG. Are induced pluripotent stem cells the future of cell-based regenerative therapies for spinal cord injury? *J Cell Physiol.* 2010;222(3):515–521.

8. Mothe AJ, Tator CH. Advances in stem cell therapy for spinal cord injury. *J Clin Invest.* 2012;122(11):3824–3834.

9. Ruff CA, Wilcox JT, Fehlings MG. Cell-based transplantation strategies to promote plasticity following spinal cord injury. *Exp Neurol.* 2012;235(1):78–90.

10. McMahill BG, Borjesson DL, Sieber-Blum M, Nolta JA, Sturges BK. Stem cells in canine spinal cord injury: promise for regenerative therapy in a large animal model of human disease. *Stem Cell Rev.* 2015;11(1):180–193.

11. Gabel BC, Curtis EI, Marsala M, Ciacci JD. A review of stem cell therapy for spinal cord injury: large animal models and the frontier in humans. *World Neurosurg.* 2017;98:438–443.

12. Iwanami A, Kaneko S, Nakamura M, et al. Transplantation of human neural stem cells for spinal cord injury in primates. *J Neurosci Res.* 2005;80(2):182–190.

13. Lee SH, Chung YN, Kim YH, et al. Effects of human neural stem cell transplantation in canine spinal cord hemisection. *Neurol Res.* 2009;31(9):996–1002.

14. Nemati SN, Jabbari R, Hajinasrollah M, et al. Transplantation of adult monkey neural stem cells into a contusion spinal cord injury model in rhesus macaque monkeys. *Cell J.* 2014;16(2):117–130.

15. Gutierrez J, Lamanna JJ, Grin N, et al. Preclinical validation of multilevel intraparenchymal stem cell therapy in the porcine spinal cord. *Neurosurgery.* 2015;77(4):604–612; discussion 612.

16. Pittenger MF, Mackay AM, Beck SC, et al. Multilineage potential of adult human mesenchymal stem cells. *Science.* 1999;284(5411):143–147.

17. Friedenstein AJ, Chailakhyan RK, Latsinik NV, Panasyuk AF, Keiliss-Borok IV. Stromal cells responsible for transferring the microenvironment of the hemopoietic tissues. Cloning in vitro and retransplantation in vivo. *Transplantation.* 1974;17(4):331–340.

18. Majumdar MK, Thiede MA, Mosca JD, Moorman M, Gerson SL. Phenotypic and functional comparison of cultures of marrow-derived mesenchymal stem cells (MSCs) and stromal cells. *J Cell Physiol.* 1998;176(1):57–66.

19. Soleimani M, Nadri S. A protocol for isolation and culture of mesenchymal stem cells from mouse bone marrow. *Nat Protoc.* 2009;4(1):102–106.

20. Gronthos S, Franklin DM, Leddy HA, Robey PG, Storms RW, Gimble JM. Surface protein characterization of human adipose tissue-derived stromal cells. *J Cell Physiol.* 2001;189(1):54–63.

21. Zuk PA, Zhu M, Ashjian P, et al. Human adipose tissue is a source of multipotent stem cells. *Mol Biol Cell.* 2002;13(12):4279–4295.

22. Romanov YA, Svintsitskaya VA, Smirnov VN. Searching for alternative sources of postnatal human mesenchymal stem cells: candidate MSC-like cells from umbilical cord. *Stem Cells.* 2003;21(1):105–110.

23. Schaffler A, Buchler C. Concise review: adipose tissue-derived stromal cells—basic and clinical implications for novel cell-based therapies. *Stem Cells.* 2007;25(4):818–827.

24. Lee OK, Kuo TK, Chen WM, Lee KD, Hsieh SL, Chen TH. Isolation of multipotent mesenchymal stem cells from umbilical cord blood. *Blood.* 2004;103(5):1669–1675.

25. Barry FP, Murphy JM. Mesenchymal stem cells: clinical applications and biological characterization. *Int J Biochem Cell Biol.* 2004;36(4):568–584.

26. Lalu MM, McIntyre L, Pugliese C, et al. Safety of cell therapy with mesenchymal stromal cells (SafeCell): a systematic review and meta-analysis of clinical trials. *PLoS One.* 2012;7(10):e47559.

27. Antonic A, Sena ES, Lees JS, et al. Stem cell transplantation in traumatic spinal cord injury: a systematic review and meta-analysis of animal studies. *PLoS Biol.* 2013;11(12):e1001738.

28. Oliveri RS, Bello S, Biering-Sorensen F. Mesenchymal stem cells improve locomotor recovery in traumatic spinal cord injury: systematic review with meta-analyses of rat models. *Neurobiol Dis.* 2014;62:338–353.

29. Hofstetter CP, Schwarz EJ, Hess D, et al. Marrow stromal cells form guiding strands in the injured spinal cord and promote recovery. *Proc Natl Acad Sci USA.* 2002;99(4):2199–2204.

30. Ankeny DP, McTigue DM, Jakeman LB. Bone marrow transplants provide tissue protection and directional guidance for axons after contusive spinal cord injury in rats. *Exp Neurol.* 2004;190(1):17–31.

31. Lu P, Jones LL, Tuszynski MH. BDNF-expressing marrow stromal cells support extensive axonal growth at sites of spinal cord injury. *Exp Neurol.* 2005;191(2):344–360.

32. Ohta M, Suzuki Y, Noda T, et al. Bone marrow stromal cells infused into the cerebrospinal fluid promote functional recovery of the injured rat spinal cord with reduced cavity formation. *Exp Neurol.* 2004;187(2):266–278.

33. Wright KT, El Masri W, Osman A, Chowdhury J, Johnson WE. Concise review: bone marrow for the treatment of spinal cord injury: mechanisms and clinical applications. *Stem Cells.* 2011;29(2):169–178.

34. Prockop DJ, Youn Oh J. Mesenchymal stem/stromal cells (MSCs): role as guardians of inflammation. *Mol Ther.* 2012;20(1):14–20.

35. Singer NG, Caplan AI. Mesenchymal stem cells: mechanisms of inflammation. *Annu Rev Pathol.* 2011;6:457–478.

36. Uccelli A. Mesenchymal stem cells exert a remarkable regenerative effect requiring minimal CNS integration: commentary on: "Mesenchymal stem cells protect CNS neurons against glutamate excitotoxicity by inhibiting glutamate receptor expression and function" by Voulgari-Kokota, et al. *Exp Neurol.* 2013;247:292–295.

37. von Bahr L, Batsis I, Moll G, et al. Analysis of tissues following mesenchymal stromal cell therapy in humans indicates limited long-term engraftment and no ectopic tissue formation. *Stem Cells.* 2012;30(7):1575–1578.

38. Weiss S, Reynolds BA, Vescovi AL, Morshead C, Craig CG, van der Kooy D. Is there a neural stem cell in the mammalian forebrain? *Trends Neurosci.* 1996;19(9):387–393.

39. McKay R. Stem cells in the central nervous system. *Science.* 1997;276(5309):66–71.

40. Gage FH. Mammalian neural stem cells. *Science.* 2000;287(5457):1433–1438.

41. Temple S. Division and differentiation of isolated CNS blast cells in microculture. *Nature.* 1989;340(6233):471–473.

42. Reynolds BA, Weiss S. Generation of neurons and astrocytes from isolated cells of the adult mammalian central nervous system. *Science.* 1992;255(5052):1707–1710.

43. Palmer TD, Takahashi J, Gage FH. The adult rat hippocampus contains primordial neural stem cells. *Mol Cell Neurosci.* 1997;8(6):389–404.

44. Buc-Caron MH. Neuroepithelial progenitor cells explanted from human fetal brain proliferate and differentiate in vitro. *Neurobiol Dis.* 1995;2(1):37–47.

45. Svendsen CN, Clarke DJ, Rosser AE, Dunnett SB. Survival and differentiation of rat and human epidermal growth factor-responsive precursor cells following grafting into the lesioned adult central nervous system. *Exp Neurol.* 1996;137(2):376–388.

46. Kalyani A, Hobson K, Rao MS. Neuroepithelial stem cells from the embryonic spinal cord: isolation, characterization, and clonal analysis. *Dev Biol.* 1997;186(2):202–223.

47. Johansson CB, Momma S, Clarke DL, Risling M, Lendahl U, Frisen J. Identification of a neural stem cell in the adult mammalian central nervous system. *Cell.* 1999;96(1):25–34.

48. Kabatas S, Teng YD. Potential roles of the neural stem cell in the restoration of the injured spinal cord: review of the literature. *Turk Neurosurg.* 2010;20(2):103–110.

49. Sandner B, Prang P, Rivera FJ, Aigner L, Blesch A, Weidner N. Neural stem cells for spinal cord repair. *Cell Tissue Res.* 2012;349(1):349–362.

50. Lu P, Woodruff G, Wang Y, et al. Long-distance axonal growth from human induced pluripotent stem cells after spinal cord injury. *Neuron.* 2014;83(4):789–796.

51. Mothe AJ, Tator CH. Review of transplantation of neural stem/progenitor cells for spinal cord injury. *Int J Dev Neurosci.* 2013;31(7):701–713.

52. Ogawa Y, Sawamoto K, Miyata T, et al. Transplantation of in vitro-expanded fetal neural progenitor cells results in neurogenesis and functional recovery after spinal cord contusion injury in adult rats. *J Neurosci Res.* 2002;69(6):925–933.

53. Tarasenko YI, Gao J, Nie L, et al. Human fetal neural stem cells grafted into contusion-injured rat spinal cords improve behavior. *J Neurosci Res.* 2007;85(1):47–57.

54. Yousefifard M, Rahimi-Movaghar V, Nasirinezhad F, et al. Neural stem/progenitor cell transplantation for spinal cord injury treatment: a systematic review and meta-analysis. *Neuroscience.* 2016;322:377–397.

55. Iyer NR, Wilems TS, Sakiyama-Elbert SE. Stem cells for spinal cord injury: strategies to inform differentiation and transplantation. *Biotechnol Bioeng.* 2017;114(2):245–259.

56. Bonner JF, Steward O. Repair of spinal cord injury with neuronal relays: from fetal grafts to neural stem cells. *Brain Res.* 2015;1619:115–123.

57. Lu P, Kadoya K, Tuszynski MH. Axonal growth and connectivity from neural stem cell grafts in models of spinal cord injury. *Curr Opin Neurobiol*. 2014;27:103–109.

58. Dell'Anno MT, Strittmatter SM. Rewiring the spinal cord: direct and indirect strategies. *Neurosci Lett*. 2017;652:25–34.

59. Cao QL, Zhang YP, Howard RM, Walters WM, Tsoulfas P, Whittemore SR. Pluripotent stem cells engrafted into the normal or lesioned adult rat spinal cord are restricted to a glial lineage. *Exp Neurol*. 2001;167(1):48–58.

60. Nori S, Okada Y, Yasuda A, et al. Grafted human-induced pluripotent stem-cell-derived neurospheres promote motor functional recovery after spinal cord injury in mice. *Proc Natl Acad Sci USA*. 2011;108(40):16825–16830.

61. Lu P, Wang Y, Graham L, et al. Long-distance growth and connectivity of neural stem cells after severe spinal cord injury. *Cell*. 2012;150(6):1264–1273.

62. Cummings BJ, Uchida N, Tamaki SJ, et al. Human neural stem cells differentiate and promote locomotor recovery in spinal cord-injured mice. *Proc Natl Acad Sci USA*. 2005;102(39):14069–14074.

63. Hofstetter CP, Holmstrom NA, Lilja JA, et al. Allodynia limits the usefulness of intraspinal neural stem cell grafts: directed differentiation improves outcome. *Nat Neurosci*. 2005;8(3):346–353.

64. Falnikar A, Li K, Lepore AC. Therapeutically targeting astrocytes with stem and progenitor cell transplantation following traumatic spinal cord injury. *Brain Res*. 2015;1619:91–103.

65. Cusimano M, Biziato D, Brambilla E, et al. Transplanted neural stem/precursor cells instruct phagocytes and reduce secondary tissue damage in the injured spinal cord. *Brain*. 2012;135(Pt 2):447–460.

66. Domen J, Wagers A, Weissman IL. Bone marrow (hematopoietic) stem cells. NIH stem cell information home page. In *Stem Cell Information* http://stemcells.nih.gov/info/Regenerative_Medicine/2006Chapter2002.htm. Published 2016.

67. Takahashi H, Koda M, Hashimoto M, et al. Transplanted peripheral blood stem cells mobilized by granulocyte colony-stimulating factor promoted hindlimb functional recovery after spinal cord injury in mice. *Cell Transplant*. 2016;25(2):283–292.

68. Chua SJ, Bielecki R, Yamanaka N, Fehlings MG, Rogers IM, Casper RF. The effect of umbilical cord blood cells on outcomes after experimental traumatic spinal cord injury. *Spine (Phila Pa 1976)*. 2010;35(16):1520–1526.

69. Saporta S, Kim JJ, Willing AE, Fu ES, Davis CD, Sanberg PR. Human umbilical cord blood stem cells infusion in spinal cord injury: engraftment and beneficial influence on behavior. *J Hematother Stem Cell Res*. 2003;12(3):271–278.

70. Nishio Y, Koda M, Kamada T, et al. The use of hemopoietic stem cells derived from human umbilical cord blood to promote restoration of spinal cord tissue and recovery of hindlimb function in adult rats. *J Neurosurg Spine*. 2006;5(5):424–433.

71. Zhao ZM, Li HJ, Liu HY, et al. Intraspinal transplantation of CD34+ human umbilical cord blood cells after spinal cord hemisection injury improves functional recovery in adult rats. *Cell Transplant*. 2004;13(2):113–122.

72. Sasaki H, Ishikawa M, Tanaka N, et al. Administration of human peripheral blood-derived CD133+ cells accelerates functional recovery in a rat spinal cord injury model. *Spine (Phila Pa 1976)*. 2009;34(3):249–254.

73. Thomson JA, Itskovitz-Eldor J, Shapiro SS, et al. Embryonic stem cell lines derived from human blastocysts. *Science.* 1998;282(5391):1145–1147.

74. Takahashi K, Yamanaka S. Induction of pluripotent stem cells from mouse embryonic and adult fibroblast cultures by defined factors. *Cell.* 2006;126(4):663–676.

75. Takahashi K, Tanabe K, Ohnuki M, et al. Induction of pluripotent stem cells from adult human fibroblasts by defined factors. *Cell.* 2007;131(5):861–872.

76. Ronaghi M, Erceg S, Moreno-Manzano V, Stojkovic M. Challenges of stem cell therapy for spinal cord injury: human embryonic stem cells, endogenous neural stem cells, or induced pluripotent stem cells? *Stem Cells.* 2010;28(1):93–99.

77. Lee-Kubli CA, Lu P. Induced pluripotent stem cell-derived neural stem cell therapies for spinal cord injury. *Neural Regen Res.* 2015;10(1):10–16.

78. Khazaei M, Ahuja CS, Fehlings MG. Induced pluripotent stem cells for traumatic spinal cord injury. *Front Cell Dev Biol.* 2016;4:152.

79. Nagoshi N, Okano H. Applications of induced pluripotent stem cell technologies in spinal cord injury. *J Neurochem.* 2017;141(6):848–860.

80. Bretzner F, Gilbert F, Baylis F, Brownstone RM. Target populations for first-in-human embryonic stem cell research in spinal cord injury. *Cell Stem Cell.* 2011;8(5):468–475.

81. Nakamura M, Okano H. Cell transplantation therapies for spinal cord injury focusing on induced pluripotent stem cells. *Cell Res.* 2013;23(1):70–80.

82. Tsuji O, Miura K, Okada Y, et al. Therapeutic potential of appropriately evaluated safe-induced pluripotent stem cells for spinal cord injury. *Proc Natl Acad Sci USA.* 2010;107(28):12704–12709.

83. McDonald JW, Liu XZ, Qu Y, et al. Transplanted embryonic stem cells survive, differentiate and promote recovery in injured rat spinal cord. *Nat Med.* 1999;5(12):1410–1412.

84. Fujimoto Y, Abematsu M, Falk A, et al. Treatment of a mouse model of spinal cord injury by transplantation of human induced pluripotent stem cell-derived long-term self-renewing neuroepithelial-like stem cells. *Stem Cells.* 2012;30(6):1163–1173.

85. Keirstead HS, Nistor G, Bernal G, et al. Human embryonic stem cell-derived oligodendrocyte progenitor cell transplants remyelinate and restore locomotion after spinal cord injury. *J Neurosci.* 2005;25(19):4694–4705.

86. Cigognini D, Silva D, Paloppi S, Gelain F. Evaluation of mechanical properties and therapeutic effect of injectable self-assembling hydrogels for spinal cord injury. *J Biomed Nanotechnol.* 2014;10(2):309–323.

87. Johnson PJ, Tatara A, McCreedy DA, Shiu A, Sakiyama-Elbert SE. Tissue-engineered fibrin scaffolds containing neural progenitors enhance functional recovery in a subacute model of SCI. *Soft Matter.* 2010;6(20):5127–5137.

88. Ide C, Kanekiyo K. Points regarding cell transplantation for the treatment of spinal cord injury. *Neural Regen Res.* 2016;11(7):1046–1049.

89. Feng SQ, Kong XH, Guo SF, et al. Treatment of spinal cord injury with co-grafts of genetically modified Schwann cells and fetal spinal cord cell suspension in the rat. *Neurotox Res.* 2005;7(1–2):169–177.

90. Takami T, Oudega M, Bates ML, Wood PM, Kleitman N, Bunge MB. Schwann cell but not olfactory ensheathing glia transplants improve hindlimb locomotor performance in the moderately contused adult rat thoracic spinal cord. *J Neurosci.* 2002;22(15):6670–6681.

91. Armati PJ, Mathey EK. An update on Schwann cell biology—immunomodulation, neural regulation and other surprises. *J Neurol Sci.* 2013;333(1–2):68–72.

92. Kanno H, Pearse DD, Ozawa H, Itoi E, Bunge MB. Schwann cell transplantation for spinal cord injury repair: its significant therapeutic potential and prospectus. *Rev Neurosci.* 2015;26(2):121–128.

93. Barnabe-Heider F, Goritz C, Sabelstrom H, et al. Origin of new glial cells in intact and injured adult spinal cord. *Cell Stem Cell.* 2010;7(4):470–482.

94. Horner PJ, Power AE, Kempermann G, et al. Proliferation and differentiation of progenitor cells throughout the intact adult rat spinal cord. *J Neurosci.* 2000;20(6):2218–2228.

95. Stenudd M, Sabelstrom H, Frisen J. Role of endogenous neural stem cells in spinal cord injury and repair. *JAMA Neurol.* 2015;72(2):235–237.

96. Sabelstrom H, Stenudd M, Frisen J. Neural stem cells in the adult spinal cord. *Exp Neurol.* 2014;260:44–49.

97. Barnabe-Heider F, Frisen J. Stem cells for spinal cord repair. *Cell Stem Cell.* 2008;3(1):16–24.

98. Ohori Y, Yamamoto S, Nagao M, et al. Growth factor treatment and genetic manipulation stimulate neurogenesis and oligodendrogenesis by endogenous neural progenitors in the injured adult spinal cord. *J Neurosci.* 2006;26(46):11948–11960.

99. Chen G, Wernig M, Berninger B, Nakafuku M, Parmar M, Zhang CL. In vivo reprogramming for brain and spinal cord repair. *eNeuro.* 2015;2(5).

100. Niu W, Zang T, Zou Y, et al. In vivo reprogramming of astrocytes to neuroblasts in the adult brain. *Nat Cell Biol.* 2013;15(10):1164–1175.

101. Mehta T, Feroz A, Thakkar U, Vanikar A, Shah V, Trivedi H. Subarachnoid placement of stem cells in neurological disorders. *Transplant Proc.* 2008;40(4):1145–1147.

102. Vaquero J, Zurita M, Rico MA, et al. An approach to personalized cell therapy in chronic complete paraplegia: the Puerta de Hierro phase I/II clinical trial. *Cytotherapy.* 2016;18(8):1025–1036.

103. Park HC, Shim YS, Ha Y, et al. Treatment of complete spinal cord injury patients by autologous bone marrow cell transplantation and administration of granulocyte-macrophage colony stimulating factor. *Tissue Eng.* 2005;11(5–6):913–922.

104. Dai G, Liu X, Zhang Z, Yang Z, Dai Y, Xu R. Transplantation of autologous bone marrow mesenchymal stem cells in the treatment of complete and chronic cervical spinal cord injury. *Brain Res.* 2013;1533:73–79.

105. Kumar AA, Kumar SR, Narayanan R, Arul K, Baskaran M. Autologous bone marrow derived mononuclear cell therapy for spinal cord injury: a phase I/II clinical safety and primary efficacy data. *Exp Clin Transplant.* 2009;7(4):241–248.

106. Oh SK, Choi KH, Yoo JY, Kim DY, Kim SJ, Jeon SR. A phase III clinical trial showing limited efficacy of autologous mesenchymal stem cell therapy for spinal cord injury. *Neurosurgery.* 2016;78(3):436–447; discussion 447.

107. Yoon SH, Shim YS, Park YH, et al. Complete spinal cord injury treatment using autologous bone marrow cell transplantation and bone marrow stimulation with granulocyte macrophage-colony stimulating factor: Phase I/II clinical trial. *Stem Cells.* 2007;25(8):2066–2073.

108. Shin JC, Kim KN, Yoo J, et al. Clinical trial of human fetal brain-derived neural stem/progenitor cell transplantation in patients with traumatic cervical spinal cord injury. *Neural Plast.* 2015;2015:630932.

109. Curtis E, Gabel BC, Marsala M, Ciacci JD. 172 A phase I, open-label, single-site, safety study of human spinal cord-derived neural stem cell transplantation for the treatment of chronic spinal cord injury. *Neurosurgery.* 2016;63(suppl 1):168–169.

110. Trounson A, McDonald C. Stem cell therapies in clinical trials: progress and challenges. *Cell Stem Cell.* 2015;17(1):11–22.

111. Curtis E, Martin JR, Gabel B, et al. A first-in-human, phase I study of neural stem cell transplantion for chronic spinal cord injury. *Cell Stem Cell.* 2018;22:941–950.

112. Deda H, Inci MC, Kurekci AE, et al. Treatment of chronic spinal cord injured patients with autologous bone marrow-derived hematopoietic stem cell transplantation: 1-year follow-up. *Cytotherapy.* 2008;10(6):565–574.

113. Bryukhovetskiy AS, Bryukhovetskiy IS. Effectiveness of repeated transplantations of hematopoietic stem cells in spinal cord injury. *World J Transplant.* 2015;5(3):110–128.

114. Zhu H, Poon W, Liu Y, et al. Phase I-II clinical trial assessing safety and efficacy of umbilical cord blood mononuclear cell transplant therapy of chronic complete spinal cord injury. *Cell Transplant.* 2016;25(11):1925–1943.

115. Zhu H, Poon W, Liu Y, et al. Phase III clinical trial assessing safety and efficacy of umbilical cord blood mononuclear cell transplant therapy of chronic complete spinal cord injury. *Cell Transplant.* 2016;25(11):1925–1943.

116. Priest CA, Manley NC, Denham J, Wirth ED 3rd, Lebkowski JS. Preclinical safety of human embryonic stem cell-derived oligodendrocyte progenitors supporting clinical trials in spinal cord injury. *Regen Med.* 2015;10(8):939–958.

117. Li JY, Christophersen NS, Hall V, Soulet D, Brundin P. Critical issues of clinical human embryonic stem cell therapy for brain repair. *Trends Neurosci.* 2008;31(3):146–153.

118. Eaton ML, Kwon BK, Scott CT. Money and morals: ending clinical trials for financial reasons. *Curr Top Behav Neurosci.* 2015;19:297–315.

119. Aghayan HR, Arjmand B, Yaghoubi M, Moradi-Lakeh M, Kashani H, Shokraneh F. Clinical outcome of autologous mononuclear cells transplantation for spinal cord injury: a systematic review and meta-analysis. *Med J Islam Repub Iran.* 2014;28:112.

120. Forostyak S, Jendelova P, Sykova E. The role of mesenchymal stromal cells in spinal cord injury, regenerative medicine and possible clinical applications. *Biochimie.* 2013;95(12):2257–2270.

121. Anderson AJ, Piltti KM, Hooshmand MJ, Nishi RA, Cummings BJ. Preclinical efficacy failure of human CNS-derived stem cells for use in the pathway study of cervical spinal cord injury. *Stem Cell Reports.* 2017;8(2):249–263.

122. Temple S, Studer L. Lessons learned from pioneering neural stem cell studies. *Stem Cell Reports.* 2017;8(2):191–193.

123. StemCells, Inc. (former management). Reaction from StemCells, Inc. to two papers in stem cell reports on the efficacy of human NSCs in Mouse Models of Alzheimer's disease and spinal cord injury. *Stem Cell Reports.* 2017;8(2)194–195.

124. Kadoya K, Lu P, Nguyen K, et al. Spinal cord reconstitution with homologous neural grafts enables robust corticospinal regeneration. *Nat Med.* 2016;22(5):479–487.

Section VII

Common Themes Between Traumatic Brain and Spinal Cord Injury

Therapeutic Hypothermia and Targeted Temperature Management in the Treatment of Traumatic Brain and Spinal Cord Injury

W. Dalton Dietrich and Helen M. Bramlett

36

Introduction

Neurotrauma is a worldwide problem that is caused by a range of primary and secondary injury mechanisms that can lead to a spectrum of acute and chronic neurological disorders.[1–3] Each year, more than 1.5 million people in the United States sustain some type of traumatic brain injury (TBI) leading to severe sensorimotor and cognitive problems. Recently, the high incidence of concussion in our civilian and military populations has also emphasized the potential detrimental effects of mild TBI (mTBI) that have been previously underappreciated.[4] Although lower numbers of new spinal cord injuries (SCI) occur each year in the United States (10,000–11,000), SCI commonly affects younger individuals, thereby producing dramatic effects on their quality of life for years to come.[5,6] In both types of neurotrauma, education and new safety approaches have been developed and initiated to help prevent injury by promoting new safety regulation and developing new technologies to protect the brain and spinal cord from direct trauma.

The pathophysiology of neurotrauma depends on various factors including injury severity and the type of primary insult, as well as on genetic and environmental factors that can modify primary and secondary injury conditions. Research efforts by investigators throughout the world have clarified the temporal profile of various injury mechanisms activated after TBI and SCI, including excitotoxicity, ionic imbalances, and free radical generation, as well as inflammatory cascades. Each of these injury cascades represents clinically important secondary injury mechanisms that are potential targets for therapeutic interventions. Individuals who undergo neurotrauma also commonly have multiorgan damage, which can complicate the treatment strategy as well as aggravate primary injury mechanisms. Together, this makes the successful treatment of neurotrauma an extremely challenging goal. Because of these factors as well as others, there is currently a lack of efficacious treatments that can be used in the early injury setting to treat either brain or spinal cord injury.[7–9] Although various drug therapies have been tested in many animal models, these encouraging findings have consistently failed when translated to large and costly multicenter clinical trials.[10] Indeed, positive results obtained in small phase I clinical trials using relatively small patient numbers have not been replicated when larger multicenter trials are conducted.[10] For example, recent multicenter trials that have tested the beneficial effects of progesterone or erythropoietin have failed to show benefits.[11–14] Thus, there is an urgent need to continue to develop novel treatment strategies that can be tested and translated to large patient populations to improve outcome and quality of life issues.

Therapeutic hypothermia has been studied as a potential neuroprotective strategy in many preclinical models of central nervous system injury as well as in the clinical arena.[15,16] In the area of SCI, profound levels of local hypothermia produced by cold solutions can be administered to the exposed spinal cord and used to reduce edema formation and protect tissues.[17] In the area of TBI, early studies provided additional information that profound hypothermia had the capacity in some patients to reduce intracranial pressure (ICP) and brain swelling and improve mortality and morbidity. However, many of these studies were difficult to replicate and the techniques that were available at the time to induce hypothermia were relatively crude and difficult to utilize.

Over the past several decades, many investigators have demonstrated the ability of small variations in temperature introduced at various periods following brain injury to significantly limit secondary injury mechanisms and improve functional outcomes.[18,19] Indeed, it has been suggested that hypothermia may be the most powerful cytoprotectant known in terms of protecting the brain from an ischemic insult. Current research has been expanded to better understand the cellular and molecular mechanism by which mild hypothermia protects against secondary injury processes as well as what critical levels of hypothermia are most protective in specific patient populations.[20,21] Thus, the therapeutic window for hypothermic protection and the duration of cooling, as well as the importance of initiating a slow rewarming phase, have been introduced into the scientific field. With the introduction of effective surface, intravascular, and more regional cooling technologies, more acute and robust cooling approaches are being tested clinically to help advance this important field of research. The general purpose of this chapter is to provide a review on the past, present, and future use of therapeutic hypothermia and targeted temperature management in preclinical and clinical models of brain and spinal cord injury. Although much has been accomplished regarding this important area of research, there remain many unanswered questions that need to be researched as we continue to advance this important field.

Spinal Cord Injury

In the 1950s, profound levels of hypothermia were utilized to protect the spinal cord from periods of cerebral ischemia and hypoxia during surgical procedures to repair blood vessels.[15] The success of these procedures ultimately led to investigators examining whether profound levels of hypothermia introduced to localized areas of the spinal cord would also be protective. Several studies in the 1960s, for example, reported that the administration of cold fluids including saline to the exposed injured spinal cord region during surgical repairs also produced variable degrees of spinal protection.[17] As a direct consequence of new positive studies in the area of brain injury, investigations were also initiated in several laboratories to test whether milder levels of systemic or focal hypothermia would also be protective in reproducible models of moderate and severe SCI.[22–27]

Preclinical Hypothermia Studies

The pathophysiology of traumatic SCI is complicated and involves the activation of multiple injury cascades that are similar to processes activated after ischemic stroke or TBI. Because therapeutic hypothermia was known to target multiple pathomechanisms including glutamate toxicity, free radical generation, apoptosis, and inflammatory cascades, it was the hypothesis that mild systemic hypothermia could be beneficial in models of traumatic SCI. In 2000, the first rodent studies of moderate to severe thoracic SCI were conducted to determine whether mild hypothermia (33°C) introduced early after trauma would be beneficial in terms of reducing contusion volume and improving locomotor function.[25,26] In the initial studies, a thoracic (T10) contusive SCI was produced and systemic hypothermia was introduced as early as 30 minutes after injury. Over the next several weeks, locomotor activity was quantitatively assessed using the open locomotor score (Basso, Beattie, Bresnahan) (BBB). Compared to normothermic (37°C) animals, posttraumatic hypothermia significantly improved locomotor function up to 6 weeks after SCI. In addition, histopathological analysis demonstrated that posttraumatic hypothermia significantly reduced overall contusion volume, preserving both gray and white matter structures. Similar findings were reported in other laboratories using different or similar models of SCI with variable cooling protocols and outcome measures including histopathological, immunocytochemical, and electrophysiological.[28–30] In one preclinical study, for example, Grulova and colleagues[31] tested the beneficial effects of hypothermia in a standardized model of SCI compression. Therapeutic hypothermia produced a beneficial effect on urinary bladder activity and on locomotor function recovery while increasing the number of NeuN-positive neurons in the dorsal and ventral horns. Also, in a study by Ok and colleagues,[32] both epidural and systemic hypothermia improved locomotor scores as compared to the normothermic group at 6 weeks.

SCI is a very heterogeneous clinical problem, and a large number of patients sustain cervical injuries that lead to severe deficits affecting both upper and lower extremities. To determine whether therapeutic hypothermia would be protective following severe cervical SCI, animal studies were initiated that utilized a newly developed cervical SCI model that reproducibly produced a consistent contusive injury at high cervical levels and allowed for long-term survival and behavioral testing. In one study, therapeutic hypothermia introduced 30 minutes after moderate cervical SCI was shown to improve forelimb grasping and strength.[33] Also, compared to normothermia, posttraumatic hypothermia reduced contusion volumes and protected the cervical motor neuron pool. The behavioral improvements with hypothermia in this cervical model were clinically relevant since upper extremity use after cervical SCI is considered an important quality of life issue. In summary, the early induction of systemic hypothermia was highly beneficial following thoracic as well as cervical SCI, leading to improvements in chronic functional outcomes. Importantly, other investigations in the field of SCI also showed that hypothermia provided protection after SCI when moderate levels of local hypothermia were introduced.[15]

One important challenge in the SCI field has been the lack of successful replication of positive findings.[34] In this regard, several replication studies of published data for pharmacological treatments reported to be protective failed. In research on SCI and other neurological conditions, it is considered important to successfully replicate findings by an independent investigator laboratory before such therapy is considered for clinical translation. In reference to the present discussion, the beneficial effects of therapeutic hypothermia after SCI needs to also be replicated. In 2013, Batchelor and colleagues[28] conducted a systematic review and meta-analysis of the therapeutic hypothermia literature in SCI. Results showed that both systemic as well as regional hypothermia significantly improved behavioral outcomes compared to normothermia. Importantly, a number of factors were reported to influence the efficacy of hypothermia including depth and duration of hypothermia, animal species, and neural behavioral assessment strategies. In a more recent study, the systematic review of the hypothermia literature also concluded that although variability exists in the literature, therapeutic hypothermia most likely confers neuroprotection after SCI by diminishing destructive secondary cascades.[35] It was also concluded that because there are currently no pharmacologic interventions to prevent secondary mechanisms of injury after SCI, clinical studies were required to test safety and efficacy.[36]

Clinical SCI

Based on supportive experimental studies showing the beneficial effects of systemic hypothermia in multiple laboratories, clinical studies have been initiated in select patient populations.[37,38] Over the past decade, our own SCI clinical group has performed a retrospective analysis of a subgroup of patients with acute, complete cervical SCI using a moderate intravascular hypothermia protocol.[39,40] In these initial clinical studies, neurological examination was first conducted in the absence of sedative muscle relaxants or head injury and classified according to American Spinal Injury Association (ASIA) score. In patients who did not receive methylprednisolone, an intravascular cooling catheter was inserted into the femoral vein using a sterile technique. Patients were cooled to target temperature (33°C) at a maximum rate of 0.5°C per hour. The goal of these studies was to maintain target temperature for 48 hours followed by a slow, controlled rewarming phase occurring at 1°C per 8 hours. This rewarming phase took an average of 24–32 hours to achieve a core temperature of 37°C. The specific exclusion criteria were age greater than 65 years, hypothermia on admission (temperature >38.5°C), severe multisystem injury, active bleeding, pregnancy, coagulopathy, thrombocytopenia, or known cardiac history.

In this first series, a total of 14 patients with acute SCI were studied.[40] All patients received cervical surgery for either decompression and/or stabilization as part of their treatment. Catheter insertion was 7.40 +/− 0.7 hours, and target temperature was achieved within 3 hours of cooling. Importantly, there were no apparent adverse effects of temperature modification related to coagulation or intraoperative hemostasis or the development of postoperative hematomas. At 6 months after the injury, six patients were shown to convert from ASIA grade A to another grade, including three patients who converted to ASIA B, two to ASIA C, and one to ASIA D. Importantly, no patient appeared to worsen as a result of hypothermia, such as descending in neurological level.

This series of single institutional studies was important because it demonstrated that the application of the intravascular cooling catheter could be safely used to achieve a reduced core target temperature, including a controlled rewarming phase. Subsequent studies have been conducted in which focal cooling strategies have also been utilized in severe spinal cord injured patients. These studies have also reported some degree of efficacy.[15,41] In the future, a larger prospective randomized multicenter trial will be required to determine the potential benefits in regard to neuroprotection recovery from SCI. In this regard, a recent multicenter trial has been funded by the Department of Defense (Levi, PI) to test the efficacy of therapeutic hypothermia in a large number of spinal cord injured subjects. For this study, ASIA A, B, and C patients will be targeted for this experimental protocol.

Traumatic Brain Injury

Preclinical Hypothermia Studies

In the early 1990s, several laboratories initiated investigations to clarify the beneficial effects of mild-to-moderate reductions in brain temperature in experimental models of TBI.[42–44] Clifton and colleagues[44] first reported that pre- and posttraumatic hypothermia significantly improved beam walking using a rat model of moderate fluid percussion injury (FPI). Compared to normothermia, improvements in mortality rates and the attenuation of deficits in beam balance and body weight loss were seen with hypothermia reduced to 30°C. These results were replicated by Lyeth and colleagues,[45] who again evaluated the beneficial effects of hypothermia (30°C) on behavioral outcome compared to normothermic treatment. In 1994, Dietrich and colleagues[43] first reported that posttraumatic hypothermia (30°C) initiated early after fluid percussion injury (FPI) significantly reduced overall contusion volume and improved neuronal survival in cortical areas overlaying the evolving contusion. Importantly, studies by Bramlett and colleagues reported that early cooling after FPI also reduced sensorimotor deficits and improved cognitive deficits using the Morris water maze.[42] These results were particularly important since cognitive deficits are an important consequence of moderate and severe TBI in patients.

Diffused axonal injury (DAI) is a common consequence of TBI and believed to participate in the functional consequences of TBI.[46,47] In several studies, investigators evaluated whether posttraumatic hypothermia would alter the degree of axonal pathology using standard markers. For example, using β-amyloid precursor protein (β-APP) immunocytochemistry to assess damaged axons, posttraumatic hypothermia was shown to reduce the overall frequency of damaged axonal profiles in specific white matter tracts compared to normothermic conditions.[48] Other studies have also demonstrated that hypothermia plus various pharmacological agents also provides variable degrees of axonal protection. In contrast, other studies have not shown that posttraumatic hypothermia benefits axonal pathology, suggesting that specific results may vary according to injury models and length of survival.[46]

To determine the therapeutic window for posttraumatic hypothermia, Markgraf and colleagues evaluated the beneficial effects of hypothermia when the cooling was initiated at different periods after the traumatic insult.[49] That study showed that if hypothermia (3 hours at 30°C) was initiated 60 minutes but not 90 minutes after TBI, beneficial effects were observed. These results indicated that hypothermia may have a clinically relevant therapeutic window that could be initiated in the clinic.

An important phase of therapeutic hypothermia treatment is the rewarming phase. Following a prolonged period of induced hypothermia, researchers identified the importance of the rewarming phase when rapid rewarming was investigated.[47] Several laboratories determined that relatively controlled, slow rewarming is necessary to provide beneficial effects. For example, in a study where axonal pathology was targeted, Suehiro and Povlishock[50] reported an augmentation of traumatically induced axonal pathology using a rapid post-hypothermic rewarming protocol. However, if posttraumatic hypothermia was followed by a slow rewarming protocol, protection of axons was demonstrated. In the clinical situation, severe TBI is commonly accompanied by multiorgan damage. To replicate this clinical condition, therapeutic hypothermia was also tested in a complicated model of TBI associated with a secondary hypoxic insult. Matsushita and colleagues (2001) showed that the hypothermia period combined with a slow rewarming protocol was neuroprotective by reducing contusion volumes when the posttraumatic hypothermia period was followed by slow but not rapid rewarming.[51] Controlled rewarming periods are now a common practice in clinical situations where therapeutic hypothermia is used. Taken together, these studies show that early and prolonged systemic hypothermia followed by a slow rewarming phase is required to produce chronic benefits in outcomes.

Clinical TBI

In the 1960s, several groups investigated profound levels of hypothermia with severe TBI with beneficial but variable results.[16] However, when new pharmacological agents appeared in the clinical scene, including barbiturates and later calcium channel blockers and N-methyl-d-aspartate (NMDA) antagonists, testing of hypothermia was mostly discontinued for treatment of severe TBI. However, based on newer preclinical data showing that relatively mild levels of hypothermia were protective in ischemic and TBI models, several groups initiated clinical studies based on these encouraging findings. Marion and colleagues first reported that 62% of patients who underwent hypothermic treatment demonstrated good outcomes 12 months after injury.[52] In 2000, Jiang and colleagues[53] showed that an extensive period of mild hypothermia (3–14 days) strikingly reduced ICP and inhibited hyperglycemia. Recent studies have also reported that the duration of cooling as well as the period of initiation after the injury are important factors in determining whether successful outcomes are seen based on these encouraging single-center studies.[54]

Clifton and colleagues[55,56] next initiated a large multicenter trial (the National Acute Brain injury Study: Hypothermia, NABISH) targeting severely injured TBI patients. In contrast to several single-center studies, mortality rates were reported not to differ between the hypothermic and normothermic groups, and no beneficial effects on neurological outcomes were reported. Potential limitations of those original multicenter trials were identified and discussed, including inconsistencies in patient care between recruitment sites and delays in initiating hypothermic treatment.[56–58] More recently, several studies have reevaluated the effects of systemic hypothermia in severe TBI patients (Polderman 2004.[59–62] The European study of therapeutic hypothermia (32–35°C) trial, an international multicenter randomized control trial, examined the effects of titrated therapeutic hypothermia on ICP and neuronal outcome.[63,64] This completed study reported that while hypothermia reduced ICP, the treatment did not improve long-term outcome. Reasons for the lack of translation from the animal models to the clinic in this situation may be due to several factors, including when the hypothermia was initiated after the injury as well as duration of hypothermia and rewarming protocols. Thus, it might not be too surprising that starting hypothermia treatments many hours or days after a severe injury may limit its beneficial effects.

It is well known that TBI produces a highly heterogeneous patient population, and therefore more precision or specialized treatments for select patient populations may be needed. One explanation of recent failures of hypothermia trials is that the therapeutic treatment needs to be initiated early after the injury and maintained for an extensive duration. Such an approach would have the advantage of targeting both acute as well as more progressive neuronal injury cascades, including later elevations in ICP that commonly occur in patients after severe TBI. The fact that, in the Eurotherm 32–35 TBI trial, hypothermia was shown to normalize ICP but not improve neurological outcomes indicates that, in some patients, ICP elevations may not be the dominant or only injury mechanisms responsible for long-term deficits.[65] Indeed, based on a wealth of preclinical data, it is clear that the early initiation of hypothermia may be needed to target secondary injury consequences of TBI which can be active hours to days after injury. In this regard, the Prophylactic Hypothermia Trial to Lessen Brain Injury (POLAR) study may provide valuable data to support this hypothesis.[11] In addition, the Long-Term Mild Hypothermia (LTH-1) for severe TBI trial to test whether hypothermia for 5 days is beneficial is currently ongoing.[59]

As previously noted, patient heterogeneity may be another factor that could impact the ability of various therapeutic interventions to be protective. Recent data have indicated that therapeutic hypothermia may be more protective only in select patient populations.[66] Postanalysis of the NABISH hypothermia multicenter trials indicated beneficial effects of therapeutic hypothermia in patients undergoing surgical decompression surgery for focal insults where early cooling was initiated. To test the hypothesis that early cooling may be most protective in animal models of decompression surgery, Yokobori and colleagues (2015) tested the benefits of systemic hypothermia for the first time in an animal model of subdural hematoma associated with decompression.[67] This group reported that mild hypothermia introduced immediately prior to decompression surgery produced the best protection and reduced biomarker indicators of tissue damage. These findings indicate that therapeutic approaches may be more appropriate for selective types of severe TBI and has led to the initiation of the Hypothermia for Patients Requiring Evacuation of Subdural Hematoma (HOPES) trial. This trial is currently being conducted in sites within the United States, Japan, and China. Recent systematic reviews regarding the benefits of therapeutic hypothermia for adult TBI are supportive.[68–71]

Detrimental Consequences of Hyperthermia

Posttraumatic Hyperthermia

Clinical studies have shown that a large percentage of patients who sustain different types of brain or spinal cord injuries demonstrate periods of hyperthermia.[72–75] These abnormal elevations in temperature can result from infection as well as from damage to thermoregulatory centers in the brain. Importantly, recent clinical findings have shown that periods of hyperthermia may actually worsen outcomes due to temperature-dependent effects on secondary injury mechanisms. In experimental models of cerebral ischemia and trauma, periods of post-injury hyperthermia significantly worsen outcomes and aggravate injury processes including glutamate neurotoxicity, apoptosis, free radical generation, and inflammation.[76,77]

Indeed, targeted temperature management strategies that prevent these periods of reactive hyperthermia are now routinely used in intensive care units.[78,79] Experimentally, investigations have shown that artificially increasing brain temperature at various periods after nervous system injury significantly aggravates histopathological damage that can include increasing contusion volumes and aggravating DAI and blood–brain barrier (BBB) function. Recent clinical studies have emphasized the detrimental consequences of periods of hyperthermia and, in some cases, concluded that inducing normothermia or ultra-mild hypothermia may be beneficial to patients.[78]

Importance of Hyperthermia in Concussion or Mild TBI

To date, the importance of brain temperature has been extensively studied only in experimental and clinical conditions of moderate to severe TBI. However, another major clinical problem is the increasing incidence of mild TBI or concussion due to sports-related events and injuries sustained by military personnel.[80–82] Recent data have for the first time also emphasized the importance of small variations in brain temperature in the clinical condition of concussion.[83,84,85] These studies are important because many athletes and military personnel who undergo single or repetitive concussions may have elevated brain temperatures at the time of injury due to elevated ambient temperatures and high levels of activity. In this regard, previous clinical studies have reported that athletes who exercise under different ambient temperatures or degrees of humidity can show significant elevations in core temperatures that reach over 39°C.[86–88]

In this regard, preclinical data show that if brain temperature is artificially elevated to 39°C at the time of a mild TBI or concussion, histopathological damage is significantly aggravated compared to normothermic conditions (37°C). In this condition, raising brain temperature 15 minutes prior to the mild TBI aggravates damage to gray and white matter structures. In terms of functional outcomes, other studies have also reported that hyperthermic mild TBI leads to an appearance of chronic cognitive deficits that are not seen under normothermic conditions. Interestingly, if brain temperature is normalized soon after the hyperthermic mild TBI insult, these cognitive deficits are significantly reduced. This would suggest that one factor that may affect the long-term consequences of mild TBI includes variations in brain temperature at the time of the injury, including small elevations in temperature that are expected to aggravate outcome. Current studies are evaluating the beneficial effects of normalizing temperature in athletes using new technologies that can selectively normalize mildly elevated temperatures using noninvasive approaches.

Conclusion

Over the past three decades, many laboratories and centers throughout the world have initiated studies testing the beneficial effects of hypothermia and targeted temperature management in models of brain and spinal cord injury. In the preclinical setting, therapeutic hypothermia produces beneficial effects on a wide spectrum of behavioral tasks as well as on structural outcomes. Indeed, therapeutic hypothermia continues to be one of the most powerful neuroprotective strategies known in the field of central nervous system injury. Nevertheless, research is needed to continue to clarify factors that may be important to the beneficial effects of therapeutic hypothermia, including how best to deliver this powerful therapy. Optimal levels of hypothermic therapy may vary from patient to patient based on injury severity and other variables now known to be present in neurotrauma. The heterogeneity of patient populations in both spinal cord and brain injury represents a major challenge in terms of determining which patients may best benefit from hypothermic therapy.

In parallel with these investigations, understanding the detrimental effects of posttraumatic hyperthermia on the pathophysiology of TBI and SCI is an active area of research. Recent studies have emphasized the beneficial effects of inhibiting periods of reactive hyperthermia after injury in terms of improving patient outcomes. It is now clear that targeted temperature management is a critical factor in the treatment of many intensive care neurological patients that commonly experience abnormal elevations in temperature. It appears reasonable that while some patients may benefit from maintaining normothermic levels and inhibiting periods of hyperthermia, others may require different levels of induced hypothermia to limit secondary injury mechanisms. Ongoing research in the area of biomarker technology will hopefully allow treating clinicians to develop more precisely targeted therapeutic interventions, such as temperature modifications, to reduce secondary injury mechanisms that can lead to long-term deficits.[67,89,90]

Recent studies have also shown that a combination of interventions including therapeutic hypothermia and pharmacological treatments may produce additive or synergistic effects. An interesting area of research therefore includes investigating what drugs should be added to therapeutic hypothermia or targeted temperature management protocols that could promote better outcomes. Various drug therapies have been reported to induce hypothermia.[91] Thus, an existing area of research continues to be the discovery and clarification of drug-induced hypothermia as a strategy to improve functional outcomes.

In addition to protection, several research groups are now concentrating on how best to repair the nervous system after damage with cell therapies or other regenerative strategies. Recent studies in this regard have emphasized that targeted temperature management may be beneficial to the injured microenvironment by promoting reparative conditions. In one study, posttraumatic hypothermia after TBI, for example, enhanced hippocampal neurogenesis that was associated with improved cognitive function.[92] Strategies that incorporate hypothermia and newly emerging compounds that enhance repair may be another exciting direction for future experimentation and translation to the clinic. In this regard, cellular therapies are being tested in patients with TBI and SCI. It will be interesting in the future to combine targeted temperature strategies with cell transplantation to determine if together they provide better outcomes. As the field continues to conduct preclinical and clinical studies on hypothermia research, it will be even more important to promote effective communication among different researchers to ensure that lessons learned are freely shared. This practice will certainly help improve the continued advancement of this exciting research area. Only through such communication among researchers and treating physicians will improved outcomes be demonstrated in our patients.

Acknowledgments

We thank Erika Suazo for excellent editorial support. The work was partially supported by NINDS R01 042133.

References

1. Bramlett HM, Dietrich WD. Long-term consequences of traumatic brain injury: Current status of potential mechanisms of injury and neurological outcomes. *J Neurotrauma*. 2015;32(23):1834–1848.

2. Corrigan JD, Selassie AW, Orman JA. The epidemiology of traumatic brain injury. *J Head Trauma Rehabil*. 2010;25:72–80.

3. Langlois JA, Rutland-Brown W, Wald MM. The epidemiology and impact of traumatic brain injury: a brief overview. *J Head Trauma Rehabil*. 2006;21:375–378.

4. Dettwiler A, Murugavel M, Putukian M, et al. Persistent differences in patterns of brain activation after sports-related concussion: a longitudinal functional magnetic resonance imaging study. *J Neurotrauma*. 2014;31:180–188.

5. National Spinal Cord Injury Statistical Center. *Spinal Cord Injury Facts and Figures at a Glance*. Birmingham, AL: University of Alabama; 2010.

6. Tator CH. Update on the pathophysiology and pathology of acute spinal cord injury. *Brain Pathol*. 1995;5:407–413.

7. Radosevich JJ, Patanwala AE, Erstad BL. Emerging pharmacological agents to improve survival from traumatic brain injury. *Brain Inj*. 2013;27:1492–1499.

8. Anderson D, Hall E. Pathophysiology of spinal cord trauma. *Ann Emerg Med*. 1993;22:987–992.

9. Cortez R, Levi AD. Acute spinal cord injury. *Curr Treat Options Neurol*. 2007;9:115–125.

10. Geisler FH, Coleman WP, Grieco G, et al. The Sygen multicenter acute spinal cord injury study. *Spine*. 2001;26:S87–S98.

11. Nichol A, Gantner D, Presneill J, et al. Protocol for a multicentre randomised controlled trial of early and sustained prophylactic hypothermia in the management of traumatic brain injury. *Crit Care Resusc*. 2015;17:92–100.

12. Skolnick BE, Maas AI, Narayan RK, et al. A clinical trial of progesterone for severe traumatic brain injury. *N Engl J Med*. 2014;371:2467–2476.

13. Wright DW, Yeatts SD, Silbergleit R., et al. Very early administration of progesterone for acute traumatic brain injury. *N Engl J Med*. 2014;371:2457–2466.

14. Robertson CS, Hannay HJ, Yamal JM, et al. Effect of erythropoietin and transfusion threshold on neurological recovery after traumatic brain injury: a randomized clinical trial. *JAMA*. 2014;312:36–47.

15. Dietrich WD, Levi AD, Wang M, Green BA. Hypothermic treatment for acute spinal cord injury. *Neurotherapeutics*. 2011;8(2):229–239.

16. Dietrich WD, Bramlett HM. The evidence for hypothermia as a neuroprotectant in traumatic brain injury. *Neurotherapeutics*. 2010;7:43–50.

17. Albin MS, White RJ, Acosta-Rua G, Yashon D. Study of functional recovery produced by delayed localized cooling of spinal cord injury in primates. *J Neurosurg*. 1968;29:113–120.

18. Busto R, Dietrich WD, Globus MY, Valdes I, Scheinberg P, Ginsberg MD. Small differences in intraischemic brain temperature critically determine the extent of ischemic neuronal injury. *J Cereb Blood Flow Metab*. 1987;7:729–738.

19. Yokobori S, Frantzen J, Bullock R, et al. The use of hypothermia therapy in traumatic is-chemic/reperfusional brain injury: review of the literatures. *Ther Hypothermia Temp Manag.* 2011;1:185–192.

20. Karnatovskaia LV, Wartenberg KE, Freeman WD. Therapeutic hypothermia for neuroprotection: history, mechanisms, risks, and clinical applications. *Neurohospitalist.* 2014;4:153–163.

21. Silasi G, Colbourne F. Therapeutic hypothermia influences cell genesis and survival in the rat hippocampus following global ischemia. *J Cereb Blood Flow Metab.* 2011;31:1725–1735.

22. Dietrich WD. Therapeutic hypothermia for spinal cord injury. *Crit Care Med.* 2009;27:S238–S242.

23. Kwon BK, Mann C, Sohn HM, et al.; NASS Section on Biologics. Hypothermia for spinal cord injury. Spine J. 2008;8(6):859–874.

24. Martinez-Arizala A, Green BA. Hypothermia in spinal cord injury. *J Neurotrauma.* 1992;9(suppl 2):S497–S505.

25. Lo TP Jr, Cho KS, Garg MS, et al. Systemic hypothermia improves histological and functional outcome after cervical spinal cord contusion in rats. *J Comp Neurol.* 2009;514(5):433–448.

26. Yu CG, Jimenez O, Marcillo AE, et al. Beneficial effects of modest systemic hypothermia on locomotor function and histopathological damage following contusion-induced spinal cord injury in rats. *J Neurosurg.* 2000;93:85–93.

27. Westergren H, Holtz A, Farooque M, Yu WR, Olsson Y. Systemic hypothermia after spinal cord compression injury in the rat: does recorded temperature in accessible organs reflect the intramedullary temperature in the spinal cord? *J Neurotrauma.* 1998;15:943–954.

28. Batchelor PE, Skeers P, Antonic A, et al. Systematic review and meta-analysis of therapeutic hypothermia in animal models of spinal cord injury. *PLoS One.* 2013;8(8):e71317.

29. Yu WR, Westergren H, Farooque M, Holtz A, Olsson Y. Systemic hypothermia following com-pression injury of the rat spinal cord: reduction of plasma protein extravasation demonstrated by immunohistochemistry. *Acta Neuropathol.* 1999;98:15–21.

30. Westergren H, Yu WR, Farooque M, Holtz A, Olsson Y. Systemic hypothermia following spinal cord compression injury in the rat: axonal changes studied by beta-APP, ubiquitin, and PGP 9.5 immunohistochemistry. *Spinal Cord.* 1999;37:696–704.

31. Grulova I, Slovinska L, Nagyova M, Cizek M, Cizkova D. The effect of hypothermia on sensory-motor function and tissue sparing after spinal cord injury. *Spine J.* 201313(12):1881–1891.

32. Ok JH, Kim YH, Ha KY. Neuroprotective effects of hypothermia after spinal cord injury in rats: comparative study between epidural hypothermia and systemic hypothermia. *Spine* (Phila Pa 1976). 2012;37(25):E1551–1559.

33. Yu CG, Jagid J, Ruenes G, Dietrich WD, Marcillo AE, Yezierski RP. Detrimental effects of systemic hyperthermia on locomotor function and histopathological outcome after traumatic spinal cord injury in the rat. *Neurosurgery.* 2001;49(152-8):158–159.

34. Steward O, Popovich PG, Dietrich WD, Kleitman N. Replication and reproducibility in spinal cord injury research. *Exp Neurol.* 2012;233(2):597–605.

35. Alkabie S, Boileau AJ. The role of therapeutic hypothermia after traumatic spinal cord injury a systematic review. *World Neurosurg.* 2016;86:432–449.

36. Resnick D, Kaiser M, Fehlings M, McCormick P. Hypothermia and human spinal cord in-jury: position statement and evidence based recommendations. AANS/CNS Joint Section on Disorders of the Spine and the AANS/CNS Joint Section on Trauma. http://www.spinesection.org/hypothermia.php. Accessed July 7, 2018.

37. Ahmad FU, Wang MY, Levi AD. Hypothermia for acute spinal cord injury: a review. *World Neurosurg.* 2014;82(1-2):207–214.

38. Cappuccino A, Bisson LJ, Carpenter B, Marzo J, Dietrich WD, Cappuccino H. The use of systemic hypothermia for the treatment of an acute cervical spinal cord injury in a professional football player. *Spine.* 2010;35:E57–E62.

39. Levi AD, Casella G, Green BA, et al. Clinical outcomes using modest intravascular hypothermia after acute cervical spinal cord injury. *Neurosurgery.* 2010;66:670–677.

40. Levi AD, Green BA, Wang MY, et al. Spinal cord injury and modest hypothermia. *J Neurotrauma.* 2009;26(3):407–415.

41. Dimar JR 2nd, Shields CB, Zhang YP, Burke DA, Raque GH, Glassman SD. The role of directly applied hypothermia in spinal cord injury. *Spine.* 2000;25:2294–2302.

42. Bramlett HM, Green EJ, Dietrich WD, Busto R, Globus MY, Ginsberg MD. Posttraumatic brain hypothermia provides protection from sensorimotor and cognitive behavioral deficits. *J Neurotrauma.* 1995;12:289–298.

43. Dietrich, WD, Alonso, O., Busto, R., Globus, MY, Ginsberg, MD Post-traumatic brain hypothermia reduces histopathological damage following concussive brain injury in the rat. *Acta Neuropathol.* 1994;87:250–258.

44. Clifton GL, Jiang JY, Lyeth BG, Jenkins LW, Hamm RJ, Hayes RL. Marked protection by moderate hypothermia after experimental traumatic brain injury. *J Cereb Blood Flow Metab.* 1991;11:114–121.

45. Lyeth BG, Jianj JY, Liu S. Behavioral protection by moderate hypothermia initiated after experimental traumatic brain injury. *J Neurotrauma.* 1993;10:57–64.

46. Bramlett, HM, Dietrich, WD The effects of posttraumatic hypothermia on diffuse axonal injury following parasaggital fluid percussion brain injury in rats. *Ther Hypothermia Temp Manag.* 2012;2:14–23.

47. Povlishock, JT, Wei, EP Posthypothermic rewarming considerations following traumatic brain injury. *J Neurotrauma.* 2009;26:333–340.

48. Ma M, Matthews BT, Lampe JW, Meaney DF, Shofer FS, Neumar RW. Immediate short-duration hypothermia provides long-term protection in an in vivo model of traumatic axonal injury. *Exp Neurol.* 2009;215:119–127.

49. Markgraf, CG, Clifton, GL, Moody, MR Treatment window for hypothermia in brain injury. *J Neurosurg.* 2001;95:979–983.

50. Suehiro E, Povlishock JT. Exacerbation of traumatically induced axonal injury by rapid posthypothermic rewarmig and attenuation of axonal change by cyclosporin A. *J Neurosurg.* 2001;94:493–498.

51. Matsushita Y, Bramlett HM, Alonso O, Dietrich WD. Posttraumatic hypothermia is neuroprotective in a model of traumatic brain injury complicated by a secondary hypoxic insult. *Crit Care Med.* 2001;29:2060–2066.

52. Marion DW, Penrod LE, Kelsey SF, et al. Treatment of traumatic brain injury with moderate hypothermia. *N Engl J Med.* 1997;336:540–546.

53. Jiang J, Yu M, Zhu C. Effect of long-term mild hypothermia therapy in patients with severe traumatic brain injury: 1-year follow-up review of 87 cases. *J Neurosurg.* 2000;93:546–549.

54. Shiozaki T, Nakajima Y, Taneda M, et al. Efficacy of moderate hypothermia in patients with severe head injury and intracranial hypertension refractory to mild hypothermia. *J Neurosurg.* 2003;99:47–51.

55. Clifton GL, Allen S, Barrodale P, et al. A phase II study of moderate hypothermia in severe brain injury. *J Neurotrauma*. 1993;10:263–271

56. Clifton GL, Choi SC, Miller ER, et al. Intercenter variance in clinical trials of head trauma–experience of the National Acute Brain Injury Study: Hypothermia. *J Neurosurg*. 2001a;95:751–755.

57. Clifton GL, Miller ER, Choi SC, et al. Lack of effect of induction of hypothermia after acute brain injury. *N Engl J Med*. 2001b;344:556–563.

58. Clifton GL, Valadka A, Zygun D, et al. Very early hypothermia induction in patients with severe brain injury (the National Acute Brain Injury Study: Hypothermia II): a randomised trial. *Lancet Neurol*. 2001;10:131–139.

59. Lei J, Gao G, Mao Q, et al. Rationale, methodology, and implementation of a nationwide multicenter randomized controlled trial of long-term mild hypothermia for severe traumatic brain injury (the LTH-1 trial). *Contemp Clin Trials* 2015;40:9–14.

60. Nichol A, Gantner D, Presneill J, et al. Protocol for a multicentre randomised controlled trial of early and sustained prophylactic hypothermia in the management of traumatic brain injury. *Crit Care Resusc*. 2015;17:92–100.

61. Polderman KH, Tjong Tjin Joe R, Peerdeman SM, Vandertop WP, Girbes AR. Effects of therapeutic hypothermia on intracranial pressure and outcome in patients with severe head injury. *Intensive Care Med*. 2002;28:1563–1573.

62. Polderman KH. Application of therapeutic hypothermia in the ICU: opportunities and pitfalls of a promising treatment modality. Part 1: Indications and evidence. *Intensive Care Med*. 2004;30:556–575.

63. Andrews PJ, Sinclair HL, Rodriguez A, et al. Eurotherm3235 Trial Collaborators. Hypothermia for intracranial hypertension after traumatic brain injury. *N Eng J Med*. 2015;374:2403–2412.

64. Flynn LM, Rhodes J, Andrews PJ. Therapeutic hypothermia reduces intracranial pressure and partial brain oxygen tension in patients with severe traumatic brain injury: preliminary data from the Eurotherm3235 Trial. *Ther. Hypothermia Temp Manag*. 2015;5:143–151.

65. Robertson CS, Ropper AH. Getting warmer on critical care for head injury. *N Engl J Med*. 2015;373:2469–2470.

66. Clifton GL, Valadka A, Zygun D, et al. Very early hypothermia induction in patients with severe brain injury (the National Acute Brain Injury Study: Hypothermia II): a randomized trial. *Lancet Neurol*. 2011;10:131–139.

67. Yokobori S, Zhang Z, Moghieb A, et al. Acute diagnostic biomarkers for spinal cord injury: review of the literature and preliminary research report. *World Neurosurg*. 2015;83(5):867–878.

68. Crossley S, Reid J, McLatchie R, et al. A systematic review of therapeutic hypothermia for adult patients following traumatic brain injury. *Crit Care*. 2014;18(2):R75.

69. Li P, Yang C. Moderate hypothermia treatment in adult patients with severe traumatic brain injury: a meta-analysis. *Brain Inj*. 2014;28(8):1036–1041.

70. Dunkley S, McLeod A. Therapeutic hypothermia in patients following traumatic brain injury: a systematic review. *Nurs Crit Care*. 2016;22:150–160.

71. Crompton EM, Lubomirova I, Cotlarciuc I, Han TS, Sharma SD, Sharma P. Meta-analysis of therapeutic hypothermia for traumatic brain injury in adult and pediatric patients. *Crit Care Med*. 2016;45:575–583.

72. Diringer MN; Neurocritical Care Fever Reduction Trial Group. Treatment of fever in the neurologic intensive care unit with a catheter-based heat exchange system. *Crit Care Med*. 2004;32:559–564.

73. Gaither JB, Galson S, Curry M, et al. Environmental hyperthermia in prehospital patients with major traumatic brain injury. *J Emerg Med*. 2015;49:375–381.

74. Kilpatrick MM, Lowry DW, Firlik AD, Yonas H, Marion DW. Hyperthermia in the neurosurgical intensive care unit. *Neurosurgery*. 2000;47 (850-5):855–856.

75. Bao L, Chen D, Ding L, Ling W, Xu F. Fever burden is an independent predictor for prognosis of traumatic brain injury. *PLoS One*. 2014;9(3):e90956.

76. Dietrich WD, Bramlett HM. Hyperthermia and central nervous system injury. *Prog Brain Res*. 2007;162:201–217.

77. Dietrich WD, Alonso O, Halley M, Busto R. Delayed posttraumatic brain hyperthermia worsens outcome after fluid percussion brain injury: a light and electron microscopic study in rats. *Neurosurgery*. 1996;38:533–541; discussion 541.

78. Hifumi T, Kuroda Y, Kawakita K, et al. Fever control management is preferable to mild therapeutic hypothermia in traumatic brain injury patients with abbreviated injury scale 3-4: a multi-center, randomized controlled trial. *J Neurotrauma*. 2016;33(11):1047–1053.

79. Maekawa T, Yamashita S, Nagao S, Hayashi N, Ohashi Y; Brain-Hypothermia Study Group. Prolonged mild therapeutic hypothermia versus fever control with tight hemodynamic monitoring and slow rewarming in patients with severe traumatic brain injury: a randomized controlled trial. *J Neurotrauma*. 2015;32(7):422–429.

80. Chen JK, Johnston KM, Frey S, Petrides M, Worsley K, Ptito A. Functional abnormalities in symptomatic concussed athletes: an fMRI study. *Neuroimage*. 2004;22:68–82.

81. Collins MW, Grindel SH, Lovell MR, et al. Relationship between concussion and neuropsychological performance in college football players. *JAMA*. 1999;282:964–970.

82. De Beaumont L, Henry LC, Gosselin N. Long-term functional alterations in sports concussion. *Neurosurg Focus*. 2012;33:E81–E87.

83. Titus DJ, Furones C, Atkins CM, Dietrich WD. Emergence of cognitive deficits after mild traumatic brain injury due to hyperthermia. *Exp Neurol*. 2015;263:254–262.

84. Kochanek, PM, Jackson, TC. It might be time to let cooler heads prevail after mild traumatic brain injury or concussion. *Exp Neurol*. 2015;267:13–17.

85. Sakurai A, Atkins CM, Alonso OF, et al. Mild hyperthermia worsens the neuropathological damage associated with mild traumatic brain injury in rats. *J Neurotrauma*. 2012;29(2):313–321.

86. Cadarette BS, Levine L, Staab JE, et al. Heat strain imposed by toxic agent protective systems. *Aviat Space Environ Med*. 2001;72:32–37.

87. Goosey-Tolfrey V, Swainson M, Boyd C, Atkinson G, Tolfrey K. The effectiveness of hand cooling at reducing exercise-induced hyperthermia and improving distance-race performance in wheelchair and able-bodied athletes. J Appl Physiol. 2008;105:37–43.

88. Nybo L. Brain temperature and exercise performance. *Exp Physiol*. 2012;97:333–339.

89. Mondello S, Shear DA, Bramlett HM, et al. Insight into pre-clinical models of traumatic brain injury using circulating brain damage biomarkers: operation brain trauma therapy. *J Neurotrauma*. 2016;33(6):595–605.

90. Moghieb A, Bramlett HM, Das JH, et al. Differential neuroproteomic and systems biology analysis of spinal cord injury. *Mol Cell Proteomics*. 2016;15(7):2379–2395.

91. Gu X, Wei ZZ, Espinera A, et al. Pharmacologically induced hypothermia attenuates traumatic brain injury in neonatal rats. *Exp Neurol*. 2015;267:135–142.

92. Bregy A, Nixon R, Lotocki G, et al. Posttraumatic hypothermia increases doublecortin expressing neurons in the dentate gyrus after traumatic brain injury in the rat. *Exp Neurol*. 2012;233:821–828.

Autoimmunity Responses in Traumatic Brain Injury and Spinal Cord Injury

Zhihui Yang, Hisham F. Bahmad, Tian Zhu, Aaron T. Wong, Isha Kothari, Firas Kobeissy, and Kevin K. W. Wang

37

Introduction

Central nervous system (CNS) trauma remains the leading cause of death and disability for people under 40 years of age throughout the world. CNS injury can be divided into brain and spinal injuries. It is estimated that, in the United States, around 5.3 million people are living with a TBI-related disability, and, in the European Union, approximately 7.7 million people who have experienced a TBI have disabilities.[1] Socioeconomically advanced countries probably have an annual traumatic spinal cord injury (SCI) rate of 10–90 per 100,000 persons. CNS injury is a growing public health concern, impacting on a patient's physical, psychological, and social well-being and placing a substantial financial burden on healthcare systems. More importantly, even mild TBI has been linked to serious long-term complications, including chronic traumatic encephalopathy (CTE), neuropsychiatric and movement disorders, and early-onset dementia. The pathology of CNS trauma is a highly complex process with both initial mechanical injury and delayed mechanisms. Primary injuries directly damage the neurons, axons, dendrites, glia, and blood vessels in a focal, multifocal, or diffuse pattern. A secondary injury is initiated by a dynamic series of complex cellular, inflammatory, mitochondrial, neurochemical, and metabolic alterations.[2,3] To date, there are no standardized therapeutic and management protocols dealing with brain and spinal trauma. Consequently, a major quest is under way to better identify diagnostic tools and direct neurotherapeutic strategies in assessing CNS trauma.

In recent years, there has been considerable interest in studies of the emerging role of autoantibodies—which have long been identified—as a new generation of biomarkers in the areas of CNS trauma, neuropsychiatric disorders, and neurotoxicity. Animal experimental studies and clinical data both indicate that an initial brain pathology appears to be the dysfunction or disruption of the blood–brain barrier (BBB).[4,5] Disruption of the BBB leads to the release of TBI-induced intracellular proteins in either intact or cleaved fragments from protease activation into the cerebrospinal fluid (CSF) or bloodstream. Currently, identified CNS-specific proteins and proteolytic fragments have been observed in both TBI and SCI studies. The leakage of such entities into the circulatory system may trigger an autoimmune response that produces antibodies to target the body's own tissues instead of fighting infections. In this chapter, we discuss the genesis of autoimmunity in TBI and SCI and summarize the current identified self-antigens as well as their potential characteristics in CNS trauma. In addition, we will focus on the possibility of using biofluid-based strategies for CNS trauma diagnosis and therapeutic approaches.

Immune System, CNS Special Barriers, and B Lymphocytes

The interaction between the CNS and the systemic immune system is delicate because it is limited by the presence of special CNS barriers such as the BBB and the blood–spinal cord barriers (BSCB), which keep CNS immune homeostasis in a dormant self-tolerant state.[6] Selective permeability of the BBB/BSCB plays a crucial role in regulating the entry of specific molecules into the CNS and excluding most macromolecules from passing into the brain.[7,8] This unique feature of the BBB/BSCB also prevents leakage of neurotransmitters into the circulation. After sustaining CNS trauma, breakdown of the BBB/BSCB frequently follows,[9] instigating the entry of typically nonpermeating molecules into the brain and thus altering the normal neural functions of the CNS.[10] Likewise, BBB/BSCB compromise causes macromolecules of proteins and their breakdown products to be released into the CSF and therefore into the peripheral circulation, including attractive candidates that may serve as signature biomarkers indicative of injury modalities within the CNS.

However, even in nonpathological states, CNS immune system components were found to be incorporated in a diversity of processes that are specific to the CNS itself and not to other body tissues.[11] For instance, cytokines, which have proinflammatory roles in peripheral organs, exhibit essential roles in regulating synaptic plasticity and activity within the CNS[12–14]; these include tumor necrosis factor-α (TNFα) and interleukin-1 (IL-1).[15] Surprisingly, although activation of the complement system and release of its components is well-known to trigger an inflammatory response in many body organs including the brain, experimental evidence reveals a potential role for some of these molecules, such as terminal C5b-9 complexes, in enhancing myelin and oligodendrocytes functions.[16] Other complement proteins were also proved to maintain a neuroprotective function through supporting the development and maturation of glia and neurons while preventing CNS toxicity and cellular apoptosis. This includes C3, C3a, C5, C5a, and the membrane attack complex (MAC).[14]

The distinctiveness of CNS immunity is denoted by the fact that the brain parenchyma has limited interaction with blood vessels, meninges, and ventricles.[17] Hence, it either expresses unique antigens that are not realized in other body tissues, or it expresses other common antigens to an appreciable degree in other tissues. The CNS-reactive antibodies that may be present in the circulation are generally harmless to the host. Nevertheless, in the context of TBI or SCI, and upon breakdown of the BBB or BSCB under pathologic conditions, an autoantibody-mediated pathology may occur.[11] In post-CNS trauma, B lymphocytes are assumed to contribute to part of the injury encountered in addition to the systemic disturbances[18] by releasing specific neural autoantibodies and several other systemic antibodies, such as serum rheumatoid factor (RF) in cases of SCI. The underlying process behind this is differentiation of B lymphocytes via antigen-specific T cells, which occurs once former cells encounter their cognate antigens, into antibody-secreting plasma cells,[19] where immunoglobulin genes undergo class-switch recombination and somatic hypermutation. In CNS injury, and upon disruption of the BBB, neural cells are exposed to the circulating antibodies and serum proteins. These molecules, particularly autoantibodies, produce their cytotoxic effects on neurons and glial cells through activation of the complement system, as previously mentioned, after which cytokine-mediated phagocytosis stimulation occurs and activation of several proteases from microglia and macrophages ensues.[20–23]

Among the several other major mechanisms anticipated that explain the self-antigen–autoantibody response is the molecular mimicry mechanism. This proposed process reckons on the cross-reactivity between a foreign antigen/protein that mimics a self-antigen and induces an abnormal autoimmune response against the host antigens themselves.[24] For instance, nonenzymatic lipid peroxidation within the CNS[25] has been shown to play a role in altering the immunogenicity of the released proteins in the context of injury.[26,27] Hence, autoantibodies recognize proteins cross-linked to lipid peroxidation in the injured neural cells and elicit circulating immunoglobulins that can recognize these proteins.

Mechanisms of Autoantibodies Secretion and Genesis in CNS

CNS-specific antigens or immune cells crossing CNS barriers is the major requirement for triggering an autoimmune response, which is characterized by autoantibody generation. Neurons, astrocytic glia, pericytes, microglia, and microvessels are critical BBB/BSCB elements that maintain the normal function of the BBB/BSCB and protect the CNS from various harmful blood substances.[28–31] The primary CNS injury leads to a mechanically broken vascular system associated with cell damage.[5] After initial trauma, neuroinflammation forces the neurons or glia cells to undergo death cascade processes resulting in consistent increased permeability of the BBB/BSCB.[32] Functional BBB changes cause potential brain antigens to enter the systemic circulation as "foreigners" that lead to the initiation of an autoimmune response. When an adaptive immune response against self-antigens is perpetuated over time due to ongoing self-antigen exposure, autoreactive B cells are activated and differentiate into plasma cells that begin producing antibodies (Figure 37.1).

Increasing evidence shows that TBI, whether it is a single mild, moderate, severe, or repetitive injury, leads to dysfunction of the BBB.[33] Earlier studies based on animal modeling suggest that acute BBB disruption is an early event following TBI.[34,35] Recently, researchers observed BBB disruption persisting up to several months after an early-phase issue with evidence of immunoglobulin G (IgG) deposition at 3 months post-injury around ipsilateral corpus callosum in TBI mice.[26] In clinical studies, increases in the CSF–serum albumin quotient, which is thought to predict a population of patients with poor long-term outcomes, suggest passive BBB dysfunction in patients with severe TBI.[15,33,36] Aside from traditional measurements, new translational studies using neuroimaging techniques also show BBB permeability in TBI patients even after mild or moderate injury. In some cases, BBB disruption can persist for years at the site of focal injury and with greater frequency among individuals with posttraumatic epilepsy.[37,38] Similar evidence is reported in SCI studies.[39,40] BSCB disruption following traumatic CNS injury generates neurotoxic products that impair synaptic and neuronal functions followed by inflammatory cell invasion that contributes to permanent neurological disability. BSCB disruption occurs within 5 minutes after SCI, lasts for up to 28 days after the initial injury, and spreads along the entire length of the cord.[41] The extended time

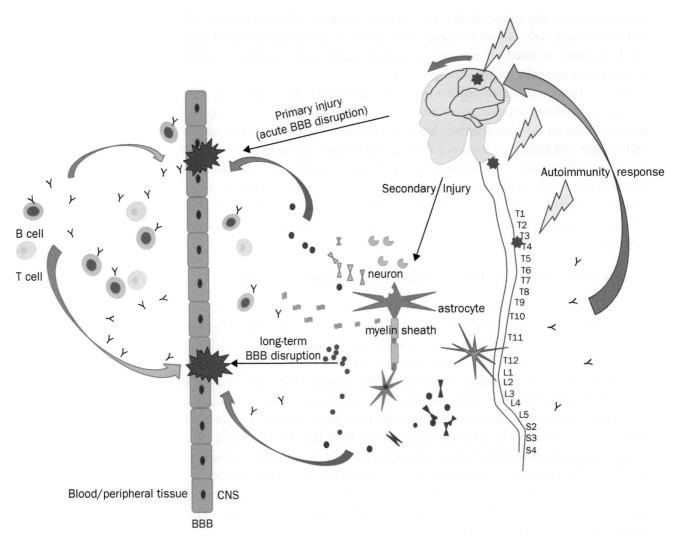

Figure 37.1 Schematic of mechanisms of autoantibody genesis and potential impacts after central nervous system injury.

course of BSCB has been confirmed by magnetic resonance imaging (MRI) analyses at 56 days after SCI.[42] The abnormal leakage occurs within several hours after injury, whereas the second peak is evident between 3 and 7 days post-injury.[43]

Generally, CNS-specific autoantibodies target brain/spinal cord cells and/or tissues not limited to neurons and glia. Neuronal or glial death exhibits either apoptotic or necrotic morphologies and contributes to the overall pathology of CNS injury.[44] Brain or spinal cord cell apoptosis and necrosis have been observed within the injury site in the acute period and in regions remote from the site of impact in the days and weeks following trauma. Accompanying BBB/BSCB disruption and traumatic insult, cell death promotes the release of brain proteins and their fragments cleaved by hyperactive proteinases. Neuronal-specific (neuron-specific enolase [NSE], ubiquitin C-terminal hydrolase-L1 [UCH-L1]), glial-specific (glial fibrillary acidic protein [GFAP]; calcium binding protein B [S100β]), and axonal-related proteins (microtubule associated tau protein, neurofilament protein-light and heavy chains) were identified in the peripheral circulation bloodstream (Figure 37.1).[45–48] Such proteins from the injured cells/tissues are exposed to the immune system and trigger the autoimmune response described earlier. Autoimmunity may result in lesion formation in areas affected and unaffected by trauma. However, depending on subtype, antibodies can be maintained within the bloodstream for years.[49–51]

Autoantibodies in TBI

Neural autoantibodies have been widely detected in CNS diseases such as Alzheimer disease, stroke, multiple sclerosis, neuromyelitis optica, and autoimmune movement disorders.[52–57] However, autoimmunity in CNS trauma (TBI and SCI) has only been examined in a limited way. Autoantigens targeting extracellular domains of neuronal cell surface receptors or synaptic proteins include N-methyl-D-aspartate receptor (NMDAR), α-amino-3-hydroxy-5-methyl-4-isoxazolepropionic acid receptor (AMPAR), glycine receptor (GlyR), S100β, GFAP, myelin basic protein (MBP), and neurofascin (NF). Furthermore, a number of different autoantigens have been discovered.

Pituitary and Hypothalamus

Hypothalamic-pituitary autoimmunity (HPA) is hypothesized as one of the mechanisms involving secondary hypopituitarism following TBI in children and adults. Currently, three original articles demonstrating an association between hypothalamus- or pituitary-related autoantibodies and TBI-induced HPA were published by the same group.[58,59] In longer term studies on 25 patients and prospective follow-up, high titers of anti-pituitary antibodies (APA) and/or anti-hypothalamus antibodies (AHA) are associated with hypopituitarism at the fifth year after TBI.[58–60] This suggests that these autoantibodies might be associated with the development of TBI-induced pituitary dysfunction. In another study, positivity for AHA, but not for APA, has been found to be associated with hypopituitarism in boxers. The authors suggested that hypothalamic damage might be more important than pituitary damage in sport-related repetitive mild trauma.[61] However, there is lack of direct data evaluating the correlation between autoantibody levels and hypopituitarism. In fact, even though the exact antigens or specific autoantibodies have not been fully identified, several candidates have been proposed: prolactin-secreting cells, growth hormone (GH), α-enolase, pituitary gland-specific factors 1a and 2 transcripts, secretogranin II, chorionic somatomammotropin, and TPIT, a corticotroph-specific transcription factor.[61–65]

Glial Fibrillary Acidic Protein

GFAP is highly expressed in astrocytes that constitute the BBB and BSCB. Autoantibodies against GFAP, along with byproducts of the breakdown of glial cells, may reflect BBB dysfunction that is associated with TBI. Two main studies have been published by our group; our studies have shown the presence of anti-GFAP autoantibodies in both severe and mild to moderate TBI patients across the acute (within 10 days of injury) and the chronic phases (average 6.2 month post-injury).[66,67] Human IgG subtype autoantibodies showed prominent immune reactivity to a cluster of bands in the 38–50 kDa region by 7–10 days post-injury, which were identified as GFAP and its breakdown products

(GBDP) that had been cleaved by calpain.[66,67] Our hypothesis is that TBI induces release of GBDPs in substantive quantities throughout the compromised BBB, resulting in an influx of these molecules in circulation. These are then recognized by the immune system as non–self-proteins, thereby triggering an autoantibody response in these individuals. These autoantibodies that specifically target a major brain protein may trigger a persistent CNS autoimmune response, possibly affecting TBI patients' long-term recovery. In addition, our other finding suggests acute plasma levels of autoantibody against GFAP is associated with a history of past exposure to TBI. The plasma levels of autoantibody against GFAP in patients with previous TBI experience is higher than in those without TBI history.[66,67] Thus, we hypothesize that repetitive injury can produce an autoimmunity-boosting effect among those with greater anti-GFAP IgG production.[66,67]

S100β

S100β is another astrocyte-specific protein. Elevated levels of autoantibodies against S100β are correlated with repeated concussive events, which are characterized by BBB disruption.[68] A recent analysis on serum samples (within 24 hours after games) from 67 football players revealed that responses in serum titers of anti-S100β antibodies were directly proportional to both number and severity of hits experienced; this also correlated with changes in brain structure detected by diffusion tensor imaging. S100β appears to be specific for mild TBI, especially sports-related TBI, when compared to the individual's baseline value.[69] Another study involving children with TBI demonstrated that the autoantibody against S100β was present in serum immediately after TBI, regardless of TBI severity. However, in cases with favorable outcomes, it dropped to a normal level within the first few days. High levels of S100β autoantibody indicate that the autoimmune response was due to repetitive disruption of the BBB and release of S100β with subsequent immune activation.[70]

Peroxiredoxin 6

Another highly expressed antigen in astrocytes—the antioxidant enzyme peroxiredoxin 6—acts as a target for evoked autoantibodies in response to TBI. Like GFAP and S100β, which are highly expressed in astrocytes, peroxiredoxin 6 may share similar mechanisms of BBB disruption, possibly involving an alteration in protein structure and a reversal of peripheral immune tolerance. In a recent study involving both an experimental TBI model and also TBI patients, circulating levels of peroxiredoxin 6 were elevated fourfold over control values 4 to 24 hours following mild to moderate TBI.[71]

Myelin Basic Protein

Aside from BBB-related antigen release, other proteins have also been identified in serum as being related to TBI. MBP is associated with the process of myelination of nerves in the nervous system. The autoantibody against MBP in CSF from TBI patients was identified to be strongly correlated with scores on the Glasgow Coma Scale in the first day after TBI.[72] The level of MBP autoantibody also indicated the recovery degree when evaluated for associations with neurological status at day 21 post-TBI.

Cytokine-regulated autoantibodies' responses to MBP have been identified in both healthy individuals and in patients with multiple sclerosis.[73] In addition, autoreactive T cells showed a response to myelin antigens that is associated with improved neuronal survival and functional recovery after TBI.[74]

Glutamate Receptors

The level of autoantibodies to AMPA glutamate receptors and NMDA glutamate receptors (NR2A subunit) were examined in serum sampled from 60 children aged 7–16 years with chronic posttraumatic headaches.[75] Serum analysis was conducted at 6 months and 1 year after the TBI. Increased autoantibody levels against AMPA demonstrated hyperstimulation of glutamate receptors and overdevelopment of the autoimmune process post-TBI while increased NR2A autoantibody levels reflected hypoxic–ischemic brain lesions. The authors hypothesized that NR2b levels may be a predictive factor or a quantitative biomarker for stroke, independent of patient recall, compliance, or moment-to-moment variability. Autoimmune response to NMDA receptor has also been confirmed in patients with a stroke or transient ischemic attack.[76] Since TBI may cause regional cerebral ischemia, which has been reported to facilitate antibody development against NMDA receptor, TBI may also share a similar mechanism in triggering these autoantibodies.[77]

Autoantibodies in SCI

Results presented by several research groups clearly demonstrated that, in animal models of SCI, trauma leads to a surprisingly robust B-cell response, with evidence of antibody-secreting B cells and IgGs present in the CSF after SCI[49]; the specific antigens are poorly identified. In one study using serum from SCI mice, the authors found oligoclonal IgG reactivity against multiple CNS proteins. Aside from this, SCI-induced synthesis of autoantibodies that bind nuclear antigens (DNA and RNA) were also present.[78] However, no exact antigen was identified in this study. K. C. Hayes et al. demonstrated autoantibodies specific for GM1 ganglioside, a myelin-associated glycoprotein, in the serum of 24 traumatically injured SCI patients with stable medical condition and long-standing central conduction deficits (>12 months).[78] Another identified target in more recent clinical research is GFAP. Autoantibody against GFAP was identified by a recent study on SCI in which 18 patients were enrolled; 78% of the patients showed GFAP autoantibody in plasm at both the acute (<48 hours post-injury) and subacute (2–4 weeks post-injury) phases.[79]

Implication of Autoantibodies in TBI as Biomarkers

Immunologic responses during the transition from acute to chronic stages of recovery after TBI could influence an individual patient's outcome. However, most human and animal model studies are limited to the trauma-induced autoimmunity measured during the acute response. It is unknown whether such autoimmune response promotes tolerance to be beneficial. Thus, it is still unclear whether these antibodies are relevant to neuropathological and functional outcomes associated with TBI. Autoantibodies may not cause harm if produced as a part of a "natural" autoantibody response.[80,81] At early stages, naïve B cells express IgM on their cell surface and synthesize natural IgM autoantibodies; such IgM antibodies, which bind multiple self-antigens, are of low affinity. Natural IgM autoantibodies that can clear damaged cells, prevent neuronal apoptosis, and reverse inflammatory effects in other neurological autoimmune diseases have been identified.[82–84] Activated B cells are able to undergo antibody class switching to express IgG on their cell surfaces and produce IgG antibodies. In another experimental study, naturally occurring IgG autoantibody binding may participate in the phagocytosis and removal of damaged neurons following a cortical lesion.[85] In addition, autoreactive T cells have shown a response to myelin antigens that was associated with improved neuronal survival and functional recovery.[86] By contrast, other studies have revealed that antibody–antigen complexes that have activated complements or have bound to fragment crystallizable (Fc) regions of Ig on myeloid or lymphoid cells may have caused cell death.[18,87–89] The recruitment and activation of complement and Fc receptor-bearing cells has been reported after traumatic SCI. Activated B cells and autoantibodies that caused neuropathology in SCI were observed in a published study. SCI can induce the synthesis of autoantibody-binding nuclear antigens including DNA and RNA. Anti-DNA antibodies are able to cross-react with neuronal antigens, followed by induction of neuropathology.[90] Although similar data confirming a pathological role for B-cell activation and autoantibody synthesis after TBI is not currently available, complement activation has been identified in experimental TBI mice brains and in patients with TBI.[91–94] Autoantibody production induced by TBI may be affected by the antigen type, antibody titer, antibody specificity, lesion location, primary injury severity, time post-injury, and many other cofactors. Both antibody actions and local titer may determine the antibody-mediated symptoms. Some antibodies may modulate cellular functions when present at a certain concentration while causing apoptosis at greater concentrations. It should be noted that, in some situations, autoantibodies do not act alone: T cells—possibly specific for the same autoantigen—may also cause tissue damage or secrete cytokines that synergize with autoantibodies in causing cell damage.[6] In addition, ongoing BBB leakage also allows other antigens to enter the CNS, potentially resulting in antibodies cross-reacting with an identical or structurally homologous antigen in the brain.[6]

Implication of Autoantibodies in Spinal Cord Injury: Pathogenic Versus Neuroprotective

Following SCI, antibody-producing B lymphocytes are activated along with other immune cells, such as T lymphocytes, neutrophils, and monocytes/macrophages.[95–99] This neuroinflammatory cascade presents a major pillar of the immune response accompanying any injury to the spinal cord. Ankeny and colleagues meticulously elaborated on the effect of B-lymphocyte activation and associated autoantibodies in the setting of SCI pathogenesis.[18,49] In one study, they showed that, in mice that are B-lymphocyte–deficient and incapable of producing antibodies, spontaneous recovery of locomotor function occurred and SCI lesion was reduced. In addition, upon injection of antibodies purified from SCI mice into uninjured spinal cord, consistent paralysis ensued.[49] Another study by the same group showed that experimental spinal contusion injury provokes long-lasting systemic and intraspinal activation of B lymphocytes. This is due to SCI-dependent stimulation of cognate B and T lymphocytes in response to the released autoantigens.[52] Notably, immunoblots of sera from injured mice revealed that these autoantibodies possess similar neurotoxic potentials via cross-reactivity with glutamine receptors (GluRs) that cause neuronal excitotoxicity.[52]

It has been postulated that several factors influence the magnitude of B-lymphocyte cell activation and autoantibody synthesis, including the level and severity of a SCI. Also, activation of the complement system cascade contributes to the pathology by enhanced intraspinal autoantibodies accumulation and activation and recruitment of myeloid lineage cells (e.g., microglia/macrophages) bearing complement receptors. On the other hand, elevated levels of myelin-reactive antibodies were recognized in serum and CSF of SCI patients and were identified as autoantigens.[78,100,101] In experimental studies, both the spleen and bone marrow show chronic B-lymphocyte activation along with increased IgG and IgM serum levels.[52] Those activated B lymphocytes reside in the injured spinal cord and are accompanied by de novo mRNA expression encoding a range of autoantibodies.[102]

Davies et al. assessed the role of inflammatory serum cytokines in 56 patients with SCIs presenting with different clinical scenarios in comparison to control subjects. Several parameters were studied including levels of the proinflammatory cytokines (TNF-α, IL-1, and IL-6), the anti-inflammatory cytokines (IL-4 and IL-10), the regulatory cytokine IL-2, the IL-1 receptor antagonist (IL-1RA), and autoantibodies against myelin-associated glycoprotein and GM1 ganglioside (anti-GM1) immunoglobulins (IgG and IgM). Results showed an elevation in circulating proinflammatory cytokines and autoantibodies in SCI subjects who presented without complications and further elevation in patients with neuropathic pain, urinary tract infection, or pressure ulcers, relative to healthy control individuals. These findings suggest either a potential protective role for autoimmunity in the released cytokines, or they may simply be a consequence of occult or evident infection.[29] Future research studies are needed to unveil the exact role of autoantibodies and their implications in neurotrauma.

Autoantibodies and B Lymphocytes: Novel Therapeutic Targets in Neural Injury

Although released autoantibodies elicit a cytotoxic effect on neural cells in head trauma, a neuroprotective role of natural autoreactive monoclonal antibodies has also been studied. Wright and colleagues proposed an emerging role of natural IgM autoantibodies in stimulating neurite outgrowth and inhibiting neuronal apoptosis, which are hallmarks in CNS neurodegenerative diseases such as amyotrophic lateral sclerosis and SCI.[82] Binding of these autoantibodies to the surface of neurons promotes neuronal cell survival through activating intracellular signaling cascades that are altered in the setting of injury.[103–105] In the same context, lysophosphatidic acid (LPA), which is a bioactive proinflammatory lypophospholipid released by activated platelets and astrocytes, has been shown to have a potentially causative role in neurotrauma.[106] High levels of this protein were observed in CSF samples taken from patients with TBI and from mice subjected to control cortical impact (CCI) injury. Interestingly, blocking LPA with specific murine anti-LPA monoclonal antibodies improved neurological outcomes in the CCI mice.[107] Those studies provide evidence about the potential therapeutic neuroprotective roles of autoreactive monoclonal antibodies in treating TBI-associated injuries.

The B-lymphocyte cell activation process involves the release and stimulation of several factors and receptors that can eventually serve as therapeutic targets against activated immunity in SCI. Those include B-cell–activating factor (BAFF), lymphotoxin-β, and proliferation-inducing ligand (APRIL), all of which contribute to B-cell survival and functioning.[19] The produced pathogenic antibodies are derived in part from the lesion site and in part they are systemically introduced due to disruption of the BSCB.[49] Based on the results of Ankeny's work, and as previously mentioned, the activated B lymphocytes and their secreted autoantibodies can serve as potential therapeutic targets in SCI.[50]

Conclusion

CNS injury causes damaged or dying brain cells to release brain-specific proteins. This causes the release of numerous brain proteins in their intact or proteolytically modified form to go into circulation in the acute phase. Accumulating evidence has shown that a subset of patients produce autoantibodies when an autoimmunity response is triggered. When autoimmunity is triggered in CNS injury, it targets a range of brain-specific antigens in a subset of TBI or SCI patients. These autoantibody assays might be useful as a biofluid-based biomarker in identifying patients who might be at risk of limited recovery and be selected to receive immunotherapy in the future. However, further research is necessary to definitively evaluate the potential of autoantibodies serving as these significant biomarkers, as well as the characteristics that define their influence on pathology and recovery.

References

1. Roozenbeek B, Maas AIR, Menon DK. Changing patterns in the epidemiology of traumatic brain injury. *Nat Rev Neurol.* 2013;9(4):231–236.

2. Schubert A, Emory L. Cellular mechanisms of brain injury and cell death. *Curr Pharm Des.* 2012;18(38):6325–6330.

3. Daneshvar DH, Goldstein LE, Kiernan PT. Post-traumatic neurodegeneration and chronic traumatic encephalopathy. *Mol cell Neurosci.* 2015;66(Pt B):81–90.

4. Yeoh S, Bell ED, Monson KL. Distribution of blood-brain barrier disruption in primary blast injury. *Ann Biomed Eng.* 2013;41(10):2206–2214.

5. Andrews AM, Lutton EM, Merkel SF, Razmpour R, Ramirez SH. Mechanical injury induces brain endothelial-derived microvesicle release: implications for cerebral vascular injury during traumatic brain injury. *Front Cell Neurosci.* 2016;10(2):43.

6. Diamond B, Honig G, Mader S, Brimberg L. Brain-reactive antibodies and disease. *Annu Rev Immunol.* 2013;2(1):50.

7. Reiber H. Dynamics of brain-derived proteins in cerebrospinal fluid. *Clin Chim Acta.* 2001;310(2):173–186.

8. Reiber H. Proteins in cerebrospinal fluid and blood: barriers, CSF flow rate and source-related dynamics. *Restor Neurol Neurosci.* 2003;21(3-4):79–96.

9. Blyth BJ, Farhavar A, Gee C, et al. Validation of serum markers for blood-brain barrier disruption in traumatic brain injury. *J Neurotrauma*. 2009;26(9):1497–1507.

10. Banks WA. Blood-brain barrier transport of cytokines: a mechanism for neuropathology. *Curr Pharm Des*. 2005;11(8):973–984.

11. Diamond B, Honig G, Mader S, Brimberg L, Volpe BT. Brain-reactive antibodies and disease. *Annu Rev Immunol*. 2013;31(1):345–385.

12. Piton A, Michaud JL, Peng H, et al. Mutations in the calcium-related gene IL1RAPL1 are associated with autism. *Hum Mol Genet*. 2008;17(24):3965–3974.

13. Stellwagen D, Malenka RC. Synaptic scaling mediated by glial TNF-alpha. *Nature*. 2006;440(7087):1054–1059.

14. Pavlowsky A, Gianfelice A, Pallotto M, et al. A postsynaptic signaling pathway that may account for the cognitive defect due to IL1RAPL1 mutation. *Curr Biol*. 2010;20(2):103–115.

15. Khairova RA, Machado-Vieira R, Du J, Manji HK. A potential role for pro-inflammatory cytokines in regulating synaptic plasticity in major depressive disorder. *Int J Neuropsychopharmacol*. 2009;12(4):561–578.

16. Rus H, Cudrici C, David S, Niculescu F. The complement system in central nervous system diseases. *Autoimmunity*. 2006;39(5):395–402.

17. Galea I, Bechmann I, Perry VH. What is immune privilege (not)? *Trends Immunol*. 2006;28(1):12–18.

18. Ankeny DP, Popovich PG. B cells and autoantibodies: complex roles in CNS injury. *Trends Immunol*. 2010;31(9):332–338.

19. Dalakas MC. B cells as therapeutic targets in autoimmune neurological disorders. *Nat Clin Pract Neurol*. 2008;4(10):557–567.

20. Mosley K, Cuzner ML. Receptor-mediated phagocytosis of myelin by macrophages and microglia: effect of opsonization and receptor blocking agents. *Neurochem Res*. 1996;21(4):481–487.

21. Beuche W, Friede RL. Myelin phagocytosis in Wallerian degeneration of peripheral nerves depends on silica-sensitive, bg/bg-negative and Fc-positive monocytes. *Brain Res*. 1986;378(1):97–106.

22. Abdul-Majid K-B, Stefferl A, Bourquin C, et al. Fc receptors are critical for autoimmune inflammatory damage to the central nervous system in experimental autoimmune encephalomyelitis. *Scand J Immunol*. 2002;55(1):70–81.

23. Griot-Wenk M, Griot C, Pfister H, Vandevelde M. Antibody-dependent cellular cytotoxicity in antimyelin antibody-induced oligodendrocyte damage in vitro. *J Neuroimmunol*. 1991;33(2):145–155.

24. Davidson A, Diamond B. Autoimmune diseases. *N Engl J Med*. 2001;345(5):340–350.

25. Keller JN, Mattson MP. Roles of lipid peroxidation in modulation of cellular signaling pathways, cell dysfunction, and death in the nervous system. *Rev Neurosci*. 1998;9(2):105–116.

26. Uchida K, Stadtman ER. Modification of histidine residues in proteins by reaction with 4-hydroxynonenal. *Proc Natl Acad Sci USA*. 1992;89(10):4544–4548.

27. Yahya MD, Pinnas JL, Meinke GC, Lung CC. Antibodies against malondialdehyde (MDA) in MRL/lpr/lpr mice: evidence for an autoimmune mechanism involving lipid peroxidation. *J Autoimmun*. 1996;9(1):3–9.

28. Garbuzova-Davis S, Saporta S, Haller E, et al. Evidence of compromised blood-spinal cord barrier in early and late symptomatic SOD1 mice modeling ALS. *PloS One*. 2007;2(11):e1205.

29. Abbott NJ, Rönnbäck L, Hansson E. Astrocyte–endothelial interactions at the blood–brain barrier. *Nat Rev Neurosci.* 2006;7(1):41–53.

30. Ballabh P, Braun A, Nedergaard M. The blood–brain barrier: an overview: structure, regulation, and clinical implications. *Neurobiol Dis.* 2004;16(1):1–13.

31. Wolburg H, Noell S, Mack A, Wolburg K. Brain endothelial cells and the glio-vascular complex. *Cell Tissue Res.* 2009;335(1):75–96.

32. Schwarzmaier SM, Kim SW, Trabold R. Temporal profile of thrombogenesis in the cerebral microcirculation after traumatic brain injury in mice. *J Neurotrauma.* 2010;27(1):121–130.

33. Hay JR, Johnson VE, Young A. Blood-brain barrier disruption is an early event that may persist for many years after traumatic brain injury in humans. *J Neuropathol Exp Neurol.* 2015;74(12):1147–1157.

34. Li W, Watts L, Long J, et al. Spatiotemporal changes in blood-brain barrier permeability, cerebral blood flow, T 2 and diffusion following mild traumatic brain injury. *Brain Res.* 2016;1646:53–61.

35. Shen Q, Watts LT, Li W, Duong TQ. Magnetic resonance imaging in experimental traumatic brain injury. *Methods Mol Biol.* 2016;1462:645–658.

36. Saw MM, Chamberlain J, Barr M, Morgan M. Differential disruption of blood–brain barrier in severe traumatic brain injury. *Neurocrit Care.* 2014;20(2):209.

37. Winter C, Bell C, Whyte T, Cardinal J. Blood–brain barrier dysfunction following traumatic brain injury: correlation of Ktrans (DCE-MRI) and SUVR (99mTc-DTPA SPECT) but not serum S100B. *Neurol Res.* 2015;37(7):599–606.

38. Tomkins O, Feintuch A, Benifla M, Cohen A. Blood-brain barrier breakdown following traumatic brain injury: a possible role in posttraumatic epilepsy. *Cardiovasc Psychiatry Neurol.* 2011;2011:765923.

39. Kumar H, Ropper AE, Lee S-H, Han I. Propitious therapeutic modulators to prevent blood-spinal cord barrier disruption in spinal cord injury. *Mol Neurobiol.* 2017;54(5):3578–3590.

40. Lee JY, Na WH, Choi HY, Lee KH, Ju BG, Yune TY. Jmjd3 mediates blood-spinal cord barrier disruption after spinal cord injury by regulating MMP-3 and MMP-9 expressions. *Neurobiol Dis.* 2016;95(11):66–81.

41. Maikos JT, Shreiber DI. Immediate damage to the blood-spinal cord barrier due to mechanical trauma. *J Neurotrauma.* 2007;24(3):492–507.

42. Cohen DM, Patel CB, Ahobila-Vajjula P, et al. Blood-spinal cord barrier permeability in experimental spinal cord injury: dynamic contrast-enhanced MRI. *NMR Biomed.* 2008;22(3):332–341.

43. Whetstone WD, Hsu J-YC, Eisenberg M, Werb Z, Noble-Haeusslein LJ. Blood-spinal cord barrier after spinal cord injury: relation to revascularization and wound healing. *J Neurosci Res.* 2003;74(2):227–239.

44. Yang Z, Wang K. Glial fibrillary acidic protein: from intermediate filament assembly and gliosis to neurobiomarker. *Trends Neurosci.* 2015;38(6):364–374.

45. Takala RSK, Posti JP, Runtti H, et al. Glial fibrillary acidic protein and ubiquitin C-terminal hydrolase-L1 as outcome predictors in traumatic brain injury. *World Neurosurg.* 2015;87:8–20.

46. Honda M, Tsuruta R, Kaneko T. Serum glial fibrillary acidic protein is a highly specific biomarker for traumatic brain injury in humans compared with S-100B and neuron-specific enolase. *J Trauma.* 2010;69(1):104–109.

47. Csajbok LZ, Nilsson I, Blennow K, Nellgård B, Rosengren L. Increased serum-GFAP in patients with severe traumatic brain injury is related to outcome. *J Neurol Sci.* 2005;240(1-2):85–91.

48. Kavalci C, Pekdemir M, Durukan P, Ilhan N. The value of serum tau protein for the diagnosis of intracranial injury in minor head trauma. *Am J Emerg Med.* 2007;25(4):391–395.

49. Ankeny DP, Guan Z, Popovich PG. B cells produce pathogenic antibodies and impair recovery after spinal cord injury in mice. *J Clin Invest.* 2009;119(10):2990–2999.

50. Dekaban GA, Thawer S. Pathogenic antibodies are active participants in spinal cord injury. *J Clin Invest.* 2009;119(10):2881–2884.

51. Ulndreaj A, Tzekou A, Mothe AJ, et al. Characterization of the antibody response after cervical spinal cord injury. *J Neurotrauma.* 2016;34(6):1209–1226.

52. Ankeny DP, Lucin KM, Sanders VM. Spinal cord injury triggers systemic autoimmunity: evidence for chronic B lymphocyte activation and lupus-like autoantibody synthesis. *J Neurochem.* 2006;99(4):1073–1087.

53. Mruthinti S, Buccafusco JJ, Hill WD, et al. Autoimmunity in Alzheimer's disease: increased levels of circulating IgGs binding Abeta and RAGE peptides. *Neurobiol Aging.* 2004;25(8):1023–1032.

54. Yokobori S, Zhang Z, Moghieb A, et al. Acute diagnostic biomarkers for spinal cord injury: review of the literature and preliminary research report. *World Neurosurg.* 2013;83(5):867–878.

55. Gruden MA, Davudova TB, Mališauskas M. Autoimmune responses to amyloid structures of Aβ (25–35) peptide and human lysozyme in the serum of patients with progressive Alzheimer's disease. *Dement Geriatr Cogn Disord.* 2004;18(2):165–171. doi:10.1159/000079197.

56. Gee JM, Kalil A, Thullbery M, Becker KJ. Induction of immunologic tolerance to myelin basic protein prevents central nervous system autoimmunity and improves outcome after stroke. *Stroke.* 2008;39(5):1575–1582. doi:10.1161/strokeaha.107.501486.

57. Elliott C, Lindner M, Arthur A, et al. Functional identification of pathogenic autoantibody responses in patients with multiple sclerosis. *Brain.* 2012;135(Pt 6):1819–1833. doi:10.1093/brain/aws105.

58. Tanriverdi F, De Bellis A, Bizzarro A, Sinisi AA. Antipituitary antibodies after traumatic brain injury: is head trauma-induced pituitary dysfunction associated with autoimmunity? *Eur J Endocrinol.* 2008;159(1):7–13. doi:10.1530/eje-08-0050.

59. Tanriverdi F, De Bellis A, Ulutabanca H. A five year prospective investigation of anterior pituitary function after traumatic brain injury: is hypopituitarism long-term after head trauma associated with autoimmunity? *J Neurotrauma.* 2013;30(16):1426–1433. doi:10.1089/neu.2012.2752.

60. Tanriverdi F, Ulutabanca H, Unluhizarci K. Three years prospective investigation of anterior pituitary function after traumatic brain injury: a pilot study. *Clin Endocrinol (Oxf).* 2008;68(4):573–579. doi:10.1111/j.1365-2265.2007.03070.x.

61. Tanriverdi F, De Bellis A, Battaglia M, et al. Investigation of antihypothalamus and antipituitary antibodies in amateur boxers: is chronic repetitive head trauma-induced pituitary dysfunction associated with autoimmunity? *Eur J Endocrinol.* 2010;162(5):861–867. doi:10.1530/EJE-09-1024.

62. Guaraldi F, Caturegli P, Salvatori R. Prevalence of antipituitary antibodies in acromegaly. *Pituitary.* 2012;15(4):490–494. doi:10.1007/s11102-011-0355-7.

63. Smith C, Bensing S, Burns C, Robinson PJ. Identification of TPIT and other novel autoantigens in lymphocytic hypophysitis: immunoscreening of a pituitary cDNA library and development of immunoprecipation assays. *Eur J Endocrinol.* 2012;166(3):391–398. doi:10.1530/eje-11-1015.

64. Caturegli P. Autoimmune hypophysitis: an underestimated disease in search of its autoantigen (s). *J Clin Endocrinol Metab.* 2007;92(6):2038–2040. doi:10.1210/jc.2007-0808.

65. Guaraldi F, Grottoli S, Arvat E, Ghigo E. Hypothalamic-pituitary autoimmunity and traumatic brain injury. *J Clin Med*. 2015;4(5):1025–1035. doi:10.3390/jcm4051025.

66. Zhang Z, Zoltewicz JS, Mondello S, Newsom KJ. Human traumatic brain injury induces autoantibody response against glial fibrillary acidic protein and its breakdown products. *PloS One*. 2014;9(3):e92698.

67. Wang K, Yang Z, Yue JK, Zhang Z. Plasma anti-glial fibrillary acidic protein autoantibody levels during the acute and chronic phases of traumatic brain injury: a transforming research and clinical knowledge in traumatic brain injury pilot study. *J Neurotrauma*. 2016;33(13):1270–1277.

68. Sorokina EG, Semenova ZB, Granstrem OK. [S100B protein and autoantibodies to S100B protein in diagnostics of brain damage in craniocerebral trauma in children]. *Zh Nevrol Psikhiatr Im S S Korsakova*. 2010;110(8):30–35.

69. Marchi N, Bazarian JJ, Puvenna V, Janigro M. Consequences of repeated blood-brain barrier disruption in football players. *PloS One*. 2013;8(3):e56805.

70. Pinelis VG, Sorokina EG, Semenova JB, et al. [Biomarkers in children with traumatic brain injury]. *Zh Nevrol Psikhiatr Im S S Korsakova*. 2015;115(8):66–72.

71. Buonora JE, Mousseau M. Autoimmune profiling reveals peroxiredoxin 6 as a candidate traumatic brain injury biomarker. *J Neurotrauma*. 2015;32(22):1805–1814.

72. Ngankam L, Kazantseva NV. [Immunological markers of severity and outcome of traumatic brain injury]. *Zh Nevrol Psikhiatr Im S S Korsakova*. 2011;111(7):61–65.

73. Hedegaard CJ, Chen N, Sellebjerg F. Autoantibodies to myelin basic protein (MBP) in healthy individuals and in patients with multiple sclerosis: a role in regulating cytokine responses to MBP. *Immunology*. 2009;128(1 Pt 2):e451. doi:10.1111/j.1365-2567.2008.02999.x.

74. Cox AL, Coles AJ, Nortje J, Bradley PG. An investigation of auto-reactivity after head injury. *J Neuroimmunol*. 2006;174(1-2):180–186. doi:10.1016/j.jneuroim.2006.01.007.

75. Goryunova AV, Bazarnaya NA, Sorokina EG. Glutamate receptor autoantibody concentrations in children with chronic post-traumatic headache. *Neurosci Behav Physiol*. 2007;37(8):761–764. doi:10.1007/s11055-007-0079-3.

76. Weissman JD, Khunteev GA, Heath R. NR2 antibodies: risk assessment of transient ischemic attack (TIA)/stroke in patients with history of isolated and multiple cerebrovascular events. *J Neurol Sci*. 2011;300(1-2):97–102. doi:10.1016/j.jns.2010.09.023.

77. Kalev-Zylinska ML, Symes W, Little KCE, et al. Stroke patients develop antibodies that react with components of N-methyl-D-aspartate receptor subunit 1 in proportion to lesion size. *Stroke*. 2013;44(8):2212–2219.

78. Hayes KC, Hull TCL, Delaney GA, et al. Elevated serum titers of proinflammatory cytokines and CNS autoantibodies in patients with chronic spinal cord injury. *J Neurotrauma*. 2002;19(6):753–761.

79. Hergenroeder GW, Moore AN, Schmitt KM, Redell JB, Dash PK. Identification of autoantibodies to glial fibrillary acidic protein in spinal cord injury patients. *Neuroreport*. 2015;27(2):90–93.

80. Walsh JT, Zheng J, Smirnov I, Lorenz U. Regulatory T cells in central nervous system injury: a double-edged sword. *J Immunol*. 2014;193(10):5013–5022.

81. Schwartz M, Raposo C. Protective autoimmunity a unifying model for the immune network involved in CNS repair. *The Neuroscientist*. 2014;20(4):343–358.

82. Wright BR, Warrington AE. Cellular mechanisms of central nervous system repair by natural autoreactive monoclonal antibodies. *Arch Neurol*. 2009;66(12):1456–1459.

83. Ehrenstein MR, Notley CA. The importance of natural IgM: scavenger, protector and regulator. *Nat Rev Immunol.* 2010;10(11):778–786.

84. Baumgarth N. The double life of a B-1 cell: self-reactivity selects for protective effector functions. *Nat Rev Immunol.* 2011;11(1):34–46.

85. Stein TD, Fedynyshyn JP. Circulating autoantibodies recognize and bind dying neurons following injury to the brain. *J Neuropathol Exp Neurol.* 2002;61(12):1100–1108. doi:10.1093/jnen/61.12.1100.

86. Cox AL, Coles AJ, Nortje J, Bradley PG. An investigation of auto-reactivity after head injury. *J Neuroimmunol.* 2006;174(1-2):180–186.

87. Taylor S, Calder CJ, Albon J, Erichsen JT, Boulton ME, Morgan JE. Involvement of the CD200 receptor complex in microglia activation in experimental glaucoma. *Exp Eye Res.* 2011;92(5):338–343.

88. Archelos JJ, Hartung HP. Pathogenetic role of autoantibodies in neurological diseases. *J Neurol Sci.* 2000;23(7):317–327. doi:10.1016/s0022-510x(05)80393-4.

89. Strait RT, Hicks W, Barasa N, et al. MHC class I-specific antibody binding to nonhematopoietic cells drives complement activation to induce transfusion-related acute lung injury in mice. *J Exp Med.* 2011;208(12):2525–2544. doi:10.1084/jem.20110159.

90. Rich MC, Keene CN, Neher MD, Johnson K, Yu ZX. Site-targeted complement inhibition by a complement receptor 2-conjugated inhibitor (mTT30) ameliorates post-injury neuropathology in mouse brains. *Neurosci Lett.* 2016;617:188–194. doi:10.1016/j.neulet.2016.02.025.

91. Bellander BM, Singhrao SK, Ohlsson M. Complement activation in the human brain after traumatic head injury. *J Neurotrauma.* 2001;18(12):1295–1311.

92. Rich MC, Keene CN, Neher MD, Johnson K, Yu ZX. Site-targeted complement inhibition by a complement receptor 2-conjugated inhibitor (mTT30) ameliorates post-injury neuropathology in mouse brains. *Neurosci Lett.* 2016;617:188–194.

93. Bellander BM, Olafsson IH, Ghatan PH, Skejo H. Secondary insults following traumatic brain injury enhance complement activation in the human brain and release of the tissue damage marker S100B. *Acta Neurochir (Wien).* 2011;153(1):90–100.

94. Ruseva MM, Ramaglia V. An anticomplement agent that homes to the damaged brain and promotes recovery after traumatic brain injury in mice. *Proc Natl Acad Sci USA.* 2015;112(46):14319–14324.

95. Blight AR. Effects of silica on the outcome from experimental spinal cord injury: implication of macrophages in secondary tissue damage. *Neuroscience.* 1994;60(1):263–273.

96. Sroga JM, Jones TB, Kigerl KA, McGaughy VM, Popovich PG. Rats and mice exhibit distinct inflammatory reactions after spinal cord injury. *J Comp Neurol.* 2003;462(2):223–240.

97. Kigerl KA, McGaughy VM, Popovich PG. Comparative analysis of lesion development and intraspinal inflammation in four strains of mice following spinal contusion injury. *J Comp Neurol.* 2005;494(4):578–594. doi:10.1002/cne.20827.

98. Popovich PG, Guan Z, Wei P, Huitinga I, van Rooijen N, Stokes BT. Depletion of hematogenous macrophages promotes partial hindlimb recovery and neuroanatomical repair after experimental spinal cord injury. *Exp Neurol.* 1999;158(2):351–365.

99. Fleming JC, Norenberg MD, Ramsay DA, et al. The cellular inflammatory response in human spinal cords after injury. *Brain.* 2006;129(Pt 12):3249–3269. doi:10.1093/brain/awl296.

100. Mizrachi Y, Ohry A, Aviel A, Rozin R, Brooks ME, Schwartz M. Systemic humoral factors participating in the course of spinal cord injury. *Paraplegia.* 1983;21(5):287–293. doi:10.1038/sc.1983.48.

101. Kil K, Zang YC, Yang D, et al. T cell responses to myelin basic protein in patients with spinal cord injury and multiple sclerosis. *J Neuroimmunol*. 1999;98(2):201–207.

102. Ankeny DP, Popovich PG. Mechanisms and implications of adaptive immune responses after traumatic spinal cord injury. *Neuroscience*. 2009;158(3):1112–1121.

103. Soldán MMP, Warrington AE, Bieber AJ, et al. Remyelination-promoting antibodies activate distinct Ca2+ influx pathways in astrocytes and oligodendrocytes: relationship to the mechanism of myelin repair. *Mol Cell Neurosci*. 2003;22(1):14–24.

104. Howe CL, Bieber AJ, Warrington AE, Pease LR, Rodriguez M. Antiapoptotic signaling by a remyelination-promoting human antimyelin antibody. *Neurobiol Dis*. 2004;15(1):120–131.

105. Pirko I, Ciric B, Gamez J, et al. A human antibody that promotes remyelination enters the CNS and decreases lesion load as detected by T2-weighted spinal cord MRI in a virus-induced murine model of MS. *FASEB J*. 2004;18(13):1577–1579.

106. Frisca F, Sabbadini RA, Goldshmit Y, Pébay A. Biological effects of lysophosphatidic acid in the nervous system. *Int Rev Cell Mol Biol*. 2012;296:273–322. doi:10.1016/B978-0-12-394307-1.00005-9.

107. Crack PJ, Zhang M, Morganti-Kossmann MC, et al. Anti-lysophosphatidic acid antibodies improve traumatic brain injury outcomes. *J Neuroinflammation*. 2014;11:37.

Index

Page numbers followed by *f* and *t* indicate figures and tables, respectively.